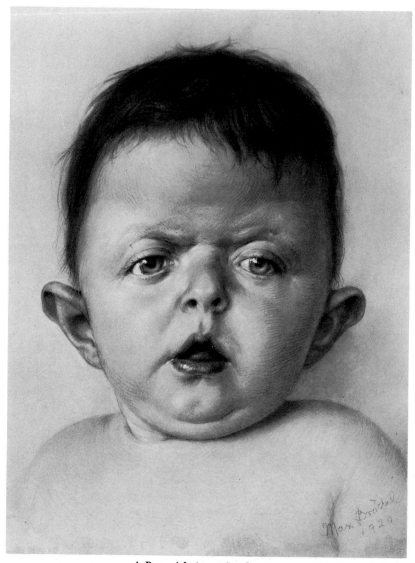

A Boy with Apert Syndrome

Original Max Brödel drawing No. 506. Property of The Johns Hopkins
University School of Medicine, Department of Art as Applied to Medicine.

Smith's Recognizable Patterns of Human Malformation

FOURTH EDITION

Kenneth Lyons Jones, M.D.

Professor of Pediatrics
Chief, Division of Dysmorphology
University of California, San Diego
School of Medicine
La Jolla, CA

W.B. SAUNDERS COMPANY
A Division of Harcourt Brace & Company

Philadelphia • London • Toronto • Montreal • Sydney • Tokyo

W.B. SAUNDERS COMPANY
A Division of
Harcourt Brace & Company

The Curtis Center
Independence Square West
Philadelphia, Pennsylvania 19106

Library of Congress Cataloging-in-Publication Data

Smith, David W., 1926–1981.

Smith's recognizable patterns of human malformation.

Rev. ed. of: Recognizable patterns of human malformation /
by David W. Smith with the assistance of Kenneth Lyons Jones.
3rd ed. 1982.

Includes bibliographies and index.

1. Abnormalities, Human—Etiology.   2. Genetic
disorders.   3. Morphogenesis.   4. Birth
injuries.   5. Growth disorders.   I. Jones, Kenneth
Lyons.   II. Title.   [DNLM: 1. Abnormalities.
QS 675 S645r 1988]

RG627.5.S58 1988   616'.043   87–35759

ISBN 0–7216–2359–X

Listed here are the latest translated editions of this book together with the
language of the translation and the publisher.

Italian (*3rd Edition*)—Piccin Nuova Libraria, Padova, Italy

Spanish (*4th Edition*)—Nueva Editorial Interamericana, Mexico, D.F., Mexico

Editor: W. B. Saunders Staff
Developmental Editor: Linda Mills
Designer: Karen Giacomucci
Production Manager: Peter Faber
Manuscript Editor: Martha Tanner
Mechanical Artist: Melissa Walter
Illustration Coordinator: Lisa Lambert
Page Layout Artist: Dorothy Chattin
Indexer: Ann Kassar

Smith's Recognizable Patterns of Human Malformation, 4/e   ISBN 0–7216–2359–X

Last digit is the print number: 9   8

Dedication of the First Edition

To my wife, Ann, beloved inspirational companion

To my father, William H. Smith,
accomplished engineer and would-be physician

To my teachers Dr. Lawson Wilkins,
molder of clinicians and humanist, and
Professor Dr. Gian Töndury,
complete anatomist, who brings embryology
into living perspective

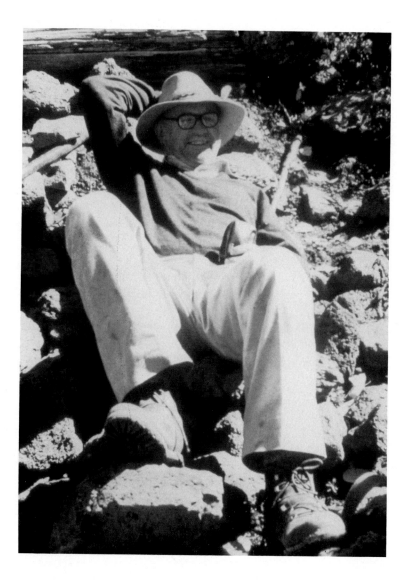

Dedicated to the Memory of

David W. Smith, M.D.
1926–1981

"Far better it is to dare mighty things, to win glorious triumphs, even though checkered by failure, than to take rank with those poor spirits who neither enjoy much nor suffer much, because they live in the great twilight that knows neither victory nor defeat."

Theodore Roosevelt, in a speech before the
Hamilton Club, Chicago, April 10, 1899

Acknowledgments

The information set forth in this book represents an amalgamation of the knowledge, contributions, and work of many individuals. In preparing the first three editions, David Smith acknowledged the following:

TEACHERS: Dr. Lawson Wilkins, Johns Hopkins University School of Medicine, whose total clinical approach served as a guide and inspiration toward the development of this book; Dr. Klaus Patau, University of Wisconsin Medical School, from whom knowledge of cytogenetics and a critical and concise approach toward writing manuscripts was gained; Dr. Gian Töndury, University of Zürich Medical School, from whom knowledge of embryology and the interpretation of errors in morphogenesis was learned; and Dr. Waldo Nelson, Temple University School of Medicine, whose editorial policy toward clinical relevance and simplicity of semantics has influenced the manner in which this book was developed.

FELLOWS AND STUDENTS: The following have been especially helpful in the development of this book.

FELLOWS: Dr. Luc Lemli, Dendermonde, Belgium; Dr. John Opitz, Helena, Montana; Dr. Robert Summitt, University of Tennessee Medical School; Dr. Arlan Rosenbloom, University of Florida Medical School; Dr. Jaime Frias, University of Nebraska Medical School; Dr. Jon Aase, University of New Mexico Medical School; Dr. Bryan Hall, University of Kentucky Medical School; Dr. Kenneth Jones, University of California Medical School (San Diego); Dr. James Hanson, University of Iowa Medical School; Dr. Sterling Clarren, University of Washington Medical School; and Dr. John Graham, Dartmouth School of Medicine. Dr. Albert Schinzel of the University of Zürich has contributed greatly to the chromosomal abnormality section in this edition.

STUDENTS: Dr. Philip Marden, at the University of Wisconsin Medical School; and Dr. John Mulvihill and Dr. Gregory Popich at the University of Washington Medical School.

ASSOCIATES: Many individuals have contributed photos and information. Especially helpful have been the following: Dr. John Opitz, Helena, Montana; Drs. Pierre Maroteaux and Maurice Lamy, Hopital des Enfants-Malades, Paris; Dr. Robert Gorlin, University of Minnesota Medical and Dental School; Dr. Victor McKusick, Johns Hopkins University Medical School; Dr. Michael Cohen, Jr., Dalhousie University; Dr. Bruce Beckwith, Denver Children's Hospital; Dr. Judith Hall, University of British Columbia; and my associates at the University of Washington, Drs. Benjamin Graham, Arno Motulsky, Thomas Shepard, David Shurtleff and Ronald Scott.

ASSISTANTS: The invaluable and dedicated secretarial and editorial assistance of Mrs. Mary Ann Sedgwick Harvey is deeply appreciated, as is the secretarial assistance of Mrs. Doris James and Mrs. Valerie Brown.

RESEARCH LIBRARIAN: Mrs. Lyle Harrah is a major contributor to the development of this book. She has made available several thousand articles, allowing for an extensive review on each syndrome, though only selected references appear in the text. Her dedication and capacity for obtaining even the most obscure references are greatly appreciated. Gerald J. Oppenheimer, Head Librarian at the University of Washington Medical School Library, has been most helpful, allowing a special room for this project.

ILLUSTRATIONS: Mrs. Phyllis Wood of the University of Washington Department of Medical Illustration prepared some of the illustrations in Chapters 1, 3, 4, and 6. Her art work, which immeasurably augments the text itself, is greatly appreciated. Mary Ann Sedgwick Harvey has been of great value in taking many of the new photos in the third edition of this text. Acknowledged for their assistance in photography and illustrations are the departments of medical photography at the University of Washington, University of Wisconsin, and the Children's Orthopedic Hospital of Washington. The C. V. Mosby Publishing Company of St. Louis deserves special acknowledgment for their permission to publish a large proportion of the photographs that appear in this text, many of which were previously published in the Journal of Pediatrics.

MEMORIAL: The Robert Gordon Schneller Memorial Fund provided funds for medical illustration and photography for the first edition of this text, which greatly enhanced the educational value of this book. Mr. and Mrs. M. R. Schneller had two sons. Robert Gordon, a student at the University of Washington, was interested in problems of malformation, at least partially because his younger brother has Down syndrome. Robert's life and his interest were cut short by a mountaineering accident at the age of 20 years. Mr. and Mrs. Schneller hope, as do I, that the contribution of his friends and relatives may assist in stimulating others to pursue the interest which Robert had in extending our knowledge about malformation problems.

In preparing the 4th edition, the invaluable assistance of the following individuals is gratefully acknowledged.

Dr. Kurt Benirschke, University of California Medical School, San Diego, whose breadth of knowledge, intellectual curiosity, and enthusiasm is a continuing stimulus.

Fellows in Dysmorphology at UCSD: Dr. Marilyn C. Jones, University of California Medical School, San Diego; Dr. H. Eugene Hoyme, University of Arizona Medical School; Dr. Luther K. Robinson, State University of New York, Buffalo; and Dr. Ronald Lacro, Boston Children's Hospital. All have made their own significant contribution to the development of this edition and have been a great inspiration to me.

Kathleen A. Johnson has steadfastly provided direction for the Division of Dysmorphology and has been a source of great support to me.

Laurie Hanessian has labored many long hours editing and transcribing the text of this edition.

Dr. David Rimoin, Cedars Sinai Medical Center, Los Angeles; Dr. Judith Hall, University of British Columbia, Vancouver; Dr. Ronan O'Rahilly, Carnegie Laboratories of Embryology and Departments of Human Anatomy and Neurology, University of California, Davis; Dr. Jon Aase, University of New Mexico Medical School, Albuquerque; and Dr. Marilyn C. Jones have been particularly helpful in preparing this edition.

Contents

Introduction
including dysmorphology approach and classification

We ought not to set them aside with idle thoughts or idle words about "curiosities" or "chances." Not one of them is without meaning; not one that might not become the beginning of excellent knowledge, if only we could answer the question—why is it rare? or being rare, why did it in this instance happen?—JAMES PAGET, LANCET, 2:1017, 1882.

The questions set forth by Paget are still applicable today. Every structural defect represents an inborn error in morphogenesis. Just as the study of inborn metabolic errors has extended our understanding of normal biochemistry, so the accumulation of knowledge concerning defects in morphogenesis may assist us in further unraveling the story of structural development.

The major portion of this text is devoted to patterns of malformation, as contrasted with patterns of deformation due to mechanical factors, which is the subject of a separate text, *Smith's Recognizable Patterns of Human Deformation*. You will also find relevant chapters on normal and abnormal morphogenesis, genetics and genetic counseling, the psychologic adaptation to the child with structural anomalies, minor anomalies and their relevance, a clinical approach toward a specific diagnosis for certain categorical problems, and normal standards of measurement for a variety of features. It is hoped that the design of the book will lend itself to practical clinical application, as well as provide a basic text for the education of those interested in a better understanding of alterations in morphogenesis. Furthermore, many of the charts have been developed for direct use in the counseling of patients and parents.

Accurate diagnosis of a specific syndrome among the 0.7 per cent of babies born with multiple malformations is a necessary prerequisite of providing a prognosis and plan of management for the affected infant, as well as genetic counseling for the parents.

DYSMORPHOLOGY APPROACH

The following is the author's approach toward the evaluation of an individual with multiple defects:

I. Gather information. The family history is an essential aspect of such an evaluation. A question such as "Are there any individuals in the family with a similar type of problem?" may be helpful. The early history should usually include information about the onset and vigor of fetal activity, gestational timing, indications of uterine constraint, mode of delivery, size at birth, neonatal adaptation, and problems in postnatal growth and development. The physical examination should be complete, with the physician searching for minor as well as major anomalies. When possible, measurements should be taken to determine whether a given feature, such as apparent ocular hypertelorism or a small-appearing ear, is truly abnormal. The charts of normal measurements in Chapter 7 are provided for this purpose. An unusual feature ideally should be interpreted in relation to the findings in other family members before its relevance is determined.

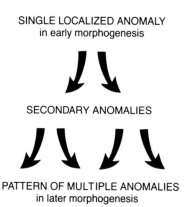

SINGLE LOCALIZED ANOMALY
in early morphogenesis

SECONDARY ANOMALIES

PATTERN OF MULTIPLE ANOMALIES
in later morphogenesis

Figure 1. Sequence designates a single localized anomaly plus its subsequently derived structural consequences, as depicted above.

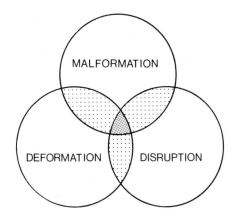

Figure 3. An initiating malformation may give rise to secondary deformation or disruption, and vice versa. The terminology, such as *malformation sequence*, refers to the *initiating* defect and its consequences. When the nature of the initiating defect is unresolved between the three types, the term *malformation* is generally utilized.

II. Interpret the patient's anomalies from the viewpoint of developmental anatomy and strive to answer the following questions:

  A. Which anomaly in the individual represents the earliest defect in morphogenesis? A table for this purpose is found in Chapter 3 (Table 3–1). From such information one can determine that the problem in development must have existed *prior* to a particular prenatal age and any factor *after* that time could not be the cause of that structural defect.

  B. Can all the anomalies in the patient be explained on the basis of a single problem in morphogenesis that leads to a cascade of subsequent defects, as shown in Figure 1? These types of patterns of structural defects, referred to as *sequences,* may be divided into three categories from the devel-

opmental pathology viewpoint, as summarized in Figure 2. The first category is the *malformation sequence* (Fig. 3), in which there has been a single localized poor formation of tissue that initiates a chain of subsequent defects. Malformation sequences occur in all gradations, the manifestations ranging from nearly normal to more severe, and have a recurrence risk that is most commonly in the 1 to 5 per cent range.

Deformation sequence is the second category, in which there is no problem in the embryo or fetus (collectively referred to as fetus in this text), but mechanical forces such as uterine constraint result in altered morpho-

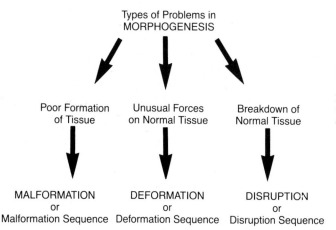

Types of Problems in
MORPHOGENESIS

Poor Formation of Tissue	Unusual Forces on Normal Tissue	Breakdown of Normal Tissue
MALFORMATION or Malformation Sequence	DEFORMATION or Deformation Sequence	DISRUPTION or Disruption Sequence

Figure 2. Three types of structural defects that can result in a chain of defects (sequence) by the time of birth.

genesis, usually of the molding type. One example is the oligohydramnios deformation sequence, due to chronic leakage of amniotic fluid; another is the breech deformation sequence, the manifold effects of prolonged breech position late in fetal life. The deformations and deformation sequences are the subject of the separate text entitled *Smith's Recognizable Patterns of Human Deformation.* Most deformations have a very good to excellent prognosis in contrast with many malformations. The recurrence risk for deformation is usually of very low magnitude, unless the cause of the deformation problem is a persisting one, such as a bicornuate uterus.

The third category is the *disruptive sequence,* in which the normal fetus is subjected to a destructive problem and its consequences. Such disruptions may be of vascular, infectious, or even mechanical origin. One example of the latter is disruption of normally developing tissues by amniotic bands. The spectra of consequences most commonly relate to the timing of the amniotic rupture, as set forth under *Early Amnion Rupture Sequence* in Chapter 1.

C. Does the patient have multiple structural defects that cannot be explained on the basis of a single initiating defect and its consequences, but rather appear to be the consequence of multiple defects in one or more tissues? These are referred to as *malformation syndromes* and are most commonly thought to be due to a single cause. The known modes of etiology for malformation syndromes include chromosomal abnormalities, mutant gene disorders, and environmental teratogens. However, there are still many for which the mode of etiology has not been resolved.

III. Attempt to arrive at a specific overall diagnosis within the five categories shown in Figure 4, confirm when possible, and counsel accordingly. When possible, counseling should include the following: an understanding of how the altered structures came to be as they are; the natural history of the condition and what measures can be utilized to

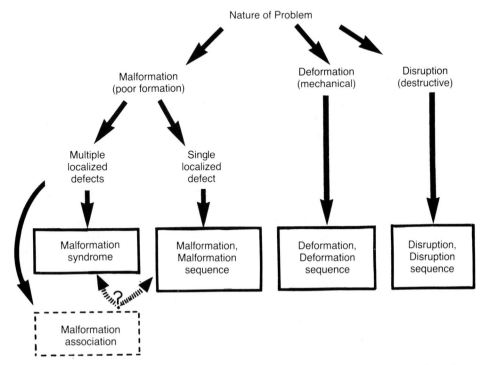

Figure 4. Most patients with multiple structural defects will fall into one of these five categories. The prognosis, management, and recurrence risk counseling may vary considerably among these categories.

assist the child; and the mode of etiology and genetic counseling (recurrence risks).

IMPORTANT GENERAL PRINCIPLES

The following are some of the important principles and information that should be appreciated in the evaluation of a patient with multiple defects.

1. Nonspecificity of Individual Defects

With rare exceptions, a clinical diagnosis of a pattern of malformation cannot be made on the basis of a single defect, as is evident in the differential diagnosis tables in the appendix. Even a rare defect may be a feature in several syndromes of variant etiology. A specific diagnosis is usually dependent on recognition of the overall *pattern of anomalies,* and the detection of minor defects may be as helpful as that of major anomalies in this regard.

2. Variance in Expression

Variance in extent of abnormality (expression) among individuals with the same etiologic syndrome is a usual phenomenon. Except for such nonspecific general features as mental deficiency and small stature, it is unusual to find a given anomaly in 100 per cent of patients with the same etiologic syndrome. For example, in full 21 trisomy Down syndrome, only mental deficiency is ubiquitous; hypotonia is a frequent feature, but most of the other individual clinical features are found in less than 80 per cent of such patients. However, a specific diagnosis of Down syndrome can generally be rendered, based on the *total pattern of anomalies.* It is especially important to appreciate that the environmentally determined disorders occur in all gradations of severity. Thus, as one example, only the more severely affected fetuses who have been heavily exposed to ethanol in utero will have sufficient features to be diagnosed as having the fetal alcohol syndrome. Many newborns will be more mildly affected, showing lesser degrees of the spectrum of fetal alcohol effects.

Intraindividual variability in expression is also frequent, with variance in the degree of abnormality on the left versus the right side of the individual.

3. Heterogeneity

Similar phenotypes (overall physical similarity) may result from *different* etiologies. Only by finer discrimination of the phenotype or mode of etiology can such similar entities be distinguished. For example, the Marfan syndrome and homocystinuria were initially discriminated on the basis of homocystinuria, next by a difference in mode of etiology (autosomal dominant for the Marfan syndrome and autosomal recessive in homocystinuria), and finally by closer scrutiny of the phenotype. As another example, achondroplasia is frequently misdiagnosed among individuals who have chondrodystrophies that only superficially resemble true achondroplasia. A diagnosis should be rendered only when there is close resemblance in the overall pattern of malformation between the patient and the disorder under consideration.

4. Etiology

Most of the disorders herein set forth have a genetic basis. Chapter 4 provides the background information relative to genetic counseling for these conditions.

Besides the following established disorders, roughly one half of the individuals with multiple defects have conditions that have not yet been recognized as specific disorders. A small percentage of such patients (8 per cent in Summitt's study)* have a structural chromosomal abnormality. In such cases, genetic counseling should be withheld until it has been determined whether either parent is a balanced translocation carrier of the chromosomal abnormality. In the absence of an evident chromosomal abnormality or familial data suggesting a particular mode of etiology, it is generally impossible to state any accurate risk of recurrence for unknown patterns of multiple malformation. It is presumptuous to inform the parents that "this is a rare

---

*R. L. Summitt: Cytogenetics in mentally defective children with anomalies: a controlled study. J. Pediatr., *74*:58, 1969.

condition and therefore unlikely to recur in your future children." Under these circumstances, the author's present approach is to inform the parents that the lowest recurrence risk is zero and the highest risk with each pregnancy would be 25 per cent. The latter figure is predicated on the possibility of recessive inheritance or a nondetectable chromosomal abnormality from a balanced translocation carrier parent.

5. Nomenclature

Some of the recommendations of an international committee on "Classification and Nomenclature of Morphologic Defects," published in *Lancet, 1*:513, 1975, are utilized in this text. The recommendations of a more recent international group, which met in Mainz, Germany, under the direction of Professor Jurgen Spranger in November 1979 and again in Seattle in February 1980, have also been utilized.

Most of the nomenclature has already been alluded to; the following recommendations relate to the naming of single defects and patterns of malformation.

Naming of Single Malformations

Utilize an adjective or descriptive term and the name of the structure or the classic equivalent in common use, for example, small mandible or micrognathia.

Naming of Patterns of Malformations

1. When the etiology is known and easily remembered, utilize the appropriate term to designate the disorder.
2. Continue time-honored designations unless there is good reason for change.
3. In the absence of a reasonably descriptive designation, eponyms, some of them multiple, may be used until the basic defect for the disorder is recognized. However, usage of an eponym should, in the future, be limited to one proper name.
4. The possessive use of an eponym should be discontinued, since the author neither had nor owned the disorder.
5. Designation of a disorder by one or more of its manifestations does not necessarily imply that they are either specific or consistent components of that disorder.
6. Avoid names that may have an unpleasant connotation for the family or affected individual.
7. The syndrome should not be designated by the initials of the originally described patients.
8. Names that are too general for a specific syndrome should be avoided.
9. Avoid acronyms unless they are extremely pertinent or appropriate.

Text continued on page 8

Nomenclature Used to Describe Chromosomal Syndromes

Many of the disorders set forth in this book are the result of chromosomal abnormalities. This section is intended to familiarize those readers who are not versed in cytogenetics with some of the basic nomenclature used in describing chromosomal syndromes. Several shorthand systems have been devised. The examples shown employ the "short system," which is the most commonly used in the recent literature. By comparing the karyotype examples with those in the text, the reader should be able to decipher the cytogenetic shorthand. No attempt has been made to include every possible abnormality. For a comprehensive discussion of nomenclature, the reader is referred to the following sources:

1. Bergsma, D. (ed.): "Paris Conference (1971): Standardization in Human Genetics." White Plains, The National Foundation—March of Dimes, BD: OAS VIII (7), 1972.
2. Bergsma, D. (ed.): "Paris Conference (1971), Supplement (1975): Standardization on Human Cytogenetics." White Plains, The National Foundation—March of Dimes, BD: OAS XI (9), 1975.
3. de Grouchy, J., and Turleau, C.: Clinical Atlas of Human Chromosomes. New York, John Wiley and Sons, 1984.
4. Schinzel, A.: Catalogue of Unbalanced Chromosome Aberrations in Man. New York, Walter de Gruyter, 1984.

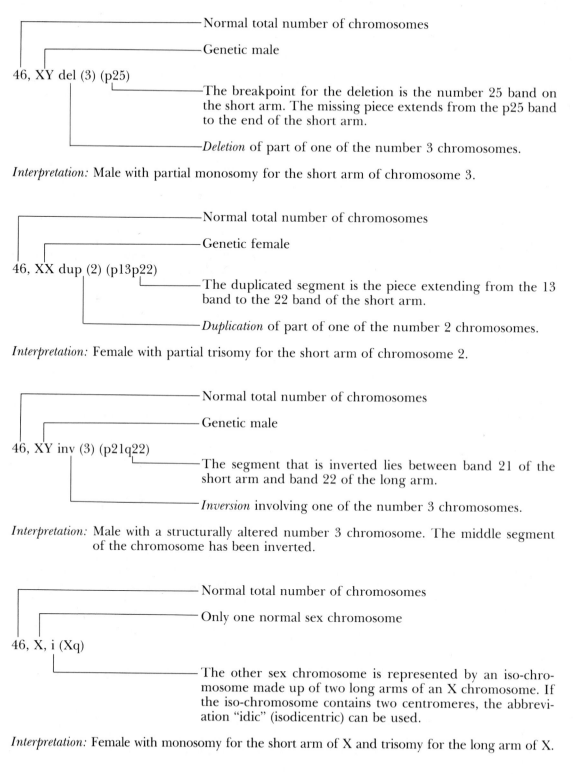

46, XY del (3) (p25)

- Normal total number of chromosomes
- Genetic male
- The breakpoint for the deletion is the number 25 band on the short arm. The missing piece extends from the p25 band to the end of the short arm.
- *Deletion* of part of one of the number 3 chromosomes.

Interpretation: Male with partial monosomy for the short arm of chromosome 3.

46, XX dup (2) (p13p22)

- Normal total number of chromosomes
- Genetic female
- The duplicated segment is the piece extending from the 13 band to the 22 band of the short arm.
- *Duplication* of part of one of the number 2 chromosomes.

Interpretation: Female with partial trisomy for the short arm of chromosome 2.

46, XY inv (3) (p21q22)

- Normal total number of chromosomes
- Genetic male
- The segment that is inverted lies between band 21 of the short arm and band 22 of the long arm.
- *Inversion* involving one of the number 3 chromosomes.

Interpretation: Male with a structurally altered number 3 chromosome. The middle segment of the chromosome has been inverted.

46, X, i (Xq)

- Normal total number of chromosomes
- Only one normal sex chromosome
- The other sex chromosome is represented by an iso-chromosome made up of two long arms of an X chromosome. If the iso-chromosome contains two centromeres, the abbreviation "idic" (isodicentric) can be used.

Interpretation: Female with monosomy for the short arm of X and trisomy for the long arm of X.

46, XY, r (6) (p24q26)

Normal total number of chromosomes

Genetic male

The breakpoints that have allowed formation of the ring are the 24 band on the short arm and the 26 band on the long arm. Genetic material distal to these breakpoints has been lost.

One of the number 6 chromosomes is represented by a *ring* chromosome.

Interpretation: Male with partial monosomy for both the distal long and distal short arms of chromosome 6.

46, XY/47, XY, + 21

One population of cells with a normal male karyotype

One population of cells with an extra chromosome 21

Interpretation: Male with *mosaic* trisomy 21.

45, XY, t (13;14) (p11;q11)

Reduced total number of chromosomes

Genetic male

The breakpoints that have allowed the translocation are the 11 band of the short arm of chromosome 13 and the 11 band of the long arm of chromosome 14. Both are adjacent to the centromeres.

Translocation between chromosomes 13 and 14. Because chromosomes 13 and 14 are composed almost exclusively of long arm material, breaks that occur adjacent to the centromere (see above) with deletion of both short arms result in an insignificant loss of genetic information. The rearrangement creates a large fused chromosome and reduces the total number of chromosomes. This particular type of translocation is called Robertsonian. The triplet "rob" may be used in place of "t" to indicate this.

Interpretation: Male with a normal amount of genetic material but reduced number of chromosomes. One of the number 13 and one of the number 14 chromosomes are represented by a large chromosome that is the fusion product of 13 and 14.

—— Normal total number of chromosomes

—— Genetic female

46, XX, t (2;5) (p21;q31)

—— The breakpoints at which the trading of material has occurred are the 21 band on the short arm of chromosome 2 and the 31 band on the long arm of 5. The material distal to the breakpoints has been involved in a 1:1 trade.

—— Reciprocal translocation between chromosomes 2 and 5.

Interpretation: Female with balanced translocation in which the distal piece of the short arm of 2 is attached to the long arm of 5 and the distal piece of the long arm of 5 is attached to the short arm of 2. No genetic material has been lost or added.

—— Normal total number of chromosomes

—— Genetic male

46, XY, der (22), t (3;22) (p23;q13) mat

—— One number 22 chromosome is abnormal, having been *derived* from a translocation.

—— This denotes that the source of the derived chromosome is a balanced *maternal* translocation.

—— The breakpoints are the 23 band on the short arm of 3 and the 13 band on the long arm of 22. The derived chromosome consists of the short arm, centromere, and proximal long arm of 22, onto which the distal part of the short arm of 3 is attached.

—— The *translocation* that produced the derived 22 involves chromosomes 3 and 22.

Interpretation: Male with trisomy for the short arm of chromosome 3 and monosomy for the distal long arm of chromosome 22.

METHOD AND UTILITY OF PRESENTATION OF PATTERNS OF MALFORMATION

The arrangement of the disorders in this book is predominantly based on the similarity in overall features or in one major feature among the patterns of malformation, as set forth in the table of contents. Thus, the order of presentation is designed to be of assistance in the diagnosis of the patient for whom a firm diagnosis has not been established. With the exception of the chromosomal abnormality syndromes, which share many features, and the disorders determined by an environ-

mental agent, the conditions are not arranged in accordance with the mode of etiology.

Each syndrome or malformation sequence has a listing of anomalies. The features that together tend to distinguish the syndrome from other known disorders are set forth in italic print. The main list consists of defects that occur in at least 25 per cent and usually more than 50 per cent of patients. Sometimes the actual percentage or number is stated for each anomaly. Below these are listed the occasional defects that occur with a frequency of 1 to 25 per cent, most commonly 5 to 10 per cent. The occurrence of these "occasional abnormalities" is of interest and has been loosely ascribed to "developmental noise." In other words, an adverse influence that usually causes a particular pattern of malformation may occasionally cause other anomalies as well. Possibly it is differences of genetic background, environment, or both that allow some individuals to express these "occasional" anomalies. The important feature is that they are not random for a particular syndrome. For example, clinicians who have seen a large number of children with the Down syndrome are not surprised to see "another" Down syndrome baby with duodenal atresia, webbed neck, or tetralogy of Fallot.

The references listed for each syndrome or malformation sequence have been selected as those that give the best account of that disorder, provide recent additional knowledge, or represent the initial description. They are arranged in chronological order.

A word of caution is indicated. This book does not contain a number of very rare syndromes, especially those reported after June 1985.

Other Sources of Information

In addition to this text, there are many others that may be of value in the recognition, management, and counseling of particular problems and patterns of malformation.

General

Bergsma, D. S.: Birth Defects Atlas and Compendium, 2nd ed. Baltimore, Williams and Wilkins Co., 1979.

Emery, A. E. H., and Rimoin, D. L.: Principles and Practice of Medical Genetics. New York, Churchill Livingstone, 1983.

Goodman, R. M., and Gorlin, R. J.: Atlas of the Face in Genetic Disorders, 2nd ed. St. Louis, C. V. Mosby Co., 1979.

Gorlin, R. J., Cohen, M. M., Jr., and Pindborg, J. J.: Syndromes of the Head and Neck, 2nd ed. New York, McGraw-Hill Book Co., 1976.

Graham, J. M.: Smith's Recognizable Patterns of Human Deformation, 2nd ed. Philadelphia, W. B. Saunders Co., 1988.

McKusick, V. A.: Mendelian Inheritance in Man: Catalogs of Autosomal Dominant, Autosomal Recessive, and X-Linked Phenotypes, 7th ed. Baltimore, The Johns Hopkins University Press, 1986.

Warkany, J.: Congenital Malformations, Chicago, Year Book Medical Publishers, 1971.

Chromosomal Abnormalities

de Grouchy, J., and Turleau, C.: Clinical Atlas of Human Chromosomes. New York, John Wiley and Sons, 1984.

Jůnis, J.: New Chromosomal Syndromes. New York, Academic Press, 1977.

Schinzel, A.: Catalogue of Unbalanced Chromosome Aberrations in Man. New York, Walter de Gruyter, 1984.

Connective Tissue, Skeletal Dysplasias, Orthopedic

Bailey, J. A.: Disproportionate Short Stature. Philadelphia, W. B. Saunders Co., 1973.

McKusick, V. A.: Heritable Disorders of Connective Tissue, 4th ed. St. Louis, C. V. Mosby Co., 1972.

Spranger, J. W., Langer, L. O., and Wiedemann, H. R.: Bone Dysplasias, An Atlas of Constitutional Disorders of Skeletal Development. Philadelphia, W. B. Saunders Co., 1974.

Temtamy, S., and McKusick, V. A.: Synopsis of hand malformations with particular emphasis on genetic factors. *In* Bergsma, D. S., and McKusick, V. A. (eds.): Clinical Delineation of Birth Defects, Vol. IV. Baltimore, Williams and Wilkins Co., 1969, pp. 125–184.

Wynne-Davies, R.: Heritable Disorders in Orthopedic Practice. Oxford, Blackwell Scientific Publications, 1973.

Mental Deficiency with Associated Anomalies

Gellis, S. S., and Feingold, M.: Atlas of Mental Retardation Syndromes. Washington, D.C., U.S. Government Printing Office, 1968.

Holmes, L. B., et al.: Mental Retardation: An Atlas of Diseases with Associated Physical Abnormalities. New York, Macmillan Publishing Co., 1972.

Hereditary Deafness With Associated Anomalies

Konigsmark, B. W., and Gorlin, R. J.: Genetic and Metabolic Deafness. Philadelphia, W. B. Saunders Co., 1976.

Ocular Abnormalities

Waardenburg, P. J.: Genetics and Ophthalmology, Vols. I and II. Oxford, Blackwell Scientific Publications, 1963.

Facial Clefting

Gorlin, R. J., Cervenka, J., and Pruzansky, S.: Facial clefting and its syndromes. *In* Bergsma, D. S., and McKusick, V. A. (eds.): Clinical Delineation of Birth Defects, Vol. VII. Baltimore, Williams and Wilkins Co., 1971, pp. 3–49.

Teratology

Briggs, G. G., Freeman, R. K., and Yaffe, S. J.: Drugs in Pregnancy and Lactation. Baltimore, Williams and Wilkins Co., 1986.

Shepard, T. H.: Catalog of Teratogenic Agents, 5th ed. Baltimore, The Johns Hopkins University Press, 1986.

1

Recognizable Patterns of Malformation

A. CHROMOSOMAL ABNORMALITY SYNDROMES

DOWN SYNDROME

(Trisomy 21 Syndrome)

*Hypotonia, Flat Facies,
Slanted Palpebral Fissures, Small Ears*

Down's report of 1866 on the ethnic classification of idiots stated that a "large number of congenital idiots are typical Mongols," and he set forth the clinical description of the Down syndrome. The textbook by Penrose and Smith provides an overall appraisal of this disease that has an incidence of 1:660 newborns, making it the most common pattern of malformation in man. *The Child with Down's Syndrome*, a book written for parents of Down syndrome children, provides them with a background as to the cause, the nature and natural history, and the adaptation of the child with Down syndrome.

ABNORMALITIES
General. Hypotonia with tendency to keep mouth open and protrude the tongue; diastasis recti.

Hyperflexibility of joints. Relatively small stature with awkward gait.
Central Nervous System. Mental deficiency.
Craniofacial. Brachycephaly with relatively flat occiput and tendency toward midline parietal hair whorl. Mild microcephaly with upslanting palpebral fissures. Thin cranium with late closure of fontanels. Hypoplasia to aplasia of frontal sinuses, short hard palate. Small nose with low nasal bridge and tendency to have inner epicanthal folds.
Eyes. Speckling of iris (Brushfield's spots) with peripheral hypoplasia of iris. Fine lens opacities by slit lamp examination (59 per cent). Refractive error.
Ears. Small; overfolding of angulated upper helix; sometimes prominent; small or absent earlobes.

Dentition. Hypoplasia, irregular placement, fewer caries than usual.

Neck. Appears short.

Hands. Relatively short metacarpals and phalanges. Fifth finger: hypoplasia of midphalanx of fifth finger (60 per cent) with clinodactyly (50 per cent), a single crease (40 per cent), or both. Simian crease (45 per cent). Distal position of palmar axial triradius (84 per cent). Ulnar loop dermal ridge pattern on all digits (35 per cent).

Feet. Wide gap between first and second toes. Plantar crease between first and second toes. Open field dermal ridge patterning in hallucal area of sole (50 per cent).

Pelvis. Hypoplasia with outward lateral flare of iliac wings and shallow acetabular angle.

Cardiac. Anomaly in about 40 per cent; atrioventricularis communis, ventricular septal defect, patent ductus arteriosus, auricular septal defect, and aberrant subclavian artery, in decreasing order of frequency.

Skin. Loose folds in posterior neck (infancy). Cutis marmorata, especially in extremities (43 per cent). Dry, hyperkeratotic skin with time (75 per cent).

Hair. Fine, soft, and often sparse; straight pubic hair at adolescence.

Genitalia. Male: relatively small penis. Hypogonadism in terms of fertility (100 per cent) and testosterone production.

OCCASIONAL ABNORMALITIES. Seizures (less than 5 per cent); strabismus (33 per cent); nystagmus (15 per cent); keratoconus (6 per cent); cataract (1.3 per cent); low placement of ears; webbed neck; two ossification centers in manubrium sterni; funnel or pigeon breast; tracheoesophageal fistula; duodenal atresia; tetralogy of Fallot; incomplete fusion of vertebral arches of lower spine (37 per cent); only 11 ribs; atlantoaxial instability (12 per cent); abnormal odontoid process (6 per cent); cryptorchidism (27 per cent from birth to nine years and 14 per cent after 15 years); syndactyly of second and third toes. The incidence of leukemia is about 1:95, or close to 1 per cent. Thyroid disorders are more common, including athyreosis, simple goiter, and hyperthyroidism.

PRINCIPAL FEATURES IN NEONATE. The diagnosis can generally be made shortly after birth, and therefore, the following ten features of Down syndrome in the neonate are presented as set forth by Hall, who found at least four of these abnormalities in all of 48 neonates with Down syndrome and six or more in 89 per cent of them.

Hypotonia	80%
Poor Moro reflex	85%
Hyperflexibility of joints	80%
Excess skin on back of neck	80%

Flat facial profile	90%
Slanted palpebral fissures	80%
Anomalous auricles	60%
Dysplasia of pelvis	70%
Dysplasia of midphalanx of fifth finger	60%
Simian crease	45%

NATURAL HISTORY. Muscle tone tends to improve with age, whereas the rate of developmental progress slows with age. For example, 23 per cent of a group of Down syndrome children under three years had a developmental quotient above 50, whereas none of those in the three to nine year group had intelligence quotients above 50. Though the I.Q. range is generally said to be 25 to 50 with an occasional individual above 50, the mean I.Q. for older patients is 24. Fortunately, social performance is usually beyond that expected for mental age, averaging three and one-third years above mental age for the older individuals. Generally "good babies" and happy children, individuals with Down syndrome tend toward mimicry, are friendly, have a good sense of rhythm, and enjoy music. Mischievousness and obstinacy may also be characteristics, and 13 per cent have serious emotional problems. Coordination is often poor, and the voice tends to be raucous.

Early developmental enrichment programs for Down syndrome children have resulted in improved rate of progress during the first four to five years of life. Whether such training programs will appreciably alter their ultimate level of performance remains to be determined.

Growth is relatively slow, and during the first eight years, secondary centers of ossification are often late in development. However, during later childhood, the osseous maturation is more "normal," and final height is usually attained around 15 years of age. Adolescent sexual development is usually somewhat less complete than normal. The girls may menstruate and can be fertile, whereas the males are considered infertile and have relatively low serum testosterone values.

The major cause for early mortality is congenital heart defects, and 44 per cent of those with cardiac anomalies die in infancy. Lower respiratory tract infections may pose a serious problem; however, between infancy and 40 years of age the mortality rate is not much greater than the normal. Low-grade problems that occur frequently are chronic rhinitis, conjunctivitis, and periodontal disease, none of which are easy to "cure."

Although asymptomatic atlantoaxial dislocation occurs in 12 to 20 per cent of individuals with Down syndrome, symptoms referable to compression of the spinal cord are rare. However, any child with Down syndrome who develops changes in bowel or bladder function, neck posturing, or loss of ambulatory skills should be evaluated carefully with plain roentgenograms of the cervical spine. The majority of patients develop symptoms before 10 years of age, when the ligamentous laxity is most severe.

ETIOLOGY. Trisomy for all or a large part of chromosome 21. The combined results of 11 unselected surveys totaling 784 cases showed the following relative frequencies of particular types of chromosomal alteration for Down syndrome:

Full 21 trisomy	94%
21 Trisomy/normal mosaicism	2.4%
Translocation cases (with about equal occurrence of D/G and G/G translocations)	3.3%

Faulty chromosome distribution leading to Down syndrome is more likely to occur at older maternal age, as shown in the following figures of incidence for Down syndrome for particular maternal ages: 15 to 29 years, 1:1500; 30 to 34 years, 1:800; 35 to 39 years, 1:270; 40 to 44 years, 1:100; and over 45 years, 1:50.

Though the general likelihood for *recurrence* of Down syndrome is 1 per cent, the principal task in giving recurrence risk figures to parents is to determine whether the Down syndrome child is a translocation case with a parent who is a translocation carrier and thereby has a relatively high risk for recurrence. The likelihood of finding a translocation in the Down syndrome child of a mother under 30 years of age is 6 per cent, and of such cases only one out of three will be found to have a translocation carrier parent. Therefore, the estimated probability that either parent of a Down syndrome patient born of a mother under 30 years is a G/D or G/G translocation carrier is 2 per cent versus 0.3 per cent when the Down syndrome patient is born of a mother over 30 years of age. Having excluded a translocation carrier parent, the risk for recurrence may be stated as about 1 per cent. Though a low figure, it is enough to justify amniocentesis for chromosome studies on any future pregnancy, allowing for early termination of a 21 trisomy abortus. The recurrence risk for the rare translocation carrier parent will depend on the type of translocation and the sex of the parent.

Mosaicism usually leads to a less severe phenotype. Any degree of intellectual ability from normal or nearly normal to severe retardation is found, and this does not always correlate with the clinical phenotype. Patients with the features of Down syndrome and relatively good performance are likely to have mosaicism (which is not always easy to demonstrate).

Cases with trisomy of only the segment 21q22 reveal the full pattern of Down syndrome indistinguishable from cases with a 47, + 21 chromosome constitution. This is especially important, as the segment 21q22 attached to any other chromosome might not be easy to detect, especially in G- or Q-banded preparations. By contrast, familial trisomy of 21pter→q21 causes an inconsistent clinical picture and mild to moderate mental retardation. Because of the uncharacteristic clinical features, de novo cases are difficult to recognize with certainty.

References

Down, J. L. H.: Observations on an ethnic classification of idiots. Clinical Lecture Reports, London Hospital, *3*:259, 1866.

Richards, B. W., et al.: Cytogenetic survey of 225 patients diagnosed clinically as mongols. J. Ment. Defic. Res., 9:245, 1965.

Hall, B.: Mongolism in newborn infants. Clin. Pediatr. (Phila.), *5*:4, 1966.

Penrose, L. S., and Smith, G. F.: Down's Anomaly. Boston, Little, Brown & Co., 1966.

Smith, D. W., and Wilson, A. C.: The Child with Down's Syndrome. Philadelphia, W. B. Saunders Co., 1973.

Williams, D. L., Summitt, R. L., et al.: Familial Down syndrome due to + (10;21) translocation. Am. J. Hum. Genet., 27:478, 1975.

Semine, A. A., et al.: Cervical-spine instability in children with Down syndrome (trisomy 21). J. Bone Joint Surg., *60-A*:649, 1978.

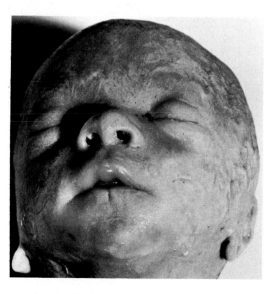

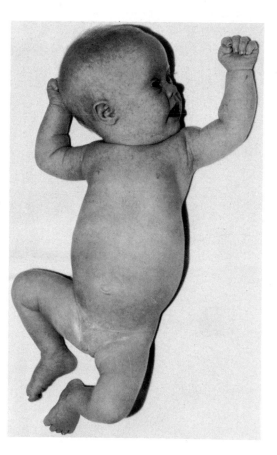

Left, At least 20% of trisomy 21 fetuses are stillborn. This 20 week fetus showed few signs of Down syndrome, the diagnosis having been made by chromosome study. *Right,* The surviving term infant shows many signs, including hypotonia. (Left photo courtesy of Dr. Renée Bernstein, University of Johannesburg, S. Africa.)

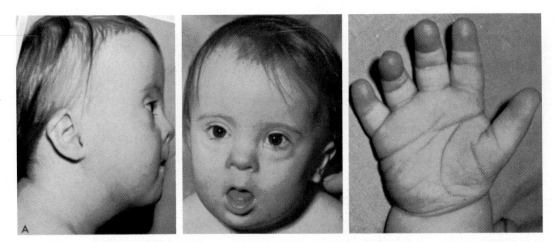

Down syndrome. *A*, Young infant. Flat facies, straight hair; protrusion of tongue; single crease on inturned fifth finger.

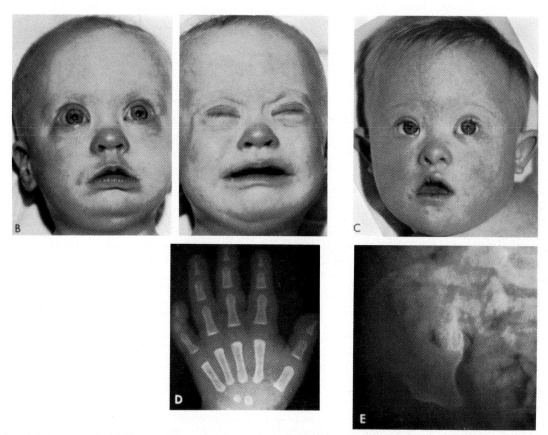

B and *C*, Inner canthal folds. Speckling of iris with lack of peripheral patterning. Small auricles, prominent at right. "Pouting" expression when crying. (*B*, *C*, from Smith, D. W.: J. Pediatr., *70*:474, 1967.) *D*, Hypoplasia, midphalanx of fifth finger. *E*, Shallow acetabular angle with small iliac wings having the shape of elephant ears.

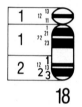

18

TRISOMY 18 SYNDROME

Clenched Hand, Short Sternum,
Low Arch Dermal Ridge Patterning on Fingertips

This condition was first recognized as a specific entity in 1960 by discovery of the extra 18 chromosome in babies with a particular pattern of malformation (Edwards et al., Patau et al., and Smith et al.). It is the second most common multiple malformation syndrome, with an incidence of about 0.3 per 1000 newborn babies. There has been a 3:1 preponderance of females to males. Several good reviews set forth a full appraisal of this syndrome.

More than 130 different abnormalities have been noted in the literature on patients with the 18 trisomy syndrome, and therefore the listing of abnormalities has been divided into those that occur in 50 per cent or more of patients, in 10 to 50 per cent of patients, and in less than 10 per cent of patients.

ABNORMALITIES FOUND IN 50 PER CENT OR MORE OF PATIENTS

General. Feeble fetal activity, weak cry. Altered gestational timing; one third premature, one third postmature. Polyhydramnios, small placenta, single umbilical artery. Growth deficiency; mean birth weight, 2340 g. Hypoplasia of skeletal muscle, subcutaneous and adipose tissue. Mental deficiency, hypertonicity (after neonatal period). Diminished response to sound.

Craniofacial. Prominent occiput, narrow bifrontal diameter. Low-set, malformed auricles. Short palpebral fissures. Small oral opening, narrow palatal arch. Micrognathia.

Hands and Feet. Clenched hand, tendency for overlapping of index finger over third, fifth finger over fourth. Absence of distal crease on fifth finger with or without distal creases on third and fourth fingers. Low arch dermal ridge pattern on six or more fingertips. Hypoplasia of nails, especially on fifth finger and toes. Short hallux, frequently dorsiflexed.

Thorax. Short sternum, with reduced number of ossification centers. Small nipples.

Abdominal Wall. Inguinal or umbilical hernia and/or diastasis recti.

Pelvis and Hips. Small pelvis, limited hip abduction.

Genitalia. Male: cryptorchidism.

Skin. Redundancy, mild hirsutism of forehead and back, prominent cutis marmorata.

Cardiac. Ventricular septal defect, auricular septal defect, patent ductus arteriosus.

ABNORMALITIES FOUND IN 10 TO 50 PER CENT OF CASES

Craniofacial. Wide fontanels, microcephaly, hypoplasia of orbital ridges. Inner epicanthal folds, ptosis of eyelid, corneal opacity. Cleft lip, cleft palate, or both.

Hands and Feet. Ulnar or radial deviation of hand, hypoplastic to absent thumb, simian crease. Equinovarus, rocker-bottom feet, syndactyly of second and third toes.

Thorax. Relatively broad, with or without widely spaced nipples.

Genitalia. Female: hypoplasia of labia majora with prominent clitoris.

Anus. Malposed or funnel-shaped anus.

Cardiac. Bicuspid aortic and/or pulmonic valves, nodularity of valve leaflets, pulmonic stenosis, coarctation of aorta.

Lung. Malsegmentation to absence of right lung.

Diaphragm. Muscle hypoplasia with or without eventration.

Abdomen. Meckel's diverticulum, heterotopic pancreatic and/or splenic tissue, omphalocele. Incomplete rotation of colon.

Renal. Horseshoe defect, ectopic kidney, double ureter, hydronephrosis, polycystic kidney.

ABNORMALITIES FOUND IN LESS THAN 10 PER CENT OF CASES

Central Nervous System. Facial palsy, paucity of myelination, microgyria, cerebellar hypoplasia, defect of corpus callosum, hydrocephalus, meningomyelocele.

Craniofacial. Wormian cranial bones, shallow elongated sella turcica. Slanted palpebral fissures, hypertelorism, colobomata of iris, cataract, microphthalmos, choanal atresia.

Hands. Syndactyly of third and fourth fingers, polydactyly, short fifth metacarpals, ectrodactyly.

Other Skeletal. Radial aplasia. Incomplete ossification of clavicle. Hemivertebrae, fused vertebrae, short neck, scoliosis, rib anomaly, pectus excavatum, dislocated hip.

Genitalia. Male: hypospadias, bifid scrotum. Female: bifid uterus, ovarian hypoplasia.

Cardiovascular. Anomalous coronary artery, transposition, tetralogy of Fallot, coarctation of aorta, dextrocardia, aberrant subclavian artery, intimal proliferation in arteries with arteriosclerotic change and medial calcification.

Abdominal. Pyloric stenosis, extrahepatic biliary atresia, hypoplastic gallbladder, gallstones, imperforate anus.

Renal. Hydronephrosis, polycystic kidney (small cysts).

Endocrine. Thyroid or adrenal hypoplasia.

Other. Hemangiomata, thymic hypoplasia, tracheoesophageal fistula, thrombocytopenia.

NATURAL HISTORY. Babies with the trisomy 18 syndrome are usually feeble and have a limited capacity for survival. Resuscitation is often performed at birth, and they may have apneic episodes in the neonatal period. Poor sucking capability may necessitate nasogastric tube feeding, but even with optimal management, they fail to thrive. Thirty per cent die within the first month and 50 per cent by two months; only 10 per cent survive the first year as severely mentally defective individuals. Once the diagnosis has been established, the author recommends limitation of all medical means for prolongation of life.

ETIOLOGY. Trisomy for all or a large part of the number 18 chromosome. The great majority of cases have full 18 trisomy, the result of faulty chromosomal distribution, which is most likely to occur at older maternal age; the mean maternal age at birth of babies with this syndrome is 32 years. Translocation cases, the result of chromosomal breakage, can only be excluded by chromosomal studies. When such a case is found, the parents should also have chromosomal studies to determine whether one of them is a balanced translocation carrier with high risk for recurrence in future offspring. Though no adequate studies of recurrence risk exist for full 18 trisomy cases, it seems safe to presume that the recurrence risk would be even lower than the 1 per cent for full 21 trisomy syndrome cases. This latter statement is predicated on the indication that most 18 trisomic individuals die in embryonic or fetal life, as suggested by the chromosomal findings in spontaneous abortuses.

Mosaicism for an additional chromosome 18 leads to a partial clinical expression of the pattern of trisomy 18, with longer survival and any degree of variation between nearly normal and the full pattern.

Partial trisomy 18: Trisomy of the short arm causes a very nonspecific clinical picture and mild or no mental deficiency. Cases with familial trisomy of the short arm, centromere, and proximal one third of the long arm show features of trisomy 18, although not the full pattern. Trisomy for the entire long arm is clinically indistinguishable from full trisomy 18. Trisomy for the distal one third to one half of the long arm leads to a partial picture of trisomy 18 with longer survival and less profound mental deficiency. In early childhood, the patients resemble trisomy 18 cases, whereas adolescents and adults display a more nonspecific pattern of malformation, including prominent orbital ridges, broad and prominent nasal bridge, everted upper lip, receding mandible, poorly modeled ears, short neck, and long, hyperextendible fingers. Muscular tone tends to be decreased, mental deficiency is severe, and about one third of the patients suffer from seizures.

References

Edwards, J. H., et al.: A new trisomic syndrome. Lancet, *1*:787, 1960.

Patau, K., et al.: Multiple congenital anomaly caused by an extra autosome. Lancet, *1*:790, 1960.

Smith, D. W., et al.: A new autosomal trisomy syndrome. J. Pediatr., *57*:338, 1960.

Smith, D. W.: Autosomal abnormalities. Am. J. Obstet. Gynecol., *90*:1055, 1964.

Taylor, A., and Polani, P. E.: Autosomal trisomy syndromes, excluding Down's. Guy's Hosp. Rep., *13*:231, 1964.

Butler, L. J., et al.: No. E (16–18) trisomy syndrome: analysis of 13 cases. Arch. Dis. Child., *40*:600, 1965.

Warkany, J., Passarge, E., and Smith, L. B.: Congenital malformations in autosomal trisomy syndromes. Am. J. Dis. Child., *112*:502, 1966.

Weber, W. W.: Survival and the sex ratio in trisomy 17–18. Am. J. Hum. Genet., *19*:369, 1967.

Turleau, C., and de Grouchy, J.: Trisomy 18 qter and trisomy mapping of chromosome 18. Clin. Genet., *12*:361, 1977.

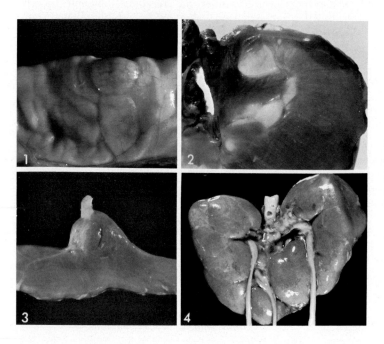

Some pathologic features of trisomy 18 syndrome. *1*, Ectopic pancreatic tissue in duodenum. *2*, Meckel's diverticulum. *3*, Defects of muscle development in diaphragm. *4*, Horseshoe fused kidneys with extra ureter.

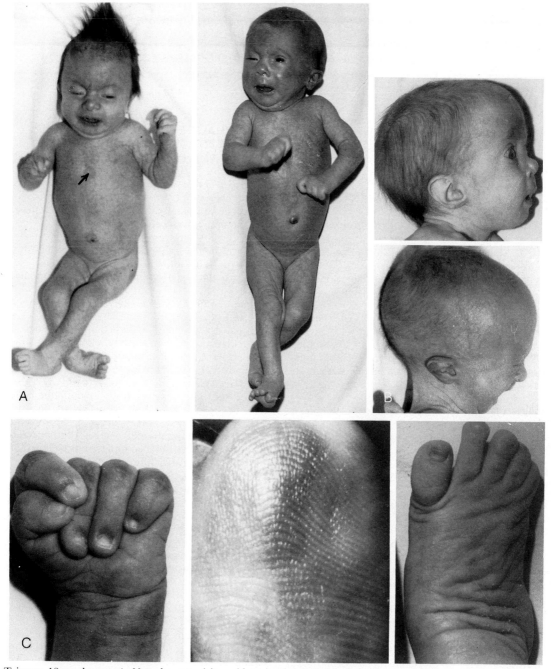

Trisomy 18 syndrome. *A*, Note hypertonicity evident in clenched hands and crossed legs; short sternum (arrow marks lower end); narrow pelvis. *B*, Prominent occiput; low-set, slanted auricle. *C*, Clenched hand with index finger overlying third; hypoplasia of fifth fingernail; low arch dermal ridge configuration on fingertip; dorsiflexed short hallux. (From Smith, D. W.: Am. J. Obstet. Gynecol., *90*:1055, 1964.)

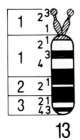

13

TRISOMY 13 SYNDROME

(D₁ Trisomy Syndrome)

*Defects of Eye, Nose, Lip, and Forebrain of
Holoprosencephaly Type; Polydactyly;
Narrow Hyperconvex Fingernails;
Skin Defects of Posterior Scalp*

Apparently described by Bartholin in 1657, this syndrome was not generally recognized until its trisomic etiology was discovered by Patau et al. in 1960. The incidence is about 1 per 5000 births.

ABNORMALITIES FOUND IN 50 PER CENT OR MORE OF PATIENTS

Central Nervous System. Holoprosencephaly type defect with varying degrees of incomplete development of forebrain and olfactory and optic nerves. Minor motor seizures, often with hypsarrhythmic electroencephalogram pattern. Apneic spells in early infancy. Severe mental defect.

Hearing. Apparent deafness (defects of organ of Corti in the two cases studied).

Cranium. Moderate microcephaly with sloping forehead. Wide sagittal suture and fontanels.

Eyes. Microphthalmia, colobomata of iris, or both. Retinal dysplasia, often including islands of cartilage.

Mouth. Cleft lip (60 to 80 per cent), cleft palate, or both.

Auricles. Abnormal helices with or without low-set ears.

Skin. Capillary hemangiomata, especially forehead. Localized scalp defects in parieto-occipital area. Loose skin, posterior neck.

Hands and Feet. Distal palmar axial triradii. Simian crease. Hyperconvex narrow fingernails. Flexion of fingers with or without overlapping and camptodactyly. Polydactyly of hands and sometimes feet. Posterior prominence of heel.

Other Skeletal. Thin posterior ribs with or without missing rib. Hypoplasia of pelvis with shallow acetabular angle.

Cardiac. Abnormality in 80 per cent with ventricular septal defect, patent ductus arteriosus, auricular septal defect, and dextroposition, in decreasing order of frequency.

Genitalia. Male: cryptorchidism, abnormal scrotum. Female: bicornuate uterus.

Hematologic. Increased frequency of nuclear projections in neutrophils. Unusual persistence of embryonic and/or fetal type hemoglobin.

Other. Single umbilical artery. Inguinal or umbilical hernia.

ABNORMALITIES FOUND IN LESS THAN 50 PER CENT OF PATIENTS

Growth. Congenital hypoplasia; mean birth weight, 2480 g.

Central Nervous System. Hypertonia, hypotonia, agenesis of corpus callosum, hydrocephalus, fusion of basal ganglia, cerebellar hypoplasia, meningomyelocele.

Eyes. Shallow supraorbital ridges, slanting palpebral fissures, absent eyebrows, hypotelorism, hypertelorism, anophthalmos, cyclopia.

Nose, Mouth, and Mandible. Absent philtrum, narrow palate, cleft tongue, micrognathia.

Hands and Feet. Retroflexible thumb, ulnar deviation at wrist, low arch digital dermal ridge pattern, fibular S-shaped hallucal dermal ridge pattern, syndactyly, cleft between first and second toes, hypoplastic toenails, equinovarus, radial aplasia.

Cardiac. Anomalous venous return, overriding aorta, pulmonary stenosis, hypoplastic aorta, atretic mitral and/or aortic valves, bicuspid aortic valve.

Abdominal. Omphalocele, heterotopic pancreatic or splenic tissue, incomplete rotation of colon, Meckel's diverticulum.

Renal. Polycystic kidney (31 per cent), hydronephrosis, horseshoe kidney, duplicated ureters.

Genitalia. Male: hypospadias. Female: duplication and/or anomalous insertion of fallopian tubes, uterine cysts, hypoplastic ovaries.

Other. Thrombocytopenia, situs inversus of lungs, cysts of thymus, calcified pulmonary arterioles, large gallbladder, radial aplasia, flexion deformity of large joints, diaphragmatic defect.

NATURAL HISTORY. Forty-four per cent of these babies die within the first month and 69 per cent by six months; only 18 per cent survive the first year. Survivors have severe mental defects, often seizures, and fail to thrive. Only one adult, 33 years of age, has been detected. Because of the high infant mortality, surgical or orthopedic corrective procedures should be withheld in early infancy to await the outcome of the first few months. Furthermore, because of the severe brain defect, it is the opinion of the author that no medical means should be utilized to prolong the life of individuals with this syndrome, as should be self-evident from the accompanying illustrations.

ETIOLOGY. Trisomy for all or a large part of a specific D group (13–15) chromosome that is tentatively referred to as number 13. Older maternal age has been a factor in the occurrence of this aneuploidy syndrome, the mean maternal age being 30.9 years. Although no accurate empiric recurrence risk data are presently available, it is presumed that the likelihood for recurrence is of very low magnitude for the full 13 trisomy cases. As with Down syndrome, chromosomal studies are indicated on 13 trisomy syndrome babies born of young mothers, in order to detect the rare translocation patient having a balanced translocation parent for whom the risk of recurrence would be of major concern.

Cases with *trisomy 13 mosaicism* most often show a less severe clinical phenotype with every degree of variation, from the full pattern of malformation seen in Trisomy 13 to a near-normal phenotype. Survival is usually longer. The degree of mental deficiency is variable.

Partial trisomy for the proximal segment (13pter→q14) is characterized by a nonspecific pattern, including a large nose, short upper lip, receding mandible, fifth finger clinodactyly, and usually severe mental deficiency. The overall picture shows little similarity to that of full trisomy 13, and survival is not significantly reduced. *Partial trisomy for the distal segment (13q14→qter)* has a characteristic phenotype associated with severe mental deficiency. The facies is marked by frontal capillary hemangiomata, a short nose with upturned tip, and elongated philtrum, synophrys, bushy eyebrows and long, incurved lashes, and a prominent antihelix. Trigonocephaly and arhinencephaly have occasionally been seen. About one fourth of the patients die during early postnatal life.

COMMENT. The defects of midface, eye, and forebrain, which occur in variable degree as a feature of this syndrome, appear to be the consequence of a single defect in the early (three weeks) development of the prechordal mesoderm, which is not only necessary for morphogenesis of the midface but also exerts an inductive role on the subsequent development of the prosencephalon, the forepart of the brain. This type of defect has been referred to as holoprosencephaly or arhinencephaly and varies in severity from cyclopia to cebocephaly to less severe forms.

References

Patau, K., et al.: Multiple congenital anomaly caused by an extra chromosome. Lancet, *1*:790, 1960.

Warburg, M., and Mikkelsen, M.: A case of 13–15 trisomy or Bartholin-Patau's syndrome. Acta Ophthalmol. (Kbh.), *41*:321, 1963.

Smith, D. W.: Autosomal abnormalities. Am. J. Obstet. Gynecol., *90*:1055, 1964.

Warkany, J., Passarge, E., and Smith, L. B.: Congenital malformations in autosomal trisomy syndromes. Am. J. Dis. Child., *112*:502, 1966.

Schinzel, A.: Autosomale Chromosomenaberationen. Arch. Genet., *52*:1, 1979.

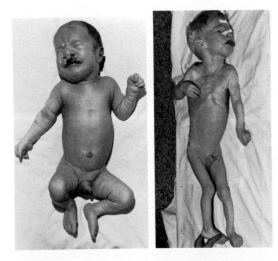

Trisomy 13 patient at six weeks (22 inches, 9 pounds) and again at two years (30 inches, 15 pounds).

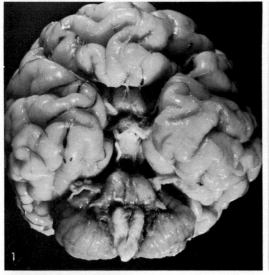

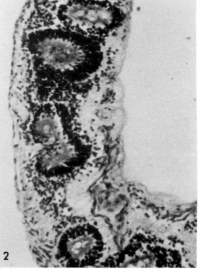

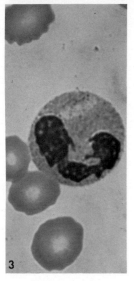

Some pathologic features of trisomy 13 syndrome. *1*, Lack of septation of forebrain (holoprosencephaly). *2*, Dysplastic retina with rosette formation. *3*, Excess nuclear projections in polymorphonuclear leukocyte.

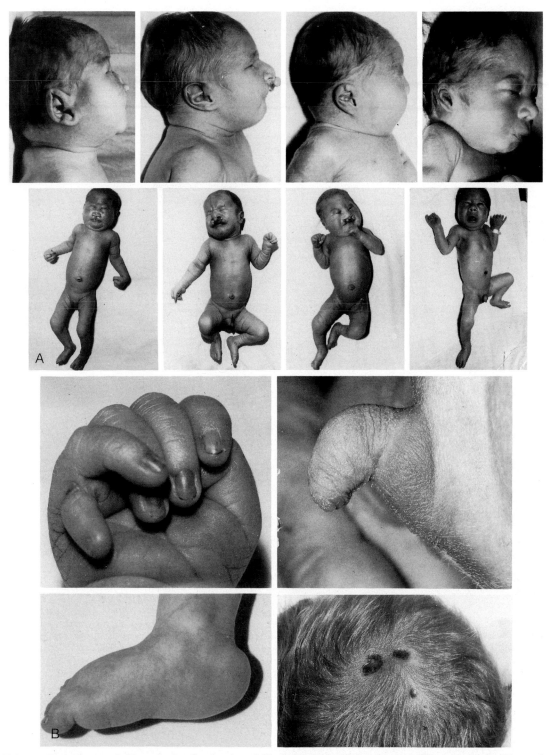

Trisomy 13 syndrome. *A*, Note sloping forehead, variable defect in facial development. (From Smith, D. W., et al: J. Pediatr., *62*:326, 1963.) *B*, Narrow hyperconvex fingernails, anomalous scrotum, prominent heel, and posterior scalp lesions. (From Smith, D. W.: Am. J. Obstet. Gynecol., *90*:1055, 1964.)

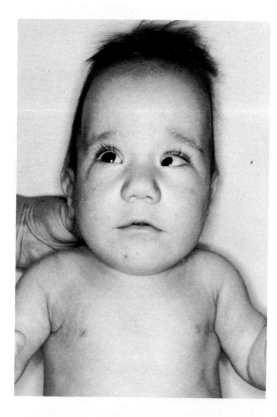

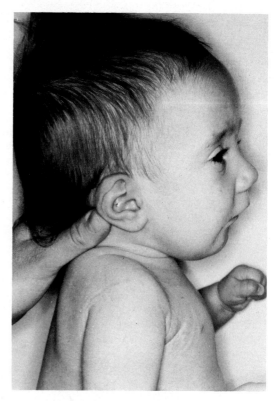

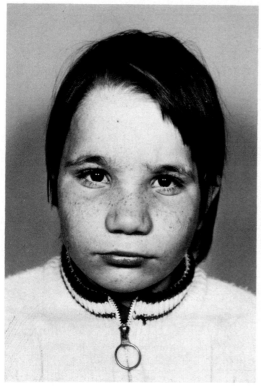

Partial 13 trisomy, proximal segment Q. *Above*, Six month old patient. High forehead; left esotropia; large, broad-based nose; receding mandible. (From Schinzel, A., et al: Humangenetik, *22*:287, 1974.) *Below*, Same patient at 11 years of age. Hypertelorism; prominent and broad-based nose; no strabismus; normal size of the mandible. (From Schinzel, A., Arch. Genet., *52*:180, 1979.)

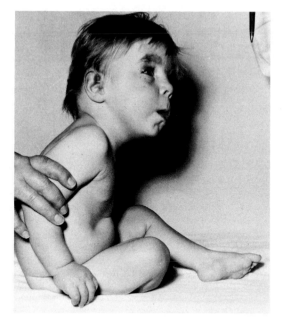

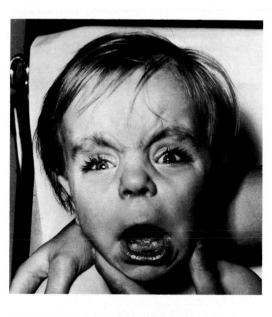

Partial 13 trisomy, distal segment Q. *Above*, One and one-half year old. Note bushy eyebrows, long and curled lashes, small nose, increased distance between nose and upper lip, and prominent antihelix. (From Schinzel, A., Arch. Genet., *52*:178, 1979.) *Below*, Same patient at 12 years of age. (From Schinzel, A., et al.: Humangenetik, *22*:287, 1974.)

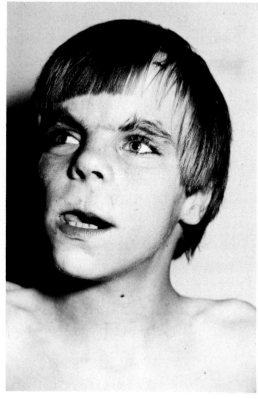

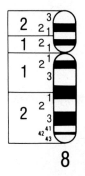

8

TRISOMY 8 SYNDROME
(Usually Trisomy 8/Normal Mosaicism)

Thick Lips, Deep-Set Eyes,
Prominent Ears, Camptodactyly

Patients with trisomy for a C-group autosome have been recognized since 1963. Most of them have been mosaics of trisomy C/normal. The phenotype tends to be similar, and, more recently, chromosomal banding techniques have identified the extra chromosome as number 8. More than 35 cases have been reported.

ABNORMALITIES
Growth. Variable, from small to tall.
Performance. Mild to severe mental deficiency with tendency to poor coordination.
Craniofacial. Tendency toward prominent forehead, deep-set eyes, strabismus, hypertelorism with broad nasal root and prominent nares, full lips, micrognathia, high arched palate, and prominent cupped ears with thick helices.
Limbs. Camptodactyly of second through fifth fingers and toes; limited elbow supination; deep creases, palms and soles; single transverse palmar crease.
Other. Long, slender trunk; narrow pelvis; widely spaced nipples.

OCCASIONAL OR UNCERTAIN INCIDENCE. Absent patellae, conductive deafness, vertebral anomaly (bifid vertebrae, extra lumbar vertebra, spina bifida occulta), cryptorchidism, agenesis of corpus callosum. Hypoplastic anemia, leukopenia.

NATURAL HISTORY. The natural history is largely dependent on the severity of mental deficiency, which is probably related to the proportion of trisomy 8 versus normal cells.

ETIOLOGY. Trisomy 8, the majority of patients being mosaics. Apparently, full trisomy 8 is usually an early lethal disorder.

References

Stalder, G. R., Buhler, E. M., and Weber, J. R.: Possible trisomy in chromosome group 6–12. Lancet, *1*:1379, 1963.

Schinzel, A., et al.: Trisomy 8 mosaicism syndrome. Helv. Pediatr. Acta, *29*:531, 1974.

Schinzel, A.: Catalogue of Unbalanced Chromosome Aberrations in Man. New York, Walter de Gruyter, 1984, p. 325.

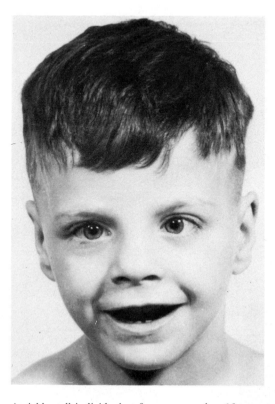

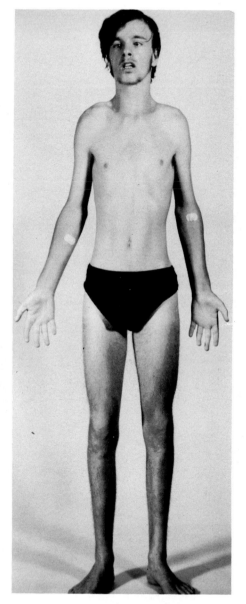

Amiable, tall individual at four years and at 16 years who has trisomy 8/normal mosaicism, with a normal karyotype from cultured leukocytes but trisomy 8 in skin fibroblast cells. He has a moderate hearing deficit and an I.Q. estimated in the 70's. He is quite active and skates, swims, and bowls. Note the facies, the small, widely spaced nipples, and the general body stance. There is some limitation of full extension of the fingers, which are partially webbed, and limited extension of the right elbow. There is hypoplasia of the supraspinatus, trapezius, and upper pectoral musculature. (Courtesy of Dr. G. Howard Valentine, War Memorial Children's Hospital, London, Ontario, Canada.)

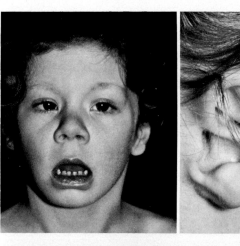

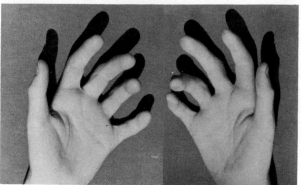

Boy with trisomy 8/normal mosaicism. (From Riccardi V. M., et al.: J. Pediatr. 77:664, 1970.)

Mentally deficient ten year old with trisomy 8/normal mosaicism. Note the prominent ears. (From De Grouchy, J., et al.: Ann. Genet. [Paris], *14*:69, 1971.)

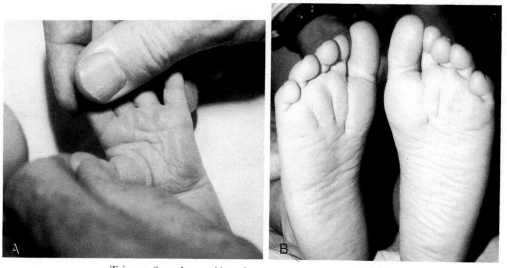

Trisomy 8 syndrome. Note deep creases on palms and soles.

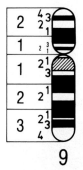

9

TRISOMY 9 MOSAIC SYNDROME

*Joint Contractures, Congenital Heart Defects,
Low-set Malformed Ears*

In 1973, Haslam et al. reported the first case of trisomy 9 mosaicism. In the same year, Feingold et al. reported the first example of a child with full trisomy 9 utilizing blood lymphocytes.

ABNORMALITIES
Growth. Prenatal onset growth deficiency.
Performance. Severe mental deficiency.
Craniofacial. Sloping forehead with narrow bifrontal diameter; upslanting, short palpebral fissures, deeply set eyes; prominent nasal bridge with short root, small fleshy tip, and slit-like nostrils; prominent upper lip covering receding lower lip; micrognathia, low-set, posteriorly rotated, and misshapen ears.
Skeletal. Joint anomalies including abnormal position and/or function of hips, knees, feet, elbows, and digits; kyphoscoliosis; narrow chest; hypoplasia of sacrum, iliac wings, and pubic arch; hypoplastic phalanges of toes.
Other. Congenital heart defects in about two thirds of cases, micropenis, cryptorchidism, renal malformations, cystic dilatation of fourth ventricle with lack of midline fusion of cerebellum.

OCCASIONAL ABNORMALITIES.
Subarachnoid cyst, microphthalmia, preauricular tags, cleft lip and/or palate, bile duct proliferation in absence of a demonstrable stenosis or atresia, punctate mineralization in developing cartilage. Diaphragmatic hernia. Meningocele. Lack of gyration of cerebral hemispheres. Absence of optic tracts. Corneal opacities.

NATURAL HISTORY. The majority of patients die during the early postnatal period. In those that survive, failure to thrive and severe motor and mental deficiency are the rule. Some patients remain bedridden throughout their lives, whereas others achieve the ability to walk and minimal speech.

ETIOLOGY. Trisomy for chromosome 9. The incidence and severity of malformations and mental deficiency correlate with the percentage of trisomic cells in the different tissues.

References

Haslam, R. H. A., et al.: Trisomy 9 mosaicism with multiple congenital anomalies. J. Med. Genet., *10*:180, 1973.

Feingold, M., et al.: A case of Trisomy 9. J. Med. Genet., *10*:184, 1973.

Bowen, P., et al.: Trisomy 9 mosaicism in a newborn infant with multiple malformations. J. Pediatr., *85*:95, 1974.

Akatsuka, A., et al.: Trisomy 9 mosaicism with punctate mineralization in developing cartilages. Eur. J. Pediatr., *131*:271, 1979.

Frohlich, G. S.: Delineation of Trisomy 9. J. Med. Genet., *19*:316, 1982.

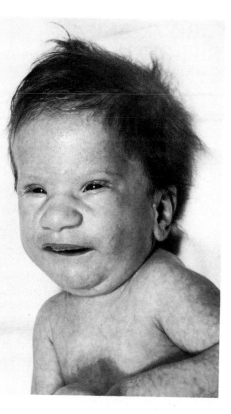

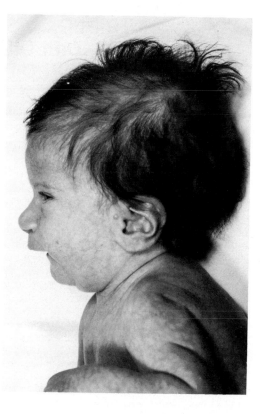

Trisomy 9 mosaic syndrome. Two month old boy. Long and narrow face with narrow eyelids in mongoloid position, broad and bulbous nose with a broad and prominent bridge, short upper lip covering the receding lower lip, small mandible, left preauricular pit, cutis marmorata, inability to lie on the back because of congenital thoracic kyphosis, and flexion position of hands and fingers. (From Schinzel, A., et al.: Humangenetik, *25*:171, 1974.)

TRIPLOIDY SYNDROME AND DIPLOID/TRIPLOID MIXOPLOIDY SYNDROME

Large Placenta with Hydatidiform Changes, Growth Deficiency, Syndactyly of Third and Fourth Fingers

Triploidy, a complete extra set of chromosomes, is estimated to occur in about 2 per cent of conceptuses. Most are lost as miscarriages, accounting for about 20 per cent of all chromosomally abnormal spontaneous abortuses. Triploid pregnancies may be accompanied by varying degrees of toxemia. Fetal wastage may be due to hydatidiform placental changes or to specific cytogenetic characteristics, with only 3 per cent of 69,XYY conceptuses surviving to be recognized. Partial hydatidiform moles are usually associated with a triploid fetus and very rarely undergo malignant changes. Classic moles show more pronounced trophoblastic hyperplasia in the absence of a fetus. These moles show a diploid karyotype and are totally androgenic in origin.

Infrequently, triploid infants survive to be born after 28 weeks' gestation with severe intrauterine growth retardation. Over 50 such infants have been described to date. Instances of diploid/triploid mixoploidy have been less frequently recognized, with only 14 cases reported thus far. Asymmetric growth deficiency with mild syndactyly and occasional genital ambiguity in 46,XX/69,XXY individuals are the key diagnostic features in mixoploid individuals.

ABNORMALITIES. Noted in 50 per cent or more of cases.
Placenta. Large, with tendency toward hydatidiform changes.
Growth. Disproportionate prenatal growth deficiency that affects the skeleton more than the cephalic region. In mixoploid individuals, skeletal growth may be asymmetric.
Craniofacial. Dysplastic calvaria with large posterior fontanel, ocular hypertelorism with eye defects ranging from colobomata to microphthalmia, low nasal bridge, low-set, malformed ears, micrognathia.
Limbs. Syndactyly of third and fourth fingers, simian crease, talipes equinovarus.
Cardiac. Congenital heart defect (atrial and ventricular septal defects).
Genitalia. Male: hypospadias, micropenis, cryptorchidism, Leydig cell hyperplasia.

Other. Brain anomalies, including hydrocephalus and holoprosencephaly; adrenal hypoplasia; and renal anomalies, including cystic dysplasia and hydronephrosis.

OCCASIONAL ABNORMALITIES. Noted in less than 50 per cent of cases. Aberrant skull shape; choanal atresia; cleft lip and/or palate; iris heterochromia; meningomyelocele; macroglossia; omphalocele or umbilical hernia; biliary tract anomalies, including aplasia of the gallbladder; incomplete rotation of colon; proximally placed thumb; clinodactyly of fifth finger; splayed toes.

NATURAL HISTORY. Partial hydatidiform molar pregnancies associated with a triploid fetus should not raise concern regarding the development of choriocarcinoma. All cases of full triploidy have either been stillborn or have died in the early neonatal period, with five months being the longest recorded survival. Individuals with diploid/triploid mixoploidy usually survive and manifest some degree of psychomotor retardation. As a result of body asymmetry, patients with mixoploidy may require a heel lift for the shorter leg to prevent compensatory scoliosis, and some of these people may resemble those having Russell-Silver syndrome. Diagnosis of mixoploidy usually requires skin fibroblast cultures, since the triploid cell line may have disappeared from among peripheral blood leukocytes. The degree of skeletal asymmetry does not appear to correspond to the proportions of triploid cells present, and triploid cells in culture grow with the same variability as diploid cells, except for those with the XYY complement, which grow much more slowly.

ETIOLOGY. In most instances, the extra set of chromosomes is paternally derived, with 66 per cent attributed to double fertilization, 24 per cent due to fertilization with a diploid sperm and 10 per cent a result of fertilization of a diploid egg (failure to shed a polar body). About 60 per cent of the cases have been XXY, with most of the remainder being XXX. It is not unusual for more than one X chromosome to remain active in triploidy. Older maternal age has not been a factor, and there are no data to indicate an increased recurrence risk, such as that seen for chromosomal disorders due to nondisjunction. In several instances, a triploid pregnancy has been followed or preceded by a molar pregnancy.

References

Book, J. A., and Santesson, B.: Malformation syndrome in man associated with triploidy (69 chromosomes). Lancet, *1*:858, 1960.

Ferrier, P., et al.: Congenital asymmetry associated with diploid-triploid mosaicism and large satellites. Lancet, *1*:80, 1964.

Niebular, E.: Triploidy in man: Cytogenetical and clinical aspects. Humangenetik, *21*:103, 1974.

Wertelecki, W., Graham, J. M., and Sergovich, F. R.: The clinical syndrome of triploidy. Obstet. Gynecol., *47*:69, 1976.

Jacobs, P. A., et al.: The origin of human triploids. Ann. Hum. Genet., *42*:49, 1978.

Poland, B. J., and Bailie, D. L.: Cell ploidy in molar placental disease. Teratology, *18*:353, 1978.

Jacobs, P. A., et al.: Late replicating X chromosomes in human triploidy. Am. J. Hum. Genet., *31*:446, 1979.

Graham, J. M., et al.: Diploid-triploid mixoploidy: Clinical and cytogenetic aspects. Pediatrics, *68*:23, 1981.

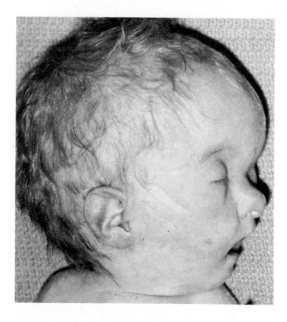

Stillborn infant with triploidy showing relatively large-appearing upper head in relation to very small face.

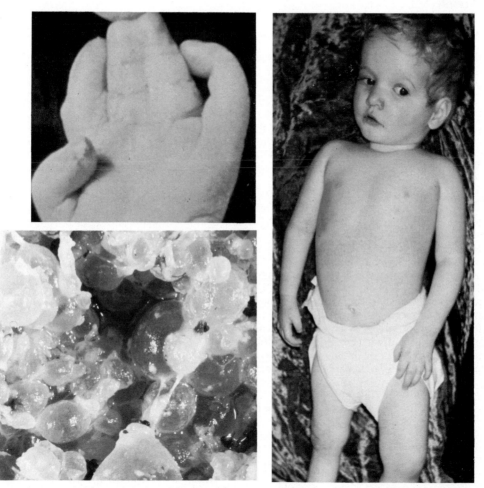

Hand (*upper left*) and placenta (*lower left*) of stillborn infant showing syndactyly and hydatidiform cystic changes, respectively. Infant (*right*) with asymmetric growth deficiency (right side smaller), syndactyly of third and fourth fingers, and mild developmental delay who has triploid/diploid mixoploidy syndrome that is evident only in cultured fibroblasts. (Courtesy of Dr. John M. Graham, Dartmouth School of Medicine, Hanover, New Hampshire.)

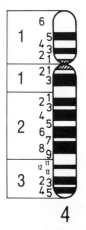

4

TRISOMY 4p SYNDROME
(Trisomy for the Short Arm of Chromosome 4)

*Characteristic Facies, Severe Mental Deficiency
with or without Seizures, Growth Deficiency*

First described by Wilson et al. in 1970, the overall pattern of malformation was more completely delineated by Gonzalez et al. in 1977. Fifty cases have now been described.

ABNORMALITIES
Growth. Prenatal onset growth deficiency. A tendency toward obesity. Adult height ranges from 145 cm to 150 cm.
Performance. Severe mental deficiency present in 100 per cent of cases. Language is more severely delayed than social and fine motor skills.
Neurologic. Hypertonia during infancy followed by hypotonia. Seizures. Abnormal EEGs.
Craniofacies. Microcephaly, prominent forehead, glabella, and supraorbital ridges. Bulbous nose with depressed or flat nasal bridge; synophrys, macroglossia, irregular teeth; small pointed mandible; frequently enlarged ears with abnormal helix and antihelix; short neck.
Limbs. Clinodactyly of fifth fingers, camptodactyly, hypoplastic fingernails and toenails.
Genitalia. Micropenis, hypospadias, cryptorchidism.
Other. Kyphoscoliosis; hypoplastic, widely spaced nipples; absent or additional ribs.

OCCASIONAL ABNORMALITIES. Microphthalmia, abnormal appearance of the retina, cleft lip, preauricular tags, cardiac defects, renal malformations and atresia, absence of corpus callosum, congenital hip dislocations, talipes equinovarus, foot position anomalies, two-three syndactyly of toes, preaxial polydactyly, vertebral anomalies.

NATURAL HISTORY. Approximately one third of reported cases died during early infancy. Without visceral anomalies, life span does not seem to be impaired. Feeding problems are frequent in the neonatal period, and respiratory difficulties are a common complication.

ETIOLOGY. Trisomy for part or most of the short arm of chromosome 4. The clinical phenotype is virtually the same in cases trisomic for the distal two thirds and for the entire short arm.

References

Wilson, M. G., et al.: Inherited pericentric inversion of chromosome No. 4. Am. J. Hum. Genet., *22*:679, 1970.
Dallapiccola, B., et al.: Trisomy 4p: Five new observations and overview. Clin. Genet., *12*:344, 1977.
Gonzalez, C. H., et al.: The trisomy 4p syndrome: Case report and review. Am. J. Med. Genet., *1*:137, 1977.
Crane, J., Sujanski, W., and Smith, A.: 4p Trisomy syndrome: Report of 4 additional cases and segregation analysis of 21 families with different translocations. Am. J. Med. Genet., *4*:219, 1979.

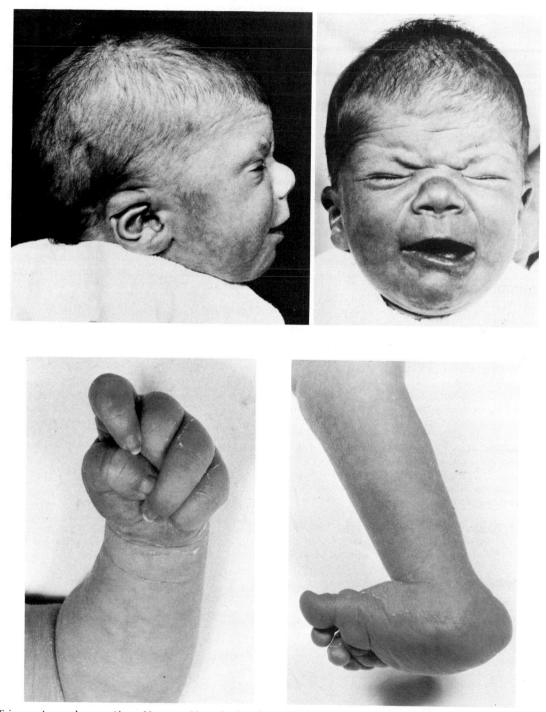

Trisomy 4p syndrome. *Above,* Neonate. Note the low frontal hairline, small pug nose with broad and depressed bridge, asymmetric crying mouth, small, misshapen ears with overfolding of the upper helix, and prominent antihelix. *Below,* Same patient. Flexion position of the fingers of the left hand and rocker-bottom foot with prominent heel. (From Schinzel, A., and Schmid, W.: Humangenetik, *15*:163, 1972.)

4p– SYNDROME

(Chromosome Number 4
Short Arm Deletion Syndrome)

*Ocular Hypertelorism with Broad or Beaked Nose,
Microcephaly and/or Cranial Asymmetry,
and Low-Set, Simple Ear with Preauricular Dimple*

After delineation of the cri du chat syndrome, occasional patients with deletions of the short arm of a B-group chromosome were found who lacked the typical cry and some other features of that condition. Autoradiographic labeling studies revealed that the deficient chromosome was a number 4 rather than a number 5, and the detection of further cases with consistent clinical findings has allowed the definition of the syndrome.

ABNORMALITIES

Growth. Marked growth deficiency, prenatal onset. Microcephaly.

Performance. Feeble fetal activity. Hypotonia. Severe mental deficiency; seizures.

Craniofacial. Strabismus, iris deformity, ocular hypertelorism, epicanthal folds; prominent glabella, cleft lip and/or palate, downturned "fishlike" mouth, short upper lip and philtrum, and micrognathia. Posterior midline scalp defects. Cranial asymmetry. Preauricular tag or pit.

Extremities. Hypoplastic dermal ridges, low dermal ridge count. Simian creases. Talipes equinovarus. Hyperconvex fingernails.

Other. Hypospadias, cryptorchidism, sacral dimple or sinus. Cardiac anomaly.

OCCASIONAL ABNORMALITIES.
Exophthalmos, defect of the medial half of the eyebrows, cardiac defect, metatarsus equinovarus, absence of pubic rami, delayed bone age, precocious puberty. Renal anomaly.

NATURAL HISTORY. These children are profoundly mentally defective and tend to have severe grand mal and minor motor seizures. Those who survive beyond early childhood have shown continued slow growth, with a propensity for respiratory tract infections.

ETIOLOGY. Partial deletion of the short arm of chromosome 4. The parents' chromosomes should be studied to determine whether either is a translocation carrier parent, which is seldom the case.

COMMENT. The missing piece may be as small as 20 per cent of the short arm of chromosome 4 and may even require prophase chromosome study for detection. The author has had experience with four cases that were missed initially on chromosomal evaluation.

References

Leao, J. C., et al.: New syndrome associated with partial deletion of short arms of chromosome no. 4. J.A.M.A., *202*:434, 1967.

Wolf, U., and Reinwein, H.: Klinische und cytogenetische Differentialdiagnose der Defizienzen an den kurzen Armen der B-Chromosomen. Z. Kinderheilkd., *98*:235, 1967.

Pfeiffer, R. A.: Neue Dokumentation zur Abgrenzung eines Syndroms der Deletion des kurzen Arms eines Chromosoms Nr. 4. Z. Kinderheilkd., *102*:49, 1968.

Guthrie, R. D., et al.: The 4p– syndrome. Am. J. Dis. Child., *122*:421, 1971.

Lurie, I. W., et al.: The Wolf-Hirschhorn syndrome. Clin. Genet., *17*:375, 1980.

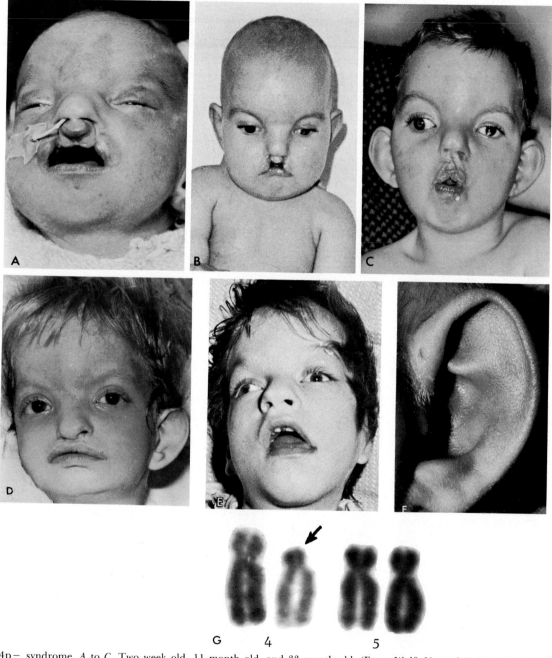

4p− syndrome. *A* to *C*, Two week old, 11 month old, and 33 month old. (From Wolf, U., and Reinwein, H.: Z. Kinderheilkd., *98*:235, 1967.) *D*, Child, five years and nine months old, with height age of ten months and intelligence quotient of less than 20. *E*, Seven year old with height age of three and one-half years and performance age of less than six months. *F*, Relatively simple form of ear with cutaneous pit. *G*, B-group chromosomes from patient shown in *E*.

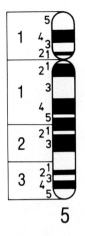

5

5p – SYNDROME

(Cri du Chat Syndrome; Partial Deletion of the Short Arm of Chromosome Number 5 Syndrome)

Cat-Like Cry in Infancy, Microcephaly, Downward Slant of the Palpebral Fissures

Lejeune et al. first described this condition in 1963. Further reports have raised to over 100 the number of cases described.

ABNORMALITIES

General
Low birth weight (less than 2.5 kg)	72%
Slow growth	100%
Cat-like cry	100%

Performance
Mental deficiency	100%
Hypotonia	78%

Craniofacial
Microcephaly	100%
Round face	68%
Hypertelorism	94%
Epicanthal folds	85%
Downward slanting of the palpebral fissures	81%
Strabismus, often divergent	61%
Low-set and/or poorly formed ears	58%
Facial asymmetry	—

Cardiac
Congenital heart disease (variable in type)	30%

Hands
Simian crease	81%
Distal axial triradius	40%
Slightly short metacarpals	—

OCCASIONAL ABNORMALITIES. Cleft lip and cleft palate, myopia, optic atrophy, preauricular skin tag, bifid uvula, dental malocclusion, short neck, clinodactyly, inguinal hernia, cryptorchidism, absent kidney and spleen, hemivertebra, scoliosis, flat feet, premature graying of hair.

NATURAL HISTORY. As babies, the patients tend to be unusually squirmy in their activity. The mewing cry, ascribed to abnormal laryngeal development, becomes less pronounced with the increasing age of the patient, thus making the diagnosis more difficult in older patients. A recent study by Wilkins et al. of 65 children with cri du chat syndrome reared in the home suggests that a much higher level of intellectual performance can be achieved than was previously suggested from studies performed on institutionalized patients. With early special schooling and a supportive home environment, some affected children attained the social and psychomotor level of a normal 5 to 6 year old. One half of the children older than ten years had a vocabulary and sentence structure adequate for communication. Scoliosis is a frequent occurrence.

ETIOLOGY. The underlying chromosomal aberration, partial deletion of the short arm of chromosome number 5, has appeared as a fresh phenomenon in the majority of the cases. A balanced translocation parent, with an increased risk for recurrence, has been found in 10 to 15 per cent of the patients.

References

Lejeune, J., et al.: Trois cas de délétion partielle du bras court du chromosome 5. C. R. Acad. Sci. [D] (Paris), 257:3098, 1963.

Berg, J. M., et al.: Partial deletion of short arm of a chromosome of the 4 and 5 group (Denver) in an adult male. J. Ment. Defic. Res., 9:219, 1965.

Breg, W. R., et al.: The cri-du-chat syndrome in adolescents and adults. J. Pediatr., 77:782, 1970.

Wilkins, L. E., Brown, J. A., and Wolf, B.: Psychomotor development in 65 home-reared children with cri-du-chat syndrome. J. Pediatr., 97:401, 1980.

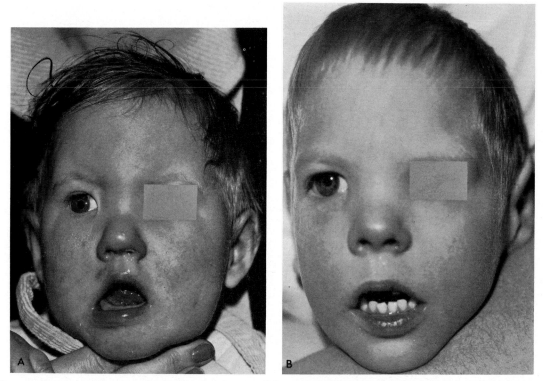

5p− syndrome. *A*, Nine month old with height age of five months; birth length, 18 inches. Note the delay in dentition. *B*, Child, three years and ten months old with height age of one and one-half years. Note the inner epicanthal fold and relatively small cranium with narrow forehead. (From Smith, D. W.: J. Pediatr., *70*:475, 1967.)

TRISOMY 9p SYNDROME

Distal Phalangeal Hypoplasia, Delayed
Closure of Anterior Fontanel, Ocular Hypertelorism

First reported in 1970 by Rethoré et al., the pattern of malformation was set forth by Centerwall and Beatty-DeSana in 1975. Approximately 100 patients have now been described.

ABNORMALITIES

Growth. Growth deficiency, primarily of postnatal onset. Delayed puberty such that some patients continue to grow up to the middle of their third decade.

Performance. Severe mental deficiency. Language tends to be most significantly delayed.

Craniofacies. Macrocephaly, hypertelorism, downslanting palpebral fissures, deep-set eyes, prominent nose, downturned corners of the mouth, cup-shaped ears.

Limbs. Short fingers and toes with dystrophic nails and short terminal phalanges; fifth finger clinodactyly with single flexion crease.

Other Skeletal. Kyphoscoliosis, usually developing during the second decade; hypoplasia of periscapular muscles with deep acromial dimples; defective ossification of the pubic bone, broad ischial tuberosity; pseudoepiphysis of metacarpals, metatarsals, and middle phalanges of fifth fingers; delayed closure of cranial sutures and fontanels.

OCCASIONAL ABNORMALITIES. Micrognathia; epicanthal folds, partial two-three syndactyly of toes and three-four syndactyly of fingers; congenital heart defects in 5 to 10 per cent of cases and cleft lip and/or palate in 5 per cent; hydrocephalus, renal malformations, micropenis, cryptorchidism, hypospadias.

NATURAL HISTORY. Approximately 5 to 10 per cent of reported patients have died in early childhood.

ETIOLOGY. In most cases, the trisomic segment comprises the entire short arm of chromosome 9 (9pter→9p12 to 9q13). If only the distal half of 9p is duplicated, the clinical picture is similar yet less severe, mental deficiency being of only moderate degree. Additional duplication of the proximal segment of 9q (up to 9q22) does not result in a significantly different clinical pattern. However, if the trisomic segment is larger than that (9pter→9q31 or 32), the clinical findings no longer fit into the trisomy 9p syndrome but rather resemble trisomy 9 mosaic syndrome.

References

Rethoré, M. O., et al.: Sur quatre cas de trisomie pour le bras court du chromosome 9. Individualisation d'une nouvelle entité morbide. Ann. Génét., *13*:217, 1970.

Centerwall, W. R., and Beatty-DeSana, J. W.: The trisomy 9p syndrome. Pediatrics, *56*:748, 1975.

Centerwall, W. R., et al.: Familial "partial 9p" trisomy: six cases and four carriers in three generations. J. Med. Genet., *13*:57, 1976.

Schinzel, A.: Trisomy 9p, a chromosome aberration with distinct radiologic findings. Radiology, *130*:125, 1979.

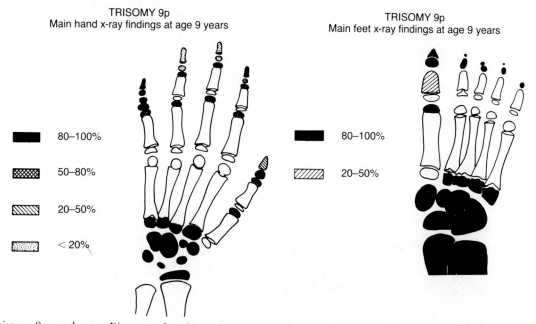

TRISOMY 9p
Main hand x-ray findings at age 9 years

TRISOMY 9p
Main feet x-ray findings at age 9 years

80–100%

50–80%

20–50%

< 20%

80–100%

20–50%

Trisomy 9p syndrome. Diagram of major radiologic findings in hand and foot of a nine year old patient. Pseudoepiphyses on metacarpals and metatarsals 2 to 5; notches on metacarpal 1, metatarsal 1, and proximal and middle phalanges of fingers; hypoplasia of the middle phalanx of fifth finger, terminal phalanges of fingers, and middle and terminal phalanges of toes; thick epiphyses, especially of terminal phalanges of big toe, thumb, and little finger; and clinodactyly of fifth finger. (From Schinzel, A.: Radiology, *130*:125, 1979.)

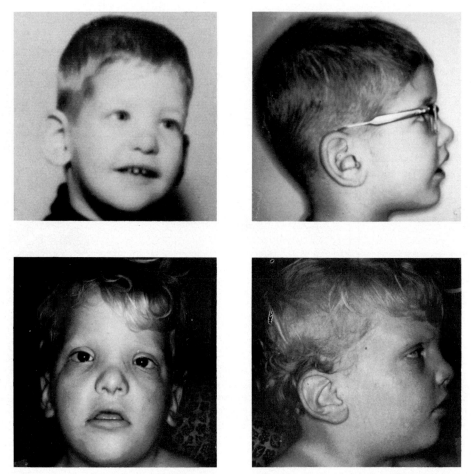

Two children with trisomy 9p syndrome. (Courtesy of Dr. Willard Centerwall, University of California, Davis.)

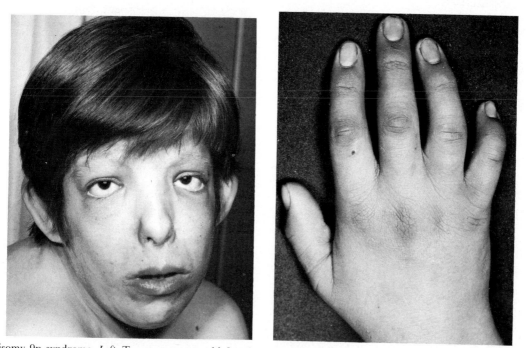

Trisomy 9p syndrome. *Left*, Twenty-one year old female patient. Note low forehead, hypertelorism, downslanting palpebral fissures, bulbous nose, short distance between nose and upper lip, thick lips, protruding ears, and short neck. *Right*, Hand from a 17 year old patient. Short hand and fingers, clinodactyly of little finger, and hypoplastic terminal phalanges of thumbs and nails of thumb and little finger. (Right photo from Schinzel, A., et al.: Hum. Genet., *30*:307, 1975.)

9p – SYNDROME

(9p Monosomy)

Craniostenosis with Trigonocephaly, Upslanting Palpebral Fissures, Hypoplastic Supraorbital Ridges

Since the initial delineation of this disorder in 1973 by Alfi et al., a number of similarly affected patients have been reported.

ABNORMALITIES

Growth. Usually normal.

Performance. Although a few affected individuals have had an intelligence quotient of 50, the majority have had severe mental deficiency.

Craniofacies. Craniostenosis involving the metopic suture leading to trigonocephaly; upslanting palpebral fissures; prominent eyes secondary to hypoplastic supraorbital ridges; midfacial hypoplasia with a short nose, depressed nasal bridge, anteverted nares, and long philtrum; micrognathia; posteriorly rotated, poorly formed ears with hypoplastic, adherent ear lobes; short neck.

Limbs. Long middle phalanges of the fingers with extra flexion creases; short distal phalanges with short nails; excess in whorl patterns on fingertips; foot positioning defects.

Cardiovascular. Ventricular septal defects, patent ductus arteriosus and/or pulmonic stenosis in one third to one half of patients.

Other. Scoliosis, widely spaced nipples, diastasis recti, inguinal and/or umbilical hernia, micropenis and/or cryptorchidism in males; hypoplastic labia majora in females.

OCCASIONAL ABNORMALITIES.
Cleft palate; postaxial polydactyly; diaphragmatic hernia; hydronephrosis; radiographic anomalies of ribs, clavicles, and vertebrae.

ETIOLOGY.
Deletion of the distal portion of the short arm of chromosome 9. In most cases, the breakpoints were located at the 9p21 or 9p22 bands.

References

Alfi, O. S., et al.; Deletion of the short arm of chromosome 9(46,9p−): A new deletion syndrome. Ann. Genet., *16*:17, 1973.

Alfi, O. S., et al.: The 9p− syndrome. Ann. Genet., *19*:11, 1976.

Mattei, J. F., et al.: Pericentric inversion, inv (9)(p22q32), in the father of a child with a duplication-deletion of chromosome 9 and gene dosage effect for adenylate kinase-I. Clin. Genet., *17*:129, 1980.

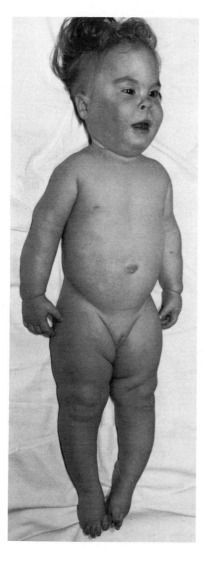

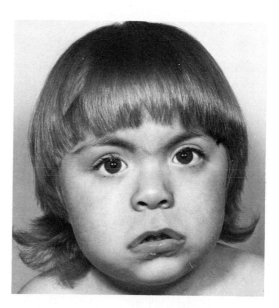

9p− syndrome. *Left,* Ten month old patient. Note trigonocephalic configuration of the skull with metopic prominence, upslanting palpebral fissures, short nose with anteverted nostrils, and short and broad neck. *Right,* One and one-half year old patient. Full, round face with low, narrow forehead, synophrys, and short nose with anteverted nostrils. (Courtesy of Dr. Albert Schinzel, University of Zürich.)

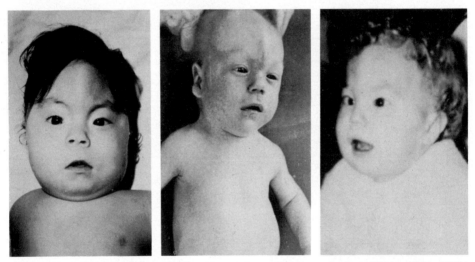

Three affected individuals with 9p− syndrome. (From Alfi, O., et al.: Ann. Génét., *19*:11, 1976.)

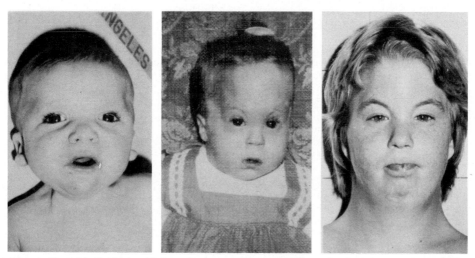

Three affected individuals with 9p– syndrome. (From Alfi, O., et al.: Ann. Génét., *19*:11, 1976.)

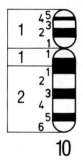

PARTIAL TRISOMY 10q SYNDROME

Ptosis, Short Palpebral Fissures, Camptodactyly

First set forth as a specific phenotype by Yunis and Sanchez in 1974, this disorder has been further delineated by Klep-de Pater et al. in 1979.

ABNORMALITIES

Growth. Prenatal onset growth deficiency; mean birth weight of 2.7 kg.

Performance. Severe mental deficiency.

Craniofacies. Microcephaly; flat face with high forehead and high, arched eyebrows; ptosis; short palpebral fissures; microphthalmia; broad and depressed nasal bridge, anteverted nares, bow-shaped mouth with prominent upper lip; cleft palate; malformed, posteriorly rotated ears.

Limbs. Camptodactyly, proximally placed thumbs, syndactyly between second and third toes, foot position anomalies, hypoplastic dermal ridge patterns.

Other. Heart and renal malformations—each occurs in approximately one half of affected patients; kyphoscoliosis; pectus excavatum; eleven pairs of ribs; cryptorchidism.

OCCASIONAL ABNORMALITIES. Brain malformations, ocular anomalies, malrotation of the gut, hypospadias, vertebral malformations, postaxial hexadactyly of hands, streak gonads.

NATURAL HISTORY. Approximately one half of reported patients died within the first year of life, usually from congenital heart defects and other malformations. Surviving children showed marked mental deficiency and usually are bedridden without the ability to communicate.

ETIOLOGY. Trisomy 10q24→qter, the distal segment of the long arm of chromosome 10.

References

Yunis, J. J., et al.: A new syndrome resulting from partial trisomy for the distal third of the long arm of chromosome 10. J. Pediatr., *84*:567, 1974.

Klep-de Pater, J. M., et al.: Partial trisomy 10q. A recognizable syndrome. Hum. Genet., *46*:29, 1979.

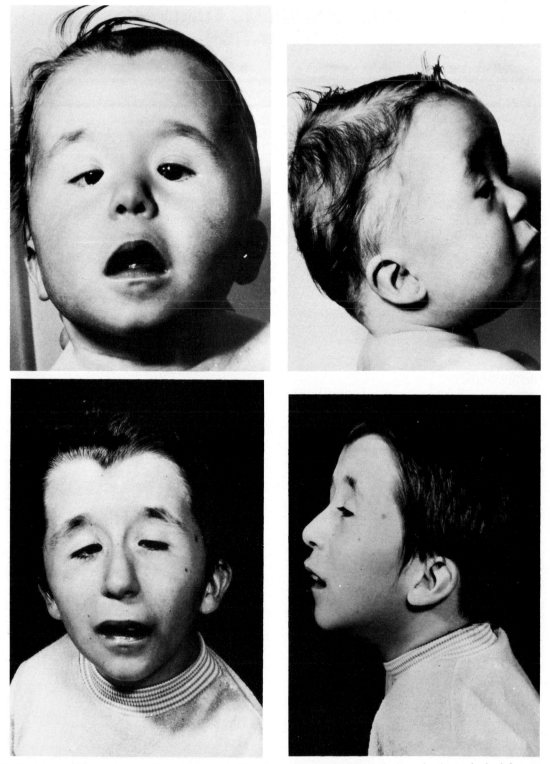

Partial trisomy 10q syndrome. *Above*, Two year old patient. Note high forehead, downslanting palpebral fissures, narrow lids, small nose, and low-set ears. *Below*, Same patient at ten years of age. (From Bühler, E., et al.:Helv. Paediatr. Acta, *22*:41, 1967.)

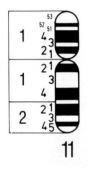

11

ANIRIDIA–WILMS TUMOR ASSOCIATION

At least 50 cases of the association of Wilms tumor and aniridia have been reported, and it is estimated that one in 70 patients with aniridia also has Wilms tumor. Many of these patients also have other defects. In 1978, Riccardi et al. identified an interstitial deletion of 11p in a group of patients with aniridia and Wilms tumor. The pattern of malformation seen in association with that chromosomal abnormality is set forth subsequently. It is important, however, to realize that 11p− is not found in all patients with the aniridia–Wilms tumor association.

ABNORMALITIES
Performance. Moderate to severe mental deficiency in most patients.
Growth. Growth deficiency and microcephaly in at least one half of the patients.
Craniofacial. Prominent lips, micrognathia, poorly formed ears.
Eyes. Aniridia in most patients; congenital cataracts, nystagmus, ptosis, blindness.
Genitalia. Cryptorchidism, hypospadias.
Wilms Tumor. In one half of the patients.

OCCASIONAL ABNORMALITIES. Glaucoma, kyphoscoliosis, inguinal hernias, ambiguous external genitalia, streak gonads, gonadoblastoma, fifth finger clinodactyly.

ETIOLOGY. For all 11 cases, the deletion includes band 11p13. Differences in the size of the deleted segment (especially distal to 11p13) in individual cases may account for the observed variability in concomitant features and in the degree of growth and mental deficiency. Deletions of segments in 11p, not including 11p13, do not cause the aniridia–Wilms tumor association. Familial occurrence resulting from unbalanced transmission of a balanced insertional translocation has been recorded. An interstitial deletion in 11p should be particularly sought in the cytogenetic investigation of mentally retarded patients with Wilms tumor and/or aniridia.

References

Anderson, S. R., et al.: Aniridia, cataract and gonadoblastoma in a mentally retarded girl with deletion of chromosome 11. Ophthalmologica, *176*:171, 1978.

Riccardi, V. M., et al.: Chromosomal imbalance in the aniridia–Wilms' tumor association: 11p interstitial deletion. Pediatrics, *61*:604, 1978.

Francke, U., et al.: Aniridia–Wilms' tumor association: evidence for specific deletion of 11p13. Cytogenet. Cell Genet., *24*:185, 1979.

Hittner, H. M., Riccardi, V. M., and Francke, U.: Aniridia caused by a heritable chromosome 11 deletion. Ophthalmology, *86*:1173, 1979.

Yunis, J. J., and Ramsay, N. K. C.: Familial occurrence of the aniridia–Wilms tumor syndrome with deletion 11p13-14.1. J. Pediatr., *96*:1027, 1980.

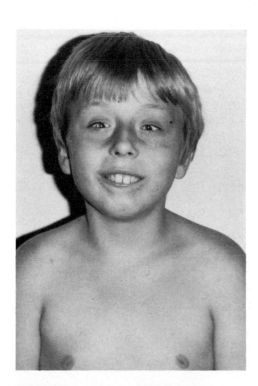

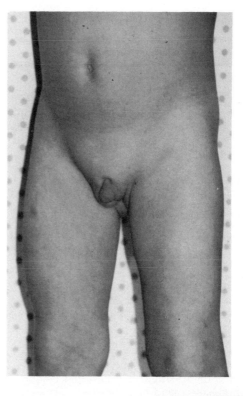

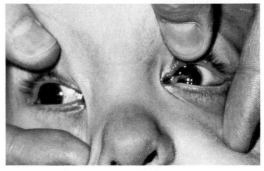

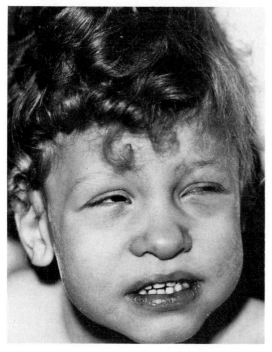

Above, Facies and micropenis in a body with aniridia–Wilms tumor association. (Courtesy of Dr. Vincent M. Riccardi, Baylor College of Medicine, Houston.) *Below*, Two year old boy with microcephaly, bilateral aniridia, ptosis, and cataract. The patient also has Wilms tumor on the right side. (Courtesy of Dr. B. Zabel, Mainz, Germany.)

13q– SYNDROME

Microcephaly with High Nasal Bridge,
Eye Defect, Thumb Hypoplasia

Partial deletion of the long arm of one of the D-group chromosomes was initially reported in 1963 by Lele et al. in a mentally deficient and growth deficient patient with retinoblastoma. Subsequently, at least 50 cases have been recorded, and the deleted chromosome has been considered to be number 13. The phenotype has been variable, but a pattern of malformation is emerging that should allow for suspicion of this disorder. A similar phenotype has been noted in 13 ring chromosome patients who are missing part of the short arm as well as part of the long arm of chromosome 13. The features listed below are those found in 13q– patients.

ABNORMALITIES. Other than mental deficiency and growth deficiency, the particular anomalies have occurred in only one third to two thirds of the cases.
Growth. Growth deficiency, usually of prenatal onset.
CNS. Mental deficiency. Microcephaly with tendency toward trigonocephaly- and holoprosencephaly-type of brain defects.
Facial. Prominent nasal bridge, hypertelorism. Ptosis, epicanthal folds, microphthalmia, colobomata. Retinoblastoma, usually bilateral. Prominent maxilla, micrognathia. Prominent ears, slanting, low placement.
Neck. Short, webbing.
Limbs. Small to absent thumbs, clinodactyly of fifth finger. Talipes equinovarus, short big toe.
Cardiac. Cardiac defect.
Genitalia. Hypospadias, cryptorchidism.
Other. Focal lumbar agenesis.

OCCASIONAL ABNORMALITIES. Found in one or two of the 11 patients. Optic nerve and retinal dysplasia, facial asymmetry, narrow palate, imperforate anus, bifid scrotum, pelvic anomaly, renal anomaly.

NATURAL HISTORY. Though the degree of mental deficiency has been variable, most patients have been severely retarded. The oldest, a 25 year old, was unable to speak or ambulate.

ETIOLOGY. Deletion of part of the long arm of a 13 chromosome. Ring 13 chromosome individuals may have a similar pattern of malformation.

COMMENT. The finding of retinoblastoma in some 13q– patients as well as in several with the 13 ring chromosome indicates a significant causal relationship between this genetic imbalance and the likelihood of developing this type of tumor. The deletion of band Q-14 on the long arm of chromosome 13 has been the specific region implicated in this particular cause for retinoblastoma. Chromosome studies would seem merited in patients with retinoblastoma who also have mental and growth deficiencies plus or minus some of the foregoing anomalies.

References

Lele, K. P., Penrose, L. S., and Stallarf, H. B.: Chromosome deletion in a case of retinoblastoma. Ann. Hum. Genet., *27*:171, 1963.

Allerdice, P. W., et al.: The 13q– deletion syndrome. Am. J. Hum. Genet., *21*:499, 1969.

Taylor, A. I.: Dq–, Dr and retinoblastoma. Humangenetik, *10*:209, 1970.

Yunis, J. J., and Ramsay, N.: Retinoblastoma and sub band deletion of chromosome 13. Am. J. Dis. Child., *132*:161, 1978.

Riccardi, V. M., et al.: Partial triplication and deletion of 13q: study of a family presenting with bilateral retinoblastoma. Clin. Genet., *18*:332, 1979.

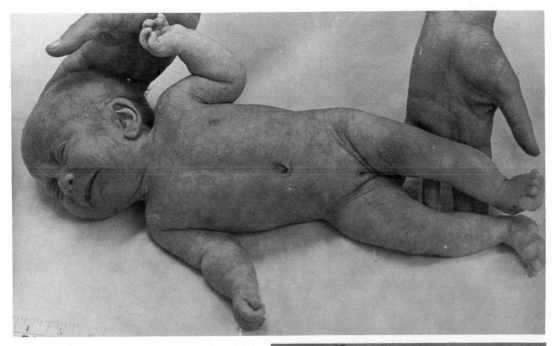

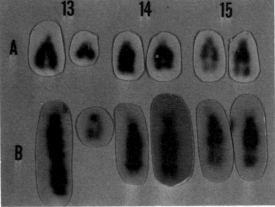

Above, Patient, who died at three months, with microcephaly, cleft palate, low-set ears, short neck with slight webbing, relatively short limbs with clenched hands, short sternum, and marked cutis marmorata. *Right*, D-group chromosomes showing 13q− deletion in the patient (*A*) and her mother (*B*), who is a 13/13 balanced translocation carrier. (Courtesy of Dr. M. Jansch, St. Joseph's Hospital, Fort Wayne, Indiana.)

18p– SYNDROME

Mental and Growth Deficiencies, Ptosis or
Epicanthal Folds, Prominent Auricles

Deletion of the short arm of chromosome 18 was first noted by de Grouchy et al. in 1963. Subsequently, more than 75 cases have been reported. There is rather broad variability in the phenotype.

ABNORMALITIES. The most consistent features are listed below.
Growth. Mild to moderate growth deficiency.
CNS. Mental deficiency, tendency toward hypotonia. Microcephaly (mild).
Facial. Ptosis, epicanthal folds, low nasal bridge, hypertelorism, rounded facies, micrognathia, wide mouth, downturning corners of mouth, large protruding ears.
Dental. High frequency of caries.
Limbs. Relatively small hands and feet.
Other. Pectus excavatum.

OCCASIONAL OR UNCERTAIN INCIDENCE

Immunologic. IgA absence or deficiency, usually asymptomatic.
CNS and Facial. Holoprosencephaly arhinencephaly-type defect (five cases).
Skin and Hair. Alopecia (three cases), hypopigmentation.
Other. Cataract, strabismus, webbed neck, broad chest, kyphoscoliosis, clinodactyly of fifth fingers, simian crease, cubitus valgus, inguinal hernia, dislocation of hip, talipes equinovarus. Development of rheumatoid arthritis–like signs and symptoms.

NATURAL HISTORY. Mild to severe mental deficiency. I.Q.s range from 25 to 75, with an average of about 45 to 50. There is a dissociation between language ability and practical performance; many do not speak even simple sentences before seven to nine years of age. Restlessness, emotional lability, fear of strangers, and lack of concentration capability are frequent features in their behavior. They can best be helped in small groups intended especially for the mentally deficient. The prognosis is poor for those patients with holoprosencephaly-type defect. Otherwise, life expectancy does not seem to be impaired. Alopecia, when a problem, develops during infancy. Adequate adaptation has occurred in some patients, and they can be capable of reproduction.

ETIOLOGY. Short arm 18 deletion, sometimes as part of the deficiency in a ring 18 chromosome. Parents should be studied to determine whether either is a balanced translocation carrier or has the unbalanced 18p– deletion. Offspring from a parent with the same deletion have been affected, who presumably would have a 50 per cent risk.

There has been a 60 per cent predominance of affected females. The mean parental ages of 31.3 years for the mothers and 35.7 for the fathers are older than average.

References

De Grouchy, J., et al.: Dysmorphie complexe avec oligophrénie: Délétion des bras courts d'un chromosome 17–18. C. R. Acad. Sci. [D] (Paris), *256*:1028, 1963.
Uchida, I. A., et al.: Familial short arm deficiency of chromosome 18 concomitant with arhinencephaly and alopecia congenita. Am. J. Hum. Genet., *17*:410, 1965.
Reinwein, H., et al.: Defizienz am kurzen Arm eines Chromosoms Nr. 18 (46,XX,18p–). Ein einheitliches Missbildungs syndrom. Monatsschr. Kinderheilkd., *116*:511, 1968.
Schinzel, A., et al.: The 18p– syndrome. Arch Genetik, *47*:1, 1974.

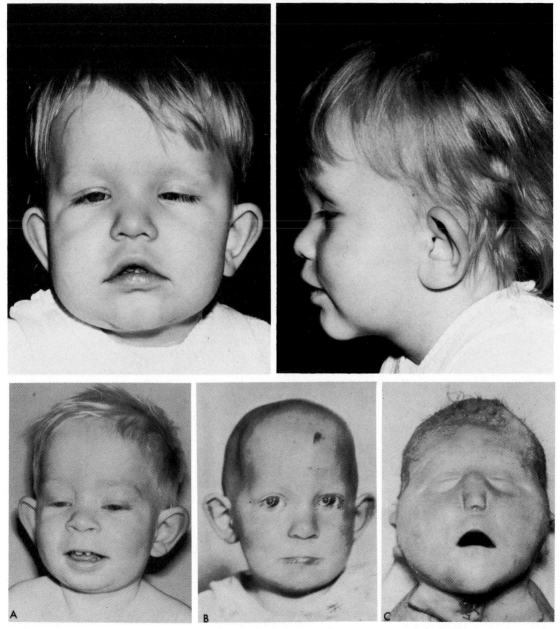

18p− syndrome. *Above*, Three year old. (From Reinwein, H., et al.: Monatsschr. Kinderheilkd., *116*:511, 1968.) *Below*, Mother (mosaic 18p−/normal) shown as a child (*B*) and two of her affected offspring (*A* and *C*), showing variability in expression for the same inherited 18p− deletion, including alopecia (*B*) and cebocephaly (*C*). (From Uchida, I. A., et al.: Am. J. Hum. Genet., *17*:410, 1965.)

18q – SYNDROME

(Long Arm 18 Deletion Syndrome)

Midfacial Hypoplasia, Prominent Antihelix, Whorl Digital Pattern

Discovered by de Grouchy et al. in 1964, this genetic imbalance syndrome has been documented in more than 29 cases.

ABNORMALITIES

Growth. Small stature.

Performance. Mental deficiency with hypotonia, poor coordination, nystagmus, conductive deafness.

Craniofacial. Microcephaly. Midfacial hypoplasia with deep-set eyes. Carp-shaped mouth, narrow palate.

Ears. Prominent antihelix, antitragus, or both. Narrow or atretic external canal.

Limbs. Long hands, tapering fingers, and short first metacarpal with proximal thumb. High-frequency whorl digital pattern, distal axial triradius, simian crease. Distal hypoplastic tapering of lower legs. Abnormal toe placement. Vertical talus with or without talipes equinovarus.

Genitalia. Female: hypoplastic labia minora. Male: cryptorchidism with or without small scrotum and penis.

Other. Skin dimples over acromion and knuckles. Cardiac defect.

OCCASIONAL ABNORMALITIES

Eyes. Inner epicanthal folds, slanted palpebral fissures, ocular hypertelorism, microphthalmia, corneal abnormality, cataract, retinal defect, abnormal optic disc.

Ears. Atretic middle ear, low-set ears.

Other. Cleft palate (30 per cent), widely spaced nipples, extra rib, horseshoe kidney, lipomata at lateral border of feet. Eczema. Absence of IgA.

NATURAL HISTORY. Mental deficiency, with I.Q.s from 40 to 85, and growth deficiency, coupled with various visual and hearing problems, may leave these individuals seriously handicapped. Behavioral problems, including obnoxious or autistic behavior, may be features. However, some patients with this deletion have not been severely affected. For example, a ten year old child studied by Wertelecki and Gerald was not obviously debilitated.

ETIOLOGY. Deletion of part of the long arm of chromosome 18; most commonly a simple deletion and occasionally as a part of a ring chromosome 18.

References

De Grouchy, J., et al.: Délétion partielle du bras long du chromosome 18. Path. Biol. (Paris), *12*:579, 1964.

Wertelecki, W., and Gerald, P. S.: Clinical and chromosomal studies of the 18q– syndrome. J. Pediatr., *78*:44, 1971.

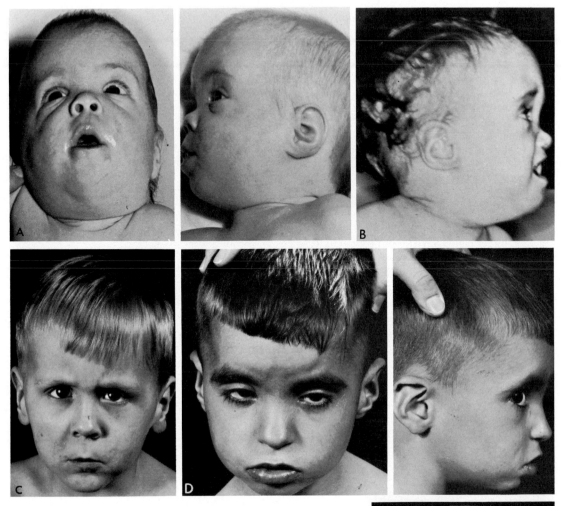

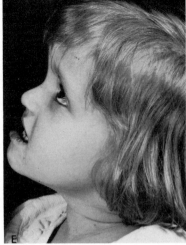

18q− syndrome. *A*, Young infant. Note shape of mouth, midfacial hypoplasia, and prominent antihelix. (Courtesy of E. Engel, Vanderbilt University.) *B*, Infant. Note prominent antihelix and absence of external auditory canal openings. *C*, Note mild slant to palpebral fissures, strabismus, and facial asymmetry. *D*, Note mouth and micrognathia. *E*, Note prominent forehead in relation to hypoplasia of midface. (*B* to *E* courtesy of W. Wertelecki, National Cancer Institute–NIH, P. S. Gerald, Boston Children's Hospital.)

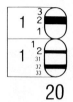

TRISOMY 20p SYNDROME

Blepharophimosis, Large and Poorly Formed Ears,
Cubitus Valgus

ABNORMALITIES

Growth. Normal in most cases.

Performance. Mild to moderate mental deficiency. Hypotonia, poor coordination, ataxia, tremor.

Craniofacies. Brachycephaly; upslanting palpebral fissures; blepharophimosis, hypotelorism or hypertelorism; flat nasal bridge with anteverted nares; large and poorly formed ears; abnormal teeth.

Limbs. Cubitus valgus, small and tapering fingers, fifth finger clinodactyly; foot position defects.

Other. Vertebral defects; unusual pelvic configuration; widely spaced and hypoplastic nipples; kyphoscoliosis, umbilical and/or inguinal hernias; genital hypoplasia with cryptorchidism.

OCCASIONAL ABNORMALITIES.
Cardiac defects including ventricular septal defect and tetralogy of Fallot, renal malformations, atretic ear canals, iridal colobomata, myopia, strabismus, cataract, hydrocephalus.

NATURAL HISTORY. Two out of 22 patients died in early infancy of congenital heart defects.

ETIOLOGY. Almost all reported cases were caused by familial rearrangements. In some cases, patients with mild mental deficiency and no major malformations were not detected before the birth of a second affected sibling.

References

Franche, U.: Partial duplication 20p. *In* Yunis, J. J. (ed.): New Chromosomal Syndromes. New York, Academic Press, 1977.

Schinzel, A.: Trisomy 20pter→q11 in a malformed boy from a t(13;20)(p11;q11) translocation carrier mother. Hum. Genet., *53*:169, 1980.

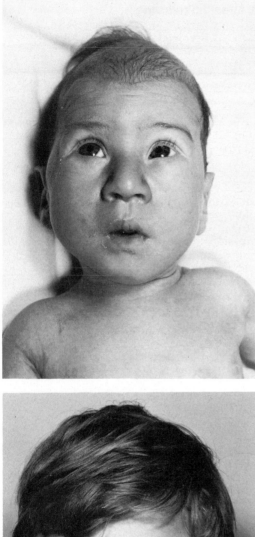

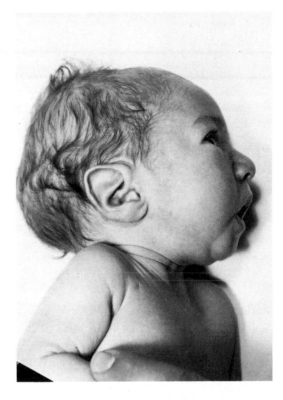

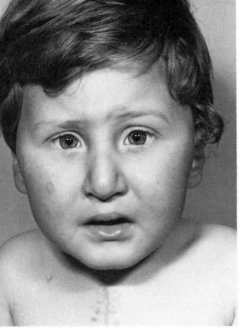

Trisomy 20p syndrome. *Above*, Two month old patient. Note sloping forehead, upslanting palpebral fissures, hypotelorism, large nose, small mouth, and posteriorly rotated ears. *Below*, Same patient at two years and ten months. Deep-set eyes; upward slant less marked than at two months. (From Schinzel, A., Hum. Genet., 53:169, 1980.)

CAT-EYE SYNDROME

(Coloboma of Iris–Anal Atresia Syndrome)

*Coloboma of Iris,
Downslanting Palpebral Fissures, Anal Atresia*

Anal atresia and colobomata of the iris, initially considered the hallmarks of this disorder, are present in combination in only a minority of the 40 patients reported.

ABNORMALITIES

Performance. Usually mild mental deficiency. Some patients have been of normal intelligence but emotionally retarded.

Growth. Normal in the majority of cases.

Craniofacial. Mild hypertelorism; downslanting palpebral fissures; inferior coloboma of iris, choroid, and/or retina; micrognathia, preauricular pits and/or tags.

Cardiac. Cardiac defects in more than one third of cases, including total anomalous pulmonary venous return and persistence of the left superior vena cava.

Anus. Anal atresia with rectovestibular fistula.

Renal. Renal agenesis.

OCCASIONAL ABNORMALITIES. Microphthalmos; low-set, malformed ears with stenotic external canals; biliary atresia; dislocation of hip; radial aplasia; cleft palate; malrotation of gut; agenesis of uterus and fallopian tubes.

ETIOLOGY. An abnormally small acrocentric extra chromosome about one half the size of a G-group autosome. Complete agreement as to the identification of the marker has not been reached. Bühler considers it to be a deleted number 22; Guanti considers it to be a chromosome 13 with an interstitial deletion; and Schinzel considers it to be a bisatellited, iso-dicentric chromosome, most probably derived from either one or both 22 chromosomes. Schinzel feels that the extra chromosome is derived from two identical segments of chromosome 22, consisting of the satellites, the entire short arm, the centromere, and a tiny piece of the long arm (22pter→22q11). That segment is thus present in quadruplicate.

One characteristic feature of the cat-eye syndrome is the high variability of clinical features noted, especially in the four instances of direct transmission of the extra chromosome from a parent to a child.

References

Schachenmann, G., et al.: Chromosomes in coloboma and anal atresia. Lancet, 2:290, 1965.

Darby, C. W., and Hughes, D. T.: Dermatoglyphics and chromosomes in cat-eye syndrome. Br. Med. J., 3:47, 1971.

Bühler, E. M., et al.: Cat-eye syndrome, a partial trisomy 22. Humangenetik, 15:150, 1972.

Balci, S., et al.: The cat-eye syndrome with unusual skeletal malformations. Acta Paediatr. Scand., 63:623, 1974.

Guanti, G.: The etiology of the cat eye syndrome reconsidered. J. Med. Genet., 18:108, 1981.

Schinzel, A., et al.: The "Cat Eye Syndrome": Dicentric small marker chromosome probably derived from a No. 22 (tetrasomy 22pter q11) associated with a characteristic phenotype. Report of 11 patients and delineation of the clinical picture. Hum. Genet., 57:148, 1981.

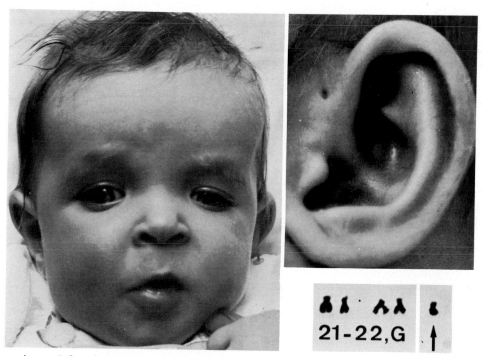

Cat-eye syndrome. Infant showing downslanting palpebral fissures, colobomata of iris, and preauricular pits. Arrow denotes extra chromosome. (From Schmid, W.: J. Genet. Hum., *16*:89, 1967.)

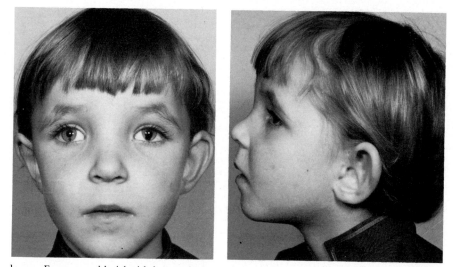

Cat-eye syndrome. Four year old girl with hypertelorism, downslanting palpebral fissures, total coloboma on left and peripheral coloboma on right iris, exotropia, and preauricular pit. (Courtesy of Dr. Albert Schinzel, University of Zürich Medical School.)

XYY SYNDROME

Tall Stature, Aberrant Behavior

Despite an incidence of one in 840 newborn males, the XYY individual is seldom detected during childhood or even in the adult. The features of the XYY syndrome are often subtle and not overtly suggestive of a chromosomal abnormality disorder. However, a pattern of variable abnormalities has come to be appreciated, which may allow for clinical suspicion of the XYY syndrome in childhood.

ABNORMALITIES. Variable features from among the following:
Growth. Acceleration in midchildhood.
Performance. Dull mentality. Explosive behavior, sometimes antisocial. Relative weakness, with poor fine motor coordination and sometimes a fine intentional tremor.
Dentition. Large teeth.
Facies. Prominent glabella, asymmetry, long ears.
Skeletal. Increased length versus breadth; evident in cranial vault, hands, and feet. Mild pectus excavatum.
Skin. Severe nodulocystic acne at adolescence.

OCCASIONAL ABNORMALITIES
Skeletal. Radioulnar synostosis.
Genital. Cryptorchidism, small penis, hypospadias.
Other. EEG abnormality. EKG showing prolonged PR interval.

NATURAL HISTORY. Though affected patients are occasionally long at birth, the tendency toward tall stature is usually not evident until they reach five to six years of age. Despite the large size, these boys are usually not strong or well-coordinated and tend to have poor development of the pectoral and shoulder girdle musculature. Behavioral problems, especially temper tantrums and aggressive or defiant activity, start in early childhood and are sometimes augmented by dull mentality. The average I.Q. is about 10 to 15 points below that of their normal siblings. Psychosexual problems are also more common. Severe acne is liable to develop at adolescence. Although the majority of 47XYY males are fertile, only rare instances of transmission of the abnormal karyotype from father to son have been documented.

Though an XYY individual may manifest no evident abnormality, the likelihood of serious behavioral problems is significant. For example, among institutionalized male juvenile delinquents, the incidence of XYY was 1:35, which is 24 times the frequency of XYY in newborn males.

ETIOLOGY. Extra Y chromosome.

References

Sandberg, A. A., et al.: XYY human male. Lancet, *2*:488, 1961.
Osborne, R.: Personal communication.
Daly, R. F.: Neurological abnormalities in XYY males. Nature, *221*:472, 1969.
Sundequist, U., and Hellstrome, E.: Transmission of 47,XYY karyotype. Lancet, *2*:1367, 1969.
Nielsen, J., Friedrich, U., and Zeuthen, E.: Stature and weight in boys with the XYY syndrome. Humangenetik, *14*:66, 1971.
Valentine, G. H., McClelland, M. A., and Sergovich, F. R.: The growth and development of four XYY infants. Pediatrics, *48*:583, 1971.
Harrison, M. J. G., and Tennent, T. G.: Neurological anomalies in XYY males. Br. J. Psychiatry, *120*:447, 1972.
Voorhees, J. J., et al.: Nodulocystic acne as a phenotypic feature of the XYY genotype. Report of five cases, review of all known XYY subjects with severe acne, and discussion of XYY cytodiagnosis. Arch. Dermatol., *105*:913, 1972.

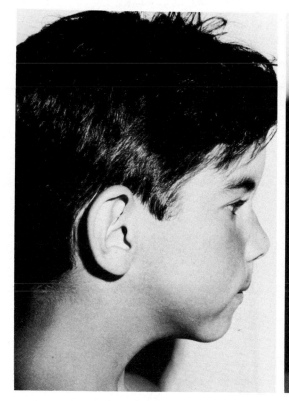

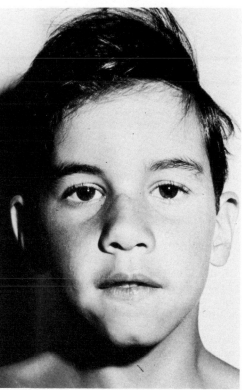

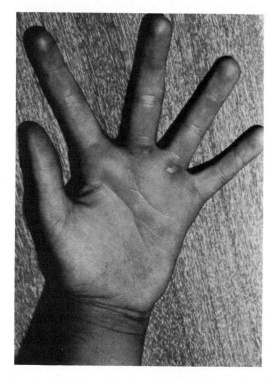

XYY syndrome. Eight year old boy, evaluated because of behavioral problems and poor school performance. Note the prominent glabella, relatively long face, and long fingers.

XXY SYNDROME, KLINEFELTER SYNDROME

Hypogenitalism and Hypogonadism,
+/− Long Legs, Dull Mentality, and/or Behavioral
Problems

This disorder, initially described by Klinefelter et al. in 1942, is now appreciated as being the most common single cause of hypogonadism and infertility, affecting about one in 500 males.

ABNORMALITIES

Performance. Tendency toward dull mentality, with about 15 to 20 per cent of patients having an I.Q. below 80. The average I.Q. is 10 to 15 points below that of their normal siblings. They tend to be late in the onset of speech and are more likely to have problems of articulation and language expression, including dysnomia. Between 20 and 50 per cent have a fine to moderate intention tremor, occasionally to the point of having difficulty in drinking a glass of water. Tendency toward behavior problems, especially immaturity, insecurity, shyness, poor judgment, and unrealistic boastful and assertive activity.

Growth. Tendency from childhood toward long limbs, with low upper to lower segment ratio and relatively tall and slim stature. Without testosterone replacement therapy, they tend to become obese as adults.

Hypogonadism with Hypogenitalism. Childhood: Relatively small penis and testes. Adolescence and adulthood: Testes remain small, usually less than 2.5 cm in length. With rare exception, testosterone production is inadequate, with the average serum testosterone values in the adult being less than one half the normal value. Infertility is the rule, with hyalinization and fibrosis of the seminiferous tubules because of excess gonadotropin. Virilization is partial and inadequate, with gynecomastia occurring in 40 per cent.

Other. Mild elbow dysplasia, fifth finger clinodactyly.

OCCASIONAL ABNORMALITIES. Genital: Cryptorchidism, hypospadias. Scoliosis during adolescent years. As adults, diabetes mellitus (8 per cent) and chronic bronchitis are more common. Mild to moderate ataxia occasionally occurs, and ulcerative breakdown of the skin over the anterior lower legs may develop.

NATURAL HISTORY. Dull mentality and/or behavioral problems are often not evident until the boy enters school. These features and relatively long limbs, small penis, and/or small testes provide the clues toward diagnosis in childhood. Subsequently, inadequate virilization, small testes, variable gynecomastia, and a worsening of behavioral problems should provide even more obvious diagnostic clues.

ETIOLOGY AND DIAGNOSIS. A buccal smear for X-chromatin is a satisfactory screening study. Any X-chromatin–positive male should have a chromosome study, ideally evaluating about 20 cells. Most will be XXY, but of X-chromatin–positive newborn males, 22 per cent have been mosaics for XXY/XY. Such mosaic individuals have a better potential prognosis for testicular function. Other variants include XXYY, in which the patient is more likely to be mentally deficient and have behavioral problems, and XXXY, an abnormality that is characterized by mental deficiency, possible growth deficiency, and multiple minor anomalies, including radioulnar synostosis at the elbow.

MANAGEMENT. Diagnosis during childhood of XXY (or XXYY or XXXY) syndrome is helpful in allowing for prospective testosterone replacement therapy beginning at the age of 11 to 12 years, if and when studies show deficient testosterone and elevated gonadotropin values for maturational age. This will bring about a more usual adolescent development and prevent many of the features of adult Klinefelter syndrome that are due to testosterone insufficiency. The author's present practice for those who show evidence of testosterone insufficiency is to give Depo-Testosterone every three weeks, starting with 25- and then 50-mg injections at about 11 years of age and increasing the dosage by 50-mg increments each year until an adult dosage of 250 mg is achieved at about 15 to 17 years of age.

References

Klinefelter, H. F., Jr., Reifenstein, E. C., Jr., and Albright, F.: Syndrome characterized by gynecomastia, aspermatogenesis without aleydigism, and increased secretion of follicle-stimulating hormone (gynecomastia). J. Clin. Endocrinol. Metab., *2*:615, 1942.

Caldwell, P. D., and Smith, D. W.: The XXY syndrome in childhood: Detection and treatment. J. Pediatr., *80*:250, 1972.

Baughman, F. H., Higgin, J. V., and Mann, J.: Sex chromosome anomalies and essential tremor. Neurology, *23*:623, 1973.

Williams, R. H., ed.: Textbook of Endocrinology, 5th ed. Philadelphia, W. B. Saunders Co., 1974.

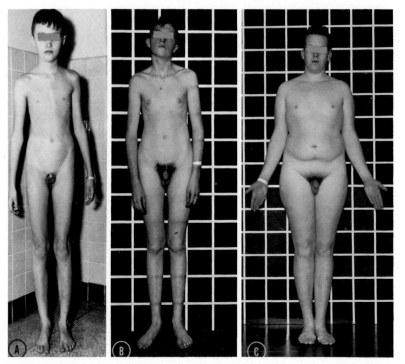

XXY syndrome. *A*, 9 year XXY child; note the small penis, long legs. *B*, 16 year untreated XXY adolescent; note the gynecomastia and scoliosis. *C*, 21 year untreated XXY adult; note the obesity, hypovirilization.

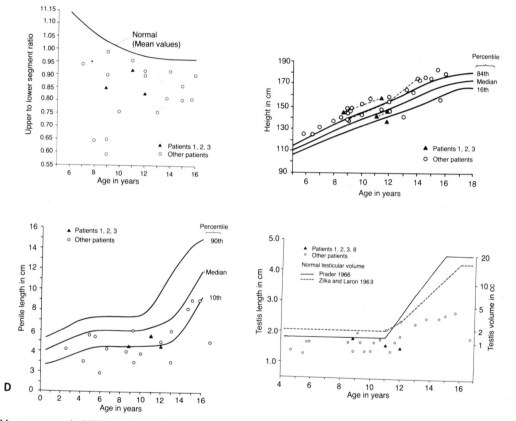

D, Measurements in XXY syndrome during childhood versus normals. (*D*, From Caldwell, P. D., and Smith, D. W.: J. Pediatr., *80*:250, 1972.)

XXXY AND XXXXY SYNDROMES

Hypogenitalism, Limited Elbow Pronation,
Low Dermal Ridge Count on Fingertips

The greater the aneuploidy, from XXY to XXXXY, the more severe the growth deficiency, mental deficiency, hypogenitalism, and other features. The abnormalities listed below are for XXXXY syndrome, and the findings for XXXY syndrome extend from the milder XXY features toward this more severe end of the spectrum.

ABNORMALITIES FOR XXXXY SYNDROME. The frequencies are based on 17 to 32 cases for each anomaly:

Performance
Mental deficiency, intelligence quotient of 19 to 57, mean I.Q. of 34. Hypotonia, joint laxity, or both, in about one third.

Growth
Tendency to low birth weight, shortness of stature, retarded osseous maturation	53%

Craniofacial
Sclerotic cranial sutures	57%
Wide-set eyes	80%
Upward slant to palpebral fissures	79%
Inner epicanthal folds	82%
Strabismus	59%
Low nasal bridge; wide or upturned nasal tip	95%
Mandibular prognathism	50%
Auricular anomaly (large, low-set, malformed)	70%

Neck
Short	72%

Thorax
Thick sternum	75%

Limbs
Limited pronation at elbow	95%
Radioulnar synostosis	42%
Clinodactyly of fifth finger	90%
Coxa valga	25%
Genu valgum	50%
Pes planus	73%
Epiphyseal dysplasia, usually mild	—

Dermal ridge patterns
High frequency of low arch pattern on fingertips, with mean total ridge count of only 50, versus the average male total ridge count of 144.

Genitalia
Small penis	80%
Small testes, hypoplastic tubules, diminished Leydig cells	94%
Cryptorchidism	28%
Hypoplastic scrotum	80%

OCCASIONAL ABNORMALITIES. Obesity, flat occiput, microcephaly, antimongoloid slant to palpebral fissures, Brushfield speckled iris, myopia, cleft palate, small peg-shaped teeth, webbed neck (12 per cent), pectus excavatum, congenital heart defect (especially patent ductus arteriosus), umbilical hernia, scoliosis, simian creases, talipes, abnormal toes, wide gap between first and second toes, hypospadias, bifid scrotum.

NATURAL HISTORY. Perinatal problems in adaptation have been frequent; linear growth is generally slow, with moderately short final height attainment. Infertility and inadequate virilization may be anticipated. Depending on the overall life situation, testosterone replacement therapy should be considered at 11 to 12 years of age.

ETIOLOGY. The XXXY or XXXXY diagnosis may be confirmed by the finding of as many as two or three X-chromatin masses in interphase nuclei (buccal smear) in a male who is found to have either 48 or 49 chromosomes with extra X chromosomes.

COMMENT. Although some of the features may initially suggest Down syndrome, the total pattern of anomalies is usually at variance with this diagnosis.

References

Fraccaro, M., Kaijser, K., and Lindsten, J.: A child with 49 chromosomes. Lancet, 2:899, 1960.
Zaleski, W. A., et al.: The XXXXY chromosome anomaly: report of three new cases and review of 30 cases from the literature. Can. Med. Ass. J., 94:1143, 1966.
Schmid, R., Pajewski, M., and Rosenblatt, M.: Epiphyseal dysplasia: a constant finding in XXXXY syndrome. J. Med. Genet., 15:282, 1978.

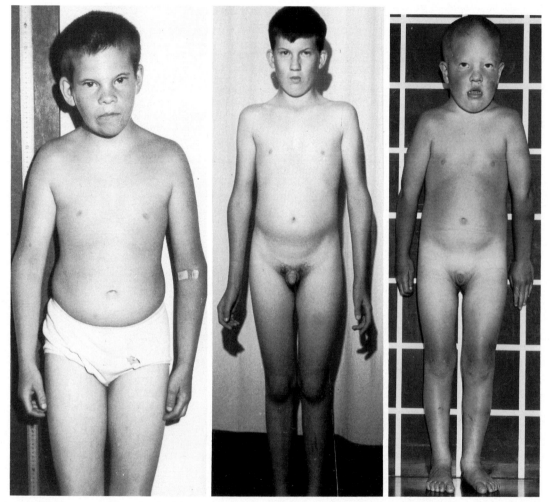

Left and middle, Preadolescent and adolescent boys with XXXY syndrome; both are short and dull of mentality. Note the facial dysmorphia, elbow aberrations, and hypogonadism *(middle)*. *Right,* Six year old with XXXXY syndrome. Note some resemblance to Down syndrome and the more severe hypogenitalism. (Right photo from Smith, D. W.: J. Pediatr., *70*:476, 1967.)

XXXX SYNDROME

Initially detected by Carr et al. in 1961, more than 20 cases have been reported. The phenotype has been quite variable, with the facies being suggestive of Down syndrome in several cases.

ABNORMALITIES. Other than mental deficiency, all of the other features have been variable. The patients are usually of normal stature.
Performance. I.Q. of 30 to 80, average of 55.
Facies. Midfacial hypoplasia, mild hypertelorism, epicanthal folds, mild micrognathia.
Limbs. Occasional fifth finger clinodactyly, radioulnar synostosis.
Other. Narrow shoulder girdle, occasional webbed neck. Variable amenorrhea, irregular menses.

NATURAL HISTORY. Besides mental deficiency, speech and behavioral problems are frequent.

ETIOLOGY. XXXX. A buccal smear for X-chromatin is an adequate screening test; only 6 to 9 per cent of the cells will show three X-chromatin masses.

References

Carr, D. H., Barr, M. L., and Plunkett, E. R.: An XXXX sex chromosome complex in two mentally defective females. Can. Med. Ass. J., *84*:131, 1961.
Telfer, M. A., et al.: Divergent phenotypes among 48,XXXX and 47,XXX females. Am. J. Hum. Genet., *22*:326, 1970.
Gardner, R. J. M., Veale, A. M. O., and Sands, V. E.: XXXX syndrome: Case report, and a note on genetic counselling and fertility. Humangenetik, *17*:323, 1973.

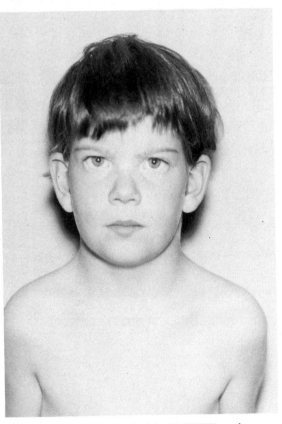

Six and one-half year old girl with XXXX syndrome.

XXXXX SYNDROME

(Penta X Syndrome)

Upward Slant to Palpebral Fissures,
Patent Ductus Arteriosus,
Small Hands with Clinodactyly of Fifth Fingers

The first description of an individual with XXXXX was by Kesaree and Wooley in 1963.

ABNORMALITIES. Mental deficiency, moderate to severe. Growth deficiency, especially postnatally. Microcephaly. Mild upward slant (mongoloid) to palpebral fissures. Low nasal bridge, short neck. Hypertelorism. Epicanthal folds. Low hairline. Dental malocclusion. Small hands with mild clinodactyly of fifth fingers. Patent ductus arteriosus.

OCCASIONAL ABNORMALITIES. Colobomata of iris, low-set ears, high frequency low arch dermal ridge patterns, simian creases, equinovarus, overlapping toes, multiple joint dislocations including shoulder, elbow, hips, wrists, and fingers. Renal dysplasia.

NATURAL HISTORY. Variable, from failure to thrive to development such as that noted in the accompanying figure.

COMMENT AND ETIOLOGY. Of interest is the occurrence in these XXXXX individuals of many of the nonspecific anomalies found in Down syndrome, a diagnosis that was initially considered in some of the patients. The finding of as many as four sex chromatin bodies in interphase nuclei in conjunction with three extra C-group chromosomes in metaphase preparations establishes the presence of five X chromosomes.

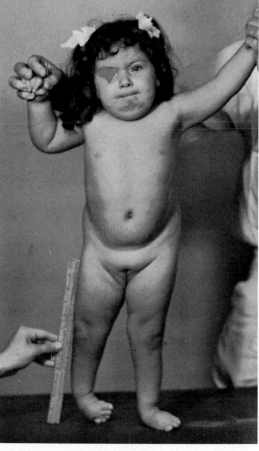

XXXXX syndrome. Twenty-eight month old with height age of 18 months and a performance level of about one year. A patent ductus arteriosus had been repaired. The hands were small, with incurved fifth fingers, and the ears were slightly low in placement. (From Brody, J., et al.: J. Pediatr., *70*:105, 1967.)

References

Kesaree, N., and Wooley, P. V.: A phenotypic female with 49 chromosomes, presumably XXXXX. A case report. J. Pediatr., *63*:1099, 1963.

Sergovich, F., Vilenberg, C., and Pozaonyi, J.: The 49,XXXXX chromosome constitution: Similarities to the 49,XXXXY condition. J. Pediatr., *78*:285, 1971.

Dryer, R. F., et al.: Pentasomy X with multiple dislocations. Amer. J. Med. Genet., *4*:313, 1979.

XO SYNDROME

(Turner Syndrome)

Short Female, Broad Chest with Wide Spacing
of Nipples, Congenital Lymphedema or Its Residua

An association between small stature and defective ovarian development had been noted as early as 1922 by Rossle, who classified the disorder under "sexagen dwarfism." A more expanded syndrome of small stature, sexual infantilism, webbed neck, and cubitus valgus in seven females was described by Turner in 1938.

Most XO conceptuses are early lethals. At birth, the incidence of sex chromatin–negative females, presumably XO individuals, is about 1:5000 newborns. Obviously, this does not include many of the XO/XX mosaics or individuals with only a partial deletion of one X, who might be sex chromatin–positive.

ABNORMALITIES. The following list of abnormalities, with the approximate percentage for each anomaly, includes those of the full monosomic XO syndrome. Patients with only a part of the cells XO (XX/XO mosaics, XY/XO mosaics with varying degrees of male-type genitalia) or in whom only a part of one X is missing (X-isochromosome X or X-deleted X) generally have a lesser degree of malformation. The most consistent features for the entire group are small stature and gonadal dysgenesis. Because the latter feature is not evident during childhood, a chromosomal study is indicated in any girl with short stature of unknown cause whose clinical phenotype is not incompatible with the XO syndrome.

Growth. Small stature, often evident by birth. Tendency to become obese.

Gonads. Ovarian dysgenesis with hypoplasia to absence of germinal elements (90 + per cent).

Lymph Vessels. Transient congenital lymphedema with residual puffiness over the dorsum of the fingers and toes (80 + per cent).

Thorax. Broad chest with widely spaced nipples that may be hypoplastic, inverted, or both (80 + per cent); often mild pectus excavatum.

Auricles. Anomalous auricles, most commonly prominent (80 + per cent).

Facies. Narrow maxilla (palate) (80 + per cent). Relatively small mandible (70 + per cent). Inner canthal folds (40 + per cent).

Neck. Low posterior hairline, appearance of short neck (80 + per cent). Webbed posterior neck (50 per cent).

Extremities. Cubitus valgus or other anomaly of elbow (70 + per cent). Knee anomalies such as medial tibial exostosis (60 + per cent). Short fourth metacarpal, metatarsal, or both (50 + per cent).

Other Skeletal. Bone dysplasia with coarse trabecular pattern, most evident at metaphyseal ends of long bones (50 + per cent). Dislocation of hip.

Nails. Narrow, hyperconvex and/or deep-set nails (70 + per cent).

Skin. Excessive pigmented nevi (50 + per cent). Distal palmar axial triradii (40 + per cent). Loose skin, especially about the neck in infancy. Tendency toward keloid formation.

Renal. Most commonly horseshoe kidney, double or cleft renal pelvis, and minor alterations (60 + per cent).

Cardiac. Cardiac defects (20 + per cent), the majority of which are bicuspid aortic valve, coarctation of aorta, and valvular aortic stenosis.

CNS. Perceptive hearing impairment (50 + per cent).

OCCASIONAL ABNORMALITIES

Skeletal. Abnormal angulation of radius to carpal bones, Madelung's deformity, short midphalanx of fifth finger, short third to fifth metacarpals and/or metatarsals, scoliosis, kyphosis, spina bifida, vertebral fusion, cervical rib, abnormal sella turcica.

Eyes. Ptosis (16 per cent), strabismus, blue sclerae, cataract.

CNS. Mental retardation. Mean intelligence quotient about 95, with performance usually below verbal score.

Other. Hemangiomata, rarely of the intestine. Long hair on arms. Idiopathic hypertension, diabetes mellitus, Crohn's disease, thyroid disorders.

NATURAL HISTORY. The congenital lymphedema usually recedes in early infancy, leaving only puffiness over the dorsum of the fingers and toes, although rarely there may be recrudescence of the lymphedema with estrogen replacement therapy. At birth, the skin tends to be loose, especially in the posterior neck where excess skin may persist as the pterygium colli. Small size is often evident at birth, the mean birth weight being 2900 g. Linear growth proceeds at about half to three fourths the usual rate; there is usually no adolescent growth spurt, and final height of 50 to 60 inches with a mean of 55 inches is achieved at a usual age, despite the roentgenographic evidence of "retarded osseous maturation."

Studies of XO abortuses have disclosed near-normal development of the ovaries in early fetal life. Apparently they usually do not make primary follicles, and the ovary degenerates rather rapidly. By adolescence there is seldom any functional ovarian tissue remaining. Gonadotropin values may be helpful before five years in early childhood and again after ten years. If they are elevated, the patient probably will not have functional ovarian tissue by adolescence.

An occasional patient may show evidence of estrogen production at adolescence, although this is generally transient; at least several XO individuals have been fertile. Generally, estrogen replacement therapy is indicated, beginning at the appropriate psychologic time for each individual. Premarin, for example, may be started at a very low dosage and gradually increased to mimic normal adolescence, and the adult dosage is reached, with cycling of therapy to allow for menstruation, at 13 to 15 years of age. In a recent study of adults with XO Turner syndrome, Sybert was unable to demonstrate an increased mean adult height in 29 individuals treated with androgens versus 37 untreated individuals with XO Turner syndrome. Furthermore, the age of initiation of estrogen therapy had no effect on adult height. She concluded that the use of anabolic steroids to increase height in XO Turner syndrome was not justified and that the postponement of estrogen therapy for the purpose of maximizing adult height is not indicated. Obesity and hypertension, if present, may be augmented by estrogen replacement. At some time between eight years and adolescence, these patients should be told that the ovaries are probably incompletely developed and that they should plan on adopting children and taking "the same kind of medicine the ovary makes" at adolescence.

The actual incidence of early mortality due to congenital heart defects is unknown because there is no large series of cases diagnosed from birth. The types of renal anomalies that occur generally pose no problem to health, which is generally good. Enhancement of physical appearance by plastic surgery for prominent inner canthal folds, protruding auricles, and especially for webbed neck should be given serious consideration prior to school age. The major psychologic problem is usually the adaptation to shortness of stature, for which there is no effective treatment currently.

At the present time, we do not have adequate information on the longevity and cause of death beyond the age of childhood for individuals with the XO syndrome. However, it is encouraging to note that Dr. Judith Hall (University of British Columbia) knows of one 90 year old woman with XO syndrome.

If the chromosomal studies show XO/XY mosaicism, an exploratory laparotomy in childhood seems indicated to remove any gonadoblastoma, which such patients have an increased risk of developing.

If the child is mentally deficient, a careful search should be made for a chromosome abnormality in addition to that of the sex chromosome. For example, X-autosome translocation patients are more likely to be mentally deficient.

ETIOLOGY. Faulty chromosomal distribution leading to XO individual with 45 chromosomes. The paternal sex chromosome is the one more likely to be missing, as indicated by studies for X-linked gene expressions in the XO individuals and their parents. There has been no significant older maternal age factor for this aneuploidy syndrome. It is generally a sporadic event in a family, although there are as yet no adequate data on risk for recurrence.

References

Rossle, R. I.: Wachstum und Altern. München, 1922.

Turner, H. H.: A syndrome of infantilism, congenital webbed neck, and cubitus valgus. Endocrinology, *23*:566, 1938.

Lindsten, J.: The nature and origin of X chromosome aberrations in Turner's syndrome. Stockholm, Almquist and Wiksell, 1963.

Weiss, L.: Additional evidence of gradual loss of germ cells in the pathogenesis of streak ovaries in Turner's syndrome. J. Med. Genet., *8*:540, 1971.

Brook, C. G. D., et al. Growth in children with 45,XO Turner syndrome. Arch. Dis. Child., *49*:789, 1974.

Chen, H., Faigenbaum, D., and Weiss, H.: Psychosocial aspects of patients with the Ullrich-Turner syndrome. Amer. J. Med. Genet., *8*:191, 1981.

Miller, M. J., et al.: Echocardiography reveals a high incidence of bicuspid aortic valve in Turner syndrome. J. Pediatr., *102*:47, 1983.

Sybert, V. P.: Adult height in Turner syndrome with and without androgen therapy. J. Pediatr., *104*:365, 1984.

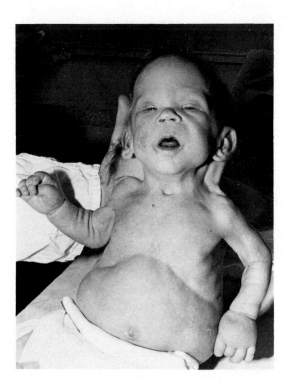

Ten day old XO patient who still has lymph-filled bilateral cysts in the posterior neck area, the cause for the webbed neck and for the prominent ears. This patient had abdominal muscle hypoplasia with bulging flanks, possibly secondary to earlier undue distention of the abdomen by fluid. Thus, this baby survived fetal life and was born with a more severe degree of lymphedema than usual.

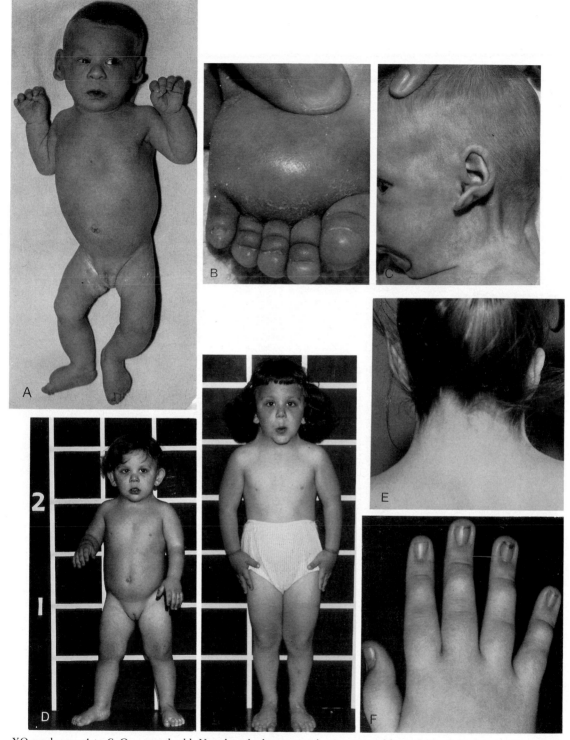

XO syndrome. *A* to *C*, One month old. Note lymphedema, prominent ears, and loose folds of skin in posterior neck with low hair line. *D*, Same girl at two years and at four years, with height ages of 17 months and three years, respectively. *E*, Low posterior hair line and residual lateral neck web. *F*, Narrow, hyperconvex, deep-set fingernails; residual puffiness. (*A* to *C*, *E*, and *F* from Lemli, L., and Smith, D. W.: J. Pediatr., *63*:577, 1963.)

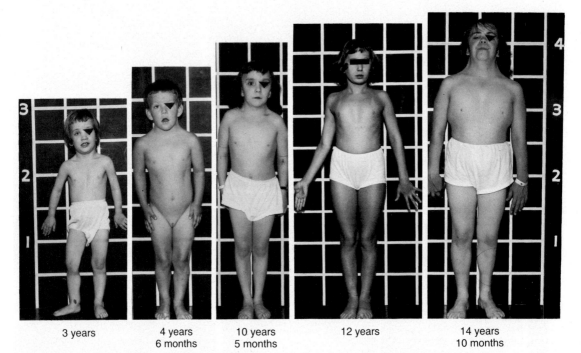

| 3 years | 4 years
6 months | 10 years
5 months | 12 years | 14 years
10 months |

Five girls with the XO syndrome. Note the variability of such features as webbed neck and broad chest.

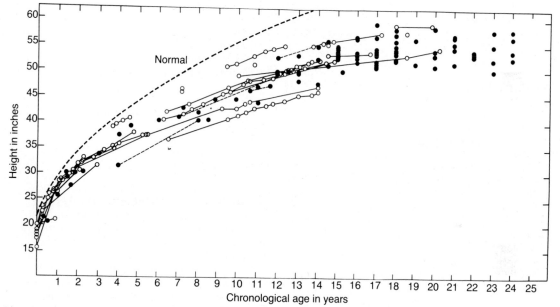

Linear growth of girls with the XO syndrome. The open dots represent patients evaluated at the University of Wisconsin; the others were taken from the literature. (From Lemli, L., and Smith, D. W.: J. Pediatr., *63*:577, 1963.)

B. VERY SMALL STATURE, NOT SKELETAL DYSPLASIA

DE LANGE SYNDROME

(Cornelia de Lange Syndrome, Brachmann–de Lange Syndrome)

Synophrys, Thin Downturning Upper Lip, Micromelia

The syndrome was originally described in 1933 by Cornelia de Lange. More than 150 cases have been reported.

ABNORMALITIES

Growth

Shortness of stature of prenatal onset	100%
Retarded osseous maturation	50%

Performance

Mental retardation and sluggish physical activity	100%
Initial hypertonicity	100%
Low-pitched, weak, growling cry in infancy	100%

Cranium

Microbrachycephaly	93%

Eyes

Bushy eyebrows and synophrys	99%
Long, curly eyelashes	100%

Nose

Small nose, anteverted nostrils	100%

Mouth

Characteristic lips and mouth*	100%
High arched palate	50%
Late eruption of widely spaced teeth	93%

Mandible

Micrognathia	97%
Spurs in the anterior angle of the mandible, prominent symphysis	66%

Skin

Hirsutism	97%
Cutis marmorata and perioral pale "cyanosis"	64%
Hypoplastic nipples and umbilicus	100%

Hands and Arms

Micromelia	69%
Phocomelia and oligodactyly	30%
Clinodactyly of fifth fingers	69%
Simian crease	84%
Proximal implantation of thumbs	81%
Flexion contracture of elbows	84%

Feet

Micromelia	99%
Syndactyly of second and third toes	81%

Male Genitalia

Hypoplasia	24%
Undescended testes	58%
Hypospadias	94%

OCCASIONAL ANOMALIES. Seizures (20 per cent), myopia, microcornea, astigmatism, optic atrophy, coloboma of the optic nerve, strabismus, proptosis, choanal atresia, low-set ears, cleft palate, congenital heart defect (29 per cent, most commonly ventricular septal defect), hiatus hernia, duplication of gut, malrotation of colon, brachyesophagus, pyloric stenosis, inguinal hernia, small labia majora, radial hypoplasia, short first metacarpal, absent second to third interdigital triradius.

NATURAL HISTORY AND MANAGEMENT. These patients show a marked retardation of growth, evident by the time of birth, and as a rule, they fail to thrive. Feeding difficulties, including regurgitation, projectile vomiting, chewing, and swallowing difficulties, often continue beyond six months. Their intellectual performance is usually severely limited, and they are seldom able to talk. Hearing loss occurs frequently. Their gait tends to be broad-based. They sometimes show autistic behavior, including self-destructive tendencies. The patients may avoid and reject social interactions and physical contact. Though rapid movement may be pleasurable, they show infrequent facial emotion and tend to have stereotypic behavior. The majority of patients followed beyond 13

---

*Thin lips with small midline beak of the upper lip and corresponding notch in the lower lip; downward curving of the angle of the mouth.

years had onset of puberty, with normal menses documented in several women. The I.Q. varies from 4 to 85, with the majority being below 35. Those with the higher I.Q.s tend to be the ones with a better birth weight and head circumference. Episodes of aspiration in infancy and increased susceptibility to infection appear to constitute the major hazards for survival in these patients.

ETIOLOGY AND RECURRENCE RISK. Unknown. Most cases are sporadic. Autosomal dominant inheritance has been suggested based on documentation of two severely affected children born to a mildly affected parent. Recurrence risk is negligible if, after careful evaluation, both parents are determined to be normal, or 50 per cent if one parent is affected. The observed low recurrence risk most likely represents the inability of more severely affected individuals to reproduce. Clinically, there appears to be a gradation in severity, and it is very difficult to be secure about a diagnosis in the more mildly affected cases. Duplication of the Q25-29 band region of chromosome 3 tends to yield a phenotype that is similar to that of the de Lange syndrome. Hence, cautious chromosome studies are indicated in some of the atypical de Lange syndrome patients.

References

de Lange, C.: Sur un type nouveau de génération (typus Amstelodamensis). Arch. Med. Engant., *36*:713, 1933.

Ptacek, L. J., et al.: The Cornelia de Lange syndrome. J. Pediatr., *63*:1000, 1963.

Vischer, D.: Typus degenerativus Amstelodamensis (Cornelia de Lange syndrome). Helv. Paediatr. Acta, *20*:415, 1965.

Barr, A. N., et al.: Neurologic and psychometric findings in Brachmann-de Lange syndrome. Neuropaediatrie, *3*:46, 1971.

Johnson, H. G., et al.: A behavioral phenotype in the de Lange syndrome. Pediatr. Res., *10*:843, 1976.

Wilson, G. N., Hieber, V. C., and Schmickel, R. D.: The association of chromosome 3 duplication and the Cornelia de Lange syndrome. J. Pediatr., *93*:783, 1978.

Hawley, P. D., Jackson, L. G., and Kurnit, D. M.: Sixty-four patients with Brachmann-de Lange syndrome: A survey. Amer. J. Med. Genet., *20*:453, 1985.

Robinson, L. K., Wolfsberg, E., and Jones, K. L.: Brachmann-de Lange syndrome: Evidence for autosomal dominant inheritance. Amer. J. Med. Genet. *22*:109, 1985.

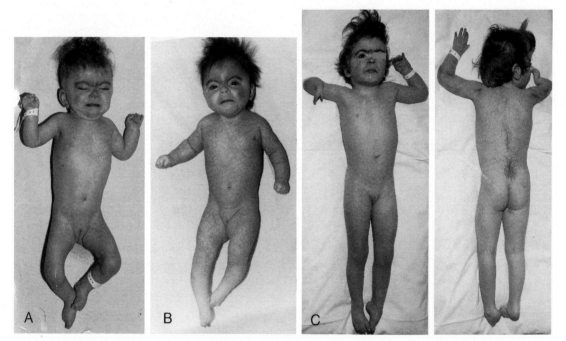

De Lange syndrome. *A*, Neonate with small hands and feet. *B*, Three month old with newborn length. *C*, Five and one half year old with height age of two years and severe defect of right distal limb.

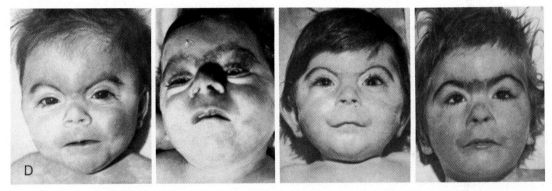

D, Similar facies of four affected individuals. (From Ptacek, L. J., et al: J. Pediatr., *63*:1000, 1963.)

RUBINSTEIN-TAYBI SYNDROME

Broad Thumbs and Toes,
Slanted Palpebral Fissures, Hypoplastic Maxilla

Rubinstein and Taybi set forth this clinical entity in 1963. More than 224 cases have been reported.

ABNORMALITIES
Growth
Short stature	94%
Retarded osseous maturation	94%

Performance
I.Q. 17 to 86	100%
EEG abnormality	60%
Stiff, unsteady gait	76%

Cranium
Small	84%

Facies
Palpebral fissures slant downward	100%
Hypoplastic maxilla with narrow palate	100%
Beaked nose with nasal septum extending below alae nasi	68%
Epicanthal folds	62%
Strabismus	79%
Refractive error	58%
Auricles low-set and/or malformed	84%

Hands and Feet
Broad thumbs with radial angulation and broad toes	100%
Other fingers and toes broad	50%
Excess dermal ridge patterning in thenar and first interdigital areas of palm	50%

Pelvis
Low acetabular angle, flare to ilia	?

Genitalia
Cryptorchidism	79%

Skin
Nevus flammeus	54%

Cardiac
Murmur (ventricular septal defect and patent ductus arteriosus most common)	33%

Renal
Variety of defects	50%

OCCASIONAL ABNORMALITIES
Skeletal. Prominent forehead, large anterior fontanel, large foramen magnum, parietal foramina, micrognathia, sternal anomalies, unfused arch of first cervical vertebra and other vertebral anomalies, scoliosis, syndactyly, polydactyly, clinodactyly of fifth finger.

Other. Cataract, colobomata, ptosis of eyelid, long eyelashes and hypertrichosis, polydactyly, simian crease, distal axial triradius, cardiac anomaly, renal anomaly, angulated penis, kyphoscoliosis, seizures, absence of corpus callosum.

NATURAL HISTORY. Respiratory infections and feeding difficulties are frequent problems in infancy. The degree of mental deficiency is variable, the most usual I.Q. being in the 40 to 50 range.

ETIOLOGY. Unknown; the disorder has occurred in one of monozygotic twins. From 112 families, there is one presumed recurrence, a crude recurrence risk of about one per cent.

COMMENT. The author has been impressed by the variability among affected individuals. Thus, presumed Rubinstein-Taybi syndrome patients have had broad thumbs but not broad toes, broad toes but not broad thumbs, and neither broad thumbs nor broad toes. The diagnosis in the latter category is, of course, a tentative one.

References

Rubinstein, J. H., and Taybi, H.: Broad thumbs and toes and facial abnormalities. A possible mental retardation syndrome. Am. J. Dis. Child., *105*:588, 1963.

Rubinstein, J. H.: The broad thumbs syndrome—Progress report 1968. Birth Defects, 5:25, 1969.

Simpson, N. E., and Brissenden, J. E.: The Rubinstein-Taybi syndrome: Familial and dermatoglyphic data. Am. J. Hum. Genet., *25*:225, 1973.

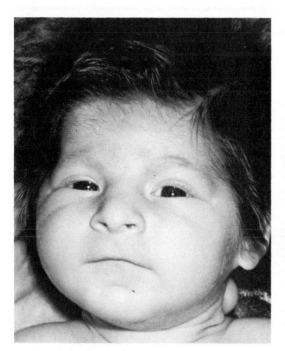

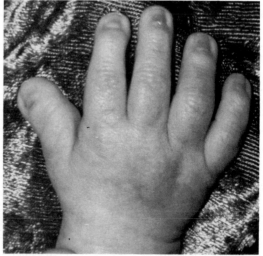

Young infant with Rubinstein-Taybi syndrome.

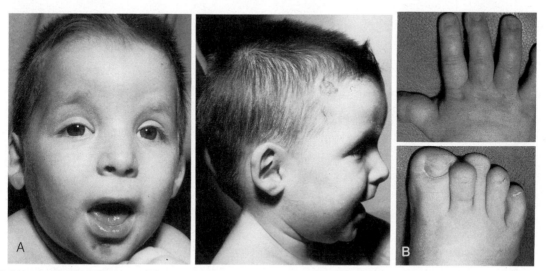

Rubinstein-Taybi syndrome. *A*, Three and one-half year old. Height age of two years. I.Q., 45. Slight downslant to palpebral fissures. *B*, Hand and foot of patient shown in *A*.

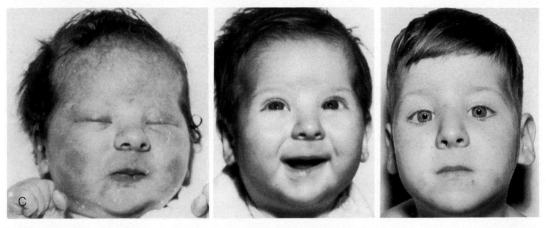

C, Changes in facies from birth to several years of age. Note broad thumb at birth.

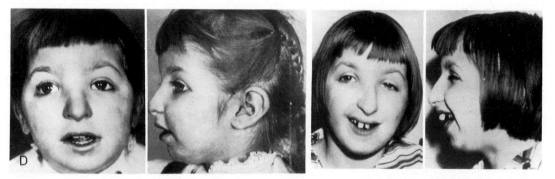

D, Changes in facies from three and one-half to 14 years. (*C* and *D* are gratefully acknowledged to J. Rubinstein, Cincinnati.)

RUSSELL-SILVER SYNDROME

(Silver Syndrome)

*Short Stature of Prenatal Onset,
Skeletal Asymmetry, Small Incurved Fifth Finger*

This pattern of malformation was independently described by Silver et al. and by Russell in 1953 and 1954. Silver emphasized the skeletal asymmetry as a feature of the disorder. This was a variable finding in the patients described by Russell. Gareis et al. have summarized the data on this syndrome and also noted that asymmetry of the prenatal onset growth deficiency is a variable feature in this disorder.

ABNORMALITIES

Growth and Skeletal. Small stature, prenatal onset. Immature osseous development in infancy and early childhood, with late closure of anterior fontanel. Asymmetry, most commonly of limbs. Short and/or incurved fifth finger.

Facies. Small, triangular facies with downturning corners of mouth. The sclerae may be bluish in early infancy.

Skin. Café au lait spots.

Other. Tendency toward excess sweating, especially on the head and upper trunk, during infancy. Liability to fasting hypoglycemia from about ten months until two to three years of age.

OCCASIONAL ABNORMALITIES. Syndactyly of second to third toes, renal anomaly, hypospadias.

NATURAL HISTORY. The patients are usually slim and underweight for length during early childhood. There tends to be a gradual improvement in growth in weight and appearance during childhood and especially during adolescence. As a result, the adult usually appears more normal than the infant with this disorder. Final height attainment can be up to five feet. During infancy, patients tend to be weak and may be slow in major motor progress. Hence there is the risk of mental deficiency being implied, whereas intelligence is usually normal. Because of the small facies, the upper head may *appear* large, though head circumference is well within the normal range. This appearance, plus the relatively large fontanels in early infancy, may give rise to a false impression of hydrocephalus—which they do not have. Somewhat frequent feedings and assurance of glucose intake during illnesses are often merited from six months of age until three years, the period of enhanced liability to fasting hypoglycemia for these patients. Documentation of growth hormone deficiency in at least six patients suggests that an endocrine evaluation should be considered if the linear growth rate reaches a plateau.

ETIOLOGY. Unknown. A recent study by Saal et al. indicates the marked heterogeneity of this disorder. Strict conformity to the diagnostic features is vital. Frequently, this disorder is utilized to designate any infant who is small for gestational age. Some of the rare chromosomal abnormalities may initially resemble Russell-Silver syndrome. Such has occurred for 18p− syndrome, for 18 trisomy/normal mosaicism, and for triploidy/normal mosaicism.

References

Silver, H. K., et al.: Syndrome of congenital hemihypertrophy, shortness of stature and elevated urinary gonadotrophins. Pediatrics, *12*:368, 1953.

Russell, A.: A syndrome of "intra-uterine" dwarfism recognizable at birth with craniofacial dysostosis, disproportionately short arms and other anomalies. Proc. R. Soc. Med., *47*:1040, 1954.

Silver, H. K.: Asymmetry, short stature, and variations in sexual development. A syndrome of congenital malformations. Am. J. Dis. Child., *107*:495, 1964.

Gareis, F. J., Smith, D. W., and Summitt, R. L.: The Russell-Silver syndrome without asymmetry. J. Pediatr., *79*:775, 1971.

Haslam, R. H. A., Berman, W., and Heller, R. M.: Renal abnormalities in the Russell-Silver syndrome. Pediatrics, *51*:216, 1973.

Christensen, M. F., and Nielsen, J.: Deletion short arm 18 and Russell-Silver syndrome. Acta Paediatr. Scand., *67*:101, 1978.

Escobar, V., Gleiser, S., and Weaver, D. D.: Phenotypic and genetic analysis of Silver-Russell syndrome. Clin. Genet., *13*:278, 1978.

Nishi, Y., et al.: Silver-Russell syndrome and growth hormone deficiency. Acta Paediatr. Scand., *71*:1035, 1982.

Saal, H. M., Pagon, R. A., and Pepin, M. G.: Reevaluation of Russell-Silver syndrome. J. Pediatr., *107*:733, 1985.

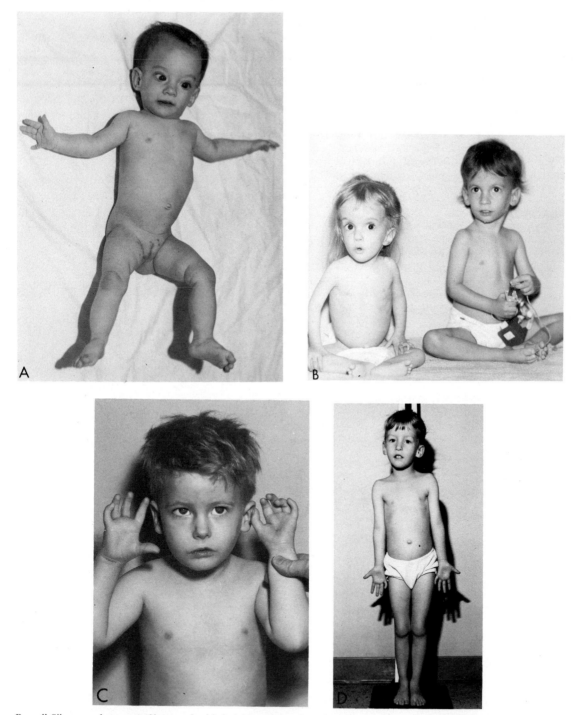

Russell-Silver syndrome. *A*, Six month old; height age, two months. Asymmetric leg length. (From Smith, D. W: J. Pediatr., *70*:483, 1967.) *B*, Seventeen month old girl with height age of six months and two year old boy with height age of fifteen months. Neither has asymmetry. Note the small facies, slimness, and "loose" sitting posture. (From Gareis, F. J., et al.: J. Pediatr., *79*:775, 1971.) *C*, Child, three years and nine months old; height age, one and one-half years. Note slight facial asymmetry. *D*, Six year old with height age of two years. Note clinodactyly of fifth fingers. (Courtesy of J. Aase, University of New Mexico.)

MULIBREY NANISM SYNDROME
(Perheentupa Syndrome)

*Small Stature, Pericardial
Constriction, Yellow Dots in Fundus*

Perheentupa et al. described the disorder in 1970, and by 1976 at least 26 cases had been reported. The term *Mulibrey* is an acronym used to denote the organs most frequently involved: muscle, liver, brain, and eyes.

ABNORMALITIES
Growth. Prenatal onset growth deficiency. Hands and feet appear relatively large in relation to body. High-pitched voice.

Craniofacies. Dolichocephaly with J-shaped sella turcica. Triangular facies. Decreased retinal pigmentation with dispersion and clusters of pigment and yellowish dots in the midperipheral region.

Other. Development of thick adherent pericardium with hepatomegaly and prominent neck veins. Variable fibrous dysplasia, especially in tibia. Muscle hypotonia.

NATURAL HISTORY. Normal intelligence. Onset of pericardial constrictive problems from infancy to late childhood. Whether the hepatomegaly is secondary to pericardial constriction remains to be resolved.

ETIOLOGY. Autosomal recessive. Twenty-four of the cases have been reported from Finland, with one from Egypt and one from the United States.

References

Perheentupa, J., et al.: Mulibrey-nanism. Dwarfism with muscle, liver, brain and eye involvement. Acta Paediatr. Scand., *59*(suppl. 206):74, 1970.

Voorhees, M. L., Husson, G. S., and Blackman, M. S.: Growth failure with pericardial constriction. Am. J. Dis. Child., *130*:1146, 1976.

Tarkkanen, A., Raitta, C., and Perheentupa, J.: Mulibrey nanism, an autosomal recessive syndrome with ocular involvement. Acta Ophthalmol., *60*:628, 1982.

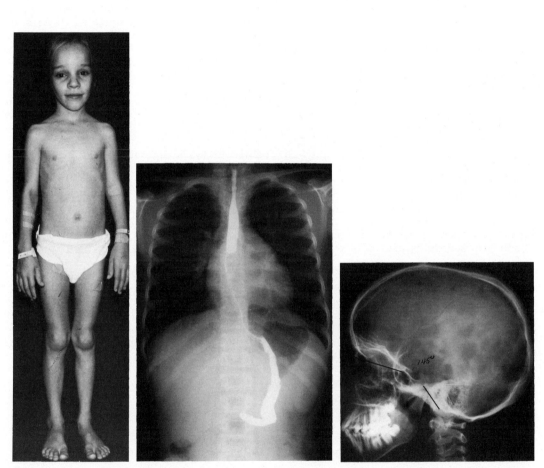

Girl with mulibrey nanism syndrome. Note the large size of the hands and feet in relation to her small stature, the aberrant cardiac silhouette and enlarged liver relating to constriction of the pericardium, and the dolicocephaly with J-shaped sella turcica. (From Voorhees, M. L., et al.: Am. J. Dis. Child., *130*:1146, 1976.)

DUBOWITZ SYNDROME

*Peculiar Facies, Infantile Eczema,
Small Stature, and Mild Microcephaly*

This disorder was initially reported by Dubowitz in 1965, and Wilroy et al. summarized 21 cases, eight of their own, in 1978.

ABNORMALITIES

Growth. Prenatal onset of growth deficiency with average birth weight of 2.3 kg and variable retarded osseous maturation.

Performance. Average intelligence to severe mental deficiency, with tendency toward hyperactivity, short attention span, stubbornness, and shyness. High-pitched, hoarse cry.

Craniofacial. Mild microcephaly, small facies, shallow supraorbital ridge with nasal bridge at about same level as forehead, short palpebral fissures with lateral telecanthus and appearance of hypertelorism, variable ptosis and blepharophimosis, prominent or mildly dysplastic ears, and micrognathia.

Skin and Hair. Eczema-like skin disorder on face and flexural areas. Sparsity of hair, especially lateral eyebrows.

Dentition. Lag in eruption, caries.

Occasional. Submucous cleft palate, pes planus, metatarsus adductus, hypospadias, cryptorchidism, clinodactyly of fifth finger, pilonidal dimple, syndactyly of toes.

NATURAL HISTORY. Eczema, noted in about one half of the patients, usually cleared by two to four years. About one third had poor feeding, and approximately the same number had chronic diarrhea in infancy. Teeth tended to become carious, and rhinorrhea and otitis media were frequent problems. Behavioral aberrations with lag in development of speech posed problems in function. Five of ten patients who had complete psychologic evaluation had low-average or average intelligence, and one had severe mental deficiency.

ETIOLOGY. Autosomal recessive, based on affected male and female siblings from unaffected parents.

COMMENT. The facies may appear similar to that of the fetal alcohol syndrome.

References

Dubowitz, V.: Familial low birth weight dwarfism with an unusual facies and a skin eruption. J. Med. Genet., *2*:12, 1965.

Opitz, J. M., et al.: The Dubowitz syndrome. Further observations. Z. Kinderheilkd., *116*:1, 1973.

Wilroy, R. S., Jr., Tipton, R. E., and Summitt, R. D.: The Dubowitz syndrome. Am. J. Med. Genet., *2*:275, 1978.

Parrish, J. M., and Wilroy, R. S.: The Dubowitz syndrome: The psychological status of ten cases at follow-up. Amer. J. Med. Genet., *6*:3, 1980.

Winter, R. M.: Dubowitz syndrome. J. Med. Genet., *23*:11, 1986.

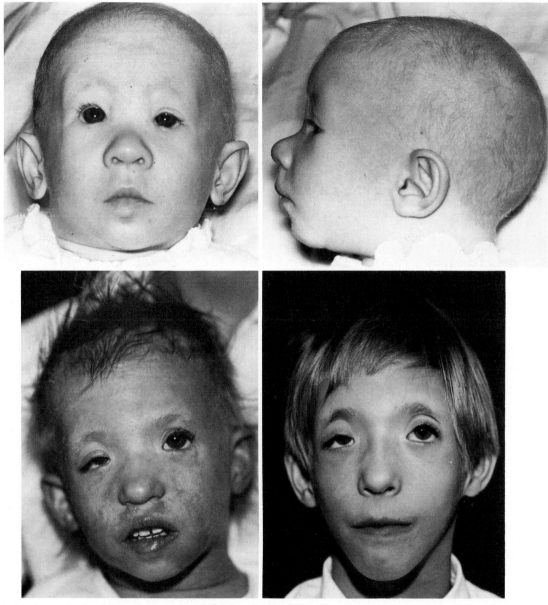

Dubowitz syndrome. *Above*, Five month old showing short palpebral fissures, asymmetric ptosis, shallow supraorbital ridges, and mild micrognathia. *Below*, Twenty month old showing eczema and above features; same patient at six and one-half years of age, at which time her I.Q. was 60. (From Grosse, R., et al.: Z. Kinderheilkd., *110*:175, 1971. Courtesy of J. M. Opitz, Helena, Montana.)

BLOOM SYNDROME

Short Stature, Malar Hypoplasia,
Telangiectatic Erythema of the Face

Since Bloom's original description in 1954, more than 100 patients with this disorder have been reported.

ABNORMALITIES

Growth. Prenatal onset growth deficiency; average adult male height, 151 cm, and adult female height, 144 cm.

Craniofacial. Mild microcephaly with dolichocephaly. Malar hypoplasia, plus or minus small nose. Facial telangiectatic erythema involves the butterfly midface region and is exacerbated by sunlight. It usually develops during the first year.

OCCASIONAL ABNORMALITIES. Mild mental deficiency. Telangiectatic erythema of the dorsa of the hands and forearms. High-pitched voice, colloid-body–like spots in Bruch membrane of the eye. Absence of upper lateral incisors. Prominent ears. Ichthyotic skin, hypertrichosis, pilonidal cyst, sacral dimple. Syndactyly, polydactyly, clinodactyly of fifth finger, short lower extremity, talipes, café au lait spots. Immunoglobulin deficiency, most particularly of IgA and IgM. Propensity to develop lymphoreticular malignancy.

NATURAL HISTORY. These patients show a consistently slow pace of growth. Feeding problems are frequent during infancy, as is otitis media. The facial erythema is very seldom present at birth, usually appearing during infancy following exposure to sunlight; it may excoriate, but improves after childhood. These are pleasant children, the majority being within the normal range in intelligence.

Malignancy has been the major known cause of death. About one in four patients has developed malignancy, the most common type being leuke-mia. Of those with malignancy, the mean age at diagnosis was 21 years, with a range from four to 44 years. Gastrointestinal malignancy is common after the age of 30.

An increased rate of chromosomal breakage and sister chromatid exchange is found in cultured leukocytes and fibroblasts from all patients studied, but not reliably so in the heterozygotes.

ETIOLOGY. Autosomal recessive, with the majority of individuals being of Ashkenazic Jewish ancestry. The frequency of the gene carrier in the Ashkenazic Jewish people is estimated at a minimum of 1 to 100. The excess of affected males to females is probably more apparent than real and relates to underdiagnosis of the disorder in females, in whom the skin lesion tends to be milder.

COMMENT. The relation of the in vitro chromosomal breakage and the development of malignancies is not well understood at present.

References

Bloom, D.: Congenital telangiectatic erythema resembling lupus erythematosus in dwarfs. Am. J. Dis. Child., *88*:754, 1954.

Bloom, D.: The syndrome of congenital telangiectatic erythema and stunted growth. J. Pediatr., *68*:103, 1966.

Sawitsky, A., Bloom, D., and German, J.: Chromosomal breakage and acute leukemia in congenital telangiectatic erythema and stunted growth. Ann. Intern. Med., *65*:487, 1966.

German, J., Bloom, D., and Passarge, E.: Bloom's syndrome VII. Progress report for 1978. Clin. Genet., *15*:361, 1979.

German, J., Bloom, D., and Passarge, E.: Bloom's syndrome XI. Progress report for 1983. Clin. Genet., *25*:166, 1984.

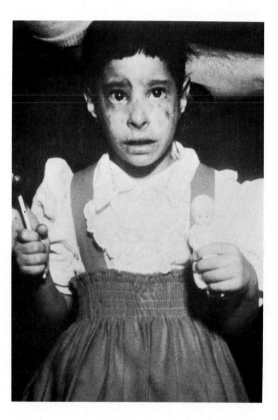

Bloom syndrome. Four and one-half year old. Height age, two and one-half years. Died of leukemia at 13 and one-half years. (Courtesy of Dr. D. Bloom.)

DE SANCTIS-CACCHIONE SYNDROME

(Xerodermic Idiocy Syndrome)

Xeroderma Pigmentosa, Microcephaly, Hypogonadism

Only about 20 cases of this disorder have been reported since its initial recognition by De Sanctis and Cacchione in 1932.

ABNORMALITIES

Growth. Moderate to severe growth deficiency, with retarded osseous maturation.

Central Nervous System. Microcephaly, mental deficiency, and deterioration with cerebral cortical and cerebellar "atrophy" and abnormal EEG. Variable spasticity, incoordination, seizures. Hypothalamic dysfunction.

Skin. Undue sun sensitivity, with progression from erythema and scaling to spotty hyperpigmentation, plus flat wart-like lesions and telangiectases to epitheliomas and atrophy with contractures to cutaneous malignancy.

Gonadal. Small testes in the male, with variable hypogonadism in both sexes, probably secondary to hypothalamic insufficiency.

NATURAL HISTORY. Slow developmental progress and growth, with variable neurologic dysfunction, including seizures, from early childhood. Progressive skin deterioration, especially related to exposure to the sun. Shortened life expectancy due to central nervous system deterioration and/or malignancy.

ETIOLOGY. Autosomal recessive. These patients have a defect in the DNA excision-repair system, the presumed basis for the deterioration of the skin following exposure to ultraviolet light (sunlight), and increased propensity to malignancy.

References

De Sanctis, C., and Cacchione, A.: L'idiozia xerodermia. Riv. Sper. Freniatr., *56*:269, 1932.

Silberstein, A. G.: Xeroderma pigmentosum with mental deficiency. A report of two cases. Am. J. Dis. Child., *55*:784, 1938.

Reed, W. B., May, S. B., and Nickel, W. R.: Xerodermapigmentosum with neurological complications. The De Sanctis-Cacchione syndrome. Arch. Dermatol., *91*:224, 1965.

Cleaver, J. E.: DNA damage and repair in light-sensitive human skin disease. J. Invest. Dermatol., *54*:181, 1970.

Shimasaki, M., et al.: Three cases of De Sanctis–Cacchione syndrome with endocrinological abnormalities. Acta Paediatr. Jap., *20*:100, 1978.

De Sanctis-Cacchione syndrome. Girl showing microcephaly, malar hypoplasia, and xeroderma pigmentosa of skin. (Courtesy of S. Myhre, Rainier State Training School, Buckley, Washington.)

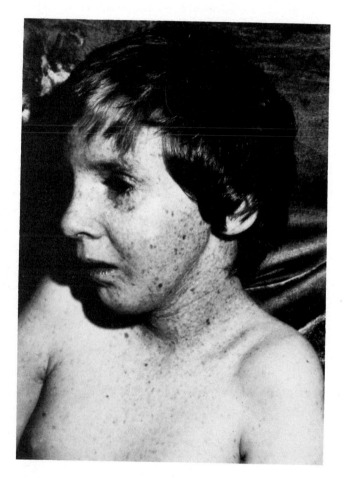

JOHANSON-BLIZZARD SYNDROME

Hypoplastic Alae Nasi, Hypothyroidism, Deafness

In 1971 Johanson and Blizzard reported three cases of this disorder and found one from the past literature. At least 18 cases have now been reported. This syndrome incorporates elements of ectodermal dysplasia with endocrine and exocrine insufficiency plus growth and mental deficiency.

ABNORMALITIES

Growth. Prenatal onset growth deficiency.

Performance. Normal intelligence to severe mental deficiency. Sensorineural deafness. Hypotonia.

Craniofacial. Mild to moderate microcephaly. Midline posterior scalp defects. Variable sparse hair with frontal upsweep. Hypoplastic to aplastic alae nasi. Nasolacrimal cutaneous fistulae. Hypoplastic deciduous teeth, absent permanent teeth.

Urorectal. Calicectasis to hydronephrosis. Imperforate anus. Vagina septate or double. Cryptorchidism. Micropenis.

Endocrine. Primary hypothyroidism.

Exocrine. Pancreatic insufficiency with malabsorption.

OCCASIONAL ABNORMALITIES.
Strabismus, small nipples and absent areolae, radiolucent skull defects, abnormal EEG, rectovaginal fistula, single urogenital orifice, abdominal and thoracic situs inversus.

NATURAL HISTORY.
Although mental deficiency is frequent, normal intelligence has clearly been documented. Hypothyroidism, occurring in about one third of cases, may progress in degree and is unusual in that the cholesterol level is not elevated; this unusual characteristic is possibly related to the concomitant malabsorption. Improvement in growth rate may occur with thyroid and pancreatin replacement therapy. However, the inadequate extent of catch-up growth implies a primary growth deficiency problem as well, as further implied by the prenatal onset of the growth deficiency.

ETIOLOGY.
Autosomal recessive.

References

Grand, R. J., et al.: Unusual case of XXY Klinefelter's syndrome with pancreatic insufficiency, hypothyroidism, deafness, chronic lung disease, dwarfism and microcephaly. Am. J. Med., *41*:478, 1966.

Johanson, A., and Blizzard, R.: A syndrome of congenital aplasia of the alae nasi, deafness, hypothyroidism, dwarfism, absent permanent teeth, and malabsorption. J. Pediatr., 79:982, 1971.

Mardini, M. K., Sakati, N. A., and Nyhan, W. L.: Johanson-Blizzard syndrome in a large inbred kindred with three involved members. Clin. Genet., *14*:247, 1978.

Daentl, D. L., et al.: The Johanson-Blizzard syndrome: Case report and autopsy findings. Am. J. Med. Genet., *3*:129, 1979.

Helin, I., and Jodal, U.: A syndrome of congenital hypoplasia of the alae nasi, situs inversus, and severe hypoproteinemia in two siblings. J. Pediatr., *99*:932, 1981.

Moeschler, J. B., and Lubinsky, M. S.: Brief clinical report: Johanson-Blizzard syndrome with normal intelligence. Amer. J. Med. Genet., *22*:69, 1985.

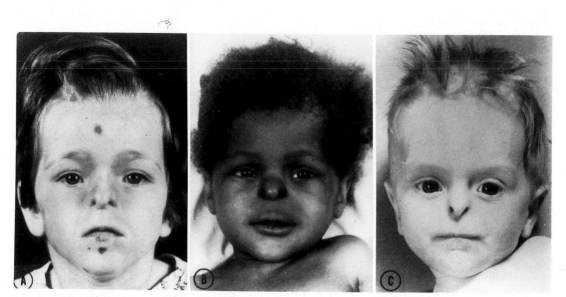

Johanson-Blizzard syndrome. Three affected children. (From Johanson, A., and Blizzard, R.: J. Pediatr., 79:982, 1971.)

SECKEL SYNDROME

Severe Short Stature, Microcephaly, Prominent Nose

Reported by Mann and Russell in 1959, this condition was extensively studied by Seckel in 1960. More precise criteria for diagnosis have recently been set forth.

ABNORMALITIES

Growth. Prenatal onset of marked growth deficiency.

CNS. Mental deficiency.

Craniofacies. Microcephaly with secondary premature synostosis. Receding forehead. Prominent nose. Micrognathia. Low-set, malformed ears with lack of lobule. Relatively large eyes with downslanting palpebral fissures.

Upper Extremities. Clinodactyly of fifth finger, simian crease, absence of some phalangeal epiphyses, hypoplasia of proximal radius with dislocation of radial head.

Lower Extremities. Dislocation of hip, hypoplasia of proximal fibula, gap between first and second toes. Inability to completely extend at knees.

Thorax. Only 11 pairs of ribs.

Genitalia. Male: cryptorchidism.

OCCASIONAL ABNORMALITIES. Facial asymmetry, strabismus, partial anodontia, enamel hypoplasia, sparse hair, scoliosis, talipes, pes planus, hypoplastic external genitalia.

NATURAL HISTORY. Gestational timing may be prolonged. Birth length, 13.5 to 17 inches; birth weight, 1 to 4.3 pounds. Final height, about 3 to 3.5 feet. Moderate to severe mental deficiency, though early motor progress may be near normal. The cerebrum is small, with a simple primitive convolutional pattern resembling that of a chimpanzee. Though they tend to be friendly and pleasant, these patients are often hyperkinetic and easily distracted. Poor joint development and support may be evident by dislocations of the hip, elbow, or both, and by later development of scoliosis, kyphosis, or both. Survival to an age of 75 years has been recorded.

ETIOLOGY. Autosomal recessive.

References

Mann, T. P., and Russell, A.: Study of a microcephalic midget of extreme type. Proc. R. Soc. Med., *52*:1024, 1959.

Seckel, H. P. G.: Bird-Headed Dwarfs. Springfield, Ill., Charles C Thomas, 1960, p. 241.

Harper, R. G., Orti, E., and Baker, R. K.: Birdheaded dwarfs (Seckel's syndrome). A familial pattern of developmental, dental, skeletal, genital, and central nervous system anomalies. J. Pediatr., *70*:799, 1967.

McKusick, V. A., et al.: Seckel's birdheaded dwarfism. N. Engl. J. Med., *277*:279, 1967.

Majewski, F., and Goecke, T.: Studies of microcephalic primordial dwarfism I: approach to a delineation of the Seckel syndrome. Am. J. Med. Genet., *12*:7, 1982.

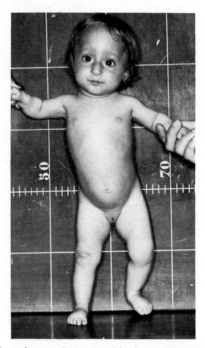

Seckel syndrome. One year old who at term birth was 1.2 kg with a length of 33.5 cm and at one year is 2.75 kg with a length of 48.5 cm and a head circumference of 34 cm. Note the disproportion of nose size to the size of the mandible and face, whereas general body proportions and adiposity are near normal for age (even though her size is still smaller than that of a neonate). (Courtesy of Dr. D. Vischer, Kinderspital, Zürich.)

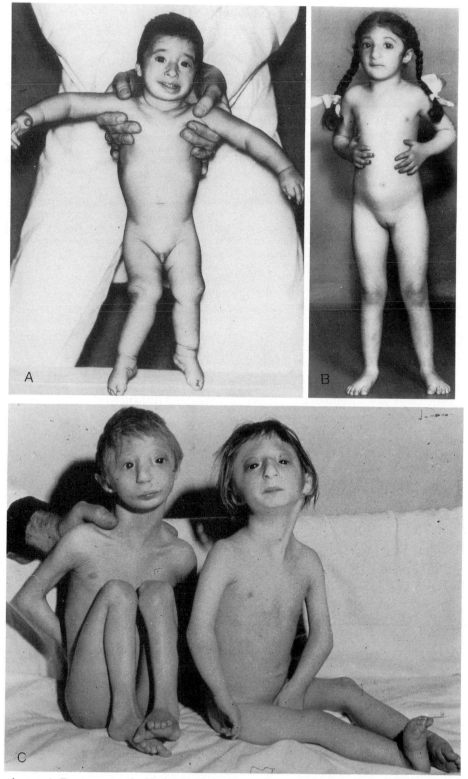

Seckel syndrome. *A*, Fourteen month old; height age, two months. *B*, Five year old; height age, 19 months. (From Seckel, H. P. G.: Bird-Headed Dwarfs. Springfield, Ill., Charles C Thomas, 1960.) *C*, Mentally deficient brother (six year old) and sister (three year old) with height ages of 11 months and four months, respectively. (From Harper, R. G., et al.: J. Pediatr., *70*:799, 1967.)

HALLERMANN-STREIFF SYNDROME

(Oculomandibulodyscephaly With Hypotrichosis Syndrome)

Microphthalmia, Small Pinched Nose, Hypotrichosis

The first report of this disorder was by Audry, who described an incomplete case in 1893. Hallermann, in 1948, and Streiff, in 1950, independently described three cases, recognizing this syndrome as a separate entity. In 1958, Francois collected all the previously published cases and emphasized the cardinal features of the condition. About 80 cases have been reported in the literature.

ABNORMALITIES

Growth. Proportionate small stature.

Craniofacial. Brachycephaly with frontal and parietal bossing, thin calvarium, and delayed ossification of the sutures. Malar hypoplasia; micrognathia, with hypoplasia of the rami and anterior displacement of the temporomandibular joint. Bilateral microphthalmia (80 per cent); cataracts (94 per cent), total or incomplete, which may resorb spontaneously. Nose is thin, small, and pointed, with hypoplasia of the cartilage, becoming parrot-like with age. Microstomia, narrow and high arched palate. Dentition: hypoplasia of the teeth and/or malimplantation, neonatal teeth, and partial anodontia. Atrophy of the skin, most prominent over the nose and sutural areas of the scalp; thin and light hair with hypotrichosis, especially of the scalp, eyebrows, and eyelashes.

OCCASIONAL ABNORMALITIES.

Scaphocephaly, microcephaly, platybasia, shallow sella turcica, absence of the mandibular condyles, double cutaneous chin. Blue sclerae, nystagmus, strabismus, downward slant to palpebral fissures, optic disc colobomata, glaucoma, and various chorioretinal pigment alterations. Syndactyly, winging of the scapulae, lordosis, scoliosis, spina bifida, funnel chest. Mental retardation (15 per cent). Hypogenitalism, cryptorchidism in the male.

NATURAL HISTORY.

Because the majority of the literature pertains to the ocular defect, there are insufficient data upon which to base the natural history in terms of the growth defect or mortality in infants. During early infancy, they may have feeding and respiratory problems, even necessitating tracheostomy. Respiratory infections may contribute to the cause of death. The peculiar physiognomy and shortness of stature may impair their psychologic adjustment, though the major handicap is the ocular defect, which usually culminates in blindness despite surgery. Though the majority of the reported patients have been of normal intelligence, motor and mental deficits, even to severe degree, have been reported.

ETIOLOGY.

Until Guyard et al. reported an apparently affected father and daughter, the etiology was undetermined. Now the most likely hypothesis is that of a single mutant gene (dominant), with most cases representing fresh mutations.

References

Audry, C.: Variété d'alopécia congénitale; alopécie suturale. Ann. Dermatol. Syph. (Ser. 3), *4*:899, 1893.

Hallermann, W.: Vogelgesicht und cataracta congenita. Klin. Monatsbl. Augenheilkd., *113*:315, 1948.

Streiff, E. B.: Dysmorphie mandibulo-faciale (tête d'oiseau) et alterations oculaires. Ophthalmologica, *120*:79, 1950.

Francois, J.: A new syndrome: dyscephalis with bird face and dental anomalies, nanism, hypotrichosis, cutaneous atrophy, microphthalmia and congenital cataract. Arch. Ophthalmol., *60*:842, 1958.

Guyard, M., Perdriel, G., and Ceruti, F.: Sur deux cas de syndrome dyscéphalizue à tête d'oiseau. Bull. Soc. Ophthalmol. Fr., *62*:443, 1962.

Hoefnagel, D., and Bernirschke, K.: Dyscephalia mandibulo-oculo-facialis. (Hallermann-Streiff syndrome). Arch. Dis. Child., *40*:57, 1965.

Judge, C., and Chalcanovskis, J. F.: The Hallermann-Streiff syndrome. J. Ment. Defic. Res., *15*:115, 1971.

Golomb, R. S., and Porter, P. S.: A distinct hair shaft abnormality in the Hallermann-Streiff syndrome. Cutis, *16*:122, 1975.

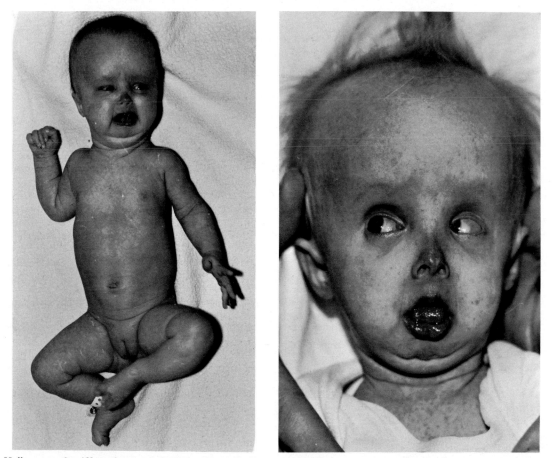

Hallermann-Streiff syndrome. *Left,* Two and one-half month old with height age of one month. *Right,* Same patient at ten months, showing changes in facies. (From Smith, D. W.: J. Pediatr., *70*:481, 1967.)

C. MODERATE SHORT STATURE, FACIAL, +/− GENITAL

SMITH-LEMLI-OPITZ SYNDROME

Anteverted Nostrils and/or Ptosis of Eyelids,
Syndactyly of Second and Third Toes,
Hypospadias and Cryptorchidism in Male

Four patients with this disorder were described by Smith et al. in 1964, and subsequently at least 43 cases have been reported.

ABNORMALITIES

Growth. Moderately small at birth, with subsequent failure to thrive.

Performance. Moderate to severe mental deficiency, with variable altered muscle tone.

Craniofacial. Microcephaly with narrow frontal area, auricles slanted or low-set, ptosis of eyelids, inner epicanthal folds, strabismus, broad nasal tip with anteverted nostrils, broad maxillary secondary alveolar ridges, micrognathia.

Limb. Simian crease, high frequency of digital whorl dermal ridge patterning, syndactyly of second and third toes.

Genitalia. Male: cryptorchidism, hypospadias, mild to severe.

OCCASIONAL ABNORMALITIES

CNS. Seizures, abnormal EEG.

Facial. Cataract, cleft palate.

Limb. Flexed fingers, asymmetrically short finger(s), distal axial triradius, polydactyly, metatarsus adductus, vertical talus, dislocation of hip, dysplasia epiphysealis punctata.

Other. Cardiac anomaly, hypoplasia of thymus, pyloric stenosis, inguinal hernia, renal anomaly, pancreatic giant cells, deep sacral dimple, pit anterior to anus. Unusually blond hair.

NATURAL HISTORY. Many of these babies are born in a breech presentation. Stillbirth and early neonatal death are not uncommon. Feeding difficulty and vomiting have been frequent problems in early infancy, and of those who survive, 20 per cent have died during the first year. Death appeared to be related to pneumonia in most of them, one of whom had a hemorrhagic necrotizing pneumonia with varicella, suggesting an impaired immune response. Necropsy studies have shown serious defects in brain morphogenesis, including micrencephaly, hypoplasia of the frontal lobes, hypoplasia of cerebellum and brain stem, dilated ventricles, irregular gyrus patterns, and irregular neuronal organization. Irritable behavior with shrill screaming may pose a problem during infancy. Muscle tone, which may be hypotonic in early infancy, tends to become hypertonic with time. The degree of mental deficiency is usually moderate to severe. Two adults described have had I.Q.s in the 20s. A number of infants with female external genitalia and a 46 XY karyotype who have multiple structural anomalies, including postaxial polydactyly, cleft palate, small tongue, eye anomalies, and cardiac defects, have died in the neonatal period. Whether this represents a distinct disorder referred to as Smith-Lemli-Opitz type II requires further delineation.

ETIOLOGY. Autosomal recessive. More than one sibling has been affected in 40 per cent of the families, and there are two recorded instances of parental consanguinity. The reported higher frequency of affected males versus females may be related to the ascertainment bias of the genital anomaly.

References

Smith, D. W., Lemli, L., and Opitz, J. M.: A newly recognized syndrome of multiple congenital anomalies. J. Pediatr., *64*:210, 1964.

Gibson, R.: A case of the Smith-Lemli-Opitz syndrome of multiple congenital anomalies in association with dysplasia epiphysealis punctata. Can. Med. Ass. J., *92*:574, 1965.

Dallaire, L., and Fraser, F. C.: The syndrome of retardation with urogenital and skeletal anomalies in siblings. J. Pediatr., *69*:459, 1966.

Nevo, S., et al.: Smith-Lemli-Opitz syndrome in an inbred family. Am. J. Dis. Child., *124*:431, 1972.

Garcia, C. A., et al.: Neurological involvement in the Smith-Lemli-Opitz syndrome. Dev. Med. Child Neurol., *15*:48, 1973.

Lowry, R. B.: Editorial comment: Variability in the Smith-Lemli-Opitz syndrome: Overlap with the Meckel syndrome. Am. J. Med. Genet., *14*:429, 1983.

Curry, C. J. R., et al.: Smith-Lemli-Opitz syndrome. Type II: Multiple congenital anomalies with male pseudohermaphroditism and frequent early lethality. Am. J. Med. Genet., *26*:45, 1987.

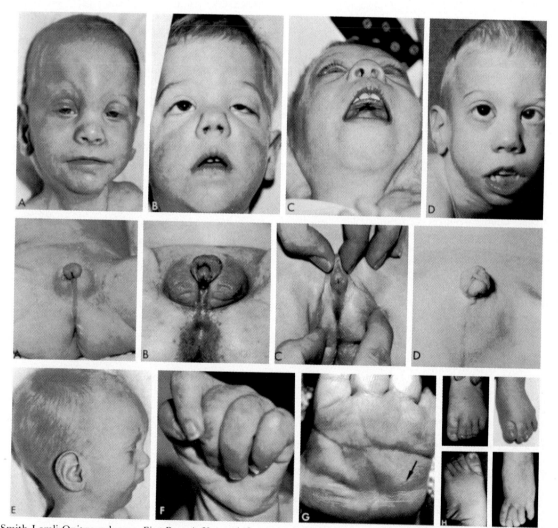

Smith-Lemli-Opitz syndrome. *First Row, A*, Young infant raised as female. *B*, Ten month old; height age, six months. *C*, Older infant. *D*, Five year old; height age, 18 months. Note ptosis, nasal configuration, and prominent lateral palatine ridges. *Second Row, A* to *D*, Genitalia of individuals pictured in first row. *E*, Lateral view of patient *A*. Note prominent midforehead (glabella), micrognathia. *F*, Clenched hand (patient *A*), a variable feature. *G*, Simian crease and distal palmar axial triradius (*arrow*). *H*, Unusual appearance of syndactyly of the second and third toes in three of four patients. (*B, C, D, G,* and *H* from Smith, D. W., et al.: J. Pediatr., *64*:210, 1964.)

WILLIAMS SYNDROME

Prominent Lips,
Hoarse Voice, Cardiovascular Anomaly

In 1961, Williams et al. described this disorder in four unrelated children with mental deficiency, an unusual facies, and supravalvular aortic stenosis. Subsequently, well over 100 cases have been described. Hypercalcemia has been an infrequent finding; cardiovascular anomalies, including supravalvular aortic stenosis, have been variable; and features such as aberrations of growth and performance and the unusual facies are more consistent relative to diagnosis.

ABNORMALITIES. Varying features from among the following:

Growth. Mild prenatal growth deficiency. Postnatal growth rate about 75 per cent of normal. Mild microcephaly.

Performance. Average I.Q. of about 56, with a range from 41 to 80. Friendly, loquacious personality, hoarse voice, hypersensitivity to sound, mild neurologic dysfunction. Perceptual and motor function more reduced (−3.0 to 3.9 SD) than verbal and memory performance (−2.0 SD).

Facies. Medial eyebrow flare, short palpebral fissures. Depressed nasal bridge. Epicanthal folds. Periorbital fullness of subcutaneous tissues. Blue eyes, stellate pattern in the iris. Anteverted nares, long philtrum, prominent lips with open mouth.

Limbs. Hypoplastic nails, hallux valgus.

Cardiovascular. Supravalvular aortic stenosis, peripheral pulmonary artery stenosis, pulmonic valvular stenosis, ventricular and atrial septal defect. There may also be renal artery stenosis with hypertension, hypoplasia of the aorta, and other arterial anomalies.

Dentition. Partial anodontia, enamel hypoplasia.

Other. Bladder diverticula, usually evident only by excretory urography.

OCCASIONAL ABNORMALITIES. Ocular hypotelorism, strabismus, malar hypoplasia, fifth finger clinodactyly, small penis, pectus excavatum, inguinal and/or umbilical hernia, hypercalcemia, autism. Degenerative renal disease has been noted in several cases by Bryan Hall, M.D., of the University of Kentucky, Lexington.

NATURAL HISTORY. In early infancy, these children tend to be fretful and have feeding problems. During childhood they tend to be outgoing and loquacious, a personality referred to as "cocktail party manner." About one sixth, however, have severe behavior problems. Of a group of ten adults evaluated by Morris et al., six were hypertensive, five were obese, and nine had limitation of joint movement. The vast majority lived in a sheltered environment.

ETIOLOGY. Unknown. All cases have been sporadic. The arterial vascular anomalies, the stromal patterning of the iris, and the bladder diverticula are all factors that suggest a problem in connective tissue development. The relationship of the calcium aberrations remains a mystery. Jensen et al. reported a 42 year old man with Williams syndrome who died of pancreatic carcinoma and had histologic evidence of calcium apatite crystals in the eyes, aorta, kidneys, and adrenals despite having a normal serum calcium level. Documentation of delayed calcium clearance after intravenous calcium loading and blunted calcitonin response after calcium infusion suggests that a deficiency of calcitonin may be responsible for the alteration in calcium metabolism.

References

Joseph, M. C., and Parrott, D.: Severe infantile hypercalcaemia with special reference to the facies. Arch. Dis. Child., *33*:385, 1958.

Williams, J. C. P., Barratt-Boyes, B. G., and Lowe, J. B.: Supravalvular aortic stenosis. Circulation, *24*:1311, 1961.

Jones, K. L., and Smith, D. W.: The Williams elfin facies syndrome. A new perspective. J. Pediatr., *86*:718, 1975.

Jensen, O. A., Marborg, M., and Dupont, A.: Ocular pathology in the elfin face syndrome. Ophthalmologica, *172*:434, 1976.

Bennett, F. C., LaVeck, B., and Sells, C. J.: The Williams elfin facies syndrome: the psychological profile as an aid in syndrome identification. Pediatrics, *61*:303, 1978.

Babbitt, D. P., Dobbs, J., and Boedecker, R. A.: Multiple bladder diverticula in Williams-elfin-facies syndrome. Pediatr. Radiol., *8*:21, 1979.

Culler, F. L., Jones, K. L., and Deftos, L. J.: Impaired calcitonin secretion in patients with Williams syndrome. J. Pediatr., *107*:720, 1985.

Daniels, S. R., et al.: Systemic hypertension secondary to peripheral vascular anomalies in patients with Williams syndrome. J. Pediatr., *106*:249, 1985.

Morris, C. A., et al.: The natural history of the Williams syndrome. Growth patterns and morbidity. Clin. Res., *35*:22A, 1987.

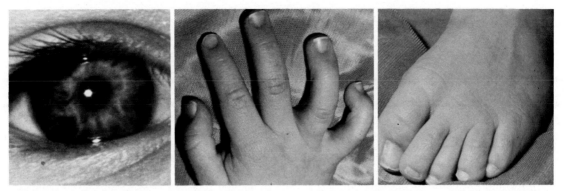

Stellate pattern to iris, relatively short nails, and valgus position of big toe—frequent features in Williams syndrome.

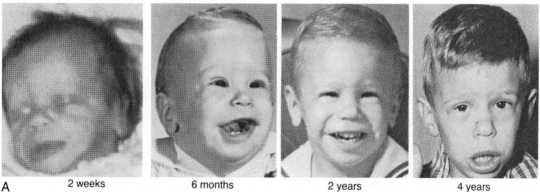

A   2 weeks   6 months   2 years   4 years

Height age—2 years and 10 months

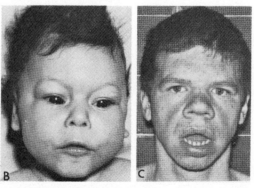

Williams syndrome. *A*, Facial appearance from the mother's photos of a boy with aortic stenosis, unusual facies, and relatively slow developmental progress. The serum calcium level is presently normal; serum calcium level during infancy is unknown. *B*, Four and one-half month old with severe hypercalcemia, whose height age was four months at seven months of age when the baby died. Necropsy showed nonspecific fibrous thickening in the intima of the aortic valve. (*B* From Joseph, M. C., and Parrott, D.: Arch. Dis. Child., *33*:385, 1958.) *C*, Seventeen year old mentally deficient boy of short stature who has evidence of supravalvular aortic stenosis. (Courtesy of A. Reichert, Rainier State Training School, Buckley, Washington.)

NOONAN SYNDROME

(Turner-like Syndrome)

Webbing of the Neck, Pectus Excavatum,
Cryptorchidism, Pulmonic Stenosis

Kobilinsky reported in 1883 a 20 year old male with webbing of the neck, incomplete folding of the ears, and low posterior hairline, but no mention was made of other physical findings. The first complete description appears to be that of Weissenberg in 1928. In 1963, Noonan and Ehmke further delineated the clinical phenotype and documented its association with valvular pulmonic stenosis. Recently, Mendez and Opitz have set forth the entire phenotype based on a review of 63 publications since 1883.

ABNORMALITIES

Growth. Short stature of postnatal onset in 50 per cent.

Performance. Mental retardation (25 per cent).

Facies. Epicanthal folds, ptosis of eyelids, hypertelorism, downslanting palpebral fissures, myopia, keratoconus, strabismus, nystagmus. Low-set and/or abnormal auricles. Anterior dental malocclusion.

Neck. Low posterior hairline, short or webbed neck.

Thorax. Shield chest and pectus excavatum or pectus carinatum or both.

Other Skeletal. Cubitus valgus. Abnormalities of vertebral column.*

Heart. Pulmonary valve stenosis due to a dysplastic or thickened valve, septal defects, patent ductus arteriosus, branch stenosis of pulmonary arteries.

Genitalia. Small penis, cryptorchidism.

OCCASIONAL ABNORMALITIES. Nerve deafness; high arched palate; large or asymmetric head; hypoplastic nipples; kyphoscoliosis; winging of scapula, cervical ribs, edema of the dorsum of the hands and feet; lymphatic vessel dysplasia; simian creases; unusual wool-like consistency of the hair (curly); skin nevi, keloids, hyperelastic skin. Hypogonadism. Malignant hyperthermia.

---

*Abnormal curvature or abnormal vertebrae (e.g., spina bifida occulta, hemivertebrae).

NATURAL HISTORY. There is no apparent propensity to any special type of illness. The degree of mental retardation is seldom severe, and the social performance is usually better than anticipated from the intelligence quotient.

Recently, Allanson et al. have documented the marked changes in the clinical phenotype from birth through adulthood.

ETIOLOGY. Unknown. Usually a sporadic occurrence within families. Apparent autosomal dominant inheritance has been documented. Because of the wide variability in expression, careful evaluation of both parents must be undertaken prior to recurrence risk counseling.

COMMENT. The differential diagnosis for patients with the Noonan syndrome is extensive. XO/XY mosaicism, fetal hydantoin syndrome, fetal mysoline syndrome, and fetal alcohol syndrome have all been considered in patients with this phenotype. Most recently, a number of patients have been described with features of both neurofibromatosis and Noonan syndrome. As of now it has been suggested that this be considered a distinct entity.

References

Kobilinsky, O.: Ueber eine flughautahnliche Ausbreitung am Halse. Arch. Anthropol., *14*:343, 1883.

Weissenberg, S.: Eine eigentumliche Hautfaltenbildung am Halse. Anthropol. Anz., *5*:141, 1928.

Noonan, J. A., and Ehmke, D. A.: Associated noncardiac malformations in children with congenital heart disease. J. Pediatr., *63*:469, 1963.

Pearl, W.: Cardiovascular anomalies in Noonan's syndrome. Chest, *71*:677, 1977.

Allanson, J. E., et al.: Noonan syndrome: The changing phenotype. Am. J. Med. Genet., *21*:507, 1985.

Mendez, H. M. M., and Opitz, J. M.: Noonan syndrome: A review. Am. J. Med. Genet., *21*:493, 1985.

Opitz, J. M., and Weaver, D. D.: Editorial comment: The neurofibromatosis-Noonan syndrome. Am. J. Med. Genet., *21*:477, 1985.

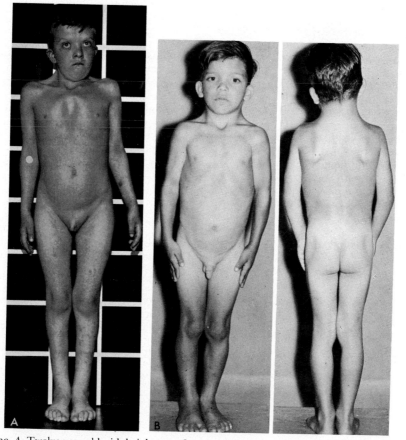

Noonan syndrome. *A*, Twelve year old with height age of seven years. Mental deficiency but a very affable personality. Cardiac defect. Cryptorchidism. (From Smith, D. W.: J. Pediatr., *70*:473, 1967.) *B*, Nine year old; height age at ten and one-half years was five years and eight months. (From Ferrier, P. E.: Pediatrics, *40*:575, 1967.)

AARSKOG SYNDROME

Hypertelorism, Brachydactyly, Shawl Scrotum

Set forth by Aarskog in 1970, there has been increasing recognition of this disorder. It can easily be misdiagnosed as the Noonan syndrome.

ABNORMALITIES

Growth. Slight to moderate short stature (71 per cent).

Facies. Rounded. Hypertelorism with variable ptosis of eyelids and slight downward slant to palpebral fissures. Small nose with anteverted nares, broad philtrum, maxillary hypoplasia, slight crease below the lower lip. Upper helices of ears incompletely outfolded. Hypodontia, retarded dental eruption, orthodontic problems.

Limbs. Brachydactyly with clinodactyly of fifth fingers, unusual position of extended fingers, simian crease, mild interdigital webbing.

Thorax. Mild pectus excavatum.

Abdomen. Prominent umbilicus, inguinal hernias.

Genitalia. "Shawl" scrotum (see figure, part *E*), cryptorchidism.

OCCASIONAL ABNORMALITIES

Skeletal. Cervical vertebral anomalies, scoliosis, cubitus valgus, splayed toes with bulbous tips, metatarsus adductus.

Genitalia. Cleft scrotum, phimosis.

Intelligence. Dull normal.

NATURAL HISTORY. Growth deficiency may be of prenatal onset but more commonly is first evident at one to three years of age and may be associated with slow maturation and a late advent of adolescence. Orthodontic correction is often necessary. Though serious mental deficiency is unusual, mild degrees have been a variable feature. Social performance is usually good, and the patients tend to have a pleasant personality. There is the suspicion of reduced fertility in some of the affected males, possibly related to the cryptorchidism.

ETIOLOGY. X-linked semidominant inheritance, with carrier females often showing some minor manifestations of the disorder, especially in the facies or hands. Full expression of the disorder in the mother of an affected son, both of whom had an X-autosome translocation, gives further credence to the concept that this is an X-linked disorder.

References

Aarskog, D.: A familial syndrome of short stature associated with facial dysplasia and genital anomalies. J. Pediatr., *77*:856, 1970.

Furukawa, C. T., Hall, B. D., and Smith, D. W.: The Aarskog syndrome. J. Pediatr., *81*:1117, 1972.

Berman, P., Desjardins, C., and Fraser, F. C.: The inheritance of the Aarskog syndrome. J. Pediatr., *86*:885, 1975.

Halse, A., Bjorvatn, K., and Aarskog, D.: Dental findings in patients with the Aarskog syndrome. Scand. J. Dent. Res., *87*:253, 1979.

Bawle, E., et al.: Aarskog syndrome: Full male and female expression associated with an X-autosome translocation. Am. J. Med. Genet., *17*:595, 1984.

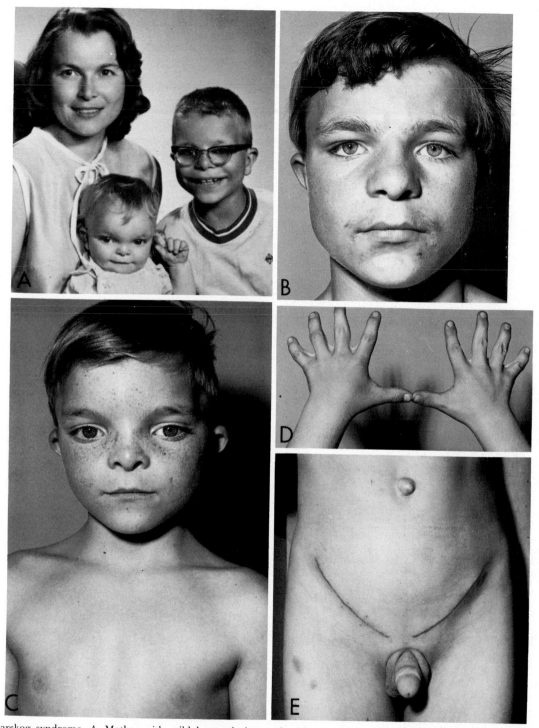

Aarskog syndrome. *A*, Mother with mild hypertelorism and widow's peak and two affected sons showing more striking hypertelorism. *B*, Sixteen year old, shown as a boy in *A*. Note the mild flare of the medial eyebrow and the less pronounced appearance of hypertelorism with age. *C*, Seven year old, shown as an infant in *A*. Note the mild overfolding of the ear helixes and the mild pectus excavatum. *D*, Mild brachyclinodactyly with mild syndactyly in patient shown in *C*. *E*, "Pouting" umbilicus, scars of inguinal hernia repairs, and "shawl" scrotum in an eight year old boy. (From Furukawa, C. T., et al.: J. Pediatr., *81*:1117, 1972.)

ROBINOW SYNDROME

(Fetal Face Syndrome)

Flat Facial Profile,
Short Forearms, Hypoplastic Genitalia

Initially reported by Robinow et al. in 1969, many additional cases of this disorder have been recognized.

ABNORMALITIES

Growth. Slight to moderate shortness of stature.

Craniofacial. Macrocephaly, large anterior fontanel, frontal bossing with apparent hypertelorism, prominent eyes, small upturned nose, long philtrum, triangular mouth with downturned angles and micrognathia, hyperplastic alveolar ridges, and crowded teeth.

Limbs. Short forearms with brachydactyly.

Spine. Hemivertebrae.

Genitalia. Small penis, clitoris, labia majora; cryptorchidism.

OCCASIONAL ABNORMALITIES

Oral-Facial. Nevus flammeus, epicanthal folds, posteriorly rotated ears, macroglossia, high arched palate, absent or bifid uvula, cleft lip and/or cleft palate, short frenulum of tongue with cleft tongue tip.

Limbs. Broad thumbs, toes, clinodactyly of fifth finger, hyperextensible fingers, short metacarpals, Madelung-like anomaly of forearm, dislocation of hip, hypoplastic interphalangeal creases, single flexion creases on third and fourth fingers, hypoplastic middle and terminal phalanges of fingers and toes.

Other. Seizures; language deficiency; atrial septal defect; pectus excavatum; rib anomaly; superiorly positioned, broad, and poorly epithelialized umbilicus; omphalocele; inguinal hernia; pilonidal dimple.

NATURAL HISTORY. The penile hypoplasia may be sufficient to initially raise the question of sex for rearing. Although partial primary hypogonadism evidenced by elevated serum FSH levels was documented in four affected males, normal pubertal virilization occurred in all three patients older than 16 years. Two adult females are 4 feet 10 inches and 5 feet, respectively, and three adult males are 5 feet 3 inches, 5 feet 7 inches, and 5 feet 10 inches in height. The facial features become less pronounced with age owing to accelerated growth of the nose at adolescence. Performance has been normal in most individuals.

ETIOLOGY. Autosomal dominant inheritance was implied in the family reported by Robinow et al. However, Wadlington et al. reported affected siblings of normal parents, and other cases have been sporadic in the family. The possibility of etiologic heterogeneity for this disorder remains open. It has been suggested that vertebral and multiple rib anomalies, as well as more severe mesomelic brachymelia, are more indicative of autosomal recessive inheritance.

References

Robinow, M., Silverman, F. N., and Smith, H. D.: A newly recognized dwarfing syndrome. Am. J. Dis. Child., *117*:645, 1969.

Wadlington, W. B., Tucker, V. L., and Schimke, R. N.: Mesomelic dwarfism with hemivertebrae and small genitalia (the Robinow syndrome). Am. J. Dis. Child., *126*:202, 1973.

Lee, P. A., et al.: Robinow's syndrome. Am. J. Dis. Child., *136*:327, 1982.

Shprintzen, R. J., et al.: Male-to-male transmission of Robinow's syndrome. Am. J. Dis. Child., *136*:594, 1982.

Bain, M. D., Winter, R. M., and Burn, J.: Robinow syndrome without mesomelic brachymelia: A report of five cases. J. Med. Genet., *23*:350, 1986.

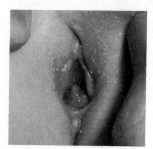

Robinow syndrome. Genitalia in an affected female, showing minute clitoris.

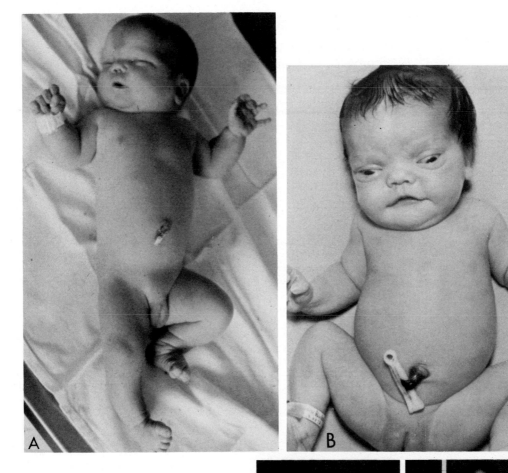

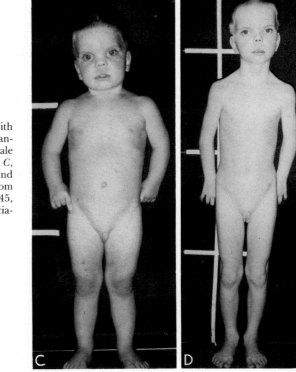

Robinow syndrome. *A*, Three day old male with micropenis, hypertelorism, and capillary hemangioma on central forehead. *B*, Two day old female with flat facies, hypertelorism, and minute clitoris. *C*, *D*, Note small nose, hypertelorism, micropenis, and variable shortness of hands. (*A*, *C*, and *D* from Robinow, M., et al.: Am. J. Dis. Child., *117*:645, 1969. Copyright 1969, American Medical Association.)

OPITZ SYNDROME

(Hypertelorism-Hypospadias Syndrome, Opitz-Frias Syndrome, G Syndrome)

Hypertelorism, Hypospadias, Swallowing Difficulties

In 1965 and again in 1969, Opitz, Smith, and Summitt reported this dominantly inherited condition, previously referred to as the BBB syndrome, in three families in which affected males usually have apparent ocular hypertelorism and hypospadias and affected females have only hypertelorism, there being no opportunity for expression of the penile malformation in the female. As the spectrum of defects in this disorder has evolved, it has become clear that the disorder described by Opitz et al. in 1969, previously referred to as the G syndrome or Opitz-Frias syndrome, is the same condition.

ABNORMALITIES

Performance. Mild to moderate mental deficiency in about two thirds of patients.
Facial. Ocular hypertelorism. Widow's peak. Posterior rotation of auricle.
Genital. Hypospadias, cryptorchidism. Bifid scrotum.
Other. Hernias.

OCCASIONAL ABNORMALITIES.

Cardiac anomaly, cleft lip plus or minus palate, short frenulum of tongue, cranial asymmetry, high nasal bridge, strabismus, downslanting palpebral fissures, diastasis recti, and imperforate anus. Laryngotracheal cleft, malformation of larynx, tracheoesophageal fistula, high carina, pulmonary hypoplasia, renal defect, agenesis of gallbladder, duodenal stricture. Increased monozygotic twinning.

NATURAL HISTORY. Swallowing problems with recurrent aspiration, stridulous respirations, intermittent pulmonary difficulty, wheezing, and a weak, hoarse cry should raise concern about a potentially lethal laryngoesophageal defect. In those cases gastrostomy or jejunostomy should be seriously considered. Initial failure to thrive may occur in more severely affected males, with improvement and normal growth if they survive.

ETIOLOGY. Autosomal dominant with sex limitation for penile malformation.

References

Opitz, J. M., Smith, D. W., and Summitt, R. L.: Hypertelorism and hypospadias. (Abstract.) J. Pediatr., 67:968, 1965.

Opitz, J. M., et al.: The G syndrome of multiple congenital anomalies. Birth Defects, 5:95, 1969.

Opitz, J. M., Summitt, R. L., and Smith, D. W.: The BBB syndrome. Familial telecanthus with associated anomalies. *In* Bergsma, D. (ed.): First Conference on Clinical Delineation of Birth Defects, Vol. 5. The National Foundation, 1969, pp. 86–94.

Gonzales, C. H., Hermann, J., and Opitz, J. M.: The hypertelorism-hypospadias (BBB) syndrome. Europ. J. Pediatr., 125:1, 1977.

Cordero, J. F., and Holmes, L. B.: Phenotypic overlap of the BBB and G syndromes. Am. J. Med. Genet., 2:145, 1978.

Stoll, C., et al.: Male-to-male transmission of the hypertelorism-hypospadias (BBB) syndrome. Am. J. Med. Genet. 20:221, 1985.

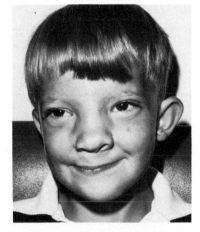

Seven year old boy with Opitz syndrome. Note hypertelorism, repaired cleft lips, and protruding auricle. Hypospadias was also present. (Courtesy of Dr. Robert Fineman, University of Utah Medical School, Salt Lake City.)

Opitz syndrome. An affected mother (mild hypertelorism) and two of her affected boys who show hypertelorism and also have hypospadias. (From the B. O. family pedigree of Opitz, J. M., et al.: Birth Defects, 5:86, 1969.)

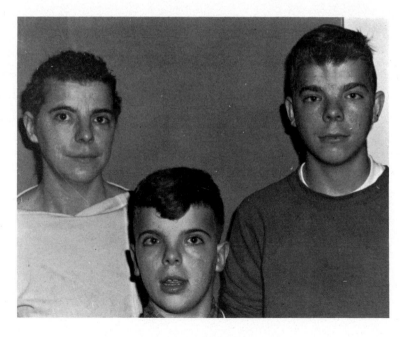

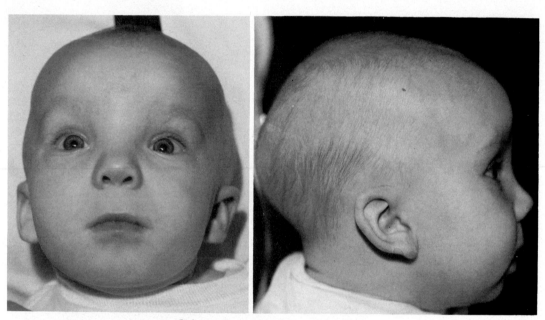

Opitz syndrome. *Above*, One month old.

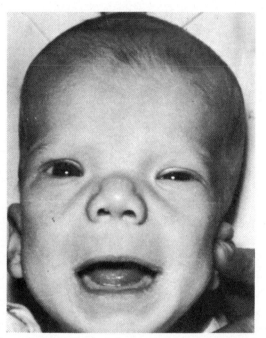

Seven and one-half month old. (From Opitz, J. M., et al.: Birth Defects, 5(2):95, 1969.)

D

D. SENILE-LIKE APPEARANCE

PROGERIA SYNDROME
(Hutchinson-Gilford Syndrome)

Alopecia, Atrophy of Subcutaneous Fat,
Skeletal Hypoplasia and Dysplasia

The following entry was recorded in the *St. James Gazette* in 1752: "March 19, 1754 died in Glamorganshire of mere old age and a gradual decay of nature at seventeen years and two months, Hopkins Hopkins, the little Welshman, lately shown in London. He never weighed more than 17 pounds but for three years past no more than twelve."

In 1886, Hutchinson described a similar patient. Later, Gilford studied this boy and another patient and termed the condition progeria, meaning premature aging. DeBusk summarized the findings in 60 cases.

ABNORMALITIES
Alopecia. Onset at birth to 18 months, with degeneration of hair follicles.

Thin Skin. Onset in early to mid-infancy.

Hypoplasia of Nails. Onset in infancy; nails may be brittle, curved, yellowish.

Loss of Subcutaneous Fat (Including Ear Lobule). Onset in infancy, last areas of adipose atrophy are cheeks and pubic area.

Periarticular Fibrosis. Onset at one to two years; stiff or partially flexed prominent joints or both; leads to "horse-riding" stance.

Skeletal Hypoplasia, Dysphasia, and Degeneration. Deficient growth, which becomes evident between six and 18 months; subsequent growth rate one-third to one-half normal. Facial hypoplasia with micrognathia, slim tubular bones and ribs with small thoracic cage, and thin calvarium with marked delay in ossification of fontanels. Skeletal dysplasia evident in coxa valga; tendency toward ovoid vertebral bodies; skeletal degeneration evident in loss of bone in clavicle and distal phalanges.

Dentition. Delayed eruption of deciduous and permanent dentition; crowding of teeth.

Atherosclerosis. As early as five years, onset of generalized atherosclerosis, especially evident in coronary arteries, aorta, and mesenteric arteries; at later age, may have cardiac murmur, left ventricular hypertrophy.

Metabolic Alterations. Mild to moderate elevation of serum cholesterol level.

OCCASIONAL ABNORMALITIES.
Scleroderma, irregular brownish-yellow skin pigmentation, perceptive hearing deficit, congenital or acquired cataract, absent breast and nipple, relatively large thymus, lymphoid and reticular hyperplasia, elevated serum lipoprotein level, aminoaciduria.

NATURAL HISTORY.
Though the onset of disease manifestations is usually stated as one to two years, there may be subtle indicators of disease within the first year. The average birth weight for 17 patients was 2.7 kg. One patient whose scalp was shaved at six weeks had no regrowth of hair. The deficit of growth becomes severe after one year of age. The tendency to fatigue easily is a factor that might limit full participation in childhood activities. The life span is shortened by the early advent of relentless arterial atheromatosis, and the usual cause of death is coronary occlusion. The life expectancy for 13 patients was seven to 27 years, with an average of 14.2 years. Since intelligence and brain development do not appear to be impaired, children with progeria should be allowed as normal a social life as possible.

At the present time, there is no effective therapy. The use of a wig is recommended for cosmetic purposes.

ETIOLOGY.
Unknown. Most cases are sporadic, and older mean paternal age suggests the possibility of a fresh mutant gene etiology. There are one or possibly two instances of affected siblings from normal parentage, suggesting autosomal re-

cessive inheritance. Possibly, there is etiologic heterogeneity for this phenotype.

COMMENT. This condition might be classified as an abiotrophic disease, since tissues that initially were fairly well developed have undergone hypoplastic, atrophic, or degenerative change. The clinical picture is different from the normal process of senile aging, and the term progeria therefore seems inappropriate.

References

Hutchinson, J.: Congenital absence of hair and mammary glands with atrophic condition of the skin and its appendages in a boy whose mother had been almost wholly bald from alopecia areata from the age of six. Trans. Med. Chir. Soc. Edinburgh, *69*:473, 1886.

Gilford, H.: Progeria: a form of senilism. Practitioner, *73*:188, 1904.

DeBusk, F. L.: The Hutchinson-Gilford progeria syndrome. J. Pediatr., *80*:697, 1972.

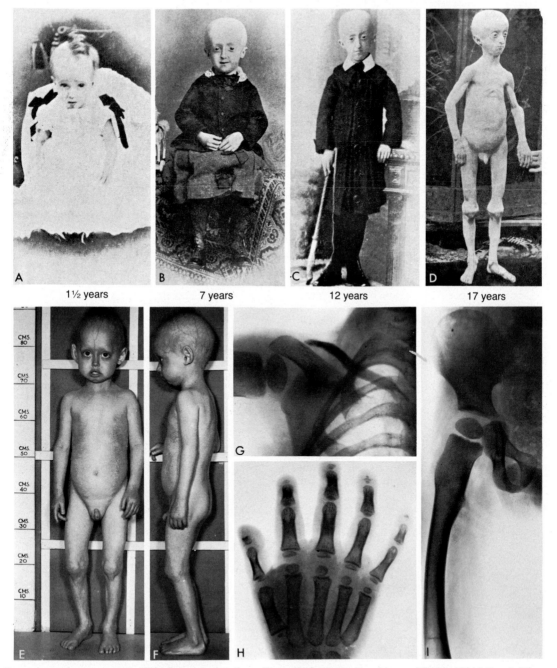

Progeria syndrome. *A* to *D*, Gilford's original patient. (From Gilford, H.: Practitioner, 73:188, 1904.) *E* to *I*, Three year old showing loss of outer clavicle, distal phalanges, and straight femur. (From Macleod, W.: Br. J. Radiol., 39:224, 1966.)

WERNER SYNDROME

*Early Adult—Cataract, Thin Skin with Thick
Fibrous Subcutaneous Tissue, Gray Sparse Hair*

The subject of Werner's doctoral thesis in 1904, this disease is usually not diagnosed until young adult life. More than 125 cases have been recorded.

ABNORMALITIES

Growth. Short stature; mean stature of affected males, 61 inches; females, 57.5 inches.

Deterioration. Loss of subcutaneous fat; slim, spindly extremities with small hands and feet; pinched facies with beak nose. Irregular dental development. Patches of stiffened skin, particularly on face and lower legs; skin ulcerations; atrophy of distal extremities. Thick, fibrous subcutaneous tissue with thin dermis. Osteoporosis, atherosclerosis with calcification. Muscle hypoplasia with patchy areas of fibrosis. Gray, sparse hair, premature balding. Cataract, retinal degeneration. Premature loss of teeth. Hypogonadism, reduced fertility. High-pitched, hoarse voice secondary to vocal chord atrophy. Liver atrophy. Adult-type diabetes (44 per cent). Mönckeberg sclerosis with organic brain syndrome. Metastatic calcifications. Excess urinary excretion of hyaluronic acid.

OCCASIONAL ABNORMALITIES.
Propensity toward malignancy (10 per cent), especially sarcoma and meningioma. Mild hyperthyroidism. Adrenal atrophy. Valvular sclerosis. Hyperkeratosis of palms and soles.

NATURAL HISTORY.
Often noted to be slim with a slow rate of growth in later childhood, these individuals have no adolescent growth spurt and reach their final height at ten to 18 years, usually at approximately 13 years. Gray hair develops at around 20 years and cataracts at about 25 years. Old age appearance is evident by 30 to 40 years, with the mean age of survival being 47 years. Calcification occurs not only in the atheromatous vessels but in the thick subcutaneous tissues as well.

ETIOLOGY.
Autosomal recessive. Epstein et al. noted a decreased rate of cell division plus a limited total number of mitotic divisions per cell in cultured fibroblasts from a patient with Werner syndrome, thereby suggesting a basic defect in cell life capacity resulting in a severe disease that resembles but is not the same as aging. Multiple stable chromosome rearrangements, including deletion of a portion of a single chromosome and translocations involving several chromosomes, as well as an increase in chromosome breakage, have been documented.

References

Werner, O.: Uber Katarakt in Verbindung mit Sklerodermie. (Doctoral dissertation, Kiel University.) Kiel, Schmidt and Klaunig, 1904.

Epstein, C. J., et al.: Werner's syndrome. Medicine, *45*:177, 1966.

Fleischmajer, R., and Nedwich, A.: Werner's syndrome. Am. J. Med., *54*:111, 1973.

Murata, K., and Nakashima, H.: Werner's syndrome: 24 cases with a review of the Japanese literature. J. Am. Geriatr. Soc., *30*:303, 1982.

Salk, D.: Werner's syndrome: A review of recent research with an analysis of connective tissue metabolism, growth control of cultured cells, and chromosome aberrations. Hum. Genet., *62*:1, 1982.

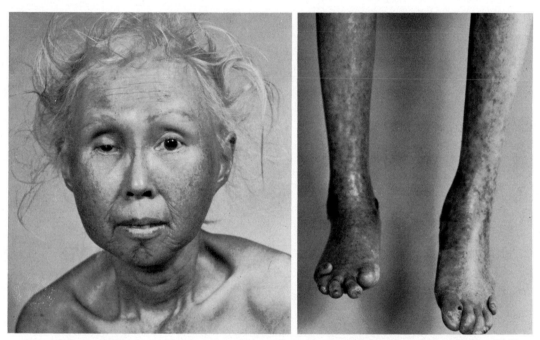

Forty-eight year old woman with Werner syndrome. (From Epstein, C. J., et al.: Medicine, *45*:177, 1966.)

COCKAYNE SYNDROME

Senile-Like Changes Beginning in Infancy,
Retinal Degeneration and Impaired Hearing,
Photosensitivity of Thin Skin

Cockayne reported this disorder in siblings in 1946. Subsequently, more than 16 other cases have been documented.

ABNORMALITIES
Growth. Growth deficiency with loss of adipose tissue by mid- to late infancy.

Performance. Mental deficiency with unsteady gait; sometimes tremor. Weakness with peripheral neuropathy. Moderate perceptive deafness.

Craniofacial. Salt and pepper retinal pigmentation, optic atrophy. Corneal opacity, cataract. Relatively small cranium with thick calvarium; loss of facial adipose tissue with slender nose, moderately sunken eyes, and thin skin that is photosensitive. Carious teeth.

Skin. Photosensitive dermatitis.

Extremities. Cool hands and feet, sometimes cyanotic. Mild to moderate joint limitation.

Trunk. Relatively short, with biconvex flattening of vertebrae and tendency toward dorsal kyphosis.

Other. Hepatomegaly. Cryptorchidism. Hypertension. Ohno and Hirooka discovered albuminuria with hyalinization of glomeruli, atrophy of tubules, and interstitial fibrosis in renal biopsies from three affected individuals.

OCCASIONAL ABNORMALITIES. Intrauterine growth retardation. Intracranial calcification, small sella turcica, cataract, nystagmus, cloudy cornea, decreased sweating and tearing, some "marble" epiphyses in digits, asymmetric fingers, short second toes, infolding of iliac crest, cryptorchidism. Graying of sparse hair.

NATURAL HISTORY. Although prenatal growth deficiency occasionally has been documented, growth and development usually proceed at a normal rate in early infancy, and it is not until two to four years of age that the pattern of defect is clearly evident. Personality and behavior tend to correspond to the mental age, which is defective. Photosensitivity of the skin may lead to problems with exposure to sunlight. Although affected patients are not prone to the development of cancer, a defect in DNA repair following ultraviolet irradiation has been documented.

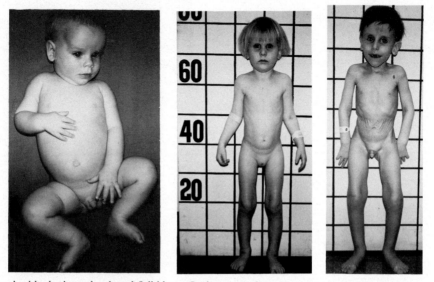

A seven month old who later developed full-blown Cockayne syndrome; a four year old and a six year old showing the dramatic changes that occur with age in this degenerative disorder. (Courtesy of Dr. Robert Summitt, University of Tennessee College of Medicine, Memphis.)

ETIOLOGY. Autosomal recessive. RNA synthesis following irradiation with ultraviolet light was abnormal in cells from one affected fetus, providing potential for prenatal diagnosis of this disorder.

References

Cockayne, E. A.: Dwarfism with retinal atrophy and deafness. Arch. Dis. Child., *21*:52, 1946.

Neill, C. A., and Dingwall, M. M.: A syndrome resembling progeria: a review of two cases. Arch. Dis. Child., *25*:213, 1950.

MacDonald, W. B., Fitch, K. D., and Lewis, I. C.: Cockayne's syndrome. An heredo-familial disorder of growth and development. Pediatrics, *25*:997, 1960.

Ohno, T., and Hirooka, M.: Renal lesions in Cockayne's syndrome. Tohoku J. Exp. Med., *89*:151, 1966.

Rainbow, A. J., and Howes, M.: A deficiency in the repair of UV and γ-ray damaged DNA in fibroblasts from Cockayne's syndrome. Mutation Research, *93*:235, 1982.

Lehman, A. R., Francis, A. J., and Giannelli, F.: Prenatal diagnosis of Cockayne's syndrome. Lancet, *1*:486, 1985.

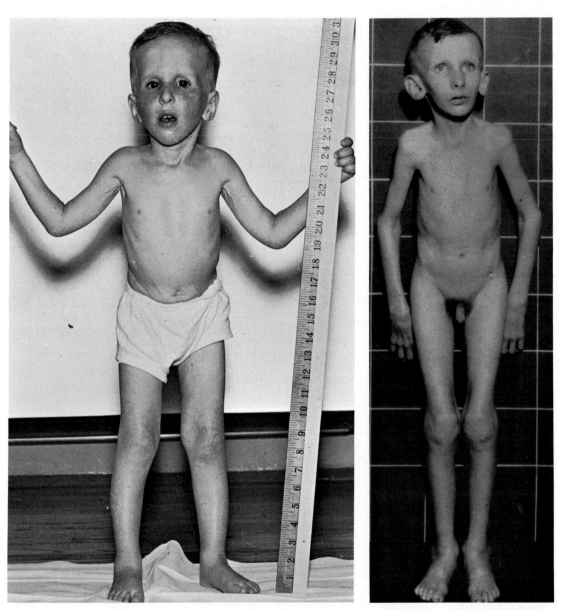

Cockayne syndrome. *Left,* Child, six years and ten months old. Height age, 16 months. (From Windmiller, J.: Am. J. Dis. Child., *105*:204, 1963.) *Right,* Fourteen and one-half year old. Height age, three and one-half years. Bone age, 16 years. (From Wilkins, L.: Diagnosis and Treatment of Endocrine Disorders in Childhood and Adolescence, 3rd ed. Springfield, Ill., Charles C Thomas, 1965. Courtesy of R. M. Blizzard.)

ROTHMUND-THOMSON SYNDROME

(Poikiloderma Congenitale Syndrome)

*Development of Poikiloderma,
Cataract with or without Other Ectodermal Dysplasia*

This condition was first described in 1868 by Rothmund, a Munich ophthalmologist who discovered multiple cases among an inbred group of people living in the nearby Alps. Over 80 cases have been reported.

ABNORMALITIES. Wide variance in expression, the most usual features being the following:
Growth. Small stature (54 per cent).
Skin. Irregular erythema progressing to telangiectasia, scarring, irregular pigmentation and depigmentation, atrophy. Photosensitivity (35 per cent).
Eyes. Juvenile zonular cataract (52 per cent), occasionally corneal dystrophy.

OCCASIONAL ABNORMALITIES
Skeletal. Small hands and feet, hypoplastic to absent thumbs, forearm reduction defects, osteoporosis and/or areas of cystic or sclerotic change.
Facial. Small saddle nose.
Teeth. Microdontia and odontia, ectopic eruption, dental caries.
Nails. Small, dystrophic (24 per cent).
Hair. Sparse, prematurely gray; occasionally alopecia.
Other Skin. Hyperkeratosis of palms and soles.
Other. Mental deficiency, osteogenic sarcoma in two patients. Growth hormone deficiency.

NATURAL HISTORY. Changes in the skin are usually evident between three months and one year of age, and the progression toward irregular "marbled" hypoplasia, termed poikiloderma, is mainly noted in the first few years. Cataract most commonly becomes evident between two and seven years of age. The principal problems for affected individuals are skin difficulties, sometimes photosensitivity; visual impairment requiring surgical intervention; and physical appearance, depending on the extent to which stature, hair, teeth, and/or nails are affected.

ETIOLOGY. Autosomal recessive, with 70 per cent of affected individuals being female, an unexplained disparity that might not be of significance because the number of reported cases is small. There may well be heterogeneity for this phenotype, since considerable variability has been noted in individuals reported as having this syndrome.

References

Rothmund, A.: Ueber Cataracten in Verbindung mit einer eigenthümlichen Hautdegeneration. Arch. Ophthalmol., *14*:159, 1868

Rook, A., Davis, R., and Stevanovic, D.: Poikiloderma congenitale. Rothmund-Thomson syndrome. Acta Derm. Venereol. (Stockh.), *39*:392, 1959.

Silver, H. K.: Rothmund-Thomson syndrome: an occulocutaneous disorder. Am. J. Dis. Child., *111*:182, 1966.

Oates, R. K., Lewis, M. B., and Walker-Smith, J. A.: The Rothmund-Thomson syndrome. Aust. Paediatr. J., 7:103, 1971.

Hall, J. G., Pagon, R. A., and Wilson, K. M.: Rothmund-Thomson syndrome with severe dwarfism. Am. J. Dis. Child., *134*:165, 1980.

Starr, D. G., McClure, J. P., and Connor, J. M.: Nondermatological complications and genetic aspects of the Rothmund-Thomson syndrome. Clin. Genet., 27:102, 1985.

Kaufman, S., et al.: Growth hormone deficiency in the Rothmund-Thomson syndrome. Am. J. Med. Genet., *23*:861, 1986.

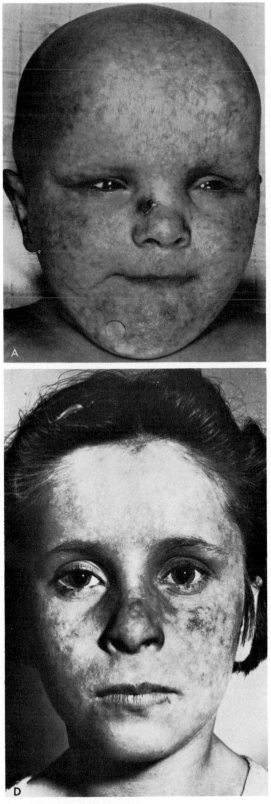

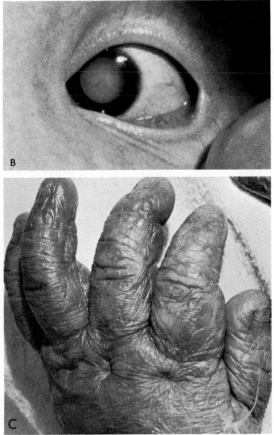

Rothmund-Thomson syndrome. *A*, Fifteen month old. (From Braun, W., and Unger, C.: Dermat. Wochenschr., *151*:1189, 1965.) *B*, Two and one-half year old. Note absence of lashes and mature cataract. *C*, Patient shown in *B*. Note severe nail dysplasia. (*B* and *C* from Wahl, J. W., et al.: Am. J. Ophthalmol., *60*:722, 1965.) *D*, Five year old. (From Rook, A. J., et al.: Acta Derm. Venereol. (Stockh.), *39*:392, 1959.)

E. EARLY OVERGROWTH WITH ASSOCIATED DEFECTS

FRAGILE X SYNDROME

(Martin-Bell Syndrome, Marker X Syndrome)

Mental Deficiency,
Mild Connective Tissue Dysplasia, Macro-orchidism

This subgroup can now be differentiated from other types of X-linked mental retardation. In 1943, Martin and Bell published the first pedigree documenting a sex-linked form of mental retardation. Lubs in 1969 showed the presence of a fragile site on the long arm of the X chromosome in affected males and some carrier females in one family. Macro-orchidism without endocrinologic abnormalities was described by Turner et al. and Cantu et al. in the affected males of a number of families. However, it was not until Sutherland demonstrated that expression of the fragile site was dependent on the nature of the cell culture medium that the association between X-linked mental retardation, macro-orchidism, and the marker X chromosome was made.

The disorder appears to be common. Among populations of mentally handicapped individuals, fragile X–positive studies have been documented in up to 5.9 per cent of males and up to 0.3 per cent of females. The phenotype is most readily identified in the male.

ABNORMALITIES
Performance. Slow mental development in 80 per cent of males; I.Q.s of 30 to 55, but sometimes extending into the mildly retarded border-line-normal range. This varies intrafamilially. Thirty per cent of females function in the borderline to mildly retarded range.
Facial. Prominent jaw, thickening of nasal bridge extending down to the nasal tip, large ears with soft cartilage, pale blue irides.

OCCASIONAL ABNORMALITIES. Nystagmus, hypotonia, lax joints, mild cutis laxa, torticollis, kyphoscoliosis, submucous cleft palate, mitral valve prolapse. Early features may suggest cerebral gigantism.

NATURAL HISTORY. Life span is normal. The patient's growth rate is slightly increased in the early years, with delayed motor milestones but no evidence of deterioration. Testicular size may be increased before puberty, but this increase becomes more obvious postpubertally. A characteristic speech pattern, referred to as "cluttering," is observed in higher functioning individuals. Psychologic profile is characterized by hyperkinetic behavior, emotional instability, hand biting, and other autistic features. All of these tend to improve at puberty. Treatment with folic acid has produced no measurable improvement in I.Q. or behavior.

ETIOLOGY. X-linked inheritance, but the molecular defect is not known. The marker on the X chromosome is a fragile site at Xq27. Phenotypically affected males generally express the marker in 10 to 40 per cent of cells. Expression is lower in heterozygous females and varies markedly in relationship to both age and intelligence. Older carrier women with normal I.Q.s tend to have low to zero expression of the marker. Frequency of expression of the fragile site is a familial characteristic. De novo mutation is extremely rare. An older paternal age effect has been demonstrated in the fathers of carrier women. Prenatal diagnosis has been successfully accomplished using cultured amniocytes and fetal blood samples obtained at fetoscopy.

References

Lubs, H. A.: A marker X chromosome. Am. J. Hum. Genet., *21*:231, 1969.
Turner, G., et al.: X-linked mental retardation associated with macro-orchidism. J. Med. Genet., *12*:367, 1975.

Cantu, J. M., et al.: Inherited congenital normofunctional testicular hyperplasia and mental deficiency. Hum. Genet., *33*:23, 1976.

Sutherland, G. R.: Fragile sites on human chromosomes: demonstration of their independence on the type of tissue culture medium. Science, *197*:265, 1977.

Turner, G., Daniel, A., and Frost, M.: X-linked mental retardation, macro-orchidism, and the Xq27 fragile site. J. Pediatr., *96*:837, 1980.

Turner, G., et al.: Conference report: Second international workshop on the fragile X and on X-linked mental retardation. Am. J. Med. Genet., *23*:11, 1986.

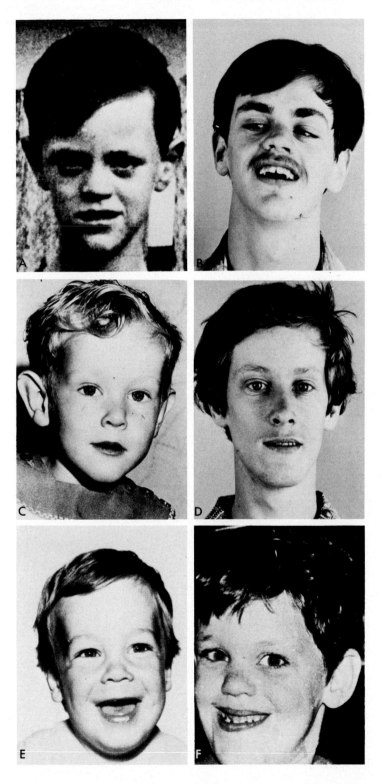

Fragile X syndrome. Increased head circumference with prominent forehead, prognathism, and big ears. *A* and *B* show the same patient at eight and 21 years; *C* and *D* show the same patient at three and 22 years; *E* shows a two year old, and *F* shows a four year old. (From Turner, G., et al.: J. Pediatr., *96*:837, 1980.)

SOTOS SYNDROME
(Cerebral Gigantism Syndrome)

Large Size, Large Hands and Feet,
Poor Coordination

Sotos et al. described five such patients in 1964, and at least 105 cases have subsequently been reported.

ABNORMALITIES

Performance. Variable mental deficiency. I.Q.s of 18 to 119, with a mean of 72. Poor coordination.

Growth. Prenatal onset of excessive size with relatively large span and large hands and feet. Advanced osseous maturation commensurate with height age. The phalangeal centers tend to be more accelerated than the carpal centers.

Craniofacial. Macrocephaly with mild dilatation of the cerebral ventricles and prominent forehead (dolichocephalic). Downslanting palpebral fissures. Hypertelorism. Prognathism with narrow anterior mandible. High, narrow palate with prominent lateral palatine ridges. Coarse-looking facies. Premature eruption of teeth.

OCCASIONAL ABNORMALITIES.
Seizures, EEG abnormalities, strabismus, facial plethora, kyphoscoliosis, abnormal glucose tolerance test (14 per cent), malignant tumors including Wilms (2 patients), vaginal carcinoma (1), hepatocarcinoma (1), cavernous hemangioma (1), mixed parotid tumor (1), osteochondroma (1), and neuroectodermal tumor (1).

NATURAL HISTORY.
The mean full-term birth length has been 55.2 cm and birth weight 3.9 kg. Growth is especially rapid in the first two to three years, after which it proceeds at a near normal rate; at ten years of age the height age is about 14 or 15 years. Neonatal problems have been frequent, including difficulties with respiration and feeding. Thereafter, general health has been good. Eighty-three per cent have had moderate to severe mental deficiency. The median age of individuals at first sitting has been nine months; walking, 17 months; and saying a few words, 25 months. The patient's excessive size, with dull mentality and poor coordination, leads to problems of social adjustment, occasionally with undue aggressiveness. Even in those patients with normal intelligence, delay of expressive language and motor development is characteristically present in infancy.

ETIOLOGY.
Unknown. Sporadic, with occasional exceptions. The majority have been males (57 per cent). At least five families have been reported in which both parent and offspring are affected, raising the question of autosomal dominant inheritance. Under this hypothesis, the great majority would represent fresh mutational cases, since the condition is most commonly a sporadic occurrence from unaffected parents. No consistent endocrine or other metabolic abnormality has been detected, and it is difficult to ascertain whether all cases have a common etiology.

References

Sotos, J. F., et al.: Cerebral gigantism in childhood. A syndrome of excessively rapid growth with acromegalic features and a nonprogressive neurologic disorder. N. Engl. J. Med., *271*:109, 1964.

Jaecken, J., van der Schueren-Lodeweyckx, and Eeckels, R.: Cerebral gigantism syndrome. Z. Kinderheilkd., *112*:332, 1972.

Zonana, J., et al.: Dominant inheritance of Sotos syndrome. J. Pediatr., *91*:251, 1977.

Dodge, P. R., Holmes, S. J., and Sotos, J. F.: Cerebral gigantism. Dev. Med. Child Neurol., *25*:248, 1983.

Maldonado, V., Gaynon, P. S., and Poznanski, A. K.: Cerebral gigantism associated with Wilms' tumor. Am. J. Dis. Child., *138*:486, 1984.

Bale, A. E., et al.: Familial Sotos syndrome (cerebral gigantism): Craniofacial and psychological characteristics. Am. J. Med. Genet., *20*:613, 1985.

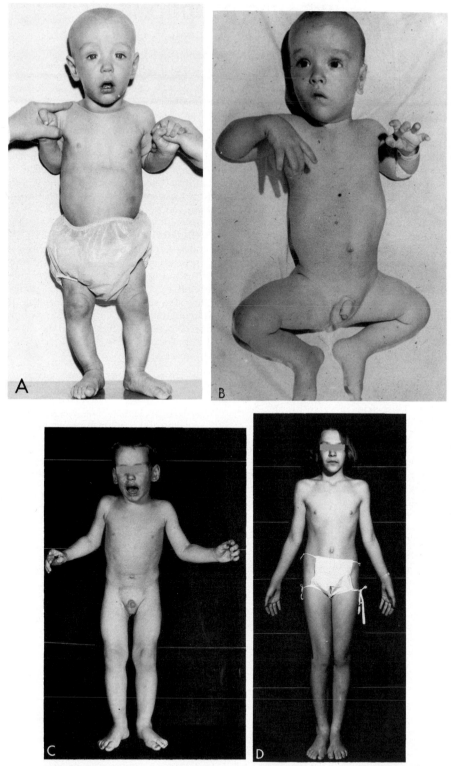

Sotos syndrome. *A*, Seven month old infant with height age of 15 months, head size at two year level, and performance at four and one-half month level. *B*, Eight and one-half month old infant with height age of 21 months and borderline mental deficiency. (*B* from Sotos, J. F., et al.: N. Engl. J. Med., *271*:109, 1964.) *C*, Twenty-five month old with height age of three years and four months and I.Q. of 70. *D*, Eleven year old with height of 5 feet, 8 inches and I.Q. of 70. (*C* and *D* are from Hook, E., and Reynolds, J. W.: J. Pediatr., *70*:900, 1967.)

WEAVER SYNDROME

Macrosomia, Accelerated Skeletal Maturation,
Camptodactyly, Unusual Facies

Weaver et al. reported two strikingly similar boys with this pattern of overgrowth. Documentation of a number of additional cases indicates that this is a distinct disorder separate from Marshall-Smith syndrome.

ABNORMALITIES
Growth. Accelerated growth and maturation, of prenatal onset.
Performance. Mild hypertonia, developmental lag, hoarse low-pitched cry. Progressive spasticity.
Craniofacial. Large bifrontal diameter, flat occiput, ocular hypertelorism, epicanthal folds, downslanting palpebral fissures, large ears, long philtrum, relative micrognathia.
Limbs. Camptodactyly, broad thumbs, thin deepset nails, prominent fingertip pads. Limited elbow and knee extension, clinodactyly of toes. Widened distal long bones, foot deformities including talipes equinovarus, calcaneovalgus, and metatarsus adductus.
Other. Relatively loose skin, inverted nipples, thin hair. Umbilical hernia.

OCCASIONAL ABNORMALITIES. Inguinal hernia, short fourth metatarsals. Hypotonia. Cyst in the septum pellucidum, cerebral atrophy, and enlarged vessels and hypervascularization in the areas of the middle and left posterior cerebral arteries.

NATURAL HISTORY. These children are usually large at birth and show accelerated growth and markedly advanced skeletal maturation during infancy, with carpal centers more advanced than phalangeal centers. In a minority of patients, overgrowth does not develop until a few months of age. The one adult who has been documented continued to grow rapidly and reached a final height greater than 2 standard deviations above the mean.

ETIOLOGY. Unknown. Two instances have been reported of mildly affected mothers giving birth to severely affected sons, raising the possibility of either autosomal dominant inheritance with sex-limited expression or X-linked recessive inheritance. However, another report has documented affected male and female siblings born to unaffected parents. Unexplained is the observation that males are affected three times as frequently as females.

References

Weaver, D. D., et al.: A new overgrowth syndrome with accelerated skeletal maturation, unusual facies, and camptodactyly. J. Pediatr., *84*:547, 1974.

Shimura, T., et al.: Marshall-Smith syndrome with large bifrontal diameter, broad distal femora, camptodactyly, and without broad middle phalanges. J. Pediatr., *94*:93, 1979.

Fitch, N.: The syndromes of Marshall and Weaver. J. Med. Genet., *17*:174, 1980.

Fitch, N.: Letter to the editor: Update on the Marshall-Smith-Weaver controversy. Am. J. Med. Genet., *20*:559, 1985.

Ardinger, H. H., et al.: Further delineation of Weaver syndrome. J. Pediatr., *108*:229, 1986.

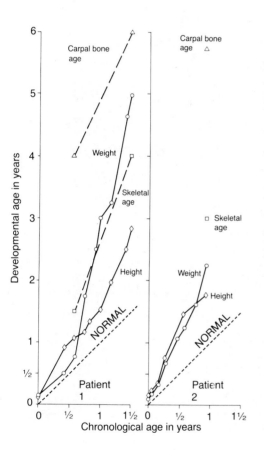

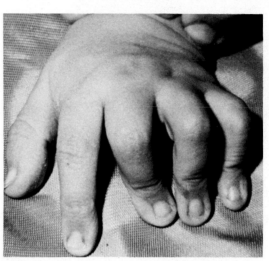

Left, Graph showing accelerated growth and maturation in two patients. *Right,* Hand showing camptodactyly.

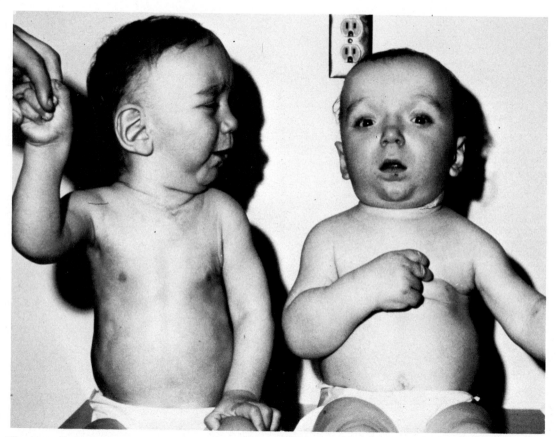

Weaver syndrome. Unrelated boys at 18 months and 11 months of age, respectively. (From Weaver, D. D., et al.: J. Pediatr., *84*:547, 1974.)

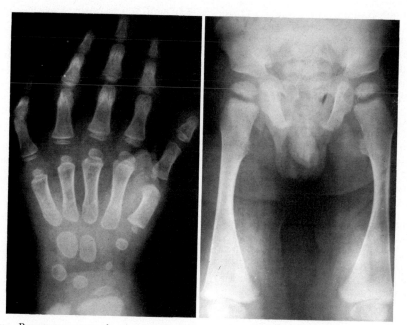

Weaver syndrome. Roentgenograms showing accelerated osseous maturation and broad distal splaying of femurs. (From Weaver, D. D., et al.: J. Pediatr., *84*:547, 1974.)

MARSHALL-SMITH SYNDROME

Accelerated Growth and Maturation,
Shallow Orbits, Broad Middle Phalanges

ABNORMALITIES

Growth. Accelerated linear growth and markedly accelerated skeletal maturation of prenatal onset. Underweight for length with failure to thrive in weight.

Performance. Motor and mental deficiency. I.Q. of 50. Hypotonia.

Craniofacial. Long cranium with prominent forehead, shallow orbits with prominent eyes, bluish sclerae, upturned nose, low nasal bridge, small mandibular ramus.

Limbs. Broad proximal and middle phalanges with narrow distal phalanges.

Other. Hypertrichosis. Umbilical hernia.

OCCASIONAL ABNORMALITIES. Choanal atresia or stenosis or both. Abnormal larynx/laryngomalacia. Brain abnormalities including macrogyria, cerebral atrophy, and absent corpus callosum. Short sternum. Rudimentary epiglottis. Omphalocele. Deep crease between hallux and second toe. Immunologic defect.

NATURAL HISTORY. These patients have failed to thrive in terms of weight. They have persistent respiratory difficulties manifested by stridor, hyperextension of the neck, and obstructing tongue. Although the majority die by 20 months with pneumonia, atelectasis, aspiration, and/or pulmonary hypertension, four children between two and five years of age are being followed by Hoyme and Bull. Aggressive management of respiratory difficulties is extremely important with respect to ultimate prognosis. The accelerated osseous maturation, of unknown cause, is of prenatal onset, as indicated by a wrist "bone age" of three to four years in one patient at two weeks of life.

ETIOLOGY. Unknown. Each has been a sporadic occurrence in the family.

References

Marshall, R. E., et al.: Syndrome of accelerated skeletal maturation and relative failure to thrive: A newly recognized clinical growth disorder. J. Pediatr., *78*:95, 1971.

Visveshwara, N., Rudolph, N., and Dragutsky, D.: Syndrome of accelerated skeletal maturation in infancy, peculiar facies and multiple congenital anomalies—An additional case. J. Pediatr., *84*:553, 1974.

Fitch, N.: The syndromes of Marshall and Weaver. J. Med. Genet., *17*:174, 1980.

Johnson, J. P., et al.: Marshall-Smith syndrome: Two case reports and a review of pulmonary manifestations. Pediatrics, *71*:219, 1983.

Fitch, N.: Letter to the editor: Update on the Marshall-Smith-Weaver controversy. Am. J. Med. Genet., *20*:559, 1985.

Hoyme, H. E., and Bull. M. J.: The Marshall-Smith syndrome: Natural history beyond infancy. Clin. Research, *35*:225A, 1987.

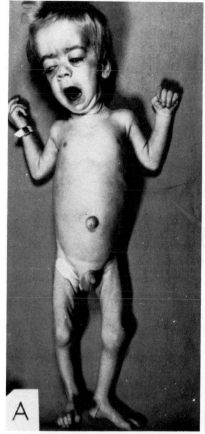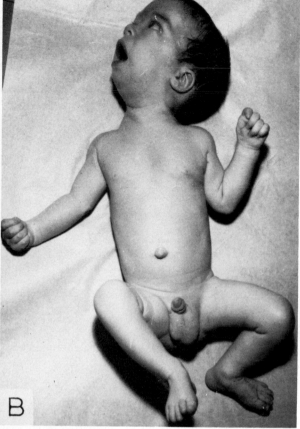

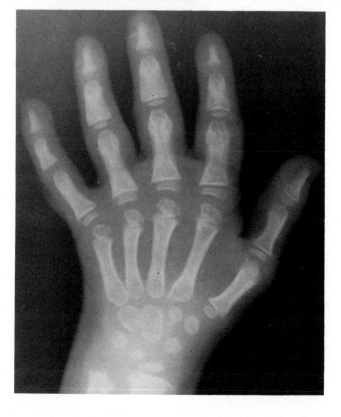

Marshall-Smith syndrome. *A*, *B*, Six and seven month old patients. *Left*, Hand of one of them (patient *A*) at 16 months, showing a carpal bone age of six years and broad middle phalanges. (From Marshall, R. E., et al.: J. Pediatr., *78*:95, 1971.)

BECKWITH-WIEDEMANN SYNDROME

(Exomphalos-Macroglossia-Gigantism Syndrome)

*Macroglossia, Omphalocele,
Macrosomia, Ear Creases*

Beckwith and Wiedemann first reported this distinct clinical entity, and about 200 cases have subsequently been reported.

ABNORMALITIES

Performance. Unknown incidence of mild to moderate mental deficiency; may be normal.

Growth. Macrosomia with large muscle mass and thick subcutaneous tissue. Accelerated osseous maturation. Metaphyseal flaring with overconstriction of diaphyses. Diminished tubulation of proximal humerus.

Craniofacial. Macroglossia. Prominent eyes with *relative* infraorbital hypoplasia. Capillary nevus flammeus, central forehead and eyelids. Metopic ridge, central forehead. Large fontanels. Prominent occiput. Malocclusion with tendency toward mandibular prognathism. Unusual linear fissures in lobule of external ear. Indentations on posterior rim of helix.

Hyperplasia and Dysplasia. Large kidneys with renal medullary dysplasia. Pancreatic hyperplasia, including excess of islets. Fetal adrenocortical cytomegaly—*a consistent feature.* Interstitial cell hyperplasia, gonads. Pituitary amphophil hyperplasia.

Other. Neonatal polycythemia. Hypoglycemia in early infancy (about one third to one half of cases). Omphalocele or other umbilical anomaly. Diastasis recti. Posterior diaphragmatic eventration. Cryptorchidism. Cardiovascular defects including isolated cardiomegaly.

OCCASIONAL ABNORMALITIES. Hepatomegaly,
mild microcephaly, hemihypertrophy, adrenal carcinoma, Wilms tumor, gonadoblastoma, hepatoblastoma, clitoromegaly, large ovaries, hyperplastic uterus and bladder, bicornuate uterus, hypospadias. Immunodeficiency. Cardiac hamartoma. Focal cardiomyopathy.

NATURAL HISTORY. Hydramnios and a relatively
high incidence of prematurity provide further indication of the rather profound prenatal alterations. Birth weight has averaged 4 kg, and length, 52.6 cm. Severe problems of neonatal adaptation may occur, with apnea, cyanosis, and seizures as symptoms. The large tongue may partially occlude the respiratory tract and lead to feeding difficulties. Placing the baby on the side or face down may help respiration, and a large, soft nipple may facilitate feeding. Detection and treatment of hypoglycemia in any neonate with features of this syndrome are critical. The hypoglycemia is responsive to hydrocortisone analogue therapy, which is usually required for only one to four months. Polycythemia might only merit therapeutic intervention during the early neonatal period. The frequency of tumor in this disorder is suggested to be 6.5 per cent. Obtaining ultrasonograms and measuring serum alpha fetoprotein every six months until the patient is six years of age to rule out Wilms tumor and hepatoblastoma, respectively, are warranted.

All of these measures are indicated, because affected individuals who survive infancy generally are healthy, and all six (of 11) surviving children in Irving's study were considered mentally normal at four to eight and one-half years of age; however, Beckwith has noted mild to moderate mental deficiency in survivors.

The excessive rate of growth often slows down after the first few years. Growth may allow adequate oral room for the large tongue. Partial glossectomy has been performed successfully in a number of cases. Evidence suggests the prognathism and dental malocclusion are secondary to the large tongue.

ETIOLOGY. Unknown. Usually sporadic. How-
ever, families in which more than one sibling is affected have been reported; severely affected children have had a mildly affected parent; and one affected member of a monozygotic twin pair has been described, making accurate recurrence risk counseling difficult. In addition, two affected children have been described recently with a partial duplication of chromosome 11p. Prenatal documentation at 19 weeks' gestation of an enlarged abdominal circumference and omphalocele has been accomplished successfully in one pregnancy monitored because of a previously affected child.

References

Wiedemann, H. R.: Complexe malformatif familial avec hernie ombilicale et macroglossie—un "syndrome nouveau"? J. Genet. Hum., *13*:223, 1964.

Irving, I.: Exomphalos with macroglossia: A study of 11 cases. J. Pediatr. Surg., 2:499, 1967.

Beckwith, J. B.: Macroglossia, omphalocele, adrenal cytomegaly, gigantism, and hyperplastic visceromegaly. Birth Defects, 5(2):188, 1969.

Filippi, G., and McKusick, V. A.: The Beckwith-Wiedemann syndrome. Medicine, 49:279, 1970.

Greenwood, R. D., et al.: Cardiovascular abnormalities in the Beckwith-Wiedemann syndrome. Am. J. Dis. Child., 131:293, 1977.

Waziri, M., et al.: Abnormality of chromosome 11 in patients with features of Beckwith-Wiedemann syndrome. J. Pediatr., 102:873, 1983.

Winter, S. C., et al.: Prenatal diagnosis of the Beckwith-Wiedemann syndrome. Am. J. Med. Genet., 24:137, 1986.

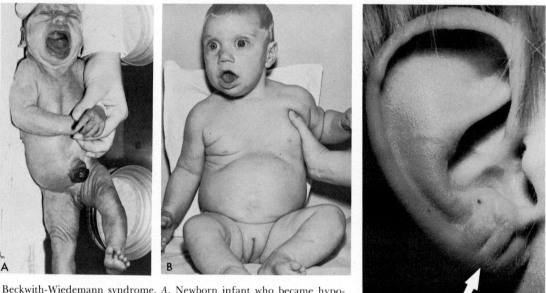

Beckwith-Wiedemann syndrome. *A*, Newborn infant who became hypoglycemic. Note clitoromegaly. *B*, Six month old large infant. Note scar of repaired omphalocele. *C*, Unusual linear creases in the lobulus of the ear.

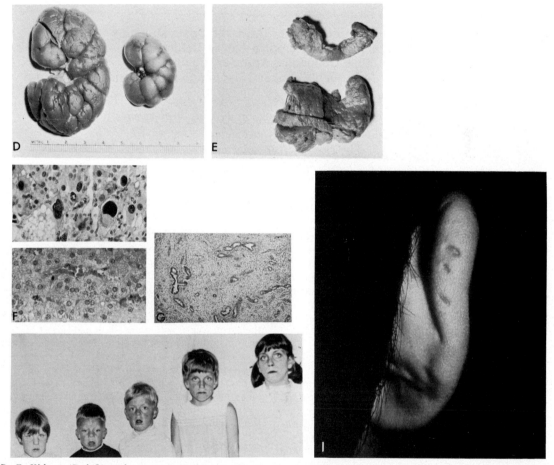

D, E, Kidney (*D,* left) and pancreas (*E,* lower) of patient compared with normal specimens. *F, G,* Fetal adrenal cytomegaly (above) compared with normal and renal medullary dysplasia (*G*). (*F* and *G* from Beckwith, J. B.: Birth Defects, 5[2]:188, 1969.) *H,* Similar facial appearance of five surviving children from four to eight years of age, who tend to be large for age, with advanced skeletal maturation. (*C* and *H* from Irving, I. M.: J. Pediatr. Surg., 2:499, 1967). *I,* Indentations on posterior rim of helix.

F. UNUSUAL BRAIN AND/OR NEUROMUSCULAR FINDINGS WITH ASSOCIATED DEFECTS

AMYOPLASIA CONGENITA DISRUPTIVE SEQUENCE

("Classic Arthrogryposis," Arthrogryposis Multiplex Congenita, Myodystrophia Fetalis Deformans, Multiple Congenital Articular Rigidities, Congenital Arthromyodysplasia, Myophagism Congenita)

Arms Extended with Flexion of Hands and Wrists, Shoulders Internally Rotated with Decreased Muscle Mass, Bilateral Equinovarus, Variable Contractures of Other Major Joints

The first report with histopathologic studies was presented in 1907 by Howard. Over 500 cases have been reported in the literature since then. Hall reported 135 cases in 350 patients with congenital contractures of the joints. Usually the contractures are symmetric and involve all four extremities, although some cases involve only the upper limbs or the lower limbs.

ABNORMALITIES
Facies. Round face with micrognathia, small upturned nose, midline capillary hemangioma.
Shoulders. Rounded and sloping with decreased muscle mass, internally rotated.
Upper Limbs. Elbows usually in extension with wrists and hands flexed ("policeman tip" position). Severe flexion contractures at metacarpophalangeal joints with mild contractures at interphalangeal joints.
Lower Limbs. Hips, usually flexed, dislocated, adducted, or abducted. Knees, flexed or extended. Feet, usually equinovarus positioning bilaterally. Many combinations of hip and knee positions observed.
Other. Stiff, straight spine.

OCCASIONAL ABNORMALITIES. Cord wrapping of limb, amniotic bands, smashed digits, cryptorchidism, hypoplastic labia, dimples at contracture sites, torticollis, and hernias. Gastroschisis, bowel atresia, and defects of muscular layer of trunk.

NATURAL HISTORY. Decreased movement in utero. Deliveries often difficult and breech presentation. Fractures of the limbs secondary to traumatic delivery. Intelligence normal unless birth trauma because of stiff joints. There is decreased bone growth of involved limbs, and there may be increased flexion and pterygium development of the large joints with time. Patients almost always become ambulatory and self-supporting with good physical therapy. Multiple orthopedic procedures are usually necessary, with functional results. It is important to begin physical therapy early to mobilize any muscle tissue present (particularly intrinsic muscles), whereas casting and splinting may lead to muscle atrophy.

ETIOLOGY. Unknown. Sporadic. Higher incidence than expected in identical twins, with only one affected. Biopsies and autopsies revealed nonspecific findings. One hypothesis is a vascular causation at a cord level for the developmental pathology.

COMMENT. It is probable that some of the associated abnormalities occasionally seen are due to a deformational process related to decreased movement in utero. Of 135 known cases, there has been no recurrence within a family. Prenatal diagnosis by serial real time ultrasonography, looking for abnormal movement, could be used in cases of parental anxiety.

References

Howard, R.: A case of congenital defect of the muscular system and its association with congenital talipes equinovarus. Proc. Roy. Soc. Med., *1*:157, 1907.

Hall, J. G., Reed, S. D., and Driscoll, E. P.: Part I. Amyoplasia: A common sporadic condition with congenital contractures. Am. J. Med. Genet., *15*:571, 1983.

Hall, J. G., et al.: Part II: Amyoplasia—A specific type of arthrogryposis with an apparent excess of discordantly affected identical twins. Am. J. Med. Genet., *15*:591, 1983.

Reid, C. O. M. V., et al.: Association of amyoplasia with gastroschisis, bowel atresia and defects of the muscular layer of the trunk. Am. J. Med. Genet., *24*:701, 1986.

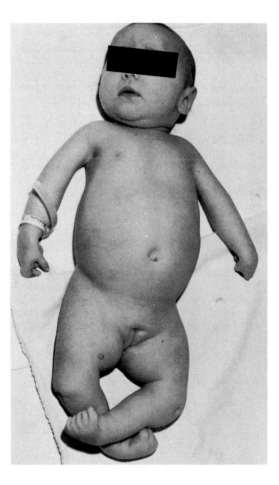

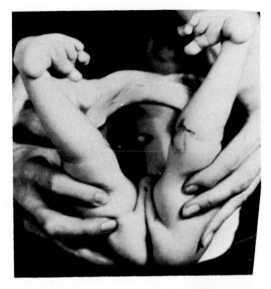

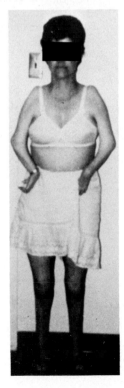

Above, Infant with amyoplasia. Note the "policeman tip" position of the arm and hand. *Below,* Adult with amyoplasia. (Courtesy of Dr. Judith Hall, University of British Columbia, Vancouver, B.C.)

DISTAL ARTHROGRYPOSIS SYNDROME

Distal Congenital Contractures, Clenched Hands
with Medial Overlapping of the Fingers at Birth,
Opening of Clenched Hands with Ulnar Deviation

In 1932, Lundblom described a mother and her son with congenital ulnar deviation and flexion of the fingers. In addition, the son had a calcaneo-valgus positioning of the feet. Hall recognized this condition as an entity in 1982 in her report of 37 patients with congenital contractures of the distal joints. Two groups of patients were recognized: type I (typical)—14 probands—and type II (atypical)—23 probands. Atypical cases may have, in various combinations, cleft palate, cleft lip, small tongue, trismus, ptosis, mild epicanthal folds, short stature, scoliosis, and dull-normal intelligence. The distinct positioning of the hands at birth (as in trisomy 18) and the autosomal dominant inheritance pattern with variable expression are the most distinguishing features.

ABNORMALITIES
Hands. The neonate's hands are clenched tightly in a fist, with thumb adduction and medially overlapping fingers. Ulnar deviation and camptodactyly occur in the adult (98 per cent).
Feet. Position deformities (88 per cent): bilateral calcaneovalgus (33 per cent), bilateral equinovarus (25 per cent), combinations (30 per cent).
Hips. Hip involvement (38 per cent): congenital dislocations, decreased abduction, mild flexion, contracture deformities.
Knees. Mild flexion contractures (30 per cent).
Shoulders. Stiff at birth (17 per cent).

OCCASIONAL ABNORMALITIES. Trismus, mild scoliosis, dimples, cryptorchidism, hernias.

NATURAL HISTORY. "Trisomy 18 position" of hand at birth. Variable talipes involvement. Patients with atypical forms of the disorder may have trouble feeding. The hands eventually unclench and may have residual camptodactyly and ulnar deviation. Intelligence is normal. There is remarkably good response to treatment in all joints.

ETIOLOGY. Autosomal dominant with extensive intrafamilial and interfamilial variability. The parent of an affected child might possibly express the gene through mild hand contractures only. Differential diagnosis includes whistling face syndrome, trismus-pseudocamptodactyly syndrome, and Beals syndrome.

COMMENT. Abnormal tendon attachments, attenuation, and tendon absence have been demonstrated in the hands and feet of some patients and may have been etiologic in producing contractures in utero. Prenatal diagnosis by serial real time ultrasonography, looking for normal movement, should be considered.

References

Lundblom, A.: On congenital ulnar deviation of the fingers of familial occurrence. Acta Orthop. Scand., *8*:393, 1932.
Hall, J. G., Reed, S. D., and Greene, D.: The distal arthrogryposes. Delineation of new entities—Review and nosologic discussion. Am. J. Med. Genet., *11*:185, 1982.

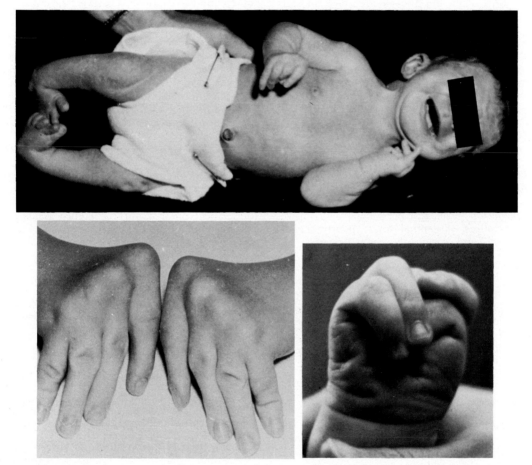

Above, Distal arthrogryposis in an infant. *Below*, The hands of an adult and the hand of an infant. (Courtesy of Dr. Judith Hall, University of British Columbia, Vancouver, B.C.)

PENA-SHOKEIR PHENOTYPE

(Fetal Akinesia/Hypokinesia Sequence)

Neurogenic Arthrogryposis, Pulmonary Hypoplasia, Hypertelorism

In 1974, Pena and Shokeir identified an early lethal disorder involving multiple joint contractures, facial anomalies, and pulmonary hypoplasia with an autosomal recessive mode of inheritance. Subsequently, a number of similar patients have been described. Hall recently suggested that this clinical phenotype is secondary to decreased in utero movement, no matter what the cause. As such, it is etiologically heterogeneous and is similar to the fetal akinesia deformation sequence, a pattern of structural defects described by Moessinger in rats who had been curarized in utero.

ABNORMALITIES

Growth. Prenatal onset growth deficiency. Head circumference is frequently spared.

Craniofacial. Prominent eyes; hypertelorism; telecanthus; epicanthal folds; poorly folded, small, and posteriorly angulated ears; depressed nasal tip; small mouth; high arched palate; micrognathia.

Limbs. Multiple ankylosis (e.g., elbows, knees, hips, and ankles); ulnar deviation of the hands; rocker-bottom feet; talipes equinovarus; camptodactyly. Absent or sparse dermal ridges, with frequent absence of the flexion creases on the fingers and palms.

Lungs. Pulmonary hypoplasia.

Genitalia. Cryptorchidism.

Other. Polyhydramnios, small or abnormal placenta, relatively short umbilical cord.

NATURAL HISTORY. Some of these babies are born prematurely. Those born at term are invariably small for the estimated dates. Approximately 30 per cent are stillborn. Although the majority of those live-born die of the complications of pulmonary hypoplasia within the first month of life, it is important to recognize that the ultimate prognosis for children with this disorder depends on the cause of the decreased fetal movement.

COMMENT. The causes of this phenotype, as well as the pathogenetic mechanisms leading to it, are heterogeneous. Muscle histology was abnormal in 15 of 17 infants (predominately neurogenic atrophy); spinal cord histology was abnormal in 5 of 8 infants; and the cerebrum was abnormal in 11 of 16 infants studied. Whatever the cause, the common denominator is decreased fetal activity. Failure of normal deglutition results in polyhydramnios, and a neuromuscular deficiency in the function of the diaphragm and intercostal muscles leads to pulmonary hypoplasia. The short umbilical cord and multiple joint contractures are due to lack of normal fetal movement. The phenotype overlaps with that of trisomy 18, from which it needs to be distinguished in the neonatal period.

ETIOLOGY. Autosomal recessive inheritance has been implied in over one half of the published cases. However, recognition that this phenotype does not have a single etiology makes accurate recurrence risk counseling difficult. A 0 per cent or 25 per cent risk for recurrence seems most appropriate in a sporadic case.

References

Pena, S. D. J., and Shokeir, M. H. K.: Syndrome of camptodactyly, multiple ankyloses, facial anomalies and pulmonary hypoplasia: A lethal condition. J. Pediatr., *85*:373, 1974.

Pena, S. D. J., and Shokeir, M. H. K.: Syndrome of camptodactyly, multiple ankyloses, facial anomalies and pulmonary hypoplasia: Further delineation and evidence of autosomal recessive inheritance. *In* Bergsma, D., and Schimke, R. M. (eds.): Cytogenetics, Environment and Malformation Syndromes. Birth Defects Original Article Series, Vol. XII. New York, Alan R. Liss, Inc., 1976, p. 201.

Dimmick, J. E., et al.: Syndrome of ankylosis, facial anomalies and pulmonary hypoplasia: A pathologic analysis of one infant. *In* Bergsma, D., and Lowry, R. B. (eds.): Embryology and Pathogenesis and Prenatal Diagnosis. Birth Defects Original Article Series, Vol. XIII. New York, Alan R. Liss, Inc., 1977, p. 133.

Chen, H., et al.: The Pena-Shokeir syndrome. Report of five cases and further delineation of the syndrome. Am. J. Med. Genet., *16*:213, 1983.

Moessinger, A. L.: Fetal akinesia deformation sequence: An animal model. Pediatrics, *72*:857, 1983.

Lindhout, D., Hageman, G., Beemer, F. A.: The Pena-Shokeir syndrome: Report of nine Dutch cases. Am. J. Med. Genet., *21*:655, 1985.

Hall, J. G.: Invited editorial comment: Analysis of Pena-Shokeir phenotype. Am. J. Med. Genet., *25*:99, 1986.

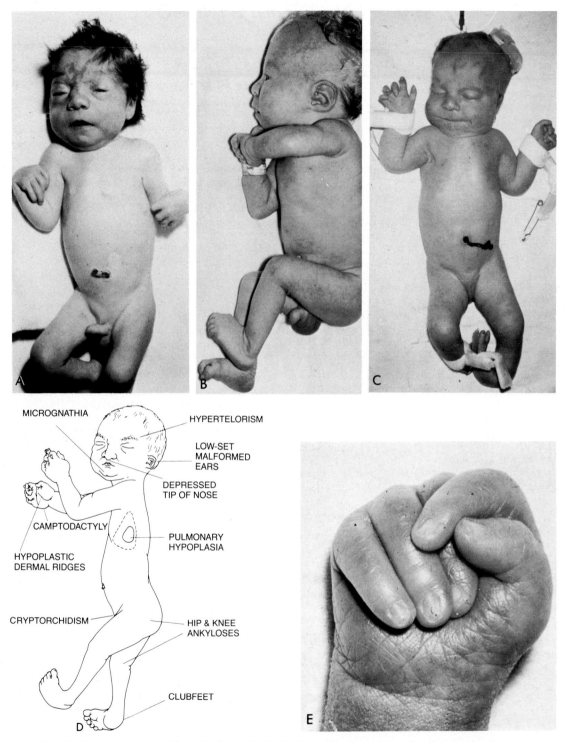

Pena-Shokeir phenotype. *A–C*, Affected infants. *D*, Predominant features of the disorder and *E*, aberrant hand position, which can be similar to that of the 18 trisomy syndrome. (*A* appears courtesy of Dr. Hope Pewnett.)

CEREBRO-OCULO-FACIO-SKELETAL (COFS) SYNDROME

*Neurogenic Arthrogryposis,
Microcephaly, Microphthalmia and/or Cataract*

Described initially by Pena and Shokeir in 1974, the disorder has been recognized as an autosomal recessive, apparently degenerative problem of the brain and spinal cord that is usually manifest before birth.

ABNORMALITIES

Brain and Neurologic. Reduced white matter of brain with gray mottling. Generalized hypotonia and hypo- or areflexia.

Craniofacial. Microcephaly, prominent root of the nose, large ear pinnae, upper lip overlapping lower lip, micrognathia (mild).

Eyes. Blepharophimosis with deep-set eyes, microphthalmia, cataracts, nystagmus.

Limbs. Camptodactyly, mild flexion contractures in the elbows and knees, rocker-bottom feet with vertical talus, posteriorly placed second metatarsal, longitudinal groove in the soles along the second metatarsal.

Other. Hirsutism, kyphosis, widely set nipples, shallow acetabular angles, coxa valga, osteoporosis, renal defects.

NATURAL HISTORY. Babies with this disorder are usually born at term with normal birth weights. In the majority, the phenotype is evident at birth. However, in a few cases, the phenotype undergoes a dramatic evolution toward the full-blown picture in a matter of weeks to months. The course of the disorder in all cases is progressive, with downhill deterioration. It is characterized by virtually no growth and increasing cachexia despite apparently adequate caloric intake, ending in death, which is usually from pulmonary infections that complicate emaciation. Survival is usually under five years.

ETIOLOGY. Autosomal recessive.

References

Pena, S. D. J., and Shokeir, M. H. K.: Autosomal recessive cerebro-oculo-facio-skeletal (COFS) syndrome. Clin. Genet., 5:285, 1974.

Preus, M., and Fraser, F. C.: The cerebro-oculo-facioskeletal syndrome. Clin. Genet., 5:294, 1974.

Scott-Emuakpor, A., Heffelfinger, J., and Higgins, J. V.: A syndrome of microcephaly and cataracts in four siblings. A new genetic syndrome? Am. J. Dis. Child., 131:167, 1977.

Surana, R. B., Fraga, J. R., and Sinkford, S. M.: The cerebro-oculo-facio-skeletal syndrome. Clin. Genet., 13:486, 1978.

Grizzard, W. S., O'Donnell, J. J., Carey, J. C.: The cerebro-oculo-facio-skeletal syndrome. Am. J. Ophthalmol., 89:293, 1980.

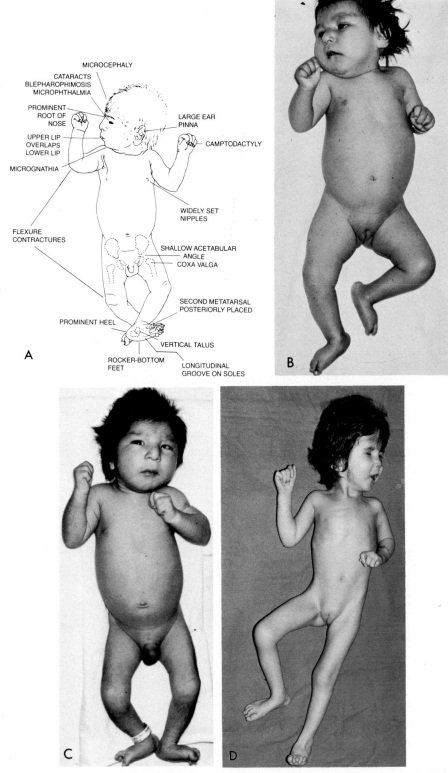

COFS syndrome. *A*, Predominant features of syndrome. *B*, *C*, Young infants with the syndrome. *D*, Eighteen month old affected infant with failure-to-thrive type of postnatal growth deficiency.

LETHAL MULTIPLE PTERYGIUM SYNDROME

Gillin and Pryse-Davis described three female siblings with this early lethal disorder in 1976. It was separated from other conditions associated with pterygia by Hall et al. in 1982. At least ten cases have been reported.

ABNORMALITIES
Growth. Deficiency of prenatal onset.
Facies. Epicanthal folds. Ocular hypertelorism. Flat nose. Midforehead hemangioma. Micrognathia. Downslanting palpebral fissures. Long philtrum.
Limbs. Flexion contractures involving elbows, shoulders, hips, knees, ankles, hands, and feet.
Pterygia. Present in the following areas: Chin to sternum, cervical, axillary, antecubital, crural, popliteal, and ankles.
Other. Small chest. Cryptorchidism. Hypoplastic dermal ridges and creases. Mild neck edema and loose skin. Thin, gracile long bones.

OCCASIONAL ABNORMALITIES.
Attenuated ascending and transverse colon. No appendix. Cardiac hypoplasia. Megaureter and hydronephrosis. Cleft palate, polyhydramnios. Hydrops.

NATURAL HISTORY.
All patients have been stillborn or have died in the immediate neonatal period, probably secondary to pulmonary hypoplasia. Decreased fetal activity and an increased incidence of breech presentation have been documented.

ETIOLOGY. Autosomal recessive.

COMMENT. Hall has distinguished three distinct lethal multiple pterygium syndromes that can be separated clinically on the basis of bony fusions and modeling errors of bones. In addition there is a usually lethal form of the popliteal pterygium syndrome that is characterized by facial clefting, a hypoplastic nasal tip, ankyloblepharon, and marked popliteal pterygium.

References

Bartsocas, C. S., and Papas, C. V.: Popliteal pterygium syndrome: Evidence for a severe autosomal recessive form. J. Med. Genet., *9*:222, 1972.

Gillin, M. E., and Pryse-Davis, J.: Pterygium syndrome. J. Med. Genet., *13*:249, 1976.

Hall, J. G., et al.: Limb pterygium syndromes. A review and report of eleven patients. Am. J. Med. Genet., *12*:377, 1982.

Hall, J. G.: Editorial comment: The lethal multiple pterygium syndromes. Am. J. Med. Genet., *17*:803, 1984.

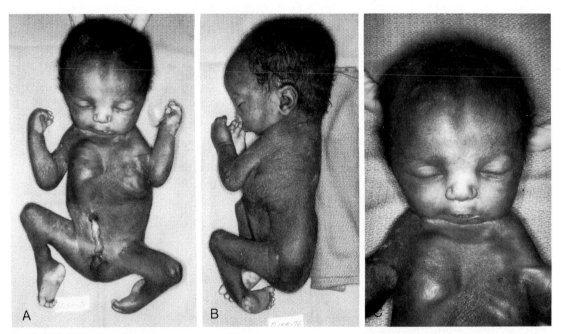

Lethal multiple pterygium syndrome. *A* to *C*, Stillborn infant with ocular hypertelorism, epicanthal folds, multiple joint contractures, and pterygia bridging virtually all joints.

NEU-LAXOVA SYNDROME

Microcephaly/Lissencephaly, Canine-facies with Exophthalmos, Syndactyly with Subcutaneous Edema

Neu et al. reported three siblings with microcephaly and multiple congenital abnormalities in 1971. An additional family with three affected siblings from a first cousin mating was reported by Laxova et al. in 1972. At least 15 cases have been reported subsequently.

ABNORMALITIES

Growth. Prenatal onset of marked growth deficiency.

Central Nervous System. Microcephaly. Lissencephaly. Absence of corpus callosum. Atrophy of cerebrum, cerebellum, pons. Absence of olfactory bulbs.

Facies. Sloping forehead. Ocular hypertelorism. Protruding eyes with absent lids. Flattened nose. Round, gaping mouth and thick everted lips. Micrognathia. Large ears. Short neck.

Skin. Yellow subcutaneous tissue covered by thin, transparent, scaling skin with edema. Ichthyosis.

Limbs. Short limbs. Syndactyly of fingers and toes, extreme puffiness of hands and feet, overlapping of digits, calcaneovalgus, vertical talus, flexion contractures of major joints with pterygia. Poorly mineralized bones.

Other. Cataracts. Microphthalmia. Persistence of some embryonic structures of eye. Absent eyelashes and head hair. Muscular atrophy with hypertrophy of fatty tissue. Polyhydramnios. Short umbilical cord. Small placenta.

OCCASIONAL ABNORMALITIES.

Hydranencephaly. Hypoplastic genitalia. Patent foramen ovale and ductus arteriosus. Atrial septal defect. Ventricular septal detect. Transposition of great vessels. Cleft lip. Cleft palate. Renal agenesis.

NATURAL HISTORY.

Most patients have been stillborn or have died in the immediate neonatal period. The oldest survivor died of pneumonia at seven weeks.

ETIOLOGY.

Autosomal recessive. Three families with two or more affected siblings born to normal parents have been reported. Consanguinity has been documented in one half of families.

COMMENT.

Recent evaluation by Curry of all reported cases plus a number of unpublished ones suggests that there may well be two types of the Neu-Laxova syndrome. Type I is associated with joint contractures, syndactyly, scaly skin, and poorly mineralized bones, and type II is characterized by massive swelling of hands and feet, ichthyosis, and hypoplastic digits. Only the type II patients have renal agenesis, congenital heart defects, and cleft lip. It is unclear at this time whether these two types simply represent variable expression of the same genetic defect or are distinct disorders.

References

Neu, R. L., et al.: A lethal syndrome of microcephaly with multiple congenital anomalies in three siblings. Pediatrics, *47*:610, 1971.

Laxova, R., Ohdra, P.T., and Timothy, J. A. D.: A further example of a lethal autosomal recessive condition in siblings. J. Ment. Def. Res., *16*:139, 1972.

Lazjuk, G. I., et al.: Brief clinical observations: The Neu-Laxova syndrome—a distinct entity. Am. J. Med. Genet., *3*:261, 1979.

Curry, C. J. R.: Letter to the editor: further comments on the Neu-Laxova syndrome. Am. J. Med. Genet., *13*:441, 1982.

Shved, I. A., Lazjuk, G. I., and Cherstvoy, E. D.: Elaboration of the phenotypic changes of the upper limbs in the Neu-Laxova syndrome. Am. J. Med. Genet., *20*:1, 1985.

Neu-Laxova syndrome. *A, B,* Thirty-eight week gestation infant with microcephaly, sloping forehead, protruding eyes with absent lids, flat nose, gaping mouth and thick lips, scaling skin with edema, and joint contractures. (From Mueller, R. F., et al.: Am. J. Med. Genet., *16:*645, 1983.)

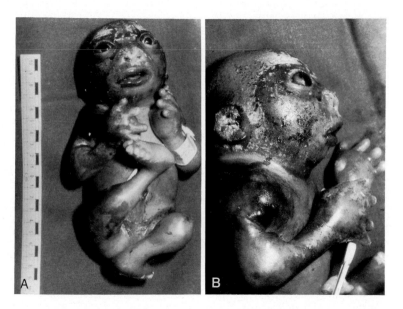

MECKEL-GRUBER SYNDROME

(Dysencephalia Splanchnocystica)

Encephalocele, Polydactyly,
Cystic Dysplasia of Kidneys

Originally described by Meckel in 1822, later by Gruber, and more recently brought to recognition by Opitz and Howe, more than 50 cases of this severe disorder have been reported.

ABNORMALITIES

Growth. Variable prenatal growth deficiency.

CNS. Posterior or dorsal encephalocele. Microcephaly with sloping forehead, cerebral and cerebellar hypoplasia.

Facial. Microphthalmia. Cleft palate. Micrognathia. Ear anomalies, especially slanting-type.

Neck. Short.

Limbs. Polydactyly (usually postaxial), talipes.

Kidney. Dysplasia with varying degrees of cyst formation.

Liver. Bile duct proliferation, fibrosis, cysts.

Genitalia. Cryptorchidism, incomplete development of external and/or internal genitalia.

OCCASIONAL ABNORMALITIES

Craniofacial. Craniosynostosis (possibly secondary). Coloboma of iris, hypoplastic optic nerve, hypotelorism or hypertelorism, hypoplastic to absent philtrum and/or nasal septum, cleft lip—sometimes midline.

Mouth. Lobulated tongue, cleft epiglottis, neonatal teeth.

Neck. Webbed.

Limbs. Relatively short bowed limbs, syndactyly, simian crease, clinodactyly.

Cardiac. Septal defect, patent ductus arteriosus, coarctation of aorta, pulmonary stenosis.

Lungs. Hypoplasia.

Other. Single umbilical artery, patent urachus, omphalocele, malrotation, accessory splenic tissue, adrenal hypoplasia, imperforate anus, missing or duplicated ureters, absence or hypoplasia of urinary bladder, enlarged placenta.

NATURAL HISTORY AND MANAGEMENT. These patients seldom survive more than a few days to weeks. Death may be related to the severe central nervous system defects and/or renal defects. Once the disorder is recognized, the parents should ideally be offered the option of no medical interference toward survival for babies with this syndrome.

COMMENT. Many of the more variable features within this syndrome may be secondary to early primary defects. For example, varying facial and brain components of the prechordal mesoderm-type anomaly occur (arhinencephaly, holoprosencephaly, and so forth), as do anomalies secondary to incomplete renal development (Potter sequence).

ETIOLOGY. Autosomal recessive, with no recognized expression in the presumed carriers of the gene. Prenatal diagnosis may be possible by an elevated alpha fetoprotein level when there is an encephalocele and/or a sonographic delineation of either the encephalocele or the dysplastic enlarged kidneys.

References

Meckel, J. R.: Beschreibung zweier durch sehr ähnliche Bildungsabweichung entsteller Geschwister. Dtsch. Arch. Physiol., 7:99, 1822.

Gruber, G. B.: Beiträge zur Frage "gekoppelter" missbildungen (Akrocephalosyndactylie und Dysencephalia splanchnocystica). Beitr. Pathol. Anat., 93:459, 1934.

Opitz, J. M., and Howe, J. J.: The Meckel syndrome (dysencephalia splanchnocystica, the Gruber syndrome). Birth Defects, 5:167, 1969.

Hsia, Y. E., Bratu, M., and Herbordt, A.: Genetics of the Meckel syndrome (dysencephalia splanchnocystica). Pediatrics, 48:237, 1971.

Meckel, S., and Passarge, E.: Encephalocele, polycystic kidneys, and polydactyly as an autosomal recessive trait simulating certain other disorders: The Meckel syndrome. Ann. Genet. (Paris), 14:97, 1971.

Fraser, F. C., and Lytwyn, A.: Spectrum of anomalies in the Meckel syndrome, or "Maybe there is a malformation syndrome with at least one constant anomaly." Am. J. Med. Genet., 9:67, 1981.

Seppänen, U., and Herva, R.: Roentgenologic features of the Meckel syndrome. Pediatr. Radiol., 13:329, 1983.

Salonen, R.: The Meckel syndrome: Clinicopathological findings in 67 patients. Am. J. Med. Genet., 18:671, 1984.

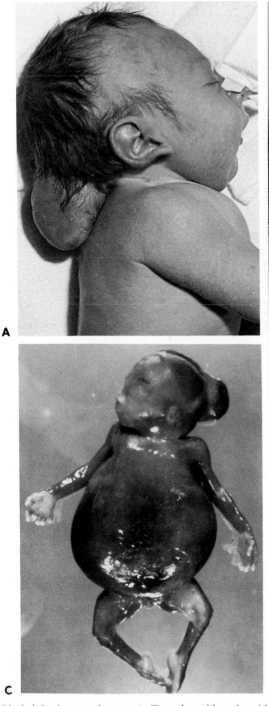

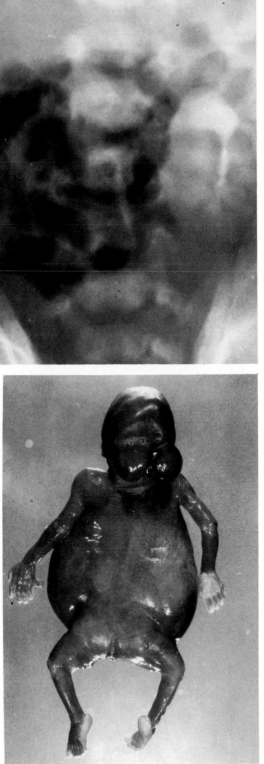

Meckel-Gruber syndrome. *A*, Two day old male with palpable enlarged kidney who was having frequent seizures and other evidence of central nervous system abnormality. *B*, IVP showed no visualization on one side and an aberrant calyceal system on the other side. The baby died at four and one-half months of age, the oldest known survivor with this syndrome. (Patient of E. Hutton, Anchorage, Alaska.) *C*, *D*, Stillborn infant with posterior encephalocele, postaxial polydactyly, and flank masses caused by massively enlarged cystic kidneys.

PALLISTER-HALL SYNDROME

*Hypothalamic Hamartoblastoma, Hypopituitarism,
Imperforate Anus, and Postaxial Polydactyly*

In 1980, Hall et al. described six unrelated newborn infants with this pattern of malformation. All died in the neonatal period. Culler and Jones subsequently described a similarly affected child, who died at the age of 19 months.

ABNORMALITIES

Growth. Mild intrauterine growth retardation.

Central Nervous System. Hypothalamic hamartoblastoma located on the inferior surface of the cerebrum, extending from the optic chiasma to the interpeduncular fossa, replacing the hypothalamus and other nuclei originating in the embryonic hypothalamic plate. Hypopituitarism with secondary hypoplasia of adrenals, occasional underdevelopment of thyroid.

Craniofacial. Flat midface with midline capillary hemangioma. Anteverted nares. Bathrocephaly. External ear anomalies. Micrognathia.

Mouth. Multiple frenuli between alveolar ridge and buccal mucosa.

Respiratory. Laryngeal cleft. Hypoplasia or absence of epiglottis. Dysplastic tracheal cartilage. Absent lung. Abnormal lung lobation.

Cardiac. Endocardial cushion defect.

Limbs. Nail dysplasia, variable degrees of syndactyly and postaxial polydactyly involving both hands and feet. Small, distally placed fourth metacarpal with one or two small fingers associated with it. Third metacarpal less frequently affected. Fourth metatarsal dysplastic.

Distal shortening of limbs, particularly the arms.

Anus. Anal defects, including imperforate anus and variable degrees of rectal atresia.

OCCASIONAL ABNORMALITIES. Holoprosencephaly with associated midline cleft lip and palate. Cleft uvula. Microphthalmia. Coloboma. Renal dysplasia. Hypoglossia. Natal teeth. Narrow cervical vertebrae. Hemivertebrae, fused ribs, and multiple manubrial ossification centers. Subluxation of the radius. Congenital hip dislocation. Subluxation of knee. Simian crease. Camptodactyly. Hypoplasia of pancreas. Micropenis.

ETIOLOGY. Unknown. All cases reported to date have been sporadic.

References

Clarren, S. K., Alvord, E. C., and Hall, J. G.: Congenital hypothalamic hamartoblastoma, hypopituitarism, imperforate anus, and postaxial polydactyly: A new syndrome? Part II: Neuropathological considerations. Am. J. Med. Genet., 7:75, 1980.

Hall, J. G., et al.: Congenital hypothalamic hamartoblastoma, hypopituitarism, imperforate anus, and postaxial polydactyly. A new syndrome? Part I: Clinical, causal, and pathogenetic considerations. Am. J. Med. Genet., 7:47, 1980.

Culler, F. L., and Jones, K. L.: Hypopituitarism in association with postaxial polydactyly. J. Pediatr., *104*:881, 1984.

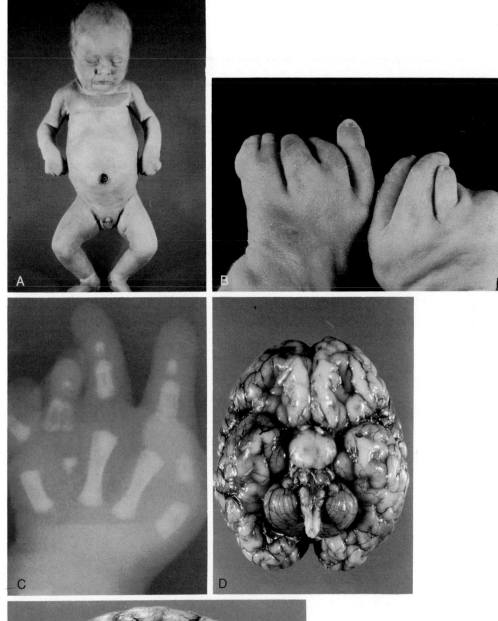

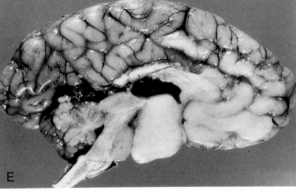

Pallister-Hall syndrome. *A* to *C*, Male infant who died at 7 days of age. He has camptodactyly, nail dysplasia, postaxial polydactyly, syndactyly, lack of ossification of distal phalanges, and a hypoplastic fourth metacarpal giving rise to two phalanges. *D, E*, Note the hamartoblastoma apparent on the inferior cerebral surface and in the sagittal section. (From Hall, J. G., et al.: Am. J. Med. Genet., 7:47, 1980.)

X-LINKED HYDROCEPHALUS SYNDROME

*Hydrocephalus, Short Flexed Thumbs,
Mental Deficiency*

Bickers and Adams first described this entity in 1949, and subsequently at least 47 cases have been reported.

ABNORMALITIES
Performance. Mental deficiency and spasticity, especially of lower extremities.
Brain. Aqueductal stenosis with hydrocephalus.
Hands. Thumb flexed over palm (cortical thumb).

OCCASIONAL ABNORMALITIES. Asymmetry of somewhat coarse facies; brain defects such as fusion of thalami, small pons, absence of septum pellucidum, hypoplasia of corticospinal tracts, porencephalic cyst, absence of corpus callosum.

NATURAL HISTORY. Prenatal hydrocephalus may be severe enough to impede delivery. However, many of the affected males have no hydrocephalus. Such individuals often have a narrow scaphocephalic cranium with an intelligence quotient in the range of 30 and tend to have spasticity. The electroencephalogram may show diffuse abnormality, and the patient may have seizures.

ETIOLOGY. X-linked recessive. The carrier female may have dull intelligence. The variability of expression includes a mentally deficient male with cortical thumbs but without hydrocephalus.

COMMENT. The gestational age at which X-linked recessive hydrocephalus can be diagnosed using prenatal ultrasonography is unknown. Ultrasonographic studies should be performed every two to four weeks from 16 through 28 weeks' gestation in order to exclude the defect with confidence.

References

Bickers, D. S., and Adams, R. D.: Hereditary stenosis of the aqueduct of Sylvius as a cause of congenital hydrocephalus. Brain, 72:246, 1949.
Edwards, J. H.: The syndrome of sex-linked hydrocephalus. Arch. Dis. Child., 36:486, 1961.
Fried, K.: X-linked mental retardation and/or hydrocephalus. Clin. Genet., 3:258, 1973.
Holmes, L. B., et al.: X-linked aqueductal stenosis. Pediatrics, 51:697, 1973.
Fairre, J., et al.: X-linked hydrocephalus. Child's Brain, 2:226, 1976.

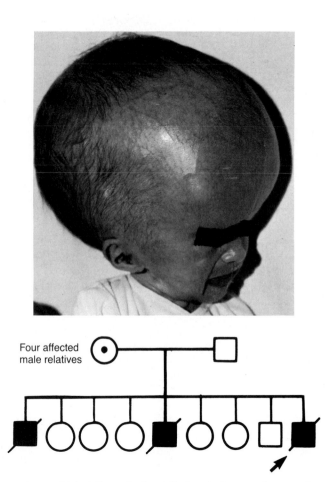

X-linked hydrocephalus syndrome. Male infant who later died and who was shown to have aqueductal stenosis as the cause for hydrocephalus. Note the family pedigree showing other affected males for whom this X-linked condition was lethal. (Courtesy of J. M. Opitz, Helena, Montana.)

WARBURG SYNDROME

(Hard ± E Syndrome)

First suggested as a distinct entity by Warburg in 1971, the first familial cases were reported by Chemke et al., and the full spectrum of associated defects was outlined by Pagon et al. and Whitley et al.

ABNORMALITIES

Brain. Agyria. Pachygyria. Cerebellar hypoplasia. Occipital encephalocele. Dandy-Walker cyst. Hydrocephalus usually due to mechanical obstruction in the posterior fossa. Ventriculomegaly even in the absence of increased intracranial pressure.

Eye. Microphthalmia. Megalocornea. The Peter anomaly. Cataract. Coloboma. Persistent hyperplastic primary vitreous. Retinal detachment with retinal dysplasia.

NATURAL HISTORY. The majority of affected children die in the neonatal period secondary to the severe defect in brain development. Of those that survive, all have had profound mental retardation.

ETIOLOGY. Autosomal recessive inheritance.

COMMENT. Because of the wide spectrum of brain and eye defects, the diagnosis is frequently not considered. Postmortem examination of the brain and eyes is often necessary.

References

Warburg, M.: The heterogenicity of microphthalmia in the mentally retarded. BD-OAS, 7:136, 1971.

Chemke, J., et al.: A familial syndrome of central nervous system and ocular malformations. Clin. Genet., 7:1, 1975.

Pagon, R. A., et al.: Autosomal recessive eye and brain anomalies: Warburg syndrome. J. Pediatr., *102*:542, 1983.

Whitley, C. B., et al.: Warburg syndrome. Lethal neurodysplasia with autosomal recessive inheritance. J. Pediatr., *102*:547, 1983.

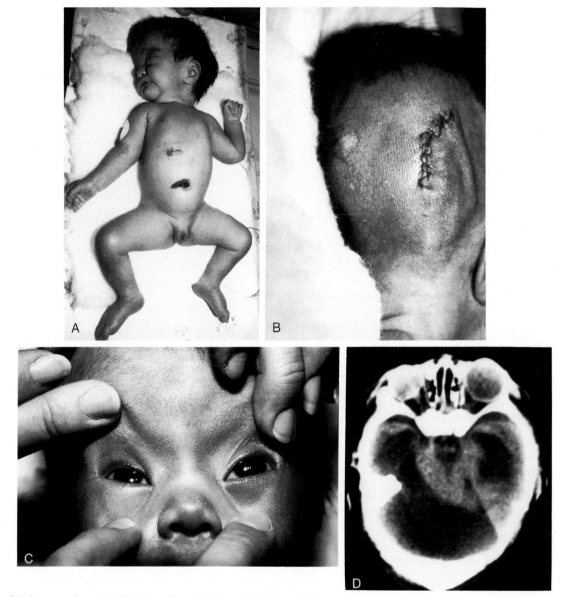

Warburg syndrome. *A*, Newborn female infant with hydrocephalus. Note the small occipital encephalocele *(B)* and unilateral microphthalmic eye *(C)*, which is better demonstrated on the CT scan *(D)*. (Courtesy of Dr. Marilyn C. Jones, Children's Hospital, San Diego, California.)

MILLER-DIEKER SYNDROME

(Lissencephaly Syndrome)

Miller in 1963 and later Dieker et al. described a specific pattern of malformation, one feature of which was lissencephaly (smooth brain). Jones et al. expanded the clinical phenotype and introduced the term Miller-Dieker syndrome to distinguish this disorder from other conditions associated with lissencephaly.

ABNORMALITIES

Brain and Performance. Incomplete development of brain, often with a smooth surface, although areas of pachygyria are often seen inferiorly. Heterotopias. Both frontal and temporal opercula fail to develop, leaving a wide-open Sylvian fossa and a figure-eight appearance on CT scan. Absent or hypoplastic corpus callosum. Small brain stem. Severe mental deficiency with initial hypoptonia, opisthotonos, failure to thrive, seizures, occasionally hypsarrhythmia by EEG.

Craniofacies. Microcephaly with bitemporal narrowing. Variable high forehead, vertical ridging and furrowing in central forehead, especially when crying. Small nose with anteverted nostrils, upslant to palpebral fissures, micrognathia. Appearance of "low-set" and/or posteriorly angulated auricles. Wide secondary alveolar ridge. Late eruption of primary teeth.

Other. Cryptorchidism, +/− pilonidal sinus. Fifth finger clinodactyly.

OCCASIONAL ABNORMALITIES. Cardiac defect. Intrauterine growth retardation. Polyhydramnios. Decreased fetal activity.

NATURAL HISTORY. Postnatal failure to thrive, with death usually before two years and often within first three months. Frequent infections.

ETIOLOGY. A deficiency in the number 17 chromosome at the p13.3 band has recently been documented in the majority of patients with this disorder. Although autosomal recessive inheritance cannot be excluded completely, all reported families with more than one affected child have had a deficiency of 17p, making autosomal recessive inheritance unlikely.

COMMENT. At least two distinct types of lissencephaly exist: Type I lissencephaly, one feature of the Miller-Dieker syndrome, associated with microcephaly and a thickened cortex with four rather than six layers; and type II, associated with obstructive hydrocephalus and additional severe brain defects (see Warburg syndrome).

References

Miller, J. Q.: Lissencephaly in two siblings. Neurology, *13*:841, 1963.

Dieker, H., et al.: The Lissencephaly Syndrome. Birth Defects, *5*:53, 1969.

Jones, K. L., et al.: The Miller-Dieker syndrome. Pediatrics, *66*:277, 1980.

Dobyns, W. B., et al.: Miller-Dieker syndrome: Lissencephaly and monosomy 17p. J. Pediatr., *102*:552, 1983.

Dobyns, W. B., Stratton, R. F., Greenberg, F.: Syndromes with lissencephaly. I: Miller-Dieker and Norman-Roberts syndrome and isolated lissencephaly. Am. J. Med. Genet., *18*:509, 1984.

Dobyns, W. B., Gilbert, E. F., and Opitz, J. M.: Letter to the editor. Further comments on the lissencephaly syndromes. Am. J. Med. Genet., *22*:197, 1985.

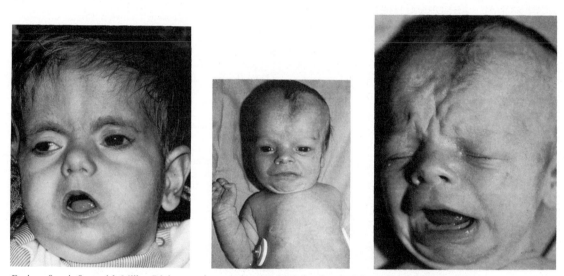

Facies of an infant with Miller-Dieker syndrome, showing high forehead with vertical soft tissue ridging and furrowing when crying and small, anteverted nose.

SJÖGREN-LARSSON SYNDROME

Ichthyosis, Mental Deficiency, Spasticity

Sjögren and Larsson reported this entity in 28 Swedish individuals in 1957, and others with the same condition have been recognized subsequently.

ABNORMALITIES

CNS. Mental retardation; I.Q.s of 30 to 60 or less. Spasticity, most pronounced in lower extremities.
Skin. Ichthyosis.
Growth. Short stature.

OCCASIONAL ABNORMALITIES.
Pigmentary retinal degeneration or flex-shaped glistening spots surrounding the macula, seizures, hypoplasia of teeth, enamal hypoplasia, hypertelorism, kyphosis. Metaphyseal dysplasia with small irregular epiphyses.

NATURAL HISTORY.
Erythema of skin in early infancy, with scaling and hyperkeratosis most apparent on lower trunk and extremities. The ichthyosiform eruption progresses during the first years of life and then stabilizes. The mental defect usually includes speech problems of dysarthria, monosyllabic speech, or no speech. Neurologic findings have their onset between four and 30 months. The electroencephalogram may show slow paroxysmal activity.

ETIOLOGY. Autosomal recessive. Sjögren and Larsson tentatively traced all the Swedish cases back to one heterozygote more than 600 years ago.

References

Sjögren, T., and Larsson, T.: Oligophrenia in combination with congenital ichthyosis and spastic disorders. Acta Psychiatr. Scand., *32*(Suppl. 113):1, 1957.

Selmanowitz, V. J., and Porter, M. J.: The Sjögren-Larsson syndrome. Am. J. Med., *42*:412, 1967.

Ozonoff, M. B., and Ogden, J. A.: Sjögren-Larsson syndrome with epiphyseal-metaphyseal dysplasia. Am. J. Roentgenol. Radium Ther. Nucl. Med., *118*:187, 1973.

Jagell, S., Polland, W., and Sandgren, O.: Specific changes in the fundus typical for the Sjögren-Larsson syndrome. An ophthalmological study of 35 patients. Acta Ophthalmol. Scand., *58*:321, 1980.

Jagell, S., and Lidén, S.: Ichthyosis in the Sjögren-Larsson syndrome. Clin. Genet., *21*:243, 1982.

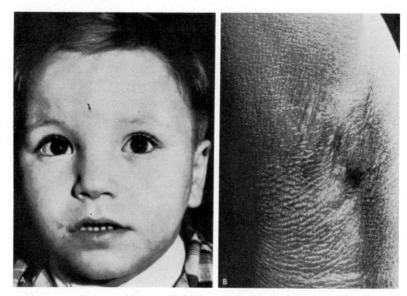

Sjögren-Larsson syndrome. *A,* Six year old. Note slight changes in skin and spacing of teeth. *B,* Fourteen year old, showing thickened, ridged skin in axillary area. (From Selmanowitz, V. J., and Porter, M. J.: Am. J. Med., *42*:412, 1967.)

MARINESCO-SJÖGREN SYNDROME

Cerebellar Ataxia, Hypotonia, Cataracts

This condition was described by Marinesco et al. in 1931 and further delineated by Sjögren in 1947. Only about 60 cases have been reported.

ABNORMALITIES

Growth. Mild to moderate growth deficiency. Microcephaly.

Performance. Moderate to severe mental deficiency with cerebellar ataxia, weakness with or without hypotonia, and tendency toward nystagmus and dysarthria.

Eyes. Cataracts, usually evident from early life.

OCCASIONAL ABNORMALITIES. Strabismus, development of kyphoscoliosis, pectus carinatum, hypogonadism.

ETIOLOGY. Autosomal recessive with high incidence of parental consanguinity.

COMMENT. Todorov's pathologic studies indicated a degenerative process, most severe in the cortical areas of the cerebellum. Electron microscope studies of four patients from two different families revealed numerous abnormally enlarged lysosomes containing whorled lamellar or amorphous inclusion bodies.

References

Marinesco, G., Draganesco, S., and Vasiliu, D.: Nouvelle maladie familiale caracterisé par une cataracte congénitale et un arrêt du développement somato-neuro-psychique. Encephale, 26:97, 1931.

Sjögren, T.: Hereditary congenital spinocerebellar ataxia combined with congenital cataract and oligophrenia. Acta Psychiatr. Scand. 46(Suppl.):286, 1947.

Andersen, B.: Marinesco-Sjögren syndrome: spinocerebellar ataxia, congenital cataract, somatic and mental retardation. Dev. Med. Child. Neurol., 7:249, 1965.

Todorov, A.: Le syndrome de Marinesco-Sjögren. Première étude anatomo-clinique. J. Genet. Hum., 14:197, 1965.

Walker, P. D., Blitzer, M.G., and Shapira, E.: Marinesco-Sjögren syndrome: Evidence for a lysosomal storage disorder. Neurology, 35:415, 1985.

ATAXIA-TELANGIECTASIA SYNDROME

(Louis-Bar Syndrome)

Ataxia, Telangiectasia, Lymphopenia, Immune Deficit

Though this disease was initially described by Louis-Bar in 1941, it has only recently received broader recognition, with well over 100 cases having been reported since 1958.

ABNORMALITIES

Growth. Deficiency, variable in age of onset.

CNS. Progressive ataxia and other evidence of degeneration of CNS function, including mental deficiency and posterior spinal column dysfunction.

Skin and Conjunctivae. Telangiectasia in bulbar conjunctivae and later over bridge of nose, auricles, and elsewhere.

Respiratory. Catarrh, frequent respiratory infections; bronchiectasis may develop.

Immune System. Deficiency in cellular immunity with thymic hypoplasia, hypoplasia of tonsil and adenoid lymphoid tissue, lymphopenia, and often low to absent gamma IgA and IgE.

OCCASIONAL FEATURES

Skin and Hair. Areas of altered skin or hair pigmentation, including café au lait spots. Sclerodermatous changes.

Lymphoreticular System. Malignancy, including leukemia, sarcoma, and Hodgkin's disease, in about 10 per cent of patients.

Gonads. Sexual immaturity. Ovarian dysgerminoma or hypoplasia.

NATURAL HISTORY. Growth deficiency, though it may be prenatal in onset, more commonly becomes evident in later infancy or in childhood. Progressive ataxia usually develops during infancy and is commonly accompanied by features of choreoathetosis and by dysrhythmic speech, drooling, aberrant ocular movements such as fixation nystagmus, stooped posture plus dull sad facies, and occasionally seizures. Instability, suggesting vestibular deficit, often becomes so severe that ambulation is no longer possible in later childhood. These children are usually affable and pleasant despite their progressive handicap. Mental deficiency, though difficult to assess, is considered a feature in about 50 per cent of cases, especially in later stages of this fatal disease. The immune deficiency probably contributes to the frequent respiratory infections and bronchiectasis. However, the persistent catarrh and the progressive generalized bronchiectasis are relatively unresponsive to antibiotic management, and there may be a basic problem in the mucous membranes besides the cellular immune deficit. Death is usually a consequence of lung infection, neurologic deficit, or both. Patients seldom survive later childhood. The oldest survivor was 37 years old, and the disease had been quiescent for 20 years.

ETIOLOGY. Autosomal recessive. Prenatal detection of an affected fetus has been performed successfully.

COMMENT. The general hypoplasia that is found in these individuals and the immune deficit with abiotrophic features of deterioration in the central nervous system, skin, and respiratory tract indicate the severe pleiotropic effect of this pair of mutant genes. No common cellular metabolic defect has yet been detected, although it has been suggested that there exists a defect in DNA repair. However, it is of interest to note certain common features among Fanconi syndrome, Bloom syndrome, and ataxia-telangiectasia. In each of these disorders, there is generalized growth deficiency, skin disorder, and a propensity to develop lymphoreticular malignancy, plus a high frequency of chromosomal breakage in cultured leukocytes.

References

Louis-Bar, D.: Sur un syndrome progressif comprenant des télangiectasies capillaires cutanées et conjonctivales, à disposition naevoide et des troubles cérébelleux. Confin. Neurol., *4*:32, 1941.

McFarlin, D. W., Strober, W., and Waldmann, T. A.: Ataxia telangiectasia. Medicine, *51*:281, 1972.

Shaham, M., et al.: Prenatal diagnosis of ataxia-telangiectasia. J. Pediatr., *100*:134, 1982.

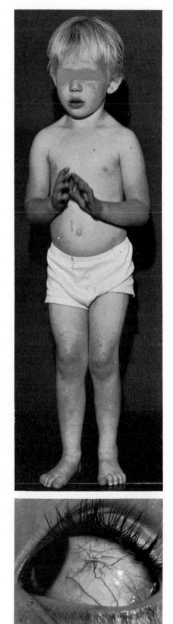

Ataxia-telangiectasia syndrome. *Top*, Nine and one-half year old. Height age, eight years. *Bottom*, Bulbar conjunctiva. (From Smith, D. W.: J. Pediatr., *70*:487, 1967.)

MENKES SYNDROME

(Menkes Kinky Hair Syndrome)

Progressive Cerebral Deterioration with Seizures,
Twisted and Fractured Hair

Menkes et al. described five related male infants with this disease in 1962, and Danks et al. have subsequently indicated that all features of the disorder are the result of copper deficiency.

ABNORMALITIES

Growth. Deficiency, sometimes small at birth.

CNS. Severe degenerative process in cerebral cortex with gliosis and atrophy. Profound and progressive neurologic deficit from one to two months with hypertonia, irritability, seizures, intracranial hemorrhage, hypothermia, and feeding difficulties.

Facies. Lack of expression movement, pudgy cheeks.

Hair. Sparse, stubby, and lightly pigmented; shows twisting and partial breakage by magnified inspection.

Skin. Occasionally thick and relatively dry. Unequal skin pigmentation at birth, particularly in darkly pigmented patients.

Skeletal. Wormian bones; metaphyseal widening, particularly of ribs and femur, with formation of lateral spurs that frequently fracture.

COMMENT. Arteriograms, as well as necropsy material, have shown widespread arterial elongation and tortuosity, most likely due to deficiency of copper-dependent cross-linking in the internal elastic membrane of the arterial wall.

NATURAL HISTORY. Progressive deterioration beginning in early infancy, with death usually by three years, although in one child as late as 12 years. Hair is normal at birth but by six weeks begins to lose pigmentation. The skeletal changes have been confused with those occurring in the battered child syndrome. Danks et al. have demonstrated a defect in intestinal copper absorption in that low levels of serum copper and ceruloplasmin have been found in all patients studied. Parenteral administration of copper has not been successful in reversing the clinical features.

ETIOLOGY. X-linked recessive. Manifestations in the carrier female include hair that is lighter than would be expected for the family, pili torti (180 degree twist of hair shaft), and increased fragility and breakage of hair. Prenatal diagnosis can be made in selected laboratories by demonstrating excessive copper uptake in cultured amniotic fluid cells.

References

Menkes, J. H., et al.: A sex-linked recessive disorder with retardation of growth, peculiar hair, and focal cerebral and cerebellar degeneration. Pediatrics, 29:764, 1962.

Danks, D. M., et al.: Menkes' kinky hair syndrome. An inherited defect in copper absorption with widespread effects. Pediatrics, 50:188, 1972.

Danks, D. M., et al.: Menkes' kinky hair syndrome. Lancet, 1:1100, 1972.

Horn, N.: Menkes X-linked disease: Prenatal diagnosis of hemizygous males and heterozygous females. Prenat. Diagn., 1:121, 1981.

Moore, C. M., and Howell, R. R.: Ectodermal manifestations in Menkes disease. Clin. Genet., 28:532, 1985.

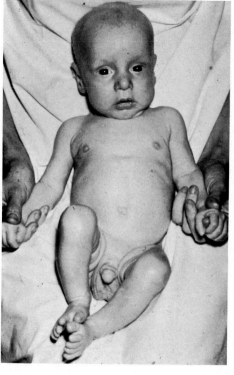

Menkes syndrome. (From Menkes, J. H., et al.: Pediatrics, 29:764, 1962.)

2 months—2.6 kg   Scalp hair × 100

ANGELMAN SYNDROME

(Happy Puppet Syndrome)

"Puppet-Like" Gait,
Paroxysms of Laughter, Characteristic Facies

This disorder, initially described in 1965 by Angelman in three unrelated children with severe mental deficiency, abnormal puppet-like gait, a characteristic facies, and frequent paroxysms of laughter, has been more completely delineated by Williams and Frias, who have documented the natural history of this disorder and have suggested that the term *happy puppet* is inappropriate.

ABNORMALITIES

Growth. Although prenatal growth deficiency is not a feature, severe postnatal growth deficiency was present in three of six adults.

Performance. Severe mental retardation with marked delay in attainment of motor milestones. Paroxysms of inappropriate laughter. Absent speech.

Craniofacial. Microbrachycephaly. Ocular anomalies including decreased pigmentation of the choroid and iris, the latter resulting in pale blue eyes. Maxillary hypoplasia, a large mouth with tongue protrusion and widely spaced teeth. Prognathia.

Neurologic. Ataxia and jerky arm movements resembling a puppet gait. Seizures varying from major motor to akinetic. EEG abnormalities consisting of high-amplitude spike and slow waves at 2 to 3 cycles per second, although electrical patterns have been variable. Hypotonia and occasionally hyperreflexia.

NATURAL HISTORY. The mental deficiency, although nonprogressive, is severe. Receptive ability may be sufficient to understand simple commands. Seizure activity may decrease with age. The laughter is not apparently associated with happiness but rather is suggestive of a defect at the brain stem level.

ETIOLOGY. Unknown. The vast majority of cases have been sporadic. Two reports of two affected siblings raise the question of autosomal recessive inheritance.

References

Angelman, H.: "Puppet" children: A report on three cases. Dev. Med. Child. Neurol., 7:681, 1965.

Kuroki, Y., et al.: The "happy puppet" syndrome in two siblings. Hum. Genet., 56:227, 1980.

Williams, C. A., and Frias, J. L.: The Angelman ("happy puppet") syndrome. Am. J. Med. Genet., 11:453, 1982.

Pashayan, H. M., et al.: The Angelman syndrome in two brothers. Am. J. Med. Genet., 13:295, 1982.

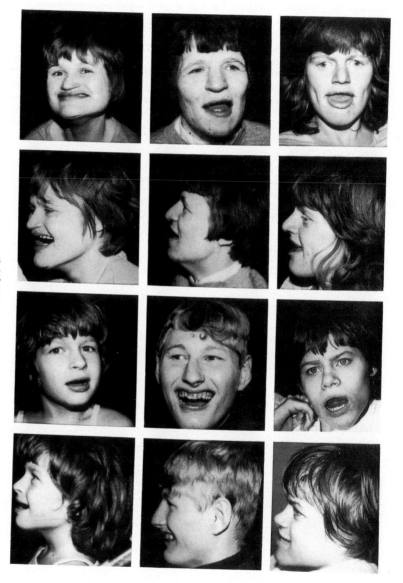

Angelman syndrome. Photographs of six affected individuals ranging from 11 years old to 33 years of age. (From Williams, C. A., and Frias, J. L.: Am. J. Med. Genet., *11*:453, 1982.)

PRADER-WILLI SYNDROME

Hypotonia, Obesity, Small Hands and Feet

Charles Dickens, in *The Pickwick Papers*, described "a fat and red-faced boy in a state of somnolency." The boy was subsequently addressed as "young dropsy," "young opium eater," and "boa constrictor," no doubt in reference to his obesity, somnolence, and excessive appetite, respectively. This may have been the first reported instance of Prader-Willi syndrome.

Prader et al. reported this pattern of abnormality in nine children in 1956, and subsequently over 200 cases have been recorded.

ABNORMALITIES. Variability in the extent and severity of features.

Small Stature. May be small at birth, occasionally normal stature until later childhood.

Obesity. Onset from infancy to six years.

Craniofacial. Almond-shaped appearance to palpebral fissures, which may be upslanting. Narrow bifrontal diameter. Strabismus.

Hair, Eye, and Skin. Blond to light brown with blue eyes and fair skin that is sun-sensitive. Picks excessively at sores.

Mental Deficiency. I.Q.s of 20 to 80, most commonly 40 to 60.

Hypotonia. Severe in early infancy.

Hands and Feet. Small. Slowing in growth of hands and/or feet, usually becoming evident in midchildhood. One patient wore size 3 shoes at 23 years.

Genitalia. Small penis and cryptorchidism. Frequent hypogonadism secondary to hypogonadotropism.

OCCASIONAL ABNORMALITIES. Poor fine and gross motor coordination. Upsweep of frontal scalp. Microcephaly, seizures, clinodactyly, syndactyly, hypoplasia of auricular cartilage. Diabetes mellitus. Scoliosis. Early dental caries.

NATURAL HISTORY. The mother may have noted feeble fetal activity, and the baby is often born in the breech position. The hypotonia is most severe in early infancy, when there may be respiratory tract and feeding problems, not uncommonly necessitating tube feeding. The degree of mental deficiency may appear to be greater in infancy than at a later age because of the severity of the hypotonia hindering developmental performance. Regarding behavior, these patients have been noted to be cheerful and good-natured. However, behavioral problems, including stubbornness and rage-type responses, tend to become more frequent in later childhood. Birth weight tends to be low, and failure to thrive is frequent in early infancy, with obesity presenting at one to three years of age, especially over the lower abdomen, buttocks, and thighs. The obesity paradoxically develops at a time when the hypotonia is improving. The caloric intake of these patients is less than usual for their height (about 80 per cent) but includes bizarre and binge-type eating. In order to control the progressive obesity, the number of calories consumed must be decreased to approximately 60 per cent of usual. This can usually be achieved only by full family cooperation and by making food inaccessible to the patient. The presence of a diabetic type of glucose tolerance curve relates to the severity of the obesity, and only an occasional patient develops diabetes mellitus during childhood. Hyperinsulinemia and blunted pituitary growth hormone responses also relate to the degree of obesity.

Early short-term testosterone therapy has resulted in enlargement of the micropenis to normal size for age. Any boy who is doing reasonably well at the age of adolescence should be considered for full testosterone replacement therapy, since his own production is usually inadequate.

ETIOLOGY. Unknown. A specific interstitial deletion in the number 15 chromosome at the Q11–13 region has been found by high-resolution prophase banding microscopy in close to one half of the cases of Prader-Willi syndrome. Usually sporadic, with occasional instances of recurrence. Empiric recurrence risk about 1.6 per cent. Possibly, the syndrome represents the consequence of a single localized defect in early hypothalamic and/or midbrain development. A recent study suggests that affected individuals who have extremely light skin and translucency of the iris have a brain defect characterized by misrouting of retinal ganglion fibers at the optic chiasm.

References

Prader, A., Labhart, A., and Willi, H.: Ein Syndrom von Adipositas, Kleinwuchs, Kryptorchismus und Oligophrenie nach myatonieartigem Zustand im Neugeborenenalter. Schweiz. Med. Wschr., *86*:1260, 1956.

Hall, B. D., and Smith, D. W.: Prader-Willi syndrome. J. Pediatr., *81*:286, 1972.

Hamilton, C. R., Scully, R. E., and Kliman, B.: Hypo-gonadotrophism in Prader-Willi syndrome. Am. J. Med., *52*:322, 1972.

Parra, A., Cervantes, C., and Schultz, R. B.: Immuno-reactive insulin and growth hormone responses in patients with Prader-Willi syndrome. J. Pediatr., *83*:587, 1973.

Pipes, P. L., and Holm, V. A.: Weight control of children with Prader-Willi syndrome. J. Am. Diet. Assoc., *62*:520, 1973.

Clarren, S. K., and Smith, D. W.: Prader-Willi syndrome. Am. J. Dis. Child., *131*:798, 1977.

Butler, M. G., Meaney, F. J., and Palmer, C. G.: Clinical and cytogenetic survey of 39 individuals with Prader-Labhart-Willi syndrome. Am. J. Med. Genet., *23*:793, 1986.

Creel, D. J., et al.: Abnormalities of the central visual pathways in the Prader-Willi syndrome associated with hypopigmentation. N. Engl. J. Med., *314*:1606, 1986.

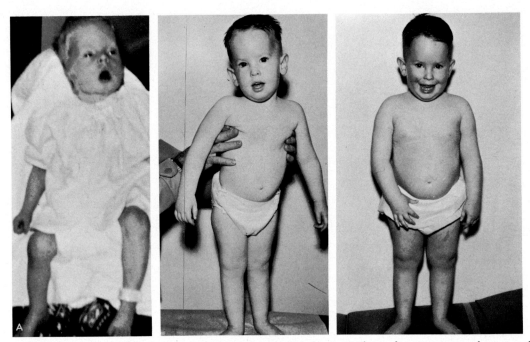

Prader-Willi syndrome. *A,* Same patient as neonate, at one year and ten months, and at two years and ten months (height age, two years and four months; developmental quotient, 60.)

Illustration continued on opposite page

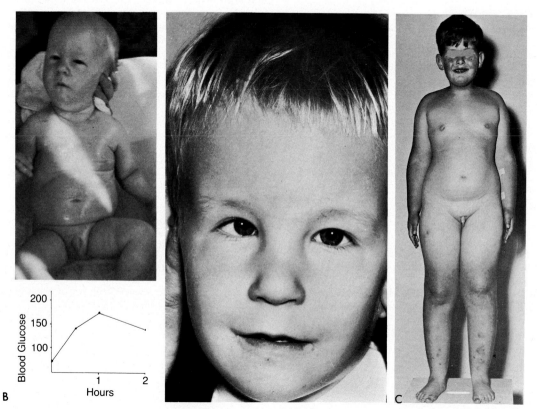

B, Same patient at five months and at four years and two months, at which time height age was three years and two months, developmental quotient was 50, and response to an oral glucose load was abnormal. *C*, Nine and one-half year old with height age of seven and one-half years and mental age of five years. (Courtesy of Prof. A. Prader, University of Kinderspital, Zurich.)

COHEN SYNDROME

Hypotonia, Obesity, Prominent Incisors

This disorder was recognized in 1973 in two affected siblings and one isolated case by Cohen et al. In excess of 25 cases have subsequently been described.

ABNORMALITIES

Growth. Truncal obesity of midchildhood onset. Low birth weight. Postnatal growth deficiency.

Performance. Persisting hypotonia and weakness. Mental deficiency; I.Q.s of 30 to 70.

Craniofacial. Microcephaly. High nasal bridge, maxillary hypoplasia with mild downslant to palpebral fissures, short philtrum, open mouth with prominent maxillary central incisors, mild micrognathia, large ears.

Eyes. Decreased visual acuity, defective vision in bright light, constricted visual fields, chorioretinal dystrophy with bull's-eye–like maculae and pigmentary deposits and optic atrophy.

Limbs. Narrow hands and feet with mild shortening of metacarpals and metatarsals, simian creases, hyperextensible joints, genu valgus, cubitus valgus.

Spine. Lumbar lordosis with mild scoliosis.

Other. Delayed puberty. Cryptorchidism.

OCCASIONAL ABNORMALITIES. Microphthalmia, colobomata, mild cutaneous syndactyly, seizures, leukopenia, ureteropelvic obstruction, tall stature, mitral valve prolapse.

NATURAL HISTORY. Weakness and hypotonia persist beyond infancy, and obesity of moderate degree has developed in midchildhood. Motor milestones are delayed. All have developed speech, although to variable extent. Despite their moderate degree of mental deficiency, the majority have a cheerful disposition.

ETIOLOGY. Autosomal recessive.

References

Cohen, M. M., Jr., et al.: A new syndrome with hypotonia, obesity, mental deficiency, and facial, oral, ocular, and limb anomalies. J. Pediatr., *83*:280, 1973.

Carey, J. C., and Hall, B. D.: Confirmation of the Cohen syndrome. J. Pediatr., *93*:239, 1978.

Kousseff, B. G.: Cohen syndrome: Further delineation and inheritance. Am. J. Med. Genet., *9*:25, 1981.

Norio, R., Christina, R., Lindahl, E.: Further delineation of the Cohen syndrome; report on chorioretinal dystrophy, leukopenia, and consanguinity. Clin. Genet., *25*:1, 1984.

North C., et al.: The clinical features of the Cohen syndrome. J. Med. Genet., *22*:131, 1985.

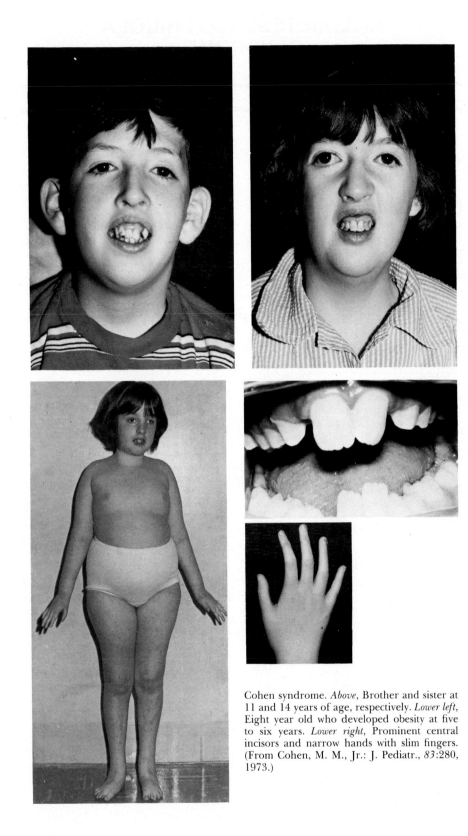

Cohen syndrome. *Above*, Brother and sister at 11 and 14 years of age, respectively. *Lower left*, Eight year old who developed obesity at five to six years. *Lower right*, Prominent central incisors and narrow hands with slim fingers. (From Cohen, M. M., Jr.: J. Pediatr., *83*:280, 1973.)

KILLIAN/TESCHLER-NICOLA SYNDROME

(Pallister Mosaic Syndrome, Tetrasomy 12p)

Teschler-Nicola and Killian described a three year old female with this disorder in 1981. A second case was reported by Schroer and Stevenson in 1983. It was subsequently recognized that two adults with a similar phenotype and mosaicism for a marker chromosome reported by Pallister et al. in 1976 had the same condition.

Recently, tetrasomy 12p, either mosaic or total, has been documented in skin fibroblasts from affected individuals, but not in peripheral blood.

ABNORMALITIES

Growth. Normal or increased birth length, weight, and head circumference, with postnatal deceleration of length and head circumference. Obesity frequently develops.

Performance. Profound mental deficiency with only minimal speech development. Seizures. Hypotonia with contractures developing with advancing age. Deafness.

Craniofacies. Sparse anterior scalp hair in infancy, with sparse eyebrows and eyelashes. Upslanting palpebral fissures. Delayed dental eruption. Prominent forehead. Ocular hypertelorism. Ptosis. Strabismus. Large ears with thick protruding lobules. Flat, broad nasal root and short nose with anteverted nostrils. Coarse face. Long philtrum with thin upper lip and distinct Cupid-bow shape. Protruding lower lip. Short neck.

Other. Streaks of hypopigmentation. Broad hands with short digits.

OCCASIONAL ABNORMALITIES. Stenosis of external auditory canal. Macroglossia. Prominent lateral palatine ridges. Bifid uvula. Micrognathia. Microcephaly. Hernias. Hypermobile joints. Kyphoscoliosis. Fifth finger clinodactyly. Congenital hip dislocation. Simian crease. Sweating abnormalities.

NATURAL HISTORY. Physical characteristics change with age. Initially sparse, anterior scalp hair grow in by two to five years; a normal-size tongue becomes macroglossic; initial micrognathia progresses to prognathism, and contractures develop between five and ten years after initial hypotonia.

ETIOLOGY. Tetrasomy 12p, either mosaic or total, in skin fibroblasts. Although most patients tested have had normal karyotype in peripheral lymphocytes, one patient had lymphocyte mosaicism for an iso-chromosome of 12p.

References

Pallister, P. D., et al.: The Pallister mosaic syndrome. Birth Defects: Original Article Series, *5XIII(3B)*:103, 1976.

Teschler-Nicola, M., and Killian, W.: Case report 72: Mental retardation, unusual facial appearance, abnormal hair. Synd. Ident., *7*(1):6, 1981.

Buyse, M. L., and Korf, B. R.: "Killian syndrome," Pallister mosaic syndrome, or mosaic tetrasomy 12p? An analysis. J. Clin. Dysmorph., *1*(3):2, 1983.

Hall, B. D.: Teschler-Nicola/Killian syndrome: A sporadic case in an 11 year old male. J. Clin. Dysmorph., *1*(3):14, 1983.

Schroer, R. J., and Stevenson, R. E.: Further clinical delineation of the syndrome of unusual facial appearance, abnormal hair and mental retardation reported by Teschler-Nicola and Killian. Proc. Greenwood Genet. Cntr., *2*:3, 1983.

Raffel, L. J., Mohaudas, T., and Rimoin, D. L.: Chromosomal mosaicism in the Killian/Teschler-Nicola syndrome. Am. J. Med. Genet., *24*:607, 1986.

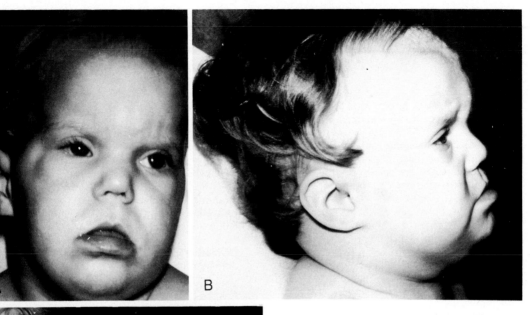

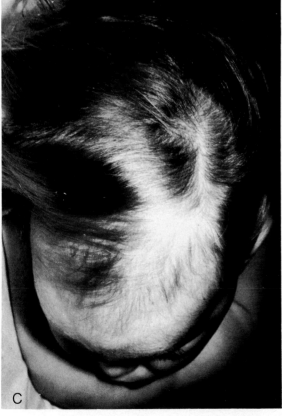

Killian/Teschler-Nicola syndrome. *A* to *C*, Two year old with sparse anterior scalp hair, eyebrows, and eyelashes. Note the prominent forehead, long philtrum with thin upper lip, and distinct Cupid-bow configuration. (Courtesy of Dr. Robert Saul, Dr. Richard Schroer, and Dr. Roger Stevenson, Greenwood Genetic Center, Greenwood, South Carolina).

ZELLWEGER SYNDROME
(Cerebro-Hepato-Renal Syndrome)

Hypotonia, High Forehead with Flat Facies,
Hepatomegaly

Bowen et al. and Smith et al. independently reported siblings with this pattern of malformation in 1964 and 1965. In 1973, Goldfischer et al. reported that peroxisomes, subcellular organelles that recently have been shown to play a role in lipid metabolism, were absent in the liver and kidneys of two affected children. More recently, lack of dihydroxyacetone phosphate acyltransferase (DHAP-AT), a peroxisomal enzyme with a major role in glycerol ether lipid synthesis, has been documented. Deficiency of this enzyme, as well as the observed increase in plasma and fibroblasts of very long chain fatty acids, provides a biochemical marker for the diagnosis of this disorder and for its potential treatment.

ABNORMALITIES
General. Growth deficiency; mean birth weight, 3300 g. Hypotonia, respiratory problems, poor sucking ability. Variable seizures.
Brain. Macrogyria and polymicrogyria noted; also, incomplete white matter and myelinization, gross defects of early brain development.
Craniofacial. Large fontanels. Flat occiput. High forehead with shallow supraorbital ridges and flat facies. Minor ear anomaly. Inner epicanthal folds. Brushfield spots. Mild micrognathia. Redundant skin of neck.
Liver. Hepatomegaly with dysgenesis, including cirrhotic changes.
Kidneys. Albuminuria. Small cysts, chiefly of glomeruli.
Cardiac. Patent ductus arteriosus, septal defect.
Limbs. Variable contractures with camptodactyly, limited extension of knee, equinovarus deformity. Simian crease.
Other. Variable elevated serum iron level and evidence of excess iron storage, pipecolic acidemia, abnormal bile acids, and absent liver peroxisomes.

OCCASIONAL ABNORMALITIES. Cataract, glaucoma, nystagmus, cubitus valgus, ulnar deviation of hands, irregular calcification of patellae, greater trochanters, and/or triradiate cartilages, deep sacral dimple, hypospadias, cryptorchidism, hypertrophied pylorus, single umbilical artery. Breech presentation.

NATURAL HISTORY. Most of these babies were born in the breech presentation and failed to thrive. Some developed icterus and some had bloody stools, possibly related to hypoprothrombinemia. All died from one day to six months after birth.

ETIOLOGY. Autosomal recessive. Prenatal diagnosis has been accomplished by documentation in amniotic fluid cells of decreased dihydroxyacetone phosphate acyltransferase or increased accumulation of unmetabolized very long chain fatty acids.

COMMENT. Several of these babies were mistakenly identified initially as having Down syndrome.

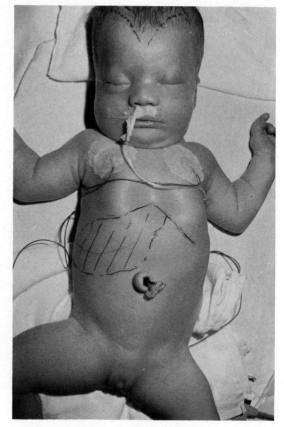

Zellweger syndrome. Affected infant showing hypotonia, enlarged fontanel, and enlarged liver.

References

Bowen, P., et al.: A familial syndrome of multiple congenital defects. Bull. Hopkins Hosp., *114*:402, 1964.

Smith, D. W., Opitz, J. M., and Inhorn, S. L.: A syndrome of multiple developmental defects including polycystic kidneys and intrahepatic biliary dysgenesis in two siblings. J. Pediatr., *67*:617, 1965.

Opitz, J. M., et al.: The Zellweger syndrome. Birth Defects: Original Article Series, *5*:144, 1969.

Goldfischer, S., et al.: Peroxisomal and mitochondrial defects in the cerebro-hepato-renal syndrome. Science, *182*:62, 1973.

Kelley, R. I.: Review: The cerebrohepatorenal syndrome of Zellweger. Morphologic and metabolic aspects. Am. J. Med. Genet., *16*:503, 1983.

Datta, N. S., Wilson, G. N., and Hajra, A. K.: Deficiency of enzymes catalyzing the biosynthesis of glycerol-ether lipids in Zellweger syndrome. N. Engl. J. Med., *311*:1080, 1984.

Hajra, A. K., et al.: Prenatal diagnosis of Zellweger cerebrohepatorenal syndrome. N. Engl. J. Med., *312*:445, 1985.

Solish, J. I., et al.: The prenatal diagnosis of the cerebro-hepato-renal syndrome of Zellweger. Prenat. Diagn., *5*:27, 1985.

Wilson, G. N., et al.: Zellweger syndrome: Diagnostic assays, syndrome delineation, and potential therapy. Am. J. Med. Genet., *24*:69, 1986.

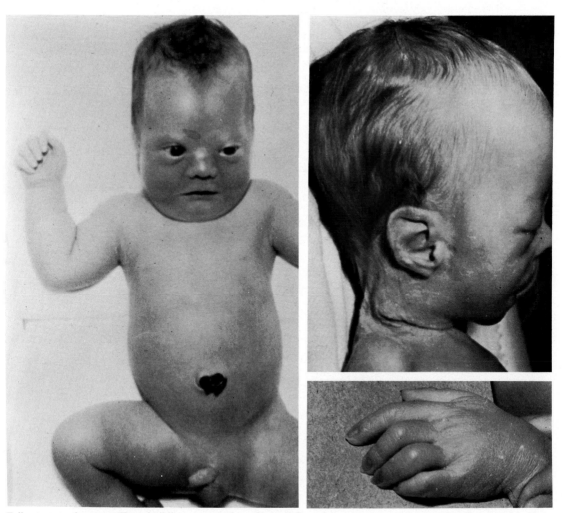

Zellweger syndrome. Affected siblings at one day of age *(left)* and post mortem at ten weeks of age *(right)*. Note camptodactyly of third, fourth, and fifth fingers. (From Smith, D. W., et al.: J. Pediatr., *67*:617, 1965.)

LOWE SYNDROME

(Oculo-Cerebro-Renal Syndrome)

Hypotonia, Cataract, Renal Tubular Dysfunction

Lowe et al. recognized this disease in 1952; subsequently, more than 50 cases have been reported.

ABNORMALITIES

General. Hypotonia and joint hypermobility progressing to joint contractures with advancing years. Diminished to absent deep tendon reflexes and muscle hypoplasia with fatty infiltration. Hyperactivity. Mental deficiency, moderate to severe, with diffuse EEG abnormality. Postnatal growth deficiency.

Eyes. Cortical cataract with or without glaucoma.

Renal and Bone. Renal tubular dysfunction with limited ammonium production and hyperchloremic acidosis, phosphaturia tending toward hypophosphatemia, and generalized aminoaciduria. Albuminuria. Moderate to severe osteoporosis and sometimes rickets. Joint swelling and effusion with synovial thickening on biopsy. There is also organic aciduria of unknown cause.

Genitalia. Cryptorchidism.

OCCASIONAL ABNORMALITIES. Seizures. Pectus excavatum. Craniosynostosis. Dental cysts. Fractures.

NATURAL HISTORY. Failure to thrive. Both growth rate and bone mineralization may improve by administration of sodium-potassium citrate in adequate quantity to correct the acidosis. The prognosis for survival with such treatment is not known. However, the prognosis for brain function is poor.

ETIOLOGY. X-linked, with many of the heterozygote females showing fine lenticular opacities by slit lamp examination and occasionally a frank cataract. Although there is an association with renal acidosis, there is increasing evidence that the basic defect may involve an alteration in connective tissue.

References

Lowe, C. U., Terrey, M., and MacLachland, E. A.: Organic-aciduria, decreased renal ammonia production, hydrophthalmos, and mental retardation. Am. J. Dis. Child., *83*:164, 1952.

Illig, R., Dumermuth, G., and Prader, A.: Das oculocerebro-renale Syndrom (Lowe). Helv. Paediatr. Acta, *18*:173, 1963.

Richards, W., et al.: The oculo-cerebro-renal syndrome of Lowe. Am. J. Dis. Child., *109*:185, 1965.

Athreya, B. H., et al.: Arthropathy of Lowe's (oculocerebrorenal) syndrome. Arthritis Rheum., *26*:728, 1983.

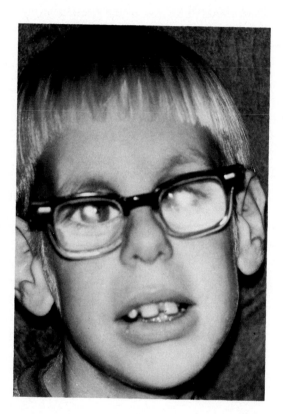

Lowe syndrome. Eleven year old who has had cataract surgery. Hypotonia with severe mental deficiency; first walked at eight years. Albuminuria. (Courtesy of Dr. Arthur Schloss, Rainier State Training School, Buckley, Washington.)

FREEMAN-SHELDON SYNDROME

(Whistling Face Syndrome)

Mask-Like "Whistling" Facies,
Hypoplastic Alae Nasi, Talipes Equinovarus

This disorder was described by Freeman and Sheldon in 1938 and at least 50 cases have been reported.

ABNORMALITIES. Most of the features are secondary to increased muscle tone.

Facies. Full forehead and mask-like facies with small mouth giving a "whistling" appearance. Deep-set eyes, broad nasal bridge, telecanthus, epicanthal folds, strabismus, blepharophimosis, small nose, hypoplastic alae nasi with coloboma, long philtrum. H-shaped cutaneous dimpling on chin. High palate, small tongue, limited palatal movement with nasal speech.

Joints and Skeletal. Ulnar deviation of hands, cortical thumbs, flexion of fingers, thick skin over flexor surface of proximal phalanges. Equinovarus with contracted toes, vertical talus, kyphosis, scoliosis. Steeply inclined anterior cranial fossa on radiographs.

Other. Postnatal growth deficiency. Inguinal hernia, incomplete descent of testes.

OCCASIONAL ABNORMALITIES. Mental deficiency, flat face, ptosis, subcutaneous ridge across lower forehead, short neck, low birth weight, dislocation of hip, spina bifida occulta, prominent mental protuberance on radiographs of facial bones.

NATURAL HISTORY. These patients are not uncommonly born in the breech position, and/or delivery may be difficult. Vomiting and dysphagia may lead to failure to thrive in infancy. There may be early mortality, often related to aspiration. Eventual intelligence is usually in the normal range.

ETIOLOGY. Autosomal dominant. A clinically indistinguishable autosomal recessive type has been reported in three separate families.

References

Freeman, E. A., and Sheldon, J. H.: Craniocarpotarsal dystrophy. An undescribed congenital malformation. Arch. Dis. Child., *13*:277, 1938.

Burian, F.: The "whistling face" characteristic in a compound cranio-facio-corporal syndrome. Br. J. Plast. Surg., *16*:140, 1963.

Antley, R. M., et al.: Diagnostic criteria for the whistling face syndrome. Birth Defects, *11*:161, 1975.

O'Connell, D. J., and Hall, C. M.: Cranio-carpotarsal dysplasia. A report of 7 cases. Radiology, *123*:719, 1977.

Kousseff, B. G., McConnachie, P., and Hadro, T. A.: Autosomal recessive type of whistling face syndrome in twins. Pediatrics, *69*:328, 1982.

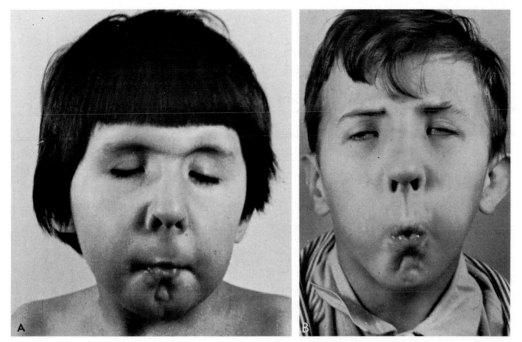

Freeman-Sheldon syndrome. *A*, Five and one-half year old girl. Note crease pattern in chin. *B*, Older boy. Note the retraction of the alae nasi. (From Burian, F.: Br. J. Plast. Surg., *16*:140, 1963.)

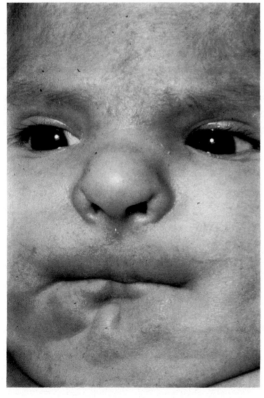

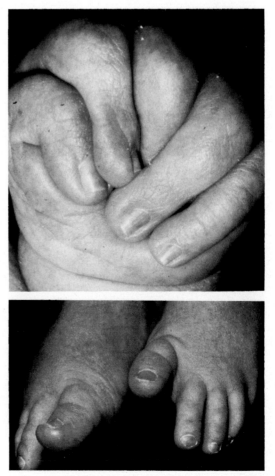

Freeman-Sheldon syndrome. Young infant showing characteristic facies and aberrant positioning in hands and feet. (Courtesy of Dr. Boris Koussef, University of South Florida, Tampa, Florida.)

STEINERT MYOTONIC DYSTROPHY SYNDROME
(Steinert Syndrome, Dystrophia Myotonica)

*Myotonia with Muscle Atrophy,
Cataract, Hypogonadism*

The text by Caughey and Myrianthopoulos presents the manifold abnormalities that may occur as features of this single mutant gene. More than 500 cases have been documented.

ABNORMALITIES
Muscle Degeneration. Myotonia (difficulty in relaxing a contracted muscle), often best appreciated in the hand or jaw or by tapping the tongue. Degeneration of swollen muscle cells giving way to thin and atrophic muscle fibers with weakness; ptosis of the eyelids is frequent. Myopathic facies.
Eyes. Cataract, often evident only as "myotonic dust" by slit lamp inspection.
Gonadal Insufficiency. Testicular atrophy (80 per cent) in males. Amenorrhea, dysmenorrhea, ovarian cyst in females.
Scalp. Premature frontal recession, especially in males.
Cardiac. Conduction defects with arrhythmias.

OCCASIONAL ABNORMALITIES.
Hypotonia in infancy, mental deficiency, microcephaly, talipes, clinodactyly, hernia, cryptorchidism, kyphoscoliosis, hyperostotic cranial bones, atrophic thin skin, macular abnormality, blepharitis, keratitis sicca, goiter, thyroid adenomata, diabetes mellitus.

NATURAL HISTORY.
The age of onset is from prenatal life to the sixth or seventh decade, with the average being in the late 20s to 30s. However, lens opacification is usually evident by slit lamp examination in the 20s. Initial signs of the disease are variable. Myotonia may be so mild as to be detected only when specifically tested for. Muscle wasting and weakness, occasionally asymmetric, most often involve the facial and temporal muscles, yielding the expressionless "myopathic facies." The most consistent evident weakness is in the orbicularis oculi muscles. Other involved muscles are the anterior cervical and those of the arms, thighs, and anterior lower leg, with progression from proximal to distal. Ptosis of the eyelids is frequent, and pseudohypertrophy is an occasional feature. One of the most sensitive early indicators of muscle dysfunction is the roentgen-

ographic evidence of partial retention of radiopaque material in the pharynx after swallowing. Mental deterioration may also be a feature. There is increasing debility, with death, usually by the fifth or sixth decade, as a consequence of pneumonia, cardiac failure, or intercurrent illness.

Pruzanski and Calderon emphasize disease manifestations in preadolescent life, and Bell and Smith note the potential prenatal manifestations. The neonatal cases are usually infants born of affected women, suggesting that a humoral factor from the mother may augment the impact of the mutant gene on the fetus. At least 18 such cases have been described. Hydramnios, due to inadequate swallowing, tends to be an ominous sign, with high early mortality due to respiratory insufficiency and/or aspiration. Growth deficiency, facial diplegia, equinovarus foot deformity, and hypotonia are frequent features of the early expression of the disorder, whereas myotonia is seldom a feature.

ETIOLOGY.
Autosomal dominant with wide variability in expression. Bundey and Carter provide evidence for genetic heterogeneity for this disorder, with at least two autosomal dominants: one in which the onset is usually in infancy and the other in which the onset is usually after 20 years of age. Although prenatal diagnosis of myotonic dystrophy should be possible by amniocentesis and analysis of secretor status, the use of these methods is only predictive of an affected fetus and is not diagnostic.

References

Caughey, J. E., and Myrianthopoulos, N. D.: Dystrophia Myotonica and Related Disorders. Springfield, Ill., Charles C Thomas, 1963.

Pruzanski, W.: Myotonic dystrophy—a multisystem disease; report of 67 cases and a review of the literature. Psychiatr. Neurol. Med. Psychol. (Leipz.), *149*:302, 1965.

Calderon, R.: Myotonic dystrophy: a neglected cause of mental retardation. J. Pediatr., *68*:423, 1966.

Pruzanski, W.: Variants of myotonic dystrophy in pre-adolescent life (the syndrome of myotonic dysembryoplasia). Brain, *89*:563, 1966.

Bell, D. B., and Smith, D. W.: Myotonic dystrophy in the neonate. J. Pediatr., *81*:83, 1972.

Bundey, S., and Carter, C. L.: Genetic heterogeneity for dystrophia myotonica. J. Med. Genet., *9*:311, 1972.

Schrott, H. G., Karp, L., and Omenn, G. S.: Prenatal prediction in myotonic dystrophy: Guidelines for genetic counseling. Clin Genet., *4*:38, 1973.

Aicardi, J., Conti, D., and Goutieres, F.: Aspects cliniques et génétiques des formes précoces de la dystrophie myotonique de Steinert. J. Génét. Hum., *23*:Suppl. 146, 1975.

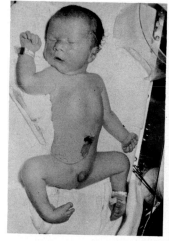

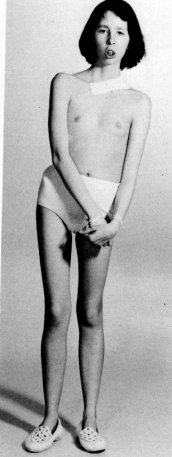

Above, Severely affected, almost immobile newborn baby of mother with myotonic dystrophy. (From Bell, D. B., and Smith, D. W.: J. Pediatr., *81*:83, 1972.) *Right*, Fourteen year old with relatively immobile facies, scoliosis, and an I.Q. of 58. *Below*, Correlation of protean features of myotonic dystrophy with age of onset, beginning with earliest age reported.

	FETAL-NEONATAL INFANCY	CHILDHOOD	ADULTHOOD
CNS	Mental deficiency – – – – – – – – – – – – – – – – – →		
OCULAR	Cataracts – – – – – – – – – – – – – – – – → Ptosis – – – – – – – – – – – – – – – – – →		
SKELETAL	Clubfeet Scoliosis/lordosis – – – – – – – → Cranial hyperostosis – – – – – – →		
RESPIRATORY	Neonatal distress Recurrent infection – – – – – – – – – – – – – – → Chronic insufficiency		
NEURO – MUSCULAR	Hypotonia/"floppy" Facial diplegia Weakness/atrophy – – – – – – – – – – – – – – – → Variable myotonia – – – – – – – – – – – – – – → Dysarthria – – – – – – – – – – →		
GI	Poor feeding Impaired deglutition – – – – – – – – – – – – – – →		
GONADAL	Cryptorchidism – – – – – – – – – – – – – – – → Hypogonadism		
CARDIAC	Disturbed conduction – – – – – →		
MISC.	Frontal baldness – – – – – – – → Decreased IgG and IgM – – – – – →		

SCHWARTZ-JAMPEL SYNDROME
(Chondrodystrophica Myotonia)

Myotonia, Blepharophimosis, Joint Limitation

Though Pinto and de Sousa were the first to report this disorder, this fact was only recently appreciated. Schwartz and Jampel described a brother and sister with this condition in 1962, and later Aberfeld et al. reported further observations on the same patients. At least 40 cases have been reported. Many, if not most, of the features appear to be secondary to a primary muscle disorder with myotonia.

ABNORMALITIES
Growth. Small stature, usually postnatal onset.
Muscle. Myotonia with sad, fixed facies and small mandible. Muscular hypertrophy in one half of patients. Hyporeflexia.
Joints. Limitation in hips, wrists, fingers, toes, and spine.
Osseous. Vertical shortness of vertebrae (platyspondyly) with short neck. Fragmentation and flattening of femoral epiphyses. Pectus carinatum.
Larynx. Small and high-pitched voice.
Eyes. Blepharophimosis, myopia. Long eyelashes in irregular rows.
Others. Low hairline, low-set ears, small testicles, flat facies.

OCCASIONAL ABNORMALITIES.
Mental deficiency. Intrauterine growth deficiency, delayed bone age, equinovarus foot deformation, hip dislocation, cataract, microcornea.

NATURAL HISTORY.
Onset of progressive myotonia, muscle wasting, and orthopedic problems during infancy, with slow linear growth. Myotonia, which usually reaches a plateau in midchildhood, is almost always recorded on electromyography, even when not present clinically. Light and electron microscopic and histochemical examinations of muscles show inconsistent myopathic abnormalities. Anesthesia may constitute a serious risk. There is slowing of growth, and there are problems of motor function, but intelligence is usually considered normal. Normal pubertal development occurs.

ETIOLOGY. Autosomal recessive.

References

Pinto, L. M., and de Sousa, J. S.: Um caso de "doenca muscular" de difícil classificacao. Rev. Port. Pediatr. Pueric., *6*:1, 1961.

Schwartz, O., and Jampel, R. S.: Congenital blepharophimosis associated with a unique generalized myopathy. Arch. Ophthalmol., *68*:52, 1962.

Aberfeld, D. C., Hinterbuchner, L. P., and Schneider, M.: Myotonia, dwarfism, diffuse bone disease and unusual ocular and facial abnormalities (a new syndrome). Brain, *88*:313, 1965.

Aberfeld, D. C.: Chondrodystrophic myotonia. Monogr. Hum. Genet., *6*:189, 1972.

Horan, F., and Beighton, P.: Orthopedic aspects of Schwartz syndrome. J. Bone Joint Surg., *57*:542, 1975.

Pavone, L., et al.: Schwartz-Jampel syndrome in two daughters of first cousins. J. Neurol. Neurosurg. Psych., *41*:161, 1978.

Edward, W. C., and Root, A. W.: Chondrodystrophic myotonia (Schwartz-Jampel syndrome): Report of a new case and follow-up of patients initially reported in 1969. Am. J. Med. Genet., *13*:51, 1982.

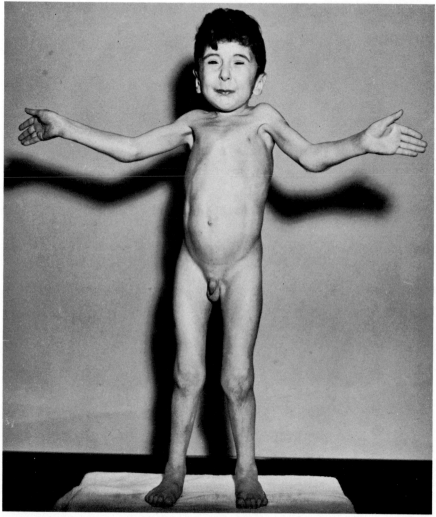

Schwartz-Jampel syndrome. Six year old male with height age of three and one-half years. A female sibling had the same disorder, and the parents appeared normal. (From Schwartz, O., and Jampel, R. S.: Arch. Ophthalmol., *68*:52, 1962.)

SCHINZEL-GIEDION SYNDROME

A brother and sister with this disorder were described in 1978 by Schinzel and Giedion. Three additional patients have been reported.

ABNORMALITIES
Growth. Postnatal growth deficiency.

Performance. Profound mental deficiency. Seizures. Opisthotonus. Spasticity. Hypsarrhythmia.

Craniofacies. Widely patent fontanels and sutures with metopic suture extending anteriorly to nasal root. High, protruding forehead. Short nose with low nasal bridge and anteverted nares. Shallow orbits with apparent proptosis. Ocular hypertelorism. Midface hypoplasia. Choanal stenosis. Attached helix with protruding lobule of low-set ear.

Limbs. Moderate shortening of forearms and legs. Talipes equinovarus. Hyperconvex nails. Hypoplastic dermal ridges. Simian crease.

Genito-Urinary. Hydronephrosis. Hydroureter. Hypospadius, short penis. Deep interlabial sulcus.

Radiologic. Steep short base of skull, wide occipital synchondrosis, multiple wormian bones, hypoplastic first ribs, broad ribs, hypoplastic/aplastic pubic bones, hypoplasia of distal phalanges.

Other. Hypertrichosis.

OCCASIONAL ABNORMALITIES. Macroglossia, facial hemangiomata, hypoplastic nipples, postaxial polydactyly, atrial septal defect, fifth toe overlapping fourth, short sternum. Bicornuate uterus.

NATURAL HISTORY. Severe postnatal growth deficiency and profound mental retardation with visual and hearing problems have occurred in all patients who have survived. Death prior to two years of age is the rule.

ETIOLOGY. Autosomal recessive inheritance is likely based on documentation of one instance of affected sibling born to unaffected parents.

References

Schinzel, A., and Giedion, A.: A syndrome of severe midface retraction, multiple skull anomalies, clubfeet, and cardiac and renal malformations in siblings. Am. J. Med. Genet., *1*:361, 1978.

Donnai, D., and Harris, R.: A further case of a new syndrome including midface retraction, hypertrichosis, and skeletal anomalies. J. Med. Genet., *16*:483, 1979.

Kelley, R. I., Zackai, E. H., and Charney, E. B.: Congenital hydronephrosis, skeletal dysplasia, and severe developmental retardation: The Schinzel-Giedion syndrome. J. Pediatr., *100*:943, 1982.

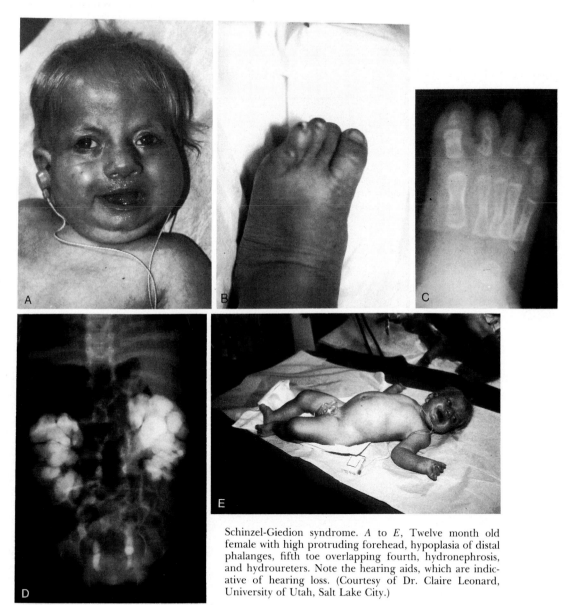

Schinzel-Giedion syndrome. *A* to *E*, Twelve month old female with high protruding forehead, hypoplasia of distal phalanges, fifth toe overlapping fourth, hydronephrosis, and hydroureters. Note the hearing aids, which are indicative of hearing loss. (Courtesy of Dr. Claire Leonard, University of Utah, Salt Lake City.)

HECHT SYNDROME
(Trismus Pseudocamptodactyly Syndrome)

This disorder of muscle development and function was first described by Hecht and Beals and by Wilson et al. in 1968. It was more recently well-delineated by Mabry et al. in a huge kindred in which the initial United States case was a young Dutch girl who arrived in this country with "crooked hands and a small mouth."

ABNORMALITIES. Appear to be based on short muscles and especially tendons.

Muscles and Tendons. Limited opening of mouth, sometimes with an enlarged coronoid process. Short flexor tendons, so that when the hand is dorsiflexed, the fingers are partially flexed. Occasionally, short flexor muscles to the feet cause such problems as downturning toes, talipes equinovarus, metatarsus adductus, and short gastrocnemius.

NATURAL HISTORY. The newborn baby may have tightly fisted hands and later usually crawls on the knuckles. These patients may have feeding problems because of the small mouth, and they tend to eat slowly. Tonsillectomy and/or intubation may present serious problems. There can be occupational handicaps relative to the military service, typing, or other situations requiring high levels of hand dexterity.

ETIOLOGY. Autosomal dominant, with an unexplained 2:1 excess of affected females.

References

Hecht, F., and Beals, R. K.: Inability to open the mouth fully. *In* Bergsma, D. (ed.): Birth Defects Original Article Series, Part III, Limb Malformation, Vol. V. New York, The National Foundation March of Dimes, 1968, p. 96.

Wilson, R. V., et al.: Autosomal dominant inheritance of shortening of flexor profundus muscle tendon. *In* Bergsma, D. (ed.): Birth Defects Original Article Series, Part III, Limb Malformation, Vol. V. New York, The National Foundation March of Dimes, 1968, p. 99.

Mabry, C. C., et al.: Trismus camptomelic syndrome. J. Pediatr., *85*:503, 1974.

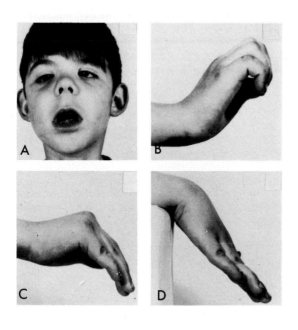

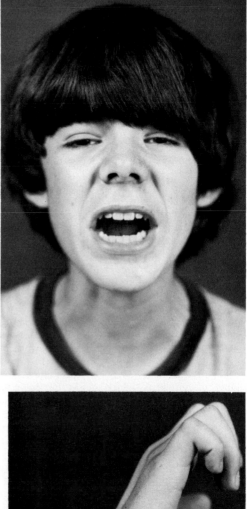

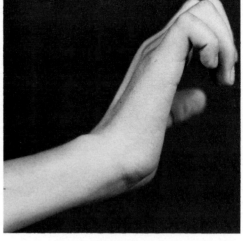

Hecht syndrome. *Left,* Boy with maximal opening of mouth *(A),* dorsiflexed hand showing flexion of fingers *(B),* extended hand with some flexion of fingers *(C),* but volar flexed hand with no finger flexion *(D). Right,* Thirteen year old boy with maximal mouth opening and flexed fingers following hand flexion. (Courtesy of Dr. C. Charlton Mabry, University of Kentucky Medical School, Louisville.)

G. FACIAL DEFECTS AS MAJOR FEATURE

MOEBIUS SEQUENCE

Sixth and Seventh Nerve Palsy

The basic features of Moebius sequence are mask-like facies with sixth and seventh nerve palsy, usually bilaterally. The necropsy cases implicate at least four modes of developmental pathology in the genesis of the problem. These are (1) hypoplasia to absence of the central brain nuclei; (2) destructive degeneration of the central brain nuclei (most common type); (3) peripheral nerve involvement; and (4) a myopathy. Thus, the Moebius sequence is but a sign and is quite nonspecific. Micrognathia, a frequent feature, may be interpreted as secondary to a neuromuscular deficit in early movement of the mandible. Some patients have more extensive cranial nerve involvement, including the third, fourth, fifth, ninth, tenth, and twelfth nerves. In the latter cases, the tongue may be limited in mobility and/or small. There may be ocular ptosis and/or a protruding auricle. About one third of the patients have talipes equinovarus, which might be the consequence of neurologic deficiency relative to early foot movement. About 15 per cent of patients have mental deficiency as a more obvious indication that the CNS defect involves more than the cranial nerve nuclei alone.

Feeding difficulties and problems of aspiration often lead to failure to thrive during infancy. The expressionless facies and speech impediments create problems in acceptance and social adaptation.

The Moebius sequence is most commonly a sporadic occurrence in an otherwise normal family, although rare instances of autosomal dominant inheritance with variable expression have been reported.

The Moebius sequence may also occur as a part of a broader pattern of malformation. Associated occasional non–CNS-related defects have included limb reduction defects, syndactyly, and the Poland sequence.

References

Moebius, P. J.: Ueber engeborene doppelseitige Abducens-Facialis-Laehmung. Munch. Med. Wochenschr., 35:91, 1888.

Henderson, J. L.: The congenital facial diplegia syndrome. Clinical features, pathology, and aetiology. A review of sixty-one cases. Brain, 62:381, 1939.

Reed, H., and Grant, W.: Möbius syndrome. Br. J. Ophthalmol., 41:731, 1957.

Van der Wiel, H. J.: Hereditary facial paralysis. Acta Genet. Statist. Med., 7:348, 1957.

Sugarman, G. I., and Stark, H. H.: Möbius anomaly with Poland's anomaly. J. Med. Genet., 10:192, 1973.

Baraitser, M.: Genetics of Möbius syndrome. J. Med. Genet., 14:415, 1977.

Myerson, M. D., and Toushee, D. R.: Speech, language and hearing in Moebius syndrome. Devel. Med. Child. Neurol., 20:357, 1978.

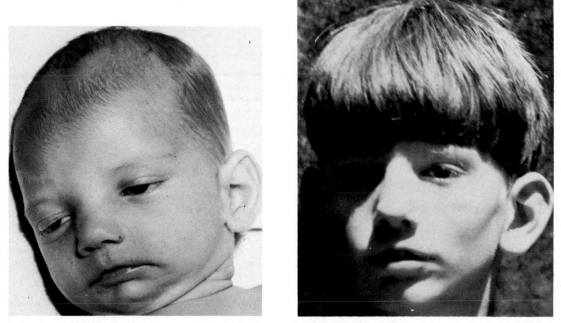

Left, Five week old with Moebius sequence, including ptosis of the eyelids. *Right*, Twelve year old whose facial appearance had improved since early childhood. Note the protruding auricle.

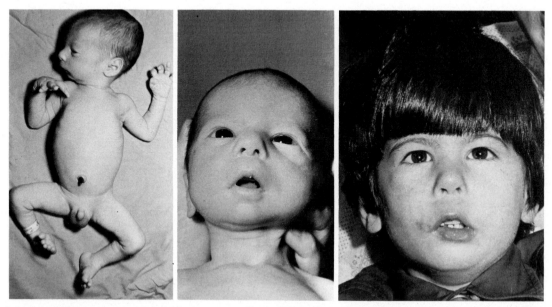

Left and *Middle*, Newborn with Moebius sequence, showing high nasal bridge, micrognathia with limited mandibular movement, small mouth with downturned corners, expressionless facies with deficit of lateral gaze, mild ptosis, mild talipes, and mild alteration in finger positioning. These clinical findings were interpreted as being the secondary neurologic consequence of a single primary defect in CNS development, especially of the nuclei of the sixth and seventh nerves. *Right*, Same patient at three years of age. He had achieved limited ability to open his mouth, was responding well to speech training, and was interpreted as having normal intelligence.

BLEPHAROPHIMOSIS SYNDROME

(Familial Blepharophimosis Syndrome)

Inner Canthal Fold,
Lateral Displacement of Inner Canthi, Ptosis

This entity, predominantly a dysplasia of the eyelids, was described by Vignes in 1889, and more than 125 cases have been reported. The existence of two types has recently been suggested: type I, associated with infertility in affected females and complete penetrance of the altered gene, and type II, transmitted by both males and females and associated with incomplete penetrance.

ABNORMALITIES

Eyes. Inverted inner canthal fold between upper and lower lid, short palpebral fissures with lateral displacement of inner canthi, low nasal bridge and ptosis of eyelids, with hypoplasia, and fibrosis of the levator palpebrae muscle. Strabismus.
Ears. Incomplete development, cupping.
Genitalia. Variable primary hypogonadism with infertility in females with type I.
Other. Variable hypotonia in early life.

OCCASIONAL ABNORMALITIES. Mental deficiency, cardiac defect.

NATURAL HISTORY. Plastic surgery is indicated both for cosmetic reasons and for improvement of ocular function.

ETIOLOGY. Autosomal dominant for both type I and type II. The importance of distinguishing between the types relates to reproductive capabilities and menstrual irregularities, including amenorrhea in females with type I. With the exception of infertility in females, the two types are indistinguishable clinically. Therefore, separating the two types can be accomplished only through a careful family history. If the affected individual, either male or female, is a member of a family in which the disorder has been transmitted only through males, it is most likely type I, whereas if transmission has occurred through both males and females, it is type II.

COMMENT. The facial appearance may initially suggest a condition with associated mental retardation; however, the affected individuals are not generally mentally deficient. Sacrez et al. reported I.Q.s from 75 to 100, with a mean value of 86.

References

Vignes: Epicanthus héréditaire. Rev. Gen. Ophtalmol. (Paris), *8*:438, 1889.
Sacrez, R., et al.: Le blépharophimosis compliqué familial. Étude des membres de la famille Blé. Ann. Pediatr. (Paris), *10*:493, 1963.
Kohn, R., and Romano, P. E.: Blepharoptosis, blepharophimosis, epicanthus inversus, and telecanthus—a syndrome with no name. Am. J. Ophthalmol. 72:625, 1972.
Zlotogora, J., Sagi, M., and Cohen, T.: The blepharophimosis, ptosis and epicanthus inversus syndrome: Delineation of two types. Am. J. Hum. Genet., *35*:1020, 1983.
Jones, C. A., and Collin, J. R. D.: Blepharophimosis and its association with female infertility. Br. J. Ophthalmol., *68*:533, 1984.

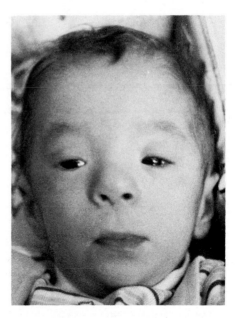

Infant with blepharophimosis syndrome.

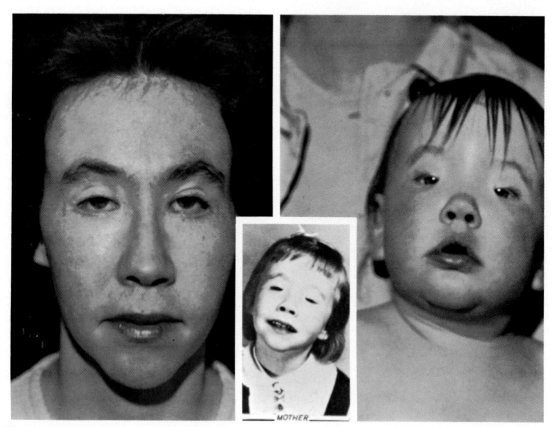

Blepharophimosis syndrome. Mother and infant daughter, with inset of the mother as a child, prior to surgical repair.

ROBIN SEQUENCE

(Pierre Robin Syndrome)

Micrognathia, Glossoptosis, Cleft Soft Palate;
Primary Defect—Early Mandibular Hypoplasia

The single initiating defect of this disorder may be hypoplasia of the mandibular area prior to nine weeks in utero, allowing the tongue to be posteriorly located and thereby impairing the closure of the posterior palatal shelves that must "grow over" the tongue to meet in the midline. The mode of pathogenesis is depicted to the right. The rounded contour of the "cleft" palate in some of these patients (see illustration) is compatible with this mode of developmental pathology and differs from the usual inverted V shape of most palatal clefts. Latham's study of a 17 week old

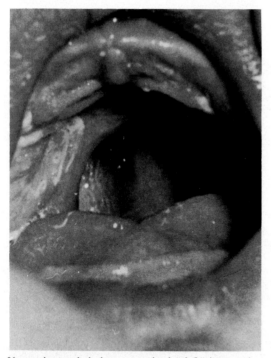

Unusual rounded shape to palatal "cleft" in a patient with the Robin sequence compatible with the incomplete closure of the palate having been secondary to the posterior displacement of the tongue.

fetus with the Robin sequence led him to the same conclusion: that early mandibular retrognathia is the primary anomaly. The posterior airway obstruction may require pulling the tongue forward and/or placing the infant in a head-down slanted position in order to allow for adequate aeration. If aeration is inadequate, the infant usually will fail to thrive and is at risk for the development of cor pulmonale. Poswillo recommends observing the growth of the palatal shelves as long as they continue to develop toward the midline before doing a surgical closure. This may occasionally mean waiting until the patient is three to four years of age to perform surgery on the palate.

The author suggests that this be termed "Robin sequence" rather than Pierre Robin syndrome. The Robin sequence is most commonly noted in otherwise normal individuals, and their prognosis is very good if they survive the early period of respiratory obstruction. Less commonly the sequence may be one feature in a multiple defect syndrome, such as the trisomy 18 syndrome, the Stickler syndrome, or a number of other disorders. It may also be a result of early in utero mechanical constraint, with the chin compressed in such a manner as to limit its growth prior to palatine closure. It is potentially quite misleading if all patients with the Robin sequence are linked together under the designation Robin syndrome, thus including those individuals with multiple primary defects of diverse etiology and prognosis.

References

Dennison, W. M.: The Pierre Robin syndrome. Pediatrics, *36*:336, 1965.
Latham, R. A.: The pathogenesis of cleft palate associated with the Pierre Robin syndrome. Br. J. Plast. Surg., *19*:205, 1966.
Hanson, J. W., and Smith, D. W.: U-shaped palatal defect in the Robin anomalad: developmental and clinical relevance. J. Pediatr., *87*:30, 1975.
Poswillo, D.: Personal communication.

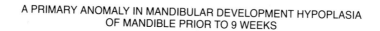

A PRIMARY ANOMALY IN MANDIBULAR DEVELOPMENT HYPOPLASIA
OF MANDIBLE PRIOR TO 9 WEEKS

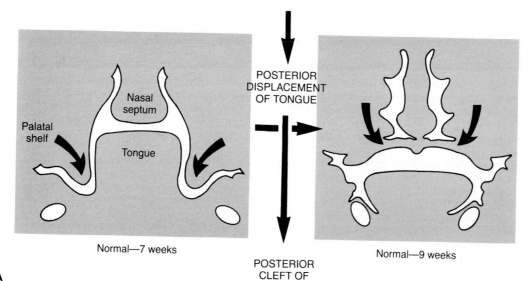

A

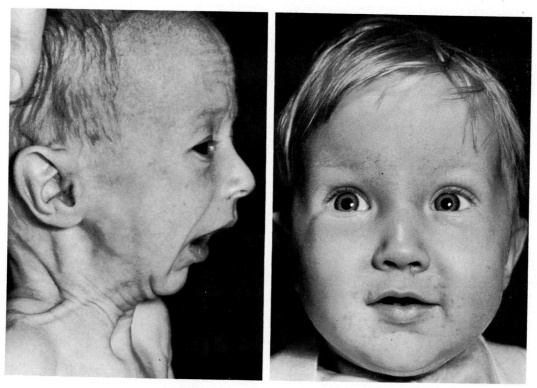

B   **C**

A, Mode of pathogenesis of the Robin sequence. B, Robin sequence with upper respiratory obstruction and failure to thrive in 3 week old (weight, 4.9 lbs [2.2 kg]). C, Same patient at 13 months, showing catch-up in mandibular growth. Patient thriving with normal growth (weight, 14.8 lbs [6.6 kg]).

CLEFT LIP SEQUENCE

Primary Defect—Closure of Lip

By 35 days of uterine age, the lip is normally fused, as illustrated in the figure. A failure of lip fusion, as shown, may impair the subsequent closure of the palatal shelves, which do not completely fuse until the eighth to ninth week. Thus, cleft palate is a frequent association with cleft lip. Other secondary anomalies include defects of tooth development in the area of the cleft lip and incomplete growth of the ala nasi on the side of the cleft. There may be mild ocular hypertelorism, the precise reason for which is undetermined. Tertiary abnormalities can include poor speech and repeated otitis media as a consequence of palatal incompetence and conductive hearing loss.

ETIOLOGY AND RECURRENCE RISK COUNSELING. Usually unknown. May have polygenic inheritance. It is several times more likely to occur in the male. The more severe the defect, the higher the recurrence risk for future siblings. For a unilateral defect, the recurrence risk is 2.7 per cent; for bilateral, it is 5.4 per cent. The following are the general risk figures: affected father, 3 per cent for offspring; affected mother, 14 per cent for offspring; one affected sibling born to unaffected parents, 4 per cent for future siblings; and two affected siblings born to unaffected parents, 10 per cent for future siblings.

COMMENT. Recent reports have documented that as many as 35 per cent of individuals with cleft lip, with or without cleft palate, have the defect as part of a broader pattern of altered morphogenesis. One should identify such individuals prior to using the above figures for recurrence risk counseling. In addition, the underlying diagnosis may well have an impact on prognosis.

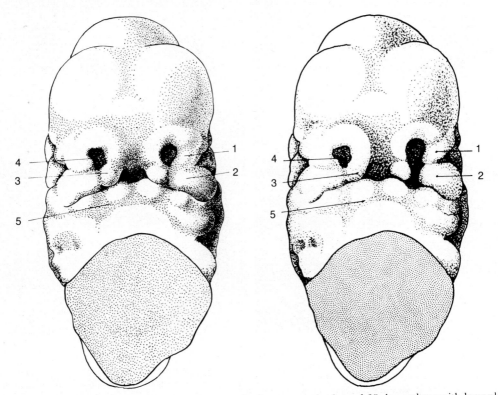

Cleft lip sequence. *Left,* Normal embryo of 35 days. *Right,* Spontaneously aborted 35 day embryo with hypoplasia of the left lateral nasal swelling and, therefore, a cleft lip. 1—lateral nasal swelling; 2—maxillary swelling; 3—medial nasal swelling; 4—nares; 5—mandibular swelling. (Courtesy of Prof. G. Töndury, University of Zurich.)

References

Bixler, D.: Heritability of clefts of the lip and palate. J. Pros. Dent., *33*:100, 1975.

Shprintzen, R. J., et al.: Anomalies associated with cleft lip, cleft palate, or both. Am. J. Med. Genet., *20*:585, 1985.

Jones, M. C.: Etiology of facial clefts: Prospective evaluation of 428 patients. Cleft Palate J. (in press).

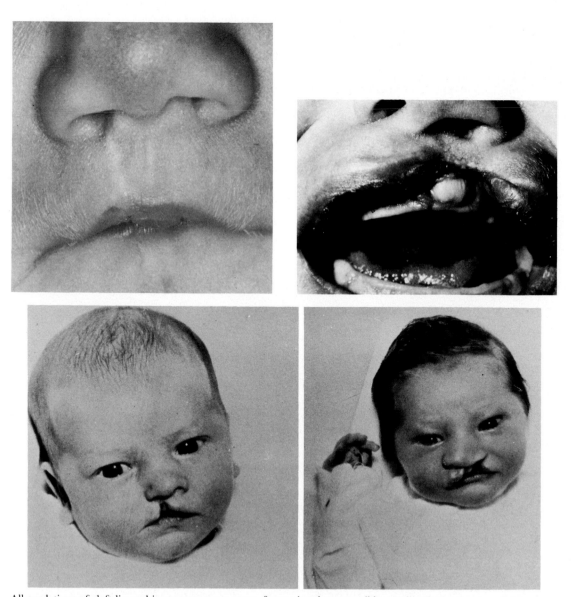

All gradations of cleft lip and its consequences occur, from a barely perceptible scar-like line at the site of closure on the right side (*above left*) to a widely open cleft with secondary consequences of cleft palate, flared ala nasi, and mild ocular hypertelorism (*lower right*). (Upper left photo courtesy of University of Arizona Medical School, Tucson.)

VAN DER WOUDE SYNDROME
(Lip Pit–Cleft Lip Syndrome)

Lower Lip Pit(s),
+/− Cleft Lip, +/− Missing Second Premolars

Originally reported by Van der Woude in 1954.

ABNORMALITIES
Oral. Lower lip pits (80 per cent). Hypodontia, missing central and lateral incisors, canines, and/or bicuspids. Cleft lip with or without cleft palate, cleft palate, cleft uvula.

NATURAL HISTORY. Surgical removal of the fistulas, which represent small accessory salivary glands, is recommended because they may produce a watery mucoid discharge that can be embarrassing for the individual.

ETIOLOGY. Autosomal dominant with about 80 per cent penetrance.

References

Van der Woude, A.: Fistula labii inferioris congenita and its association with cleft lip and palate. Am. J. Hum. Genet., *6*:244, 1954.

Cervenka, J., Gorlin, R. J., and Anderson, V. E.: The syndrome of pits of the lower lip and cleft lip or cleft palate. Genetic considerations. Am. J. Hum. Genet., *19*:416, 1967.

Janku, P., et al.: The van der Woude syndrome in a large kindred: Variability, penetrance, genetic risks. Am. J. Med. Genet., *5*:117, 1980.

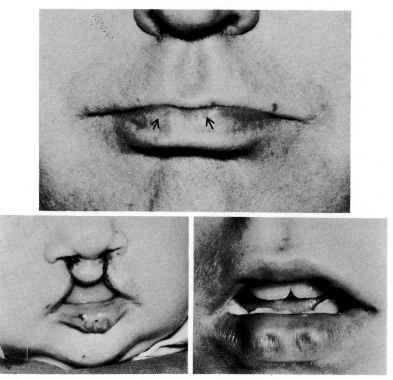

Van der Woude syndrome. Father and his two sons showing lip pits (denoted by arrows for the father), with cleft lip expression in the infant son.

FRONTONASAL DYSPLASIA SEQUENCE

(Median Cleft Face Syndrome)

*Unknown Primary Defect in Midfacial Development
With Incomplete Anterior Appositional Alignment of Eyes*

DeMyer recognized the transitional gradations in severity of this presumed single primary localized defect in 33 cases and termed the pattern of anomaly the median facial cleft syndrome. Sedano et al. subsequently extended these observations and recommended frontonasal dysplasia as a more appropriate designation for this defect. The accompanying figure sets forth a crude interpretation of the developmental pathogenesis and gradations of the sequence.

ABNORMALITIES. Defects that may occur in the more severe cases; the milder cases may have only a few of the defects.
Eyes. Ocular hypertelorism. Lateral displacement of inner canthi.
Forehead. Widow's peak. Deficit in midline frontal bone (cranium bifidum occultum).
Nose. Variability from notched broad nasal tip to completely divided nostrils with hypoplasia to absence of the prolabium and premaxilla with a median cleft lip. Variable notching of alae nasi. Broad nasal root. Lack of formation of nasal tip.

OCCASIONAL ABNORMALITIES. Accessory nasal tags. Midline dermoid lipoma. Microphthalmia.

Preauricular tags, low-set ears, conductive deafness. Mental deficiency. Lipoma of corpus callosum.

NATURAL HISTORY. Depending on the severity of the defect, radical cosmetic surgery is usually merited. The majority of affected individuals are of normal intelligence. DeMyer noted 8 per cent severe mental deficiency and 12 per cent mild impairment of intelligence.

ETIOLOGY. Unknown. Generally a sporadic occurrence; it may occasionally be familial.

References

DeMyer, W.: The median cleft face syndrome. Differential diagnosis of cranium bifidum occultum, hypertelorism, and median cleft nose, lip, and palate. Neurology [Minneap.], *17*:961, 1967.

Sedano, H. O., et al.: Frontonasal dysplasia. J. Pediatr., *76*:906, 1970.

Pascual-Castroviejo, I., Pascual-Pascual, S. I., Perez-Higueras, A.: Fronto-nasal dysplasia and lipoma of the corpus callosum. Eur. J. Pediatr., *144*:66, 1985.

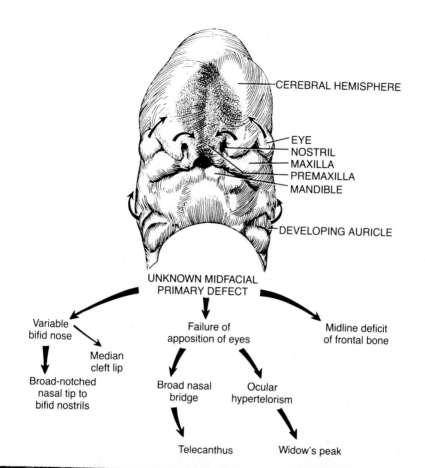

CEREBRAL HEMISPHERE

EYE
NOSTRIL
MAXILLA
PREMAXILLA
MANDIBLE

DEVELOPING AURICLE

UNKNOWN MIDFACIAL
PRIMARY DEFECT

Variable
bifid nose

Median
cleft lip

Broad-notched
nasal tip to
bifid nostrils

Failure of
apposition of eyes

Broad nasal
bridge

Ocular
hypertelorism

Telecanthus

Widow's peak

Midline deficit
of frontal bone

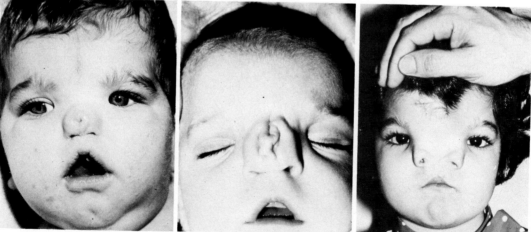

Above, Developmental pathogenesis of the frontonasal dysplasia sequence. *Below*, Affected individuals.

FRASER SYNDROME

(Cryptophthalmos Syndrome)

Cryptophthalmos,* Defect of Auricle,
Genital Anomaly

The association of other multiple malformations in patients with the rare anomaly of cryptophthalmos had been appreciated prior to 1962, when a rather distinctive syndrome found in two sets of siblings was set forth by Fraser. Over 90 patients have been reported. Since cryptophthalmos is not an obligate feature of this disorder, it is more appropriately termed Fraser syndrome.

ABNORMALITIES

Facial. Cryptophthalmos, usually with defect of eye. Hair growth on lateral forehead extending to lateral eyebrow. Hypoplastic notched nares. Broad nose with depressed bridge. Ear anomaly, most commonly cupped.

Performance. Mental deficiency.

Limbs. Partial cutaneous syndactyly.

Genitalia. Incomplete development. Male: hypospadias, cryptorchidism. Female: bicornuate uterus, vaginal atresia. Clitoromegaly.

Other. Laryngeal stenosis or atresia. Renal agenesis.

OCCASIONAL ABNORMALITIES. Midline groove toward nasal tip. Unilateral absence of a nostril. Cleft lip, with or without cleft palate, and cleft palate. Dental malocclusion and crowding. Bony skull defects. Hypertelorism, lacrimal duct defect, partial midfacial cleft, atresia of external ear, defect of middle ear, fusion of superior helix to

*Cryptophthalmos (hidden eye) fundamentally means absence of the palpebral fissure but usually includes varying absence of eyelashes and eyebrows and defects of the eye, especially the anterior part.

scalp, microtia, laryngeal stenosis or atresia, widely spaced nipples, umbilical anomaly, anal atresia, cardiac defects, thymic aplasia/hypoplasia, diastasis of symphysis pubis, partial absence of sternum, absent phalanges.

NATURAL HISTORY. This disorder should be considered in stillborn babies with renal agenesis. Because the defect of eyelid development is frequently accompanied by ocular anomaly, the likelihood of achieving adequate visual perception is small, although early surgical intervention was of value in one case.

ETIOLOGY. Autosomal recessive. There is etiologic heterogeneity for the cryptophthalmos anomaly. A number of individuals with isolated cryptophthalmos who do not have the Fraser syndrome have been reported.

References

Fraser, C. R.: Our genetical "load." A review of some aspects of genetical variation. Ann. Hum. Genet., *25*:387, 1962.

Gupta, S. P., and Saxena, R. C.: Cryptophthalmos. Br. J. Ophthalmol., *46*:629, 1962.

Azvedo, E. S., Biondi, J., and Ramaldo, L. M.: Cryptophthalmos in two families. J. Med. Genet., *10*:389, 1973.

Mortimer, G., McEwen, H. P., and Yates, J. R. W.: Fraser syndrome presenting as monozygous twins with bilateral renal agenesis. J. Med. Genet., *22*:76, 1985.

Thomas, I. T., et al.: Isolated and syndromic cryptophthalmos. Am. J. Med. Genet., *25*:85, 1986.

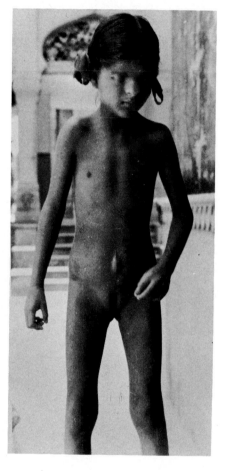

Fraser syndrome. A genetic male with cryptophthalmos, malformed ears with atresia of external auditory canals, aberrant umbilicus, and incomplete development of external genitalia. (Courtesy of S. P. Gupta, University of Lucknow, India.)

MELNICK-FRASER SYNDROME
(Branchio-Oto-Renal [BOR] Syndrome)

The association of branchial arch anomalies (preauricular pits, branchial fistulas), hearing loss, and renal hypoplasia constitutes the branchio-oto-renal syndrome first described by Melnick et al. in 1975 and further delineated by Fraser et al. The prevalence is roughly 1:40,000. The syndrome occurs in about 2 per cent of profoundly deaf children.

ABNORMALITIES

Hearing loss	89%
Preauricular pits	77%
Branchial fistulas or cysts	63%
Anomalous pinna	41%
Malformed middle and/or inner ear	? %
Lacrimal duct stenosis/aplasia	? %
Renal dysplasia	66%

OTHER ABNORMALITIES. Long, narrow face, "constricted palate," deep overbite, and facial paralysis may occur.

NATURAL HISTORY. The ear pits or branchial clefts may go unnoticed until the hearing loss appears, or they may become infected and require surgery. The hearing loss may be sensorineural (25 per cent), conductive (25 per cent), or mixed (50 per cent) and ranges from mild to severe. Age of onset can be from early childhood to young adulthood, and hearing loss is occasionally precipitous. There may be malformations of the middle ear, vestibular system, and cochlea, including displaced, malformed, or fused ossicles and the Mondini malformation of the cochlea. Defects of the external ear range from severe microtia to minor anomalies of the pinna, which is variously described as cup- or loop-shaped, flattened, or hypoplastic. The external canal can be narrow, slanted upward, or malformed, making otoscopic examination difficult.

The renal anomalies range from minor dysplasia (sharply tapered superior poles, blunting of calyces, duplication of the collecting system) to bilateral renal agenesis with renal failure in about 6 per cent of patients.

ETIOLOGY. An autosomal dominant gene with high penetrance and variable expression.

COMMENTS. The probability that a newborn child with a preauricular pit will have profound hearing loss is about 1:200. A preauricular pit or branchial cleft in a deaf child is a strong indication for renal investigation, and since renal dysplasia can be detected prenatally, carriers of the BOR gene are candidates for prenatal diagnosis.

References

Melnick, M., et al.: Autosomal dominant branchio-oto-renal dysplasia. Birth Defects Original Article Series, *XI*(5):121, 1975.

Fraser, F. C., et al.: Genetic aspects of the BOR syndrome—branchial fistulas, ear pits, hearing loss, and renal anomalies. Am. J. Med. Genet., 2:241, 1978.

Fraser, F. C., Sproule, J. R., and Halal, F.: Frequency of the branchio-oto-renal (BOR) syndrome in children with profound hearing loss. Am. J. Med. Genet., 7:341, 1980.

Heimler, A., and Lieber, E.: Branchio-oto-renal syndrome: Reduced penetrance and variable expressivity in four generations of a large kindred. Am. J. Med. Genet., *25*:15, 1986.

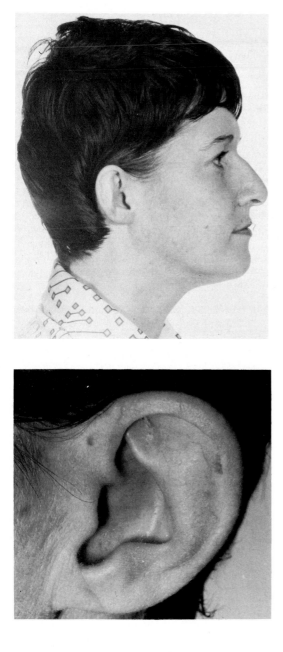

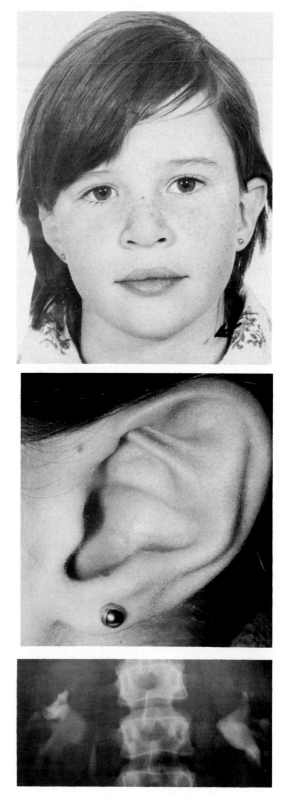

Melnick-Fraser syndrome. *Upper left*, Note mildly altered auricle. *Upper right*, Note small branchial fistula (*arrow*). *Middle*, Preauricular pits and mildly altered ear form. *Lower right*, Roentgenographic evidence of renal dysplasia. (Courtesy of Dr. F. Clarke Fraser, McGill Center for Human Genetics, Montreal, Quebec.)

WAARDENBURG SYNDROME, TYPES I AND II

Lateral Displacement of Medial Canthi, Partial Albinism, Deafness

Waardenburg set forth this pattern of malformation in 1951. He found this syndrome in 1.4 per cent of congenitally deaf children and from these data estimated the incidence to be about 1:42,000 in Holland. Among the more than 1000 cases that have been reported, Hageman and Delleman have distinguished two different disorders; in type I, there is lateral displacement of the inner canthi, whereas in type II, there is not.

ABNORMALITIES. Lateral displacement of inner canthi. Broad and high nasal bridge with hypoplastic alae nasi. Medial flare of eyebrows, which may meet in midline. Partial albinism. Deafness. Broad mandible.

OCCASIONAL ABNORMALITIES. Rounded tip of nose, full lips with accentuated "Cupid's bow" to upper lip, cleft lip and palate, cardiac anomaly (ventricular septal defect), upper limb defect, Hirschsprung aganglionosis. Sprengel's anomaly, supernumery vertebrae and ribs, spina bifida, scoliosis.

NATURAL HISTORY. The partial albinism is most commonly expressed as a white forelock and/or isochromic beautiful pale blue eyes with hypoplastic iridic stroma; however, it may be present as heterochromia of the iris, areas of vitiligo on the skin, patches of white hair other than the forelock, and/or mottled peripheral pigmentation of the retina. The white forelock may be present at birth only to become pigmented early in life; the hair may become prematurely gray or white.

Deafness is the most serious feature, and if present, is usually bilateral and severe. The defect appears to be in the organ of Corti, with atrophic changes in the spiral ganglion and nerve. Deafness is a feature in 25 per cent of type I cases (with lateral displacement of inner canthi) and in about 50 per cent of type II cases.

ETIOLOGY. Autosomal dominant for both type I and type II. Five of the 16 propositi of Waardenburg were considered to represent fresh mutations, a calculated mutation rate of 0.4×10^{-5} per gamete. Older paternal age has been a factor in the fresh mutation cases.

COMMENT. The association of dominantly inherited albinism and deafness was noted in cats as early as 1769 and subsequently in the horse and several types of dog.

References

Waardenburg, P. J.: A new syndrome combining developmental anomalies of the eyelids, eyebrows and nose root with pigmentary defects of the iris and head hair and with congenital deafness. Am. J. Hum. Genet., *3*:195, 1951.

DiGeorge, A. M., Olmsted, R. W., and Harley, R. D.: Waardenburg's syndrome. J. Pediatr., *57*:649, 1960.

Hageman, M. J., and Delleman, J. W.: Heterogeneity in Waardenburg syndrome. Am. J. Hum. Genet., *29*:468, 1977.

Klein, D.: Historical background and evidence for dominant inheritance of the Klein-Waardenburg syndrome (type III). Am. J. Med. Genet., *14*:231, 1983.

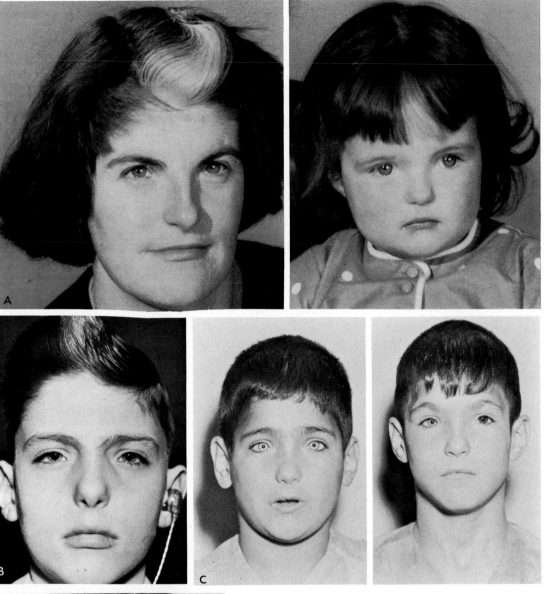

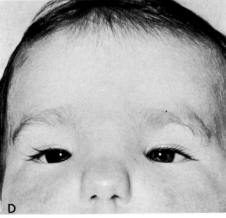

Waardenburg syndrome. *A*, Mother and daughter. Note the isochromic light iris. (From Partington, M. W.: Arch. Dis. Child., *34*:154, 1959.) *B*, Ten year old with congenital deafness. Note prominent nasal root, small alae nasi. (From DiGeorge, A. M., et al.: J. Pediatr., *57*:649, 1960.) *C*, Brothers, only one of whom has deafness. Note the lack of a white forelock. *D*, Four month old infant who had a white forelock at birth that is now pigmented. Note heterochromia of irises, lateral placement of inner canthi, and small alae nasi.

TREACHER COLLINS SYNDROME

(Mandibulofacial Dysostosis, Franceschetti-Klein Syndrome)

Malar Hypoplasia with Downslanting Palpebral Fissures, Defect of Lower Lid, Malformation of External Ear

Although Thomson reported the first case in 1846, the syndrome has been associated with Treacher Collins, who described two cases in 1900. Franceschetti and Klein made extensive reports on this condition and called it mandibulofacial dysostosis (1940s). More than 250 cases have been reported.

ABNORMALITIES

Antimongoloid slanting palpebral fissures	89%
Malar hypoplasia, +/− cleft in zygomatic bone	81%
Mandibular hypoplasia	78%
Lower lid coloboma	69%
Partial to total absence of lower eyelashes	53%
Malformation of auricles	77%
External ear canal defect	36%
Conductive deafness	40%
Cleft palate	28%
Incompetent soft palate	32%
Projection of scalp hair onto lateral cheek	26%

OCCASIONAL ABNORMALITIES. Pharyngeal hypoplasia. Coloboma of the upper lid. Microphthalmia. Macrostomia. Microstomia. Choanal atresia. Blind fistulas and skin tags between auricle and angle of the mouth. Absence of the parotid gland. Congenital heart defect. Cryptorchidism. Mental deficiency has been reported in only 5 per cent of the cases.

NATURAL HISTORY. These patients can develop early respiratory problems as a result of having a narrow airway and may occasionally require temporary tracheostomy. The narrow airway may make intubation difficult. As the great majority of these patients are of normal intelligence, the early recognition of deafness and its correction with hearing aids or surgery (when possible) are of great importance for development.

The growth of the facial bones during infancy and childhood results in some cosmetic improvement that may be enhanced by plastic surgery.

ETIOLOGY. Autosomal dominant, with 60 per cent of the cases representing presumed fresh mutations. Analysis of affected families shows a regular autosomal dominant inheritance with almost 100 per cent penetrance. An excess of affected offspring from affected females and of normal offspring from affected males has been found. There is wide variability in expression but moderate similarity within a given sibship. Prenatal diagnosis has been accomplished successfully in two instances utilizing fetoscopy.

COMMENT. The wide variance in expression that allows for different clinical forms of the condition has led to erroneous interpretations of some cases, which have been described as separate entities. Franceschetti and Klein have emphasized this phenotypic variability.

References

Thomson, A: Notice of several cases of malformation of the external ear, together with experiments on the state of hearing in such persons. Month. J. Med. Sci., 7:420, 1846.

Treacher Collins, E.: Case with symmetrical congenital notches in the outer part of each lower lid and defective development of the malar bones. Trans. Opthalmol. Soc. U.K., 20:90, 1900.

Franceschetti, A., and Klein, D.: The Mandibulofacial Dysostosis, A New Hereditary Syndrome. Copenhagen, E. Munksgaard, 1949.

Peterson-Falzone, S., and Pruzansky, S.: Cleft palate and congenital palatopharyngeal incompetency in mandibulofacial dysostosis. Cleft Palate J., 13:354, 1976.

Shprintzen, R. J., and Berkman, M. D.: Pharyngeal hypoplasia in Treacher Collins syndrome. Arch. Otolaryngol., 105:127, 1979.

Nicolaides, K. H., et al.: Prenatal diagnosis of mandibulofacial dysostosis. Prenat. Diagn., 4:201, 1984.

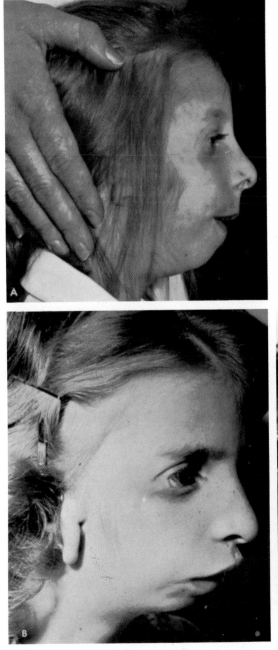

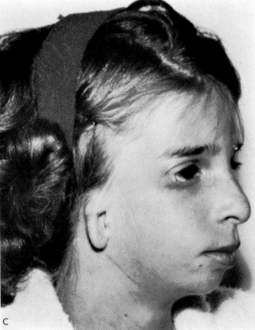

Treacher-Collins syndrome. *A*, Six year old. Note the hair extending onto the lateral cheek. *B*, Preadolescent girl. Note the defect of lower eyelid and the malar hypoplasia. *C*, Same as *B*, postadolescent. Note the improvement in cosmetic appearance after a sliding osteotomy to the mandible and plastic surgery to the rudimentary auricle.

MARSHALL SYNDROME

In 1958 Marshall described seven family members in three generations with a disorder characterized by cataracts, sensorineural deafness, and an extremely short nose with a flat bridge. Subsequently, more than 20 cases have been reported.

ABNORMALITIES

Growth. Short stature.

Facies. Short depressed nose with flat nasal bridge and anteverted nares. Appearance of large eyes. Flat midface. Prominent, protruding upper incisors. Thick lips.

Eyes. Myopia. Cataracts. Esotropia.

Hearing. Sensorineural deafness.

Skeletal. Calvarial thickening. Absent frontal sinuses. Falx, tentorial, and meningeal calcifications. Spondyloephiphyseal abnormalities including mild platyspondyly, slightly small and irregular distal femoral and proximal tibial epiphyses, outward bowing of radius and ulna, and wide tufts of distal phalanges.

OCCASIONAL ABNORMALITIES. Mental deficiency. Retinal detachment. Cleft palate.

NATURAL HISTORY. The cataracts may spontaneously resorb, leading to glaucoma and/or lens dislocation.

ETIOLOGY. Autosomal dominant.

References

Marshall, D.: Ectodermal dysplasia. Report of a kindred with ocular abnormalities and hearing defect. Am. J. Ophthalmol., *45*:143, 1958.

Zellweger, H., Smith, J. K., and Grützner, P.: The Marshall syndrome: report of a new family. J. Pediatr., *84*:868, 1974.

O'Donnell, J. J., Sirkin, S., Hall, B. D.: Generalized osseous anormalities in the Marshall syndrome. Birth Defects Original Article Series, *XII*(5):299, 1976.

Aymé, S., Preus, M.: The Marshall and Stickler syndromes: objective rejection of lumping. J. Med. Genet., *21*:34, 1984.

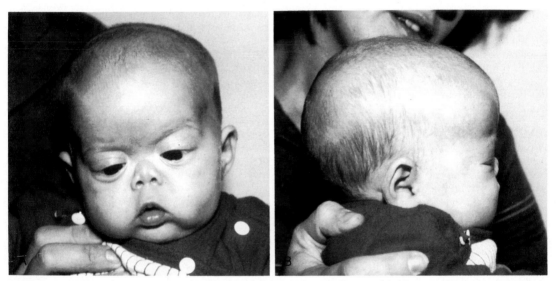

Marshall syndrome. *A, B,* One year old with short depressed nose, flat nasal bridge, anteverted nares, and the appearance of large eyes.

H

H. FACIAL-LIMB DEFECTS AS MAJOR FEATURE

MILLER SYNDROME

(Postaxial Acrofacial Dysostosis Syndrome)

Treacher Collins–Like Facies,
Limb Deficiency, Especially Postaxial

In 1979, Miller et al. brought together six cases, four of which were from the literature, and recognized this disorder as a concise entity. The facies is similar to that of Treacher Collins syndrome and, in combination with limb defects, resembles Nager syndrome. The severity of the postaxial deficiencies distinguishes it from the latter syndrome.

ABNORMALITIES. Noted in three or more of the six patients.
Craniofacial. Malar hypoplasia, sometimes with radiologic evidence of a vertical bony cleft, with downslanting palpebral fissures. Colobomata of eyelids and ectropion. Micrognathia. Cleft lip and/or cleft palate. Hypoplastic, cup-shaped ears.
Limbs. Limb deficiencies, most severe on the postaxial side of the limbs, often including the radii and ulnae as well as the digits. Syndactyly. Low arch dermal ridge patterning.
Other. Accessory nipple(s).

OCCASIONAL ABNORMALITIES. Heart defect, conductive hearing loss.

NATURAL HISTORY. These individuals are usually of normal intelligence. Multiple facial plastic surgery procedures are usually warranted on a cosmetic basis.

ETIOLOGY. Occurrence of affected siblings of opposite sex of unaffected parents in the family followed by Dr. Robert Fineman of the University of Utah Medical School has implicated autosomol recessive inheritance for this disorder.

References

Genée, E.: Une forme extensive de dysostose mandibulofaciale. J. Genet. Hum., *17*:45, 1969.
Smith, D. W., Pashayan, H., and Wildervanck, L. S.: Case Report 28. Syndrome Ident. *3*(1):7, 1975.
Miller, M., Fineman, R., and Smith, D. W.: Postaxial acrofacial dysostosis syndrome. J. Pediatr., *95*:970, 1979.

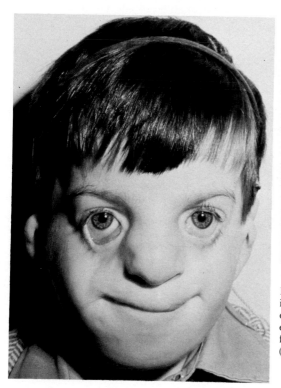

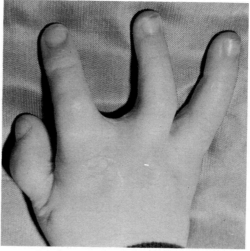

Miller syndrome. Affected individual showing striking malar and maxillary hypoplasia and lower lid defects. Note the hearing aid, required for middle ear deafness. The deficiency in the hand is complete for the fifth ray and incomplete for the other digits. (From Miller, M., et al.: J. Pediatr., *95*:970, 1979.)

NAGER SYNDROME
(Nager Acrofacial Dysostosis Syndrome)

*Radial Limb Hypoplasia, Malar Hypoplasia,
Ear Defects*

Nager and deReynier described a Treacher Collins syndrome–like patient with radial limb defects in 1948, and subsequently at least 22 cases have been recognized.

ABNORMALITIES
Performance. Intelligence normal. Conductive deafness and problems with articulation.
Craniofacial. Malar hypoplasia with downslanting palpebral fissures, micrognathia, partial to total absence of lower eyelashes, varying degrees of auricular deficiency, preauricular tags, atresia of external ear canal, cleft palate.
Limbs. Hypoplasia to aplasia of thumb, +/− radius. Proximal radioulnar synostosis and limitation of elbow extension. Short forearms.

OCCASIONAL ABNORMALITIES. Lower lid coloboma. Projection of scalp hair onto lateral cheek. Missing toe. Overlapping toes. Syndactyly of toes. Absent distal flexion creases on toes. Hip dislocation. Clubfeet. Hypoplastic first rib. Tetralogy of Fallot.

NATURAL HISTORY. The recommendations for early detection of deafness, hearing aid augmentation, and plastic surgery are similar to those for Treacher Collins syndrome. Early respiratory and feeding problems may occur. Premature delivery and perinatal mortality are relatively high, the latter perhaps related to upper airway hypoplasia, which has recently been described in one patient.

ETIOLOGY. Unknown. Walker reported one set of mildly affected siblings of unaffected parents, raising the question of autosomal recessive inheritance.

References

Nager, F. R., and deReynier, J. P.: Das Gehörogan bei den angeborenen Kopfmissbildungen. Pract. Oto-rhinolaryngol. (Basal), *10* (Suppl. 2):1, 1948.

Bowen, P., and Harley, F. Mandibulofacial dysostosis with limb malformations (Nager's acrofacial dysostosis). Birth Defects Original Article Series, *X*(5):109, 1974.

Walker, F.: Apparent autosomal recessive inheritance of Treacher-Collins syndrome. Birth Defects Original Article Series, *X*(8):0135, 1974.

Meyerson, M. D., et al.: Nager acrofacial dysostosis: early intervention and long-term planning. Cleft Palate J., *14*:35, 1977.

Halal, F., et al.: Differential diagnosis of Nager acrofacial dysostosis syndrome: Report of four patients with Nager syndrome and discussion of other related syndromes. Am. J. Med. Genet., *14*:209, 1983.

Krauss, C. M., Hassell, L. A., Gang, D. L.: Brief clinical report: Anomalies in an infant with Nager acrofacial dysostosis. Am. J. Med. Genet., *21*:761, 1985.

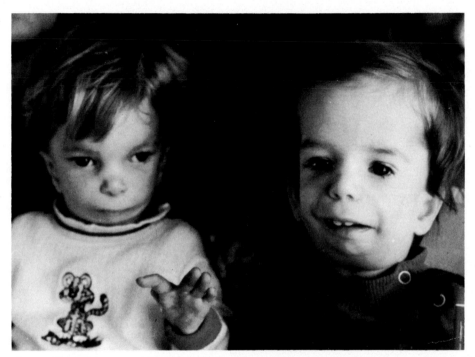

Nager syndrome. Unrelated young girl and boy showing the facies and hypoplasia of the thumb. (From Meyerson, M. D., et al.: Cleft Palate J., *14*:35, 1977.)

TOWNES SYNDROME

*Thumb Anomalies, Auricular Anomalies,
Anal Anomalies*

Townes and Brocks first described this disorder in 1972, and at least 36 affected individuals were reported by 1978.

ABNORMALITIES

Craniofacial. Auricular anomalies varying from large ears to poorly formed ears to microtia. Variable features of hemifacial microsomia. especially preauricular tags.

Limbs. Thumb anomalies varying from hypoplasia to finger-like, triphalangeal, or supernumerary thumb. Pseudoepiphysis of second metacarpals. Fusion of triquetrum and hamate. Fusion and/or short metatarsals. Prominence of distal ends of lateral metatarsals. Absent or hypoplastic third toe. Clinodactyly of fifth toe.

Anus. Anal defects including imperforate anus, anterior placement, and stenosis.

Renal. Anomalies, from renal hypoplasia to ureterovesical reflux to urethral valves.

OCCASIONAL ABNORMALITIES. Deafness. Preauricular pit. Cardiac defect. Duodenal atresia. Cystic ovary.

ETIOLOGY. Autosomal dominant with marked variability in the severity of expression for each feature.

COMMENT. It is of interest that this single gene disorder encompasses many of the features of both the VATER association and the facio-auriculo-vertebral malformation sequence.

References

Townes, P. L., and Brocks, E. R.: Hereditary syndrome of imperforate anus with hand, foot and ear anomalies. J. Pediatr., *81*:321, 1972.

Reid, I. S., and Turner, G.: Familial anal abnormality. J. Pediatr., *88*:992, 1976.

Kurnit, D. M., et al.: Autosomal dominant transmission of a syndrome of anal, ear, renal and radial congenital malformations. J. Pediatr., *93*:270, 1978.

Walpole, I. R., and Hockey, A.: Syndrome of imperforate anus, abnormalities of hands and feet, satyr ears, and sensorineural deafness. J. Pediatr., *100*:250, 1982.

Monteiro de Pino-Neto, J.: Phenotypic variability in Townes-Brocks syndrome. Am. J. Med. Genet., *18*:147, 1984.

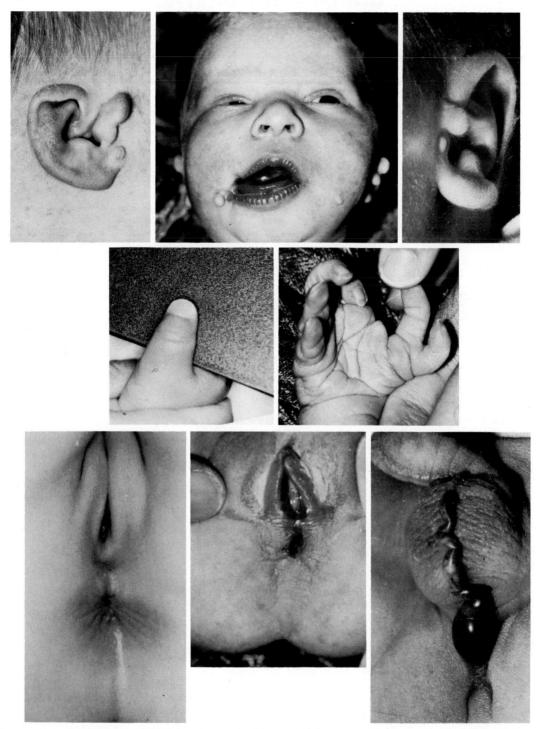

Townes syndrome. Variation of facial morphogenesis with preauricular tags and features resembling Facio-Auriculo-Vertebral sequence (Hemifacial Microsomia Goldenhar s.). Note the alterations of thumb development, from hypoplasia to supernumerary and finger-like thumb, and of anal development, from altered placement to imperforate anus. (Left side and lower right side photos are courtesy of Dr. Gillian Turner, Prince of Wales Hospital, Sydney, Australia.)

ORAL-FACIAL-DIGITAL SYNDROME

(OFD Syndrome, Type I)

Oral Frenula and Clefts,
Hypoplasia of Alae Nasi, Digital Asymmetry

Papillon-Léage and Psaume set this condition forth as a clinical entity in 1954. More than 130 cases have been reported.

ABNORMALITIES

Oral. Webbing between buccal mucous membrane and alveolar ridge. Partial clefts in mid-upper lip, tongue, alveolar ridges (at area of lateral incisors, which may be missing), between premaxilla and lateral hard palate, with or without irregular complete cleft of soft palate. Dental caries and anomalous anterior teeth. Absent lateral incisors.

Facial. Hypoplasia of alar cartilages, lateral placement of inner canthi. Milia of ears and upper face in infancy.

Digital. Asymmetric shortening of digits with clinodactyly, with or without syndactyly, brachydactyly, and/or polydactyly.

Scalp. Dry, rough, sparse hair and dry scalp.

CNS. Variable; mental deficiency in about 57 per cent, with average I.Q. of 70. Brain malformation, including absence of corpus callosum and heterotopia of gray matter, in about 20 per cent of patients.

Cranium. Increased naso-sella-basion angle at base of cranium.

Renal. Autopsy finding of microcysts (7/9).

OCCASIONAL ABNORMALITIES

Oral. Enamel hypoplasia, supernumerary teeth, hamartoma of tongue, fistula in lower lip. Choanal atresia.

Facial. Frontal bossing. Hypoplastic mandibular ramus and zygoma.

Digital. Polydactyly of the foot.

Skeletal. Nonprogressive metaphyseal rarefaction.

CNS. Trembling, hydrocephalus, seizures. Malformation of brain in 20 per cent of necropsies.

Hair. Alopecia.

Skin. Granular seborrheic skin.

Renal. Polycystic renal disease.

NATURAL HISTORY. Patients may do poorly in early infancy; as many as one third die during this period. Management is directed toward plastic surgical correction of oral clefts and dental care, including dentures when indicated. Psychometric evaluation is merited because about one half of the reported patients have mental deficiency.

ETIOLOGY. Dominant mutant gene with a lethal effect in the XY male. The ratio of female to male offspring of affected women has been 2:1, and no affected woman has been known to have a son with the OFD syndrome. Therefore, the risk for the OFD mother of having an affected offspring is one in three. Present data do not allow for a distinction between an X-linked gene, lethal in the hemizygote, and an autosomal mutant, which is an early lethal in the male.

References

Papillon-Léage, Mme., and Psaume, J.: Une malformation héréditaire de la muqueuse buccale: brides et freins anormaux. Rev. Stomatol. (Paris), 55:209, 1954.

Gorlin, R. J., and Psaume, J.: Orodigitofacial dysostosis—a new syndrome. J. Pediatr., 61:520, 1962.

Doege, T. C., et al.: Studies of a family with the oral-facial-digital syndrome. N. Engl. J. Med. 271:1073, 1964.

Majewski, F., et al.: Das oro-facio-digitale Syndrom. Symptome und Prognose. Z. Kinderheilkd., 112:89, 1972.

Whelan, D. T., Feldman, W., and Dost, I.: The oro-facial-digital syndrome. Clin. Genet., 8:205, 1975.

Jacquemart, C. J., et al.: The oral-facial-digital syndromes reviewed: The role of computerized axial tomography in management. Arizona Med., 37:261, 1980.

Annerén, G., et al.: Oro-facial-digital syndrome I and II: Radiological methods for diagnosis and the clinical variations. Clin. Genet., 26:178, 1984.

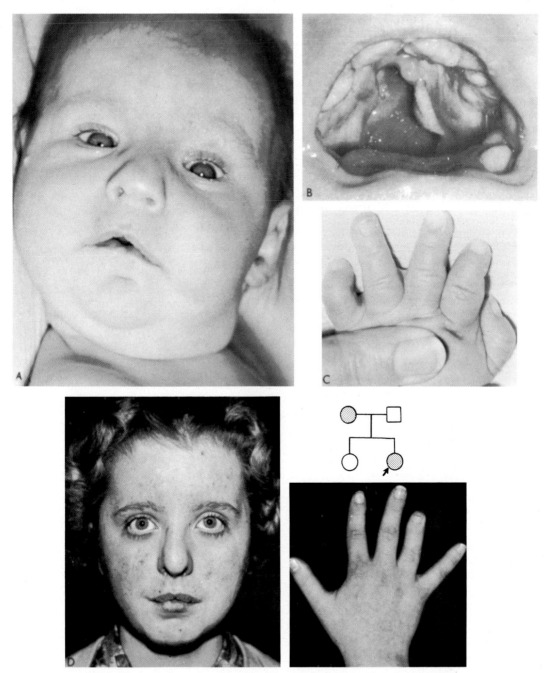

Oral-facial-digital syndrome. *A*, Young infant of a normal mother. *B*, Irregular clefts in alveolar ridge, palate, and tongue. *C*, Short third finger; partial syndactyly of third and fourth fingers. *D*, Seventeen year old daughter of affected mother.

MOHR SYNDROME

(OFD Syndrome, Type II)

*Cleft Tongue, Conductive Deafness,
Partial Reduplication of Hallux*

Mohr described this pattern in several male siblings in 1941, and at least 16 cases have been reported.

ABNORMALITIES

General. Mild shortness of stature. Conductive deafness due apparently to defect of incus.

Facies and Mouth. Low nasal bridge with lateral displacement of inner canthi. Broad nasal tip, sometimes slightly bifid. Midline partial cleft of lip. Hypertrophy of usual frenula. Midline cleft of tongue, nodules on tongue. Flare to alveolar ridge. Hypoplasia of zygomatic arch, maxilla, and body of mandible.

Limbs. Partial reduplication of hallux and first metatarsal, cuneiform and cuboid bones. Relatively short hands with clinodactyly of fifth finger. Polydactyly. Metaphyseal flaring and irregularity.

OCCASIONAL ABNORMALITIES. Wormian cranial bones, missing central incisors, cleft palate, pectus excavatum, scoliosis. Mental deficiency.

NATURAL HISTORY. These patients apparently have normal intelligence, and plastic surgery is indicated for the clefts, frenula, and partial reduplication of the hallux. A surgical attempt to reconstruct the auditory ossicles was unsuccessful in one case.

ETIOLOGY. Presumed autosomal recessive.

COMMENT. The condition may easily be confused with the oral-facial-digital syndrome.

References

Mohr, O. L.: A hereditary sublethal syndrome in man. Skr. Norske Vidensk. Akad., I. Mat. Naturv. Klasse, *14*:3, 1941.

Rimoin, D. L., and Edgerton, M. T.: Genetic and clinical heterogeneity in the oral-facial-digital syndromes. J. Pediatr., *71*:94, 1967.

Pfeiffer, R. A., Majewski, F., and Mannkopf, H.: Das syndrome von Mohr und Classen. Klin. Paediatr., *184*:224, 1972.

Levy, E. P., Fletcher, B. D., and Fraser, F. C.: Mohr syndrome with subclinical expression of the bifid great toe. Am. J. Dis. Child, *128*:531, 1974.

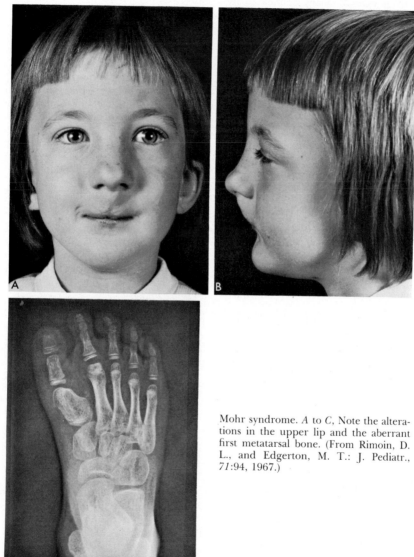

Mohr syndrome. *A* to *C*, Note the altera-tions in the upper lip and the aberrant first metatarsal bone. (From Rimoin, D. L., and Edgerton, M. T.: J. Pediatr., *71*:94, 1967.)

SHPRINTZEN SYNDROME

(Velo-Cardio-Facial Syndrome)

This syndrome was recognized by Shprintzen et al. in 1978, with at least 39 cases delineated by 1980. Since the patients were predominantly evaluated at craniofacial centers, there is a bias toward those with palatal defects.

ABNORMALITIES

Performance. Learning disabilities; mild intellectual impairment (approximately 50 per cent); I.Q. generally ranges from 70 to 90, with some slightly higher.

Growth. Smaller stature, usually below tenth percentile; microsomia in 30 to 40 per cent of patients.

Ears and Hearing. Conductive hearing loss secondary to cleft palate; minor auricular anomalies.

Craniofacial. Cleft of the secondary palate, either overt or submucous; prominent nose with squared nasal root and narrow alar base; narrow palpebral fissures; abundant scalp hair; deficient malar area; vertical maxillary excess with long face; retruded mandible with chin deficiency; microcephaly (40 to 50 per cent).

Limbs. Slender and hypotonic with hyperextensible hands and fingers.

Cardiac. Ventricular septal defect (70 to 75 per cent); right aortic arch (40 to 50 per cent); tetralogy of Fallot (15 to 20 per cent); aberrant left subclavian artery (15 to 20 per cent).

OCCASIONAL ABNORMALITIES. Robin malformation sequence; other types of cardiac defect; scoliosis; umbilical or inguinal hernia; cryptorchidism; hypospadias; laryngeal web. Small optic discs with tortuous vessels and cataracts. Holoprosencephaly.

NATURAL HISTORY. Hypotonia in infancy is frequent (70 to 80 per cent). Speech development is often delayed, and language is impaired. Speech is almost always hypernasal, with the pharyngeal musculature being hypotonic. Socialization skills may surpass intellectual skills. Personality may tend toward perseverative behavior, with concrete thinking secondary to intellectual impairment or learning disorders. Obstructive sleep apnea has been noted following pharyngeal surgery to improve speech in several patients.

ETIOLOGY. Autosomal dominant.

References

Shprintzen, R. J., et al.: A new syndrome involving cleft palate, cardiac anomalies, typical facies, and learning disabilities; velo-cardio-facial syndrome. Cleft Palate J., *15*:56, 1978.

Young, D., Shprintzen, R. J., and Goldberg, R. B.: Cardiac malformations in the velo-cardio-facial syndrome. Am. J. Cardiol., *46*:643, 1980.

Shprintzen, R. J., et al.: The velo-cardio-facial syndrome: A clinical and genetic analysis. Pediatrics, *67*:167, 1981.

Fitch, N.: Velo-cardio-facial syndrome and eye abnormality. Am. J. Med. Genet., *15*:699, 1983.

Williams, M. A., Shprintzen, R. J., and Goldberg, R. B.: Male-to-male transmission of the velo-cardio-facial syndrome: A case report and review of 60 cases. J. Craniofac. Genet. Dev. Biol., *5*:175, 1985.

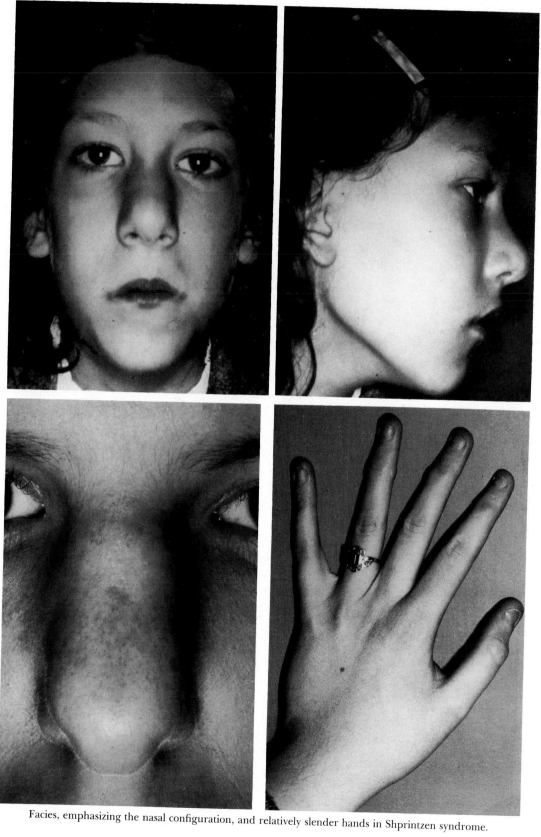

Facies, emphasizing the nasal configuration, and relatively slender hands in Shprintzen syndrome.

RUVALCABA SYNDROME

Hypoplastic Alae Nasi,
Small Mouth, Short Metacarpals

In 1971, Ruvalcaba et al. reported a striking syndrome in two brothers whose maternal female first cousins were said to be similarly affected but to a milder degree. Later, in 1977, Hunter et al. reported a " 'New' Syndrome of Mental Retardation with Characteristic Facies and Brachyphalangy" in three generations of one family that showed similar characteristics. Hunter considers that the patients he described represent a disorder different from that described by Ruvalcaba. Further recognition of affected families may allow for a better answer to this question.

ABNORMALITIES
Growth. Prenatal onset growth deficiency, with late adolescence.
Performance. Mental deficiency of variable degree; jovial personality.
Craniofacial. Microcephaly, small alae nasi, small mouth with thin lips, narrow maxilla with crowded teeth.
Limbs. Brachyphalangy with short lateral metacarpals and metatarsals, fusion of some carpal bones, fifth finger clinodactyly. Short limbs with short hands and feet. Limitation of complete joint extension.
Other Skeletal. Spondylodysplasia, pectus carinatum, narrow trunk, kyphoscoliosis.
Genitalia. Cryptorchidism. Small testes.

OCCASIONAL ABNORMALITIES. Downslanting palpebral fissures, craniosynostosis, cardiac defect, areas of hypoplastic skin, seizures, inguinal hernia. Retinal degeneration.

ETIOLOGY. Unknown. There are unaffected "carriers," and one possibility is that of a small and difficult-to-detect translocation chromosomal abnormality. Autosomal dominant with variable expression and lack of penetrance is not excluded, whereas male to male transmission excludes X-linkage.

References

Ruvalcaba, R. H. A., Reichert, A., and Smith, D. W.: A new familial syndrome with osseous dysplasia and mental deficiency. J. Pediatr., *79*:450, 1971.

Hunter, A. G. W., et al.: "New" syndrome of mental retardation with characteristic facies and brachyphalangy. J. Med. Genet., *14*:430, 1977.

Bianchi, E., et al.: Ruvalcaba syndrome. A case report. Eur. J. Pediatr., *142*:301, 1984.

Hunter, A.: Letter to the editor.: Ruvalcaba syndrome. Am. J. Med. Genet., *21*:785, 1985.

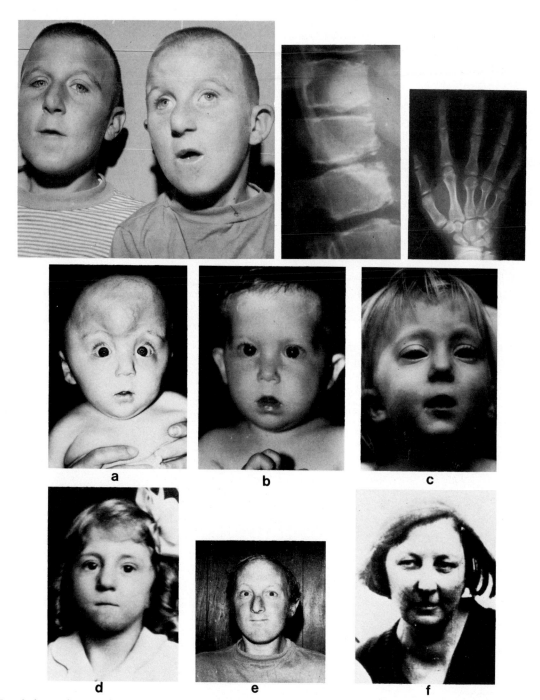

Ruvalcaba syndrome. *Above*, Two boys at 14 and 15 years, with roentgenograms showing epiphyseal dysplasia in the spine and short metacarpals (3–5) and fusion of lunate and scaphoid bones. (From Ruvalcaba, R. H. A., et al.: J. Pediatr., 79:450, 1973.) *Below*, Six affected individuals in three generations of a family. Those designated *a* and *e* are males. Note the striking similarity of *e* to the above patients. It is important to emphasize that Hunter does not consider these individuals to have the same disorder as that reported by Ruvalcaba (above). Hence this remains an open question. (From Hunter, A. G. W., et al.: J. of Med. Genet., *14*:430, 1977.)

MIETENS SYNDROME

Corneal Opacity, Narrow Nose,
Flexion Contracture at Elbow

In 1966, Mietens and Weber recorded this pattern of malformation in four of six siblings born of normal unrelated parents.

ABNORMALITIES
General. Dull mentality, with I.Q.s of 70 to 81. Small stature.

Facies. Corneal opacity, horizontal and rotary nystagmus and strabismus. Narrow nose with hypoplasia of alae nasi.

Extremities. Short forearms and dislocation of proximal radius, with flexion contracture at elbow.

OCCASIONAL ABNORMALITIES. Pes valgus, inability to extend knee fully, dislocation of hip, pectus excavatum, aneurysm.

NATURAL HISTORY. Because of the impaired vision plus the limitation of function of the arms, it is difficult to know whether the I.Q.s of 70 to 80 are a valid indicator of mental defect. Vascular anomalies may be a serious feature in this syndrome. The older girl (see illustration) died of rupture of an aneurysm of the right anterior cerebral artery.

ETIOLOGY. Undetermined. ? Autosomal recessive.

References

Mietens, C., and Weber, H.: A syndrome characterized by corneal opacity, nystagmus, flexion contracture of the elbows, growth failure, and mental retardation. J. Pediatr., *69*:624, 1966.

Mietens, C.: Personal communication.

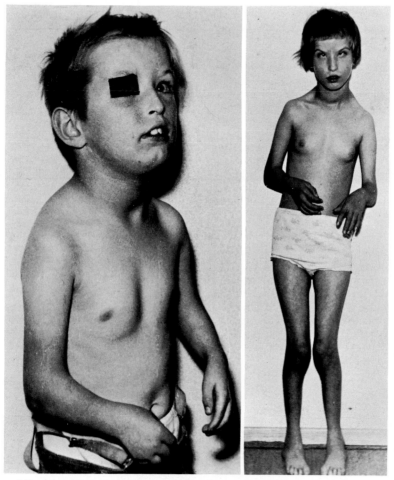

Mietens syndrome. Affected siblings. Note the hypoplasia of the alae nasi and the position of the dislocated elbows. (From Mietens, C., and Weber, H.: J. Pediatr., *69*:624, 1966.)

OCULODENTODIGITAL SYNDROME

(Oculodentodigital Dysplasia)

Microphthalmos, Enamel Hypoplasia,
Camptodactyly of Fifth Fingers

Originally described in 1920 by Lohmann, this pattern was more fully characterized by Gorlin, Meskin, and St. Geme in 1963.

ABNORMALITIES

Eyes. Microphthalmos, microcornea, fine porous iris. Short palpebral fissures.
Nose. Thin, hypoplastic alae nasi with small nares.
Teeth. Enamel hypoplasia.
Hands and Feet. Syndactyly of fourth and fifth fingers, third and fourth toes. Camptodactyly of fifth fingers. Midphalangeal hypoplasia or aplasia of one or more fingers and/or toes.
Hair. Fine, dry, and/or sparse and slow growing.
Other Skeletal. Broad tubular bones and mandible with wide alveolar ridge.

OCCASIONAL ABNORMALITIES.
Small palpebral fissures, epicanthal folds, glaucoma, cataract, bony orbital hypotelorism with normal inner canthal distance, partial anodontia, microdontia, premature loss of teeth, cleft lip and palate, conductive hearing impairment, cubitus valgus, hip dislocation, osteopetrosis, poor posture. Skull hyperostosis. Neurologic dysfunction, including hyperactive deep tendon reflexes, ataxia, and dysarthria, may become a feature.

NATURAL HISTORY. Inadequate information. Mentally normal.

ETIOLOGY. Autosomal dominant with variable expression; many cases represent fresh mutations. An affected child with severe ocular defects born to unaffected first-cousin parents suggests a rare autosomal recessive variety of this syndrome.

References

Lohmann, W.: Beitrag zur Kenntnis des reinen Mikrophthalmus. Arch. Augenh., *86*:136, 1920.
Gorlin, R. J., Meskin, L. H., and St. Geme, J. W.: Oculodentodigital dysplasia. J. Pediatr., *63*:69, 1963.
Eidelman, E., Chosack, A., and Wagner, M. L.: Orodigitofacial dysostosis and oculodentodigital dysplasia. Two distinct syndromes with some similarities. Oral Surg., *23*:311, 1967.
Judisch, G. F., et al.: Oculodentodigital dysplasia. Arch. Ophthalmol., *97*:878, 1979.
Traboulsi, E. I., Faris, B. M., and Der Kaloustian, V. M.: Persistent hyperplastic primary vitreous and recessive oculo-dento-osseous dysplasia. Am. J. Med. Genet., *24*:95, 1986.

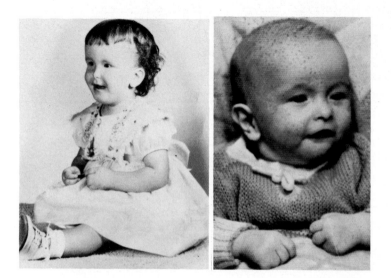

Infants with oculodentodigital syndrome. Note the small alae nasi, small mandibles, and 4–5 cutaneous syndactyly. (Courtesy of Teresa Hadro, Southern Illinois University School of Medicine [left photo] and Dr. David R. Cox, University of California Medical School in San Francisco [right photo].)

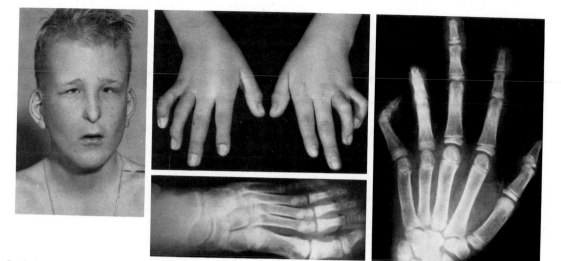

Oculodentodigital syndrome. Twelve year old. Note the microcornea, small eyes, hypoplasia of the alae nasi, camptodactyly, repaired syndactyly of the fourth and fifth fingers, and bony abnormalities. (From Gorlin, R. J., et al.: J. Pediatr., *63*:69, 1963.)

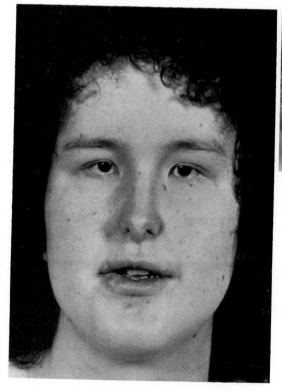

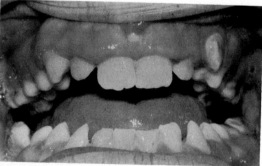

Oculodentodigital syndrome. Young woman who had shunted hydrocephalus in early childhood. Note the similar facial features and the small melanomata also present in the upper photo. (Courtesy of Dr. Boris G. Kousseff, University of South Florida, Tampa.)

OTO-PALATO-DIGITAL SYNDROME, TYPE I

(Taybi Syndrome)

*Deafness, Cleft Palate,
Broad Distal Digits with Short Nails*

Initially decribed by Taybi in 1962, many cases have been recognized subsequently.

ABNORMALITIES

Performance. Mild mental deficiency; I.Q.s of 75 to 90.

Growth. Small stature, all below tenth percentile for age.

Hearing. Moderate conductive deafness.

Cranium. Frontal and occipital prominence with thick frontal bone and thick base of skull, having a steep naso-basal angulation. Absence of frontal and sphenoid sinuses.

Facies. Facial bone hypoplasia and hypertelorism with small nose and mouth but lateral fullness of the supraorbital ridges.

Mouth. Partial anodontia, impacted teeth, or both. Cleft soft palate, small tonsils.

Midskeletal. Small trunk, pectus excavatum, failure of neural arch fusion, small iliac crests.

Limbs. Limited elbow extension, inward-bowing tibiae. Short, broad distal phalanges of thumbs and toes, to a lesser extent for other digits, with short nails. Relatively short third, fourth, fifth metacarpals. Fusion of hamate and capitate bones. Accessory ossification center at the base of the second metatarsal.

OCCASIONAL ABNORMALITIES. Delayed closure of anterior fontanel, hip dislocation, limited knee flexion, syndactyly of toes, hallucal nail dystrophy.

NATURAL HISTORY. Speech development is retarded on the basis of hearing impairment, mental deficiency, or both.

ETIOLOGY. X-linked semidominant. Females show mild to almost full expression, especially the fullness of the lateral supraorbital ridges, short nails, clinodactyly of toes, and roentgenographic abnormalities in limbs and skull.

References

Taybi, H.: Generalized skeletal dysplasia with multiple anomalies. Am. J. Roentgenol. Radium Ther. Nucl. Med., *88*:450, 1962.

Dudding, B. A., Gorlin, R. J., and Langer, L. O.: The oto-palato-digital syndrome. A new symptom-complex consisting of deafness, dwarfism, cleft palate, characteristic facies, and a generalized bone dysplasia. Am. J. Dis. Child., *113*:214, 1967.

Gorlin, R. J., Poznanski, A. K., and Hendon, I.: The oto-palato-digital (OPD) syndrome in females. Oral Surg., *35*:218, 1973.

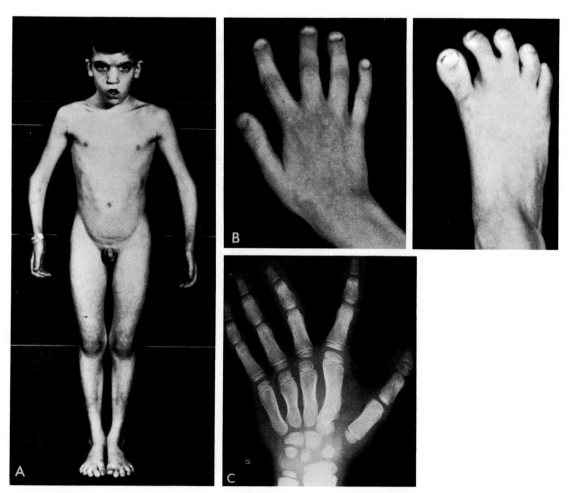

Oto-palato-digital syndrome, type I. *A* to *C*, Note irregular length and form of distal phalanges, especially thumb. (From Dudding, B. A., Gorlin, R. J., and Langer, L. O.: Am. J. Dis. Child., *113*:214, 1967.)

OTO-PALATO-DIGITAL SYNDROME, TYPE II

Fitch et al. and later Kozlowski et al. each described this pattern of malformation in two half brothers. Nine cases have been reported.

ABNORMALITIES

Growth. Postnatal growth deficiency in survivors.

Craniofacies. Late closure of large anterior fontanel. Wide sutures. Prominent forehead. Low-set ears. Ocular hypertelorism. Antimongoloid slant to palpebral fissures. Flat nasal bridge. Small mouth. Micrognathia. Cleft palate. Radiographic evidence of dense fontanels, supraorbital ridge, and skull base. Small mandible with obtuse angle.

Limbs. Flexed, overlapping fingers. Short thumbs and great toes. Polydactyly. Syndactyly. Clinodactyly of second finger. Bowing of radius, ulna, femur, and tibia. Small to absent fibula. Hypoplastic, irregular metacarpals. Nonossified fifth metatarsal. Subluxed elbows, wrists, and knees.

Other. Cryptorchidism. Conductive hearing loss. Pectus excavatum, abnormal teeth. Thin, wavy clavicles and ribs. Some flat vertebral bodies. Mental deficiency (2 patients).

NATURAL HISTORY. Six out of nine reported patients have died prior to five months of age because of, in most cases, respiratory difficulties. Two of the three survivors are developmentally delayed.

ETIOLOGY. X-linked, with mild manifestations in heterozygous females.

References

Fitch, N., Jequier, S., and Papageorgiou, A.: A familial syndrome of cranial, facial, oral and limb anomalies. Clin. Genet., *10:*226, 1976.

Kozlowski, K., et al.: Oto-palato-digital syndrome with severe x-ray changes in two half brothers. Pediatr. Radiol., *6:*97, 1977.

Fitch, N., Jequier, S., and Gorlin, R.: The oto-palato-digital syndrome, proposed type II. Am. J. Med. Genet., *15:*655, 1983.

Brewster, T. G., et al.: Oto-palato-digital syndrome, type II—an X-linked skeletal dysplasia. Am. J. Med. Genet., *20:*249, 1985.

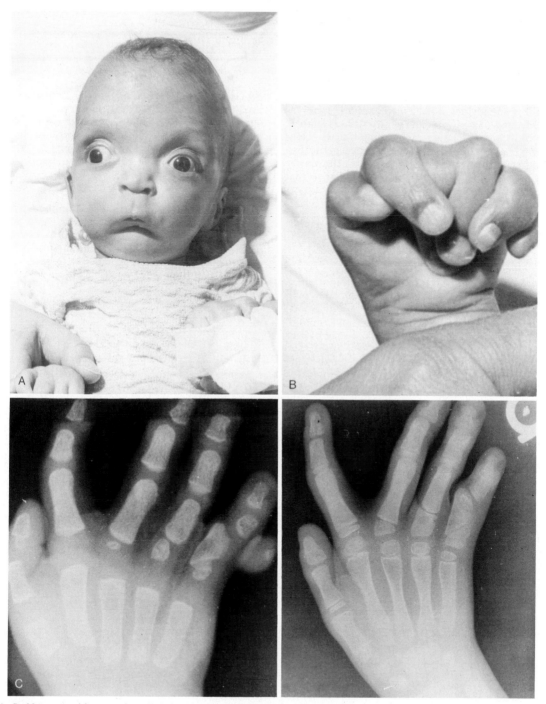

A, B, Neonate with oto-palato-digital syndrome, type II. Note the prominent forehead, ocular hypertelorism, flat nasal bridge, small mouth, micrognathia, and the flexed overlapping fingers. *C,* Radiographs of the hand at one and five years of age reveal hypoplastic irregular metacarpals, abnormal epiphyses of proximal phalanges 4 and 5, and postaxial polydactyly. (From Fitch, N., et al.: Am. J. Med. Genet, *15*:655, 1983.)

COFFIN-LOWRY SYNDROME

Downslanting Palpebral Fissures,
Bulbous Nose, Tapering Fingers

Coffin et al. in 1966 and Lowry et al. in 1971 independently described a mental retardation syndrome associated with coarse facies, short stature, and thick, soft hands with tapering fingers. Temtamy recognized the similarity between the two and referred to the disorder as the Coffin-Lowry syndrome. The facies may appear similar to that of the Williams syndrome.

ABNORMALITIES

Growth. Mild to moderate growth deficiency, apparently of postnatal onset.

Performance. Mental deficiency, usually severe. Relative weakness. Hypotonia.

Facies. Coarse appearance with downslanting palpebral fissures and maxillary hypoplasia, mild hypertelorism, prominent brow, and short, broad nose with thick alae nasi and septum. Large open mouth with thick, everted lower lip. Prominent ears.

Dental. Hypodontia, malocclusion, and wide spaced teeth.

Thorax. Short bifid sternum with pectus carinatum.

Spine. Anterior superior marginal vertebral defects, thoracolumbar scoliosis.

Limbs. Large, soft hands with tapering fingers and tufted drumstick appearance to distal phalanges on roentgenogram. Accessory transverse hypothenar crease. Flat feet. Lax ligaments.

OCCASIONAL ABNORMALITIES. Microcephaly.
Thick calvarium, dilated lateral ventricles. Hypoplastic sinuses and mastoids. Simian crease. Forearm fullness. Delayed closure of anterior fontanel. Inguinal hernia. Rectal prolapse. Uterine prolapse. Mitral insufficiency.

NATURAL HISTORY. The mental deficiency is usually of severe degree, leaving the patient without speech. Although the face coarsens with age, and the vertebral dysplasia and kyphoscoliosis generally do not develop until after six years, there is no evidence of progressive mental deterioration.

ETIOLOGY. X-linked inheritance is implied, with striking similarity between the severely affected hemizygous males. Clinical findings in carrier females include slight to moderate mental deficiency, mild facial changes, tapered fingers, and short stature, although some obligate carriers are completely normal.

References

Coffin, G. S., Siris, E., and Wegienka, L. C.: Mental retardation with osteocartilaginous anomalies. Am. J. Dis. Child., *112*:205, 1966.

Lowry, B., Miller, J. R., and Fraser, F. C.: A new dominant gene mental retardation syndrome. Am. J. Dis. Child., *121*:496, 1971.

Temtamy, S. A., et al.: The Coffin-Lowry syndrome. A simply inherited trait comprising mental retardation, facio-digital anomalies and skeletal anomalies. Birth Defects Original Article Series, XI(6):133, 1975.

Hunter, A. G. W., Partington, M. W., Evans, J. A.: The Coffin-Lowry syndrome. Experience from four centres. Clin. Genet., *21*:321, 1982.

Vles, J. S. H., et al.: Early signs in Coffin-Lowry syndrome. Clin Genet., *26*:448, 1984.

Haspeslagh, M., et al.: The Coffin-Lowry syndrome. Eur. J. Pediatr., *143*:82, 1984.

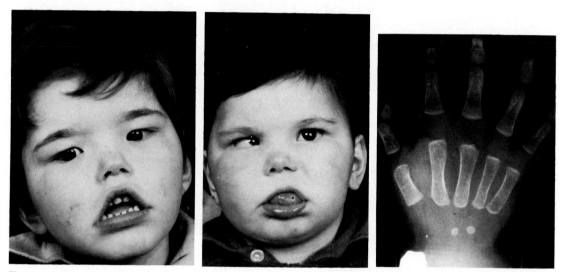

Two young boys with the Coffin-Lowry syndrome, showing aberrant facies with short noses, and radiologic evidence of lag in development of unusual epiphyses. (Courtesy of Dr. Marcus Pembrey, Institute of Child Health, University of London.)

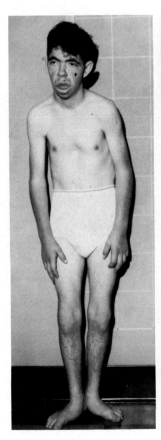

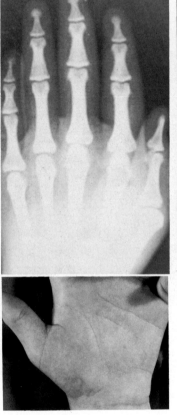

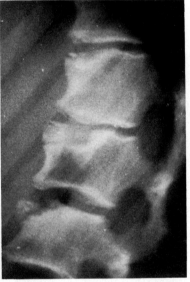

Coffin-Lowry syndrome. Seriously mentally deficient young adult patient. Note stooped posture, facies, vertebral changes, tufted terminal phalanges, and accessory transverse hypothenar crease. (Courtesy of Dr. Selma Myhre, Rainier State Training School, Buckley, Washington.)

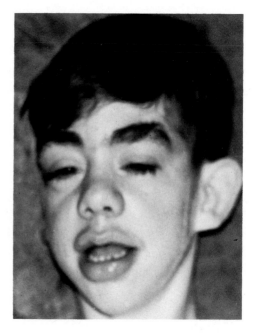

Coffin-Lowry syndrome. Fifteen year old mentally deficient boy with height of 4 feet, 9 inches, ptosis of eyelids, pectus excavatum, scoliosis, and clinodactyly of the fifth finger, in addition to the obvious facial features. (Courtesy of Dr. Selma Myhre, Rainier State Training School, Buckley, Washington.)

THE FG SYNDROME

Imperforate Anus, Hypotonia, Prominent Forehead

Initially described by Opitz and Kaveggia in three brothers and two of their male first cousins, over 30 cases of this X-linked recessive disorder now have been documented.

ABNORMALITIES

Performance. Mental deficiency. Delayed motor development. Hypotonia. EEG disturbances with seizures. Hyperactive behavior with short attention span. Affable, extroverted personality with occasional temper tantrums when frustrated.

Growth. Postnatal onset of short stature.

Craniofacies. Postnatal onset of megalencephaly. Large anterior fontanel. Prominent forehead with frontal hair upsweep. Ocular hypertelorism. Prominent lower lip. Small ears with simple structure. Facial skin wrinkling. Epicanthal folds. Short palpebral fissures. Narrow palate. Large-appearing cornea.

Gastrointestinal. Imperforate anus. Anal stenosis. Anteriorly placed anus. Constipation.

Skeletal. Broad thumbs and great toes. Multiple joint contractures. Syndactyly. Minor vertebral defects.

Other. Sacral dimple. Cryptorchidism. Low total dermal ridge count.

OCCASIONAL ABNORMALITIES. Craniosynostosis. Hydrocephalus. Absence of corpus callosum. Malrotation of cecum. Absence of mesentery. Pyloric stenosis. Dilatation of urinary tract. Cardiac defect. Sensorineural deafness.

NATURAL HISTORY. Almost one half of the original 17 patients died prior to two years of age primarily because of complications of the cardiac defect or imperforate anus. Although mental deficiency has been severe in the survivors, their generally affable personality has led to an adequate social adjustment in most cases.

ETIOLOGY. X-linked recessive inheritance. All carrier mothers have been of normal intelligence.

References

Opitz, J. M., and Kaveggia, E. G.: Studies of malformation syndromes of man XXXIII: The FG syndrome. An X-linked recessive syndrome of multiple congenital anomalies and mental retardation. Z. Kinderhlkd, *117*:1, 1974.

Keller, M. A., et al.: A new syndrome of mental deficiency with craniofacial, limb and anal abnormalities. J. Pediatr., *8*:589, 1976.

Ricardi, V. M., Hassler, E., and Lubinsky, M. S.: The FG syndrome: Further characterization. Report of a third family, and of a sporadic case. Am. J. Med. Genet., *1*:47, 1977.

Opitz, J. M., et al.: Studies of malformation syndromes of humans XXXIIIC: The FG syndrome—Further studies on three affected individuals from the FG family. Am. J. Med. Genet., *12*:147, 1982.

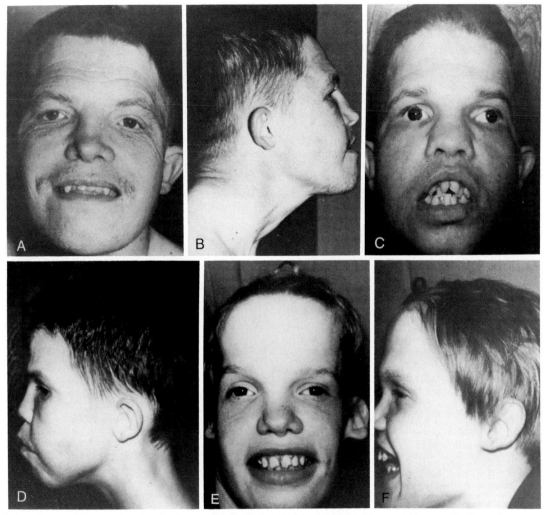

FG syndrome. Three affected male siblings; 29 *(A, B)*, 27 *(C, D)*, and 17 *(E, F)* years old. Note the frontal upsweep, lateral displacement of the medial canthi, and small ears.

STICKLER SYNDROME

(Hereditary Arthro-ophthalmopathy)

Flat Facies, Myopia, Spondyloepiphyseal Dysplasia

In 1965, Stickler et al. reported the initial observations on affected individuals in five generations of one family; the skeletal aspects have been further documented by Spranger, and the total spectrum of the disorder has been set forth by Herrmann et al.

ABNORMALITIES

Orofacial. Flat facies with depressed nasal bridge and epicanthal folds, midfacial or mandibular hypoplasia, clefts of hard and/or soft palate and occasionally of uvula, micrognathia, Robin sequence, deafness (both sensorineural and conductive), dental anomalies.

Ocular. Myopia (8 to 18 diopters) usually present before the age of ten; retinal detachment and/or cataracts.

Musculoskeletal. Hypotonia, hyperextensible joints, marfanoid habitus. Prominence of large joints may be present at birth. Severe arthropathy can occur in childhood. Lesser joint pains simulate juvenile rheumatoid arthritis. Subluxation of hip. Mild to moderate spondyloepiphyseal dysplasia, i.e., flat vertebrae with anterior wedging and underdevelopment of the distal tibial epiphyses. Long bones show disproportionately narrow shafts relative to their metaphyseal width.

OCCASIONAL ABNORMALITIES. Scoliosis, mental deficiency. Glaucoma. Mitral valve prolapse.

COMMENT. The Stickler syndrome should be considered in any neonate with the Robin sequence, particularly in those with a family history of cleft palate and in patients with dominantly inherited myopia, nontraumatic retinal detachment, and/or mild spondyloepiphyseal dysplasia.

NATURAL HISTORY. Arthritis, if present, most commonly becomes a problem after 30 years of age. Symptoms become more severe with advancing years, leading in some cases to total hip replacement. Progressive myopia may give rise to retinal detachment and lead to blindness, the most severe complication of this disorder. Although 40 per cent develop myopia prior to 10 years of age and 75 per cent by age 20, it does not occur in some patients until after age 50. Retinal detachment can occur in childhood but usually not until after 20 years of age. It is to be hoped that the detachment can be corrected surgically if recognized early.

ETIOLOGY. Autosomal dominant inheritance with highly variable expression.

References

Stickler, G. B., et al.: Hereditary progressive arthroophthalmopathy. Mayo Clin. Proc., 40:433, 1965.

Stickler, G. B., and Pugh, D. G.: Hereditary progressive arthro-ophthalmopathy. II. Additional observations on vertebral abnormalities, a hearing defect, and a report of a similar case. Mayo Clin. Proc., 42:495, 1967.

Spranger, J.: Arthro-ophthalmopathia hereditaria. Ann. Radiol. (Paris), 11:359, 1968.

Herrmann, J., et al.: The Stickler syndrome (hereditary arthroophthalmopathy). Birth Defects, 11(2):76, 1975.

Liberfarb, R. M., Hirose, T., Holmes, L. B.: The Wagner-Stickler syndrome. A study of 22 families. J. Pediatr., 99:394, 1981.

Liberfarb, R. M., and Goldblatt, A.: Prevalence of mitral-valve prolapse in the Stickler syndrome. Am. J. Med. Genet., 24:387, 1986.

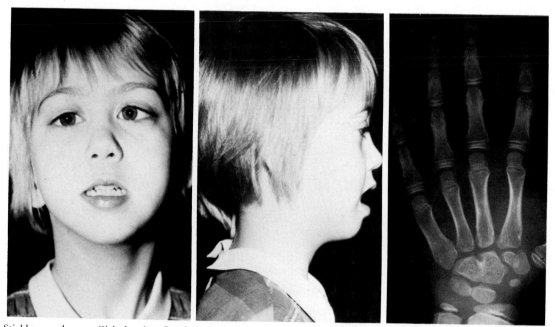

Stickler syndrome. Girl showing flat facies, inner canthal folds, relatively narrow diaphyses, and hamate-capitate carpal synostosis. (Courtesy of Dr. Judith Hall, University of British Columbia, Vancouver, B.C.)

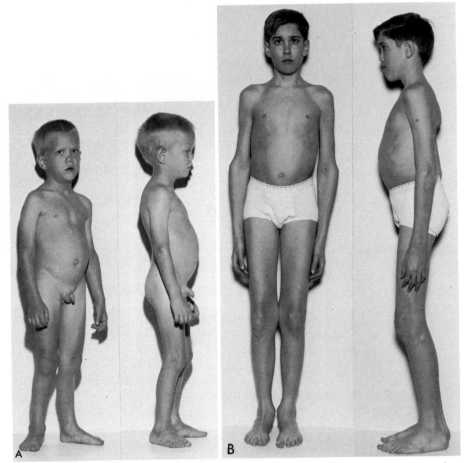

Stickler syndrome. *A, B,* Child and adolescent from a large affected kindred. Note relative arachnodactyly in adolescent boy. (From Stickler, G. B., et al.: Mayo Clin. Proc., *40*:433, 1965.)

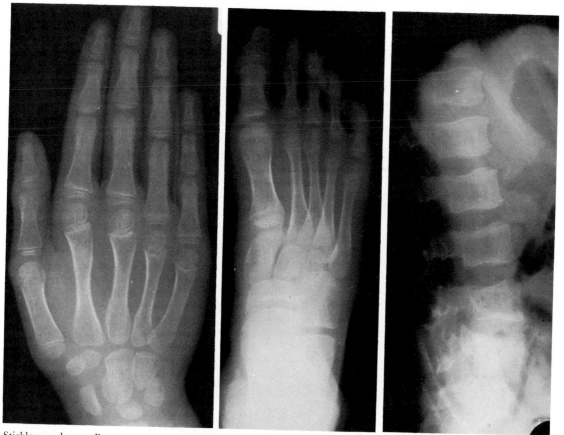

Stickler syndrome. Roentgenograms showing arachnodactyly, fusion of some carpal centers, and mild spondyloepiphyseal dysplasia.

LARSEN SYNDROME

*Multiple Joint Dislocation,
Flat Facies, Short Fingernails*

Larsen, Schottstaedt, and Bost described six sporadic cases of this condition in 1950.

ABNORMALITIES

Facies. Flat, with depressed nasal bridge and prominent forehead, hypertelorism.

Joints. Dislocations of elbows, hips, knees, and wrists, with dysplastic epiphyseal centers developing in childhood.

Hands. Long, nontapering fingers with spatulate thumbs, short nails, short metacarpals, and multiple carpal ossification centers.

Feet. Talipes equinovalgus or varus. Delayed coalescence of the two calcaneal ossification centers.

OCCASIONAL ABNORMALITIES.
Cleft palate, abnormal segmentation of cervical vertebrae, scoliosis. Hypoplastic humerus, simian crease. Cardiovascular defect. Mobile, infolding arytenoid cartilage.

NATURAL HISTORY.
Recent evaluations of adults in four generations of one family indicate that prognosis is relatively good following aggressive orthopedic management. Many patients begin walking late. Osteoarthritis involving large joints and progressive kyphoscoliosis are potential complications. Particular care should be exercised during anesthesia because of the mobile arytenoid cartilage.

ETIOLOGY.
Unknown. Autosomal dominant inheritance is indicated by one of the original patients reported by Larsen having had an affected child. However, families with both autosomal dominant and autosomal recessive inheritance have been described subsequently.

References

Larsen, L. J., Schottstaedt, E. R., and Bost, F. C.: Multiple congenital dislocations associated with characteristic facial abnormality. J. Pediatr., *37*:574, 1950.

Latta, R. J., et al.: Larsen's syndrome: A skeletal dysplasia with multiple joint dislocations and unusual facies. J. Pediatr., *78*:291, 1971.

Silverman, F. N.: Larsen's syndrome: Congenital dislocation of the knees and joints, distinctive facies, and frequently, cleft palate. Ann. Radiol. (Paris), *15*:297, 1972.

Robertson, F. W., Kozlowski, K., Middleton, R. W.: Larsen's syndrome. Clin. Pediatr., *14*:53, 1975.

Striscinglio, P., et al.: Severe cardiac anomalies in sibs with Larsen syndrome. J. Med. Genet., *20*:422, 1983.

Stanley, D., and Seymoor, N.: The Larsen syndrome occurring in four generations of one family. Int. Orthop., *8*:267, 1985.

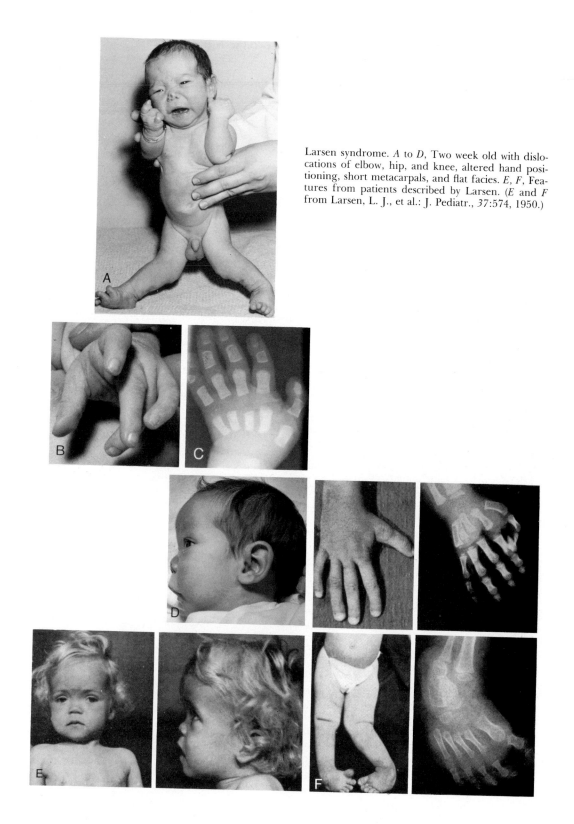

Larsen syndrome. *A* to *D*, Two week old with dislocations of elbow, hip, and knee, altered hand positioning, short metacarpals, and flat facies. *E, F*, Features from patients described by Larsen. (*E* and *F* from Larsen, L. J., et al.: J. Pediatr., *37*:574, 1950.)

LANGER-GIEDION SYNDROME

(Tricho-Rhino-Phalangeal Syndrome With Exostosis)

Multiple Exostoses, Bulbous Nose with
Peculiar Facies, Loose Redundant Skin in Infancy

Hall et al. in 1974 reported five new cases of this disorder and included two further sporadic cases from the literature. An extensive review of the literature, including data from over 30 patients, has recently been published by Langer et al. Although the facies of these patients resemble that of the tricho-rhino-phalangeal syndrome, other features allow for separation of the two syndromes.

ABNORMALITIES

Growth. Postnatal onset of mild growth deficiency.

Performance. Mild to severe mental deficiency in 70 per cent, with the remaining patients in the normal to dull-normal range.

Cranium. Microcephaly.

Facies. Large laterally protruding ears; heavy eyebrows; deep-set eyes; large bulbous nose with thickened alae nasi and septum, dorsally tented nares, and broad nasal bridge; simple philtrum, which is prominent and elongated; thin upper lip; recessed mandible.

Hair. Sparse scalp hair.

Skin. Redundancy and/or looseness in infancy, which regresses with age. Maculopapular nevi about the scalp, facies, neck, upper trunk, and upper limbs.

Hands. Cone-shaped epiphyses, which become radiologically evident at about three to four years of age; lack of normal modeling in metaphyseal regions; poor funnelization at proximal ends of phalanges; metaphyseal hooking over the lateral edges of the cone-shaped epiphyses; exostoses. Brittle nails.

Bones. Multiple exostoses of long tubular bones, with onset and distribution similar to the autosomal dominant variety of multiple cartilaginous exostoses. Exostoses can involve other areas, such as the ribs, scapulae, and pelvic bones.

Other. Syndactyly. Tendency toward fractures. Winged scapulae. Lax joints. Hypotonia. Exotropia. Recurrent upper respiratory tract infections. Disproportionate delay in the onset of speech. Deafness. Malocclusion. Dental abnormalities. Perthes-like changes in capital femoral epiphysis, segmentation defects of vertebrae with scoliosis, narrow posterior ribs.

OCCASIONAL ABNORMALITIES. Hypochromic anemia, thin hypomineralized bones, clinobrachydactyly, bowed femora, ocular hypotelorism, ptosis, prominent eyes, epicanthal folds, iris coloboma, abducens palsy, tragal skin tag, cardiac defects, small phallus, cryptorchidism, inguinal and umbilical hernia, ureteral reflux, widely spaced nipples, simian crease, delayed sexual development, premature thelarche and pubarche, hydrometrocolpos, abnormal EEG, seizures.

NATURAL HISTORY. Some of these children have such redundancy and/or looseness to their skin at birth that they are misdiagnosed as having the Ehlers-Danlos syndrome. Recurrent respiratory tract infections during the first four to five years. General health is usually good after that except for a tendency toward fractures and the usual problems of multiple exostoses with their variable effects on bone growth.

ETIOLOGY. Unknown. An affected father-daughter pair has raised the possibility of autosomal dominant inheritance with wide variability of expression. All other cases have been sporadic. Twenty-five per cent of affected patients have had a deletion of chromosome 8q most likely involving 8q23 or 8q24.

References

Hall, B. D., et al.: Langer-Giedion syndrome. Birth Defects, *10*(12):147, 1974.

Langer, L. O., et al.: The tricho-rhino-phalangeal syndrome with exostosis (or Langer-Giedion syndrome): Four additional patients without mental retardation and review of the literature. Am. J. Med. Genet., *19*:81, 1984.

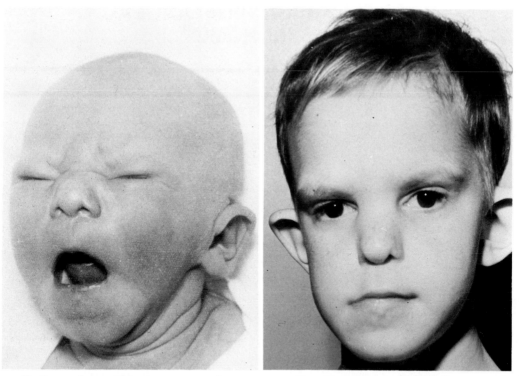

Langer-Giedion syndrome. Patient as neonate and at seven years. Note the sparseness of hair, bulbous nose, simple but prominent philtrum, redundant folds of skin on the neck, superiorly tented nares, thin upper lip, and prominent ears.

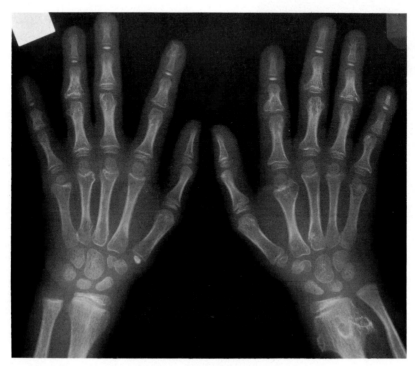

Langer-Giedion syndrome. Eleven and one-half year old, showing exostoses, cone-shaped epiphyses, and metaphyseal hooking at the proximal ends of a number of the middle phalanges.

TRICHO-RHINO-PHALANGEAL SYNDROME

Bulbous Nose, Sparse Hair, Epiphyseal Coning

Klingmuller reported two siblings with this pattern of malformation in 1956. Giedion further established the syndrome and set forth the tricho-rhino-phalangeal designation for it.

ABNORMALITIES
Growth. Mild growth deficiency (third to tenth percentiles).
Facial. Pear-shaped nose, prominent and long philtrum, narrow palate, +/− micrognathia, large prominent ears. Small, carious teeth with dental malocclusion. Horizontal groove on chin.
Hair. Sparse, thin hair with relative hypopigmentation.
Nails. Thin.
Skeletal. Short metacarpals and metatarsals, especially the fourth and fifth. Development of broadened middle phalangeal joint with cone-shaped epiphyses, especially the second through fourth fingers and toes. Aberrant angulation of tapering distal fingers. Short distal phalanges of thumbs and toes. Split distal radial epiphyses. Winged scapulae.

OCCASIONAL ABNORMALITIES. Coxa plana and coxa magna, flattening of capital femoral epiphysis, partial syndactyly, pectus carinatum, pes planus, short stature, mental deficiency, craniosynostosis, deep voice, hypotonia during infancy.

NATURAL HISTORY. The hair is usually sparse at birth. Osseous changes such as the cone-shaped epiphyses may develop in early childhood and become worse until adolescent growth is complete. Increased frequency of upper respiratory tract infections has been noted in some cases. A form of degenerative hip disease often develops in young adulthood or later life.

ETIOLOGY. Heterogeneity is suggested by autosomal dominant–type inheritance in some families (the great majority), whereas autosomal recessive inheritance is suggested in affected sibships of normal parentage.

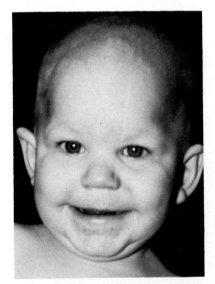

Tricho-rhino-phalangeal syndrome. One year old, showing sparse, fine hair and slight bulbous change in the nasal tip. The facial and digital aberrations change with age. (Courtesy of Dr. Jaime L. Frias, University of Nebraska Medical School, Omaha.)

References

Klingmuller, G.: Über eigentumliche Konstitutionsanomalien bei 2 Schwestern und ihre Beziehungen zu neueren entwicklungspathologischen Befunden. Hautarzt, 7:105, 1956.

Giedion, A.: Das tricho-rhino-phalangeale Syndrom. Helv. Paediatr. Acta, 21:475, 1966.

Gorlin, R. J., Cohen, M. M., and Wolfson, J.: Tricho-rhino-phalangeal syndrome. Am. J. Dis. Child., 118:585, 1969.

Fontaine, G., et al.: Le syndrome trichorhinophalangien. Arch. Fr. Pediatr., 27:635, 1970.

Felman, A. H., and Frias, J. L.: The tricho-rhino-phalangeal syndrome: Study of 16 patients in one family. Am. J. Roentgenol., 129:631, 1977.

Goodman, R. M., et al.: New clinical observations in the trichorhinophalangeal syndrome. J. Craniofac. Genet. Dev. Biol., 1:15, 1981.

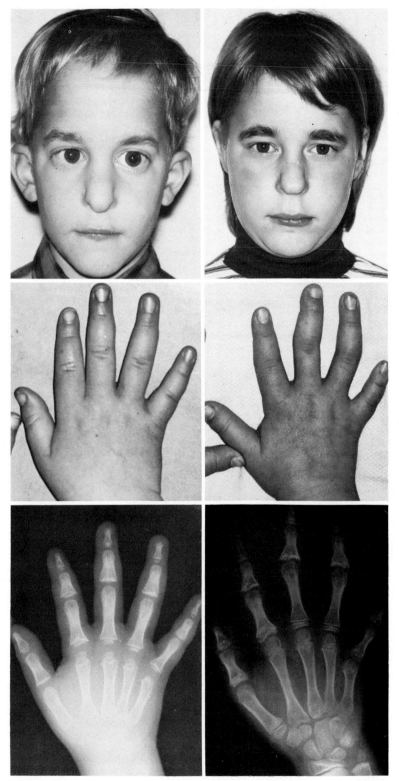

Tricho-rhino-phalangeal syndrome. Six year old son (*left*) and nine year old daughter (*right*) of an affected father who became bald at 21 years of age. The children have fine, slow-growing hair. Note the tented hypoplastic nares, prominent philtrum, and the asymmetric length of fingers related to radiographic evidence of irregular metaphyseal cupping with cone-shaped epiphyses. (Courtesy of D. Weaver, University of Indiana, Indianapolis.)

ECTRODACTYLY–ECTODERMAL DYSPLASIA–CLEFTING SYNDROME

(EEC Syndrome)

Ectrodactyly, Ectodermal Dysplasia, Cleft Lip-Palate

Although the association of ectrodactyly and cleft lip had been noted, it was not until 1970 that Rüdiger et al. appreciated that at least some of these patients also had features of ectodermal dysplasia and named the disorder the EEC syndrome. Bixler et al. added two additional cases and summarized the past observations.

ABNORMALITIES. All features are variable.

Skin. Fair and thin, with mild hyperkeratosis. Hypoplastic nipples.

Hair. Light-colored, sparse, thin, wiry.

Teeth. Partial anodontia, microdontia, caries.

Eyes. Blue irides, photophobia, blepharophimosis, atresia, defects of lacrimal duct system, blepharitis, dacryocystitis.

Face. Cleft lip, +/− cleft palate, maxillary hypoplasia, mild malar hypoplasia.

Limbs. Defects in midportion of hands and feet, varying from syndactyly to ectrodactyly. Mild nail dysplasia.

OCCASIONAL ABNORMALITIES. Deafness, small or malformed auricles, renal anomaly.

NATURAL HISTORY. These individuals are usually of normal intelligence and adapt reasonably well with surgical closure of the facial clefts plus (as needed) limb surgery, dentures, and wigs. Early and continued ophthalmologic evaluation and management for the defective lacrimal duct system are imperative, since chronic dacryocystitis with corneal scarring can be the major debilitating problem in this disorder.

ETIOLOGY. Autosomal dominant inheritance is implied, with variable expression and even lack of penetrance being noted in some families.

References

Rüdiger, R. A., Haase, W., and Passarge, E.: Association of ectrodactyly, ectodermal dysplasia, and cleft lip-palate. Am. J. Dis. Child., *120*:160, 1970.

Bixler, D., et al.: The ectrodactyly-ectodermal dysplasia-clefting (EEC) syndrome. Clin. Genet., *3*:43, 1972.

Cockayne, E. A.: Cleft palate, hare lip, dacryocystitis and cleft hand and feet. Biometrika, *28*:60, 1936.

Walker, J. C., and Clodius, L.: The syndromes of cleft lip, cleft palate and lobster-claw deformities of hands and feet. Plast. Reconstr. Surg., *32*:627, 1963.

Robinson, G. C., Wildervanck, L. S., and Chiang, T. P.: Ectrodactyly, ectodermal dysplasia, and cleft lip-palate syndrome. J. Pediatr., *82*:107, 1973.

Kaiser-Kupfer, M.: Ectrodactyly, ectodermal dysplasia and clefting syndrome. Am. J. Ophthalmol., *76*:992, 1973.

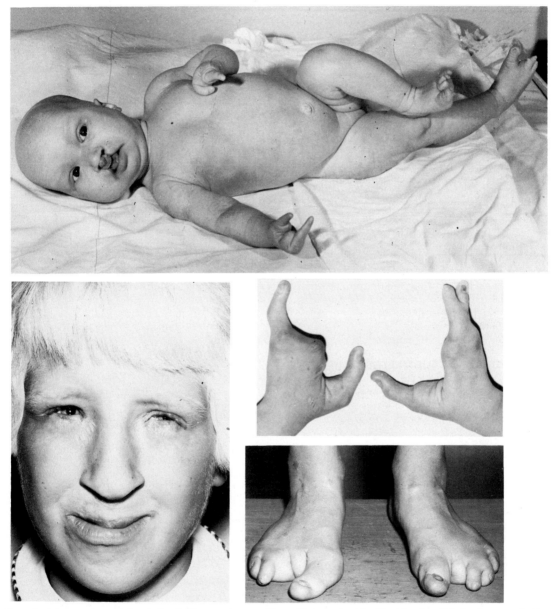

Ectrodactyly–ectodermal dysplasia–clefting syndrome. *Above,* Six month old with thin, dry, lightly pigmented skin, sparse, fine hair, photophobia with inflammation of conjunctiva, facial cleft, and small ears. Note the intraindividual variability of anomaly in the feet. (From Rüdiger, R. A., et al.: Am. J. Dis. Child., *120*:160, 1970. Courtesy of E. Passarge.) *Below,* Eighteen year old (wearing a wig) with coarse, sparse hair who has photophobia and blepharophimosis and only five poorly developed teeth. Note the small melanomata in the thin skin, which shows patchy areas of dermatitis. Studies revealed absence of the right kidney, with a double collecting system on the left.

HAY-WELLS SYNDROME OF ECTODERMAL DYSPLASIA

(Ankyloblepharon–Ectodermal Dysplasia–Clefting Syndrome, AEC Syndrome)

Ankyloblepharon, Ectodermal Dysplasia, Cleft Lip-Palate

In 1976, Hay and Wells described a specific type of ectodermal dysplasia associated with cleft lip or cleft palate and congenital filiform fusion of the eyelids. The association of facial clefting with ankyloblepharon filiforme adnatum had previously been documented in several case reports.

ABNORMALITIES

Craniofacies. Oval face. Broadened nasal bridge. Maxillary hypoplasia. Cleft lip, cleft palate, or both. Conical, widely spaced teeth. Hypodontia to partial anodontia. Ankyloblepharon filiforme adnatum.

Skin. Palmar and plantar keratoderma. Patchy, partial deficiency of sweat glands. Partial anhidrosis. Hyperpigmentation.

Nails. Absent or dystrophic.

Hair. Wiry and sparse to alopecia.

OCCASIONAL ABNORMALITIES. Deafness. Atretic external auditory canal. Cup-shaped auricles. Lacrimal duct atresia. Supernumerary nipples. Soft-tissue syndactyly. Rarely, ventricular septal defect or patent ductus arteriosus.

NATURAL HISTORY. Surgical excision of the ankyloblepharon filiforme adnatum is required during the early neonatal period. Anomalies of the eye are not associated with these tissue bands. Surgical closure of facial clefting and early ophthalmologic evaluation of the lacrimal duct system are required. Severe chronic granulomas of the scalp, which begin as infections, have been a serious problem and in one case have required multiple skin grafts. These patients have a partial capacity to produce sweat from fewer glands, so that hyperthermia is not a serious threat. Intelligence is normal.

ETIOLOGY. Autosomal dominant. Ankyloblepharon filiforme adnatum is not a simple failure of eyelid separation. The eyelid fusion bands histologically are composed of a central core of vascular connective tissue entirely surrounded by epithelium. Muscle fibers may be observed as well. These bands may represent abnormal proliferation of mesenchymal tissue at certain points on the lid margin or an ectodermal deficit allowing mesodermal union. The associated anomalies of this syndrome, with the exception of cleft lip, originate at eight to nine weeks of fetal life and can be explained as an abnormality in ectodermal development or defective ectodermal-mesodermal interaction.

References

Duke-Elder, S.: Textbook of Ophthalmology, Vol. 5. London, Kimpton, 1952, p. 4665.

Khanna, V. N.: Ankyloblepharon filiforme adnatum. Am. J. Ophthalmol., *43*:774, 1957.

Rogers, J. W.: Ankyloblepharon filiforme adnatum. Arch. Ophthalmol., *65*:114, 1961.

Long, J. C., and Blandford, S. E.: Ankyloblepharon filiforme adnatum with cleft lip and palate. Am. J. Ophthalmol., *53*:126, 1962.

Hay, R. J., and Wells, R. S.: The syndrome of ankyloblepharon, ectodermal defects, and cleft lip and palate: an autosomal dominant condition. Br. J. Dermatol., *94*:277, 1976.

Spiegel, J., and Colton, A.: AEC syndrome: Ankyloblepharon, ectodermal defects, and cleft lip and palate. J. Am. Acad. Dermatol., *12*:810, 1985.

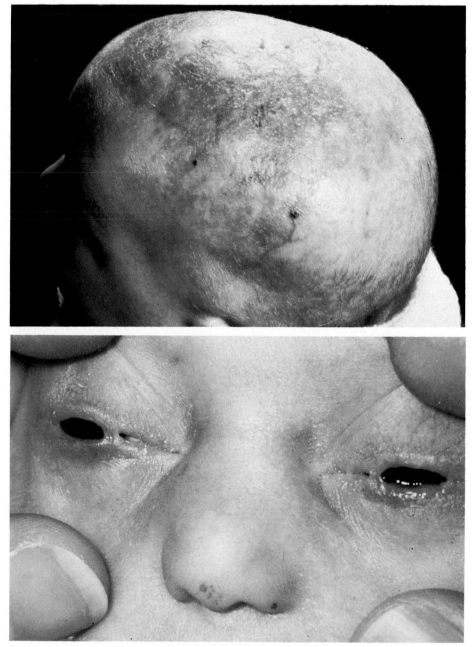

Ectodermal dysplasia with folliculitis of scalp, adhesions between eyelids, and cleft palate. (Courtesy of Dr. Mark Stephan, Madigan General Hospital, Tacoma, Washington.)

ROBERTS-SC PHOCOMELIA SYNDROME

(Pseudothalidomide Syndrome, Hypomelia-Hypotrichosis-Facial Hemangioma Syndrome)

Hypomelia, Midfacial Defect, Severe Growth Deficiency

This disorder was initially described by Roberts in 1919 and more recently by Appelt et al. Freeman et al. reported five cases and reviewed the features in the 17 previously recognized patients. The cases reported by Herrmann et al. as "pseudothalidomide or SC syndrome" and the case reported by Hall and Greenberg as "hypomelia-hypotrichosis-facial hemangioma syndrome" may be examples of this disorder, although this question is not fully resolved.

ABNORMALITIES

Performance. Microbrachycephaly. Severe mental defect in some and borderline to mild mental deficiency in others.

Growth. Profound growth deficiency of prenatal onset. Birth weight 1.5 to 2.2 kg and birth length frequently less than 40 cm.

Facial. Cleft lip with or without cleft palate and prominent premaxilla, hypertelorism, midfacial capillary hemangioma, thin nares, shallow orbits and prominent eyes with bluish sclerae, micrognathia. Malformed ears with hypoplastic lobules.

Hair. Sparse, may be silvery-blond in some survivors.

Limbs. Hypomelia, more severe in upper limbs, varying from phocomelia to lesser degrees of limb reduction, often including hypoplasia or absence of radii, first metacarpals and thumbs, fibulae, ulnae, carpals, and tibiae; syndactyly, fifth finger clinodactyly, and talipes deformity. Incomplete development of dermal ridges.

Genitalia. Cryptorchidism. Phallus may *appear* relatively large in relation to body size.

OCCASIONAL ABNORMALITIES.

Frontal encephalocele, hydrocephalus, microphthalmia, corneal clouding, cataract, lid coloboma, cranial nerve paralysis, short neck, cardiac anomaly (atrial septal defect), renal anomaly (polycystic and/or horseshoe kidney). Bicornuate uterus. Polyhydramnios. Thrombocytopenia. Hypospadius.

NATURAL HISTORY.

Most individuals born at term with birth length less than 37 cm and severe defects in midfacial and limb development have been stillborn or have died in early infancy. The survivors have had marked growth deficiency, and some have had severe mental deficiency as well. Birth length greater than 37 cm, less severe limb defects, absence of cleft palate, and presence of thin nares have been associated with a better prognosis.

ETIOLOGY. Autosomal recessive.

COMMENT.

Approximately 50 per cent of tested individuals have had premature separation of centromeric heterochromatin of many chromosomes. Included have been a number of patients exhibiting phenotypic overlap between the Roberts syndrome and the SC phocomelia syndrome, suggesting that the two are either allelic or represent variable severity of the same genetic condition.

References

Roberts, J. B.: A child with double cleft of lip and palate, protrusion of the intermaxillary portion of the upper jaw and imperfect development of the bones of the four extremities. Ann. Surg., 70:252, 1919.

Appelt, H., Gerken, H., and Lenz, W.: Tetraphokomelie mit Lippen-Kiefer-Gaumenspalte und Clitorishypertrophie—Ein Syndrom. Paediatr. Paedol., 2:119, 1966.

Herrmann, J., et al.: A familial dysmorphogenetic syndrome of limb deformities, characteristic facial appearance and associated anomalies: The pseudothalidomide or SC-syndrome. Birth Defects, 5:81, 1969.

Freeman, M. V. R., et al.: Roberts syndrome. Clin. Genet., 5:1, 1974.

Grosse, F. R., Pandel, C., and Wiedemann, H. R.: Tetraphocomelia-cleft palate syndrome. Human-genetik, 28:353, 1975.

Herrmann, J., and Opitz, J. M.: The SC phocomelia and the Roberts syndrome: Nosologic aspects. Eur. J. Pediatr., 125:117, 1977.

Waldenmaier, C., Aldenhoff, P., and Klemm, T.: The Roberts syndrome. Hum. Genet., 40:345, 1978.

Parry, D. M., et al.: SC phocomelia syndrome, premature centromere separation, and congenital cranial nerve paralysis in two sisters, one with malignant melanoma. Am. J. Med. Genet., 24:653, 1986.

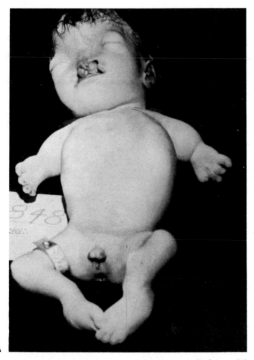

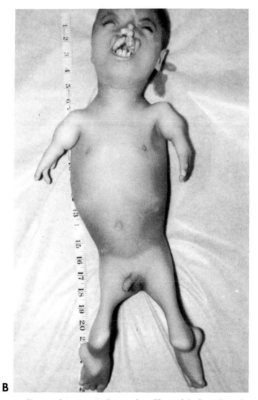

Roberts-SC phocomelia syndrome. *A*, Severely affected infant female at autopsy and, *B*, her severely growth deficient and mentally deficient ten year old brother. (From Freeman, M. V., et al.: Clin. Genet., 5:1, 1974.)

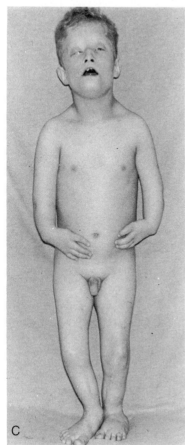

C, Eight year old severely mentally deficient boy with silvery-blond hair and a height age of three and one-half years. (From S. Jurenka, St. Amant Wards, Winnipeg, Canada.) *D*, Same patient, as an infant and at eight years of age. Note capillary hemangioma on forehead in infancy and sparse scalp hair as a child. (From Hall, B. D., and Greenberg, M. H.: Am. J. Dis. Child., *123*:602, 1972.)

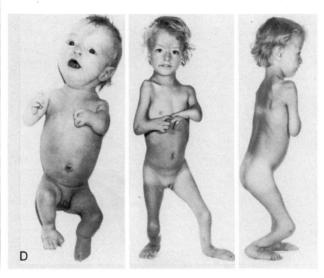

I. LIMB DEFECT AS MAJOR FEATURE

GREBE SYNDROME

*Marked Distal Limb Reduction, Polydactyly,
Normal Facies*

Grebe described this disorder in 1952, Quelce-Salgado reported 47 cases in five kindreds in an inbred Brazilian population, and Scott more recently summarized the findings. Over 50 cases have been described.

ABNORMALITIES
Growth. Small stature due to limb deficiency.
Limbs. Reduction, most striking distally, with very short digits. Fingers resemble toes. Missing or hypoplastic bones. Legs shorter than arms. Valgus position of feet. Obese limbs. Polydactyly.
Radiographic. Short radii and ulnae, the latter most severe. Rudimentary carpal bones and phalanges. Short tibiae, with increased severity from proximal to distal segments. Short feet in valgus, with rudimentary phalanges.

NATURAL HISTORY. Many of the patients have been stillborn or have died in infancy. Survivors are said to be of normal intelligence, develop normal secondary sexual characteristics, and walk without difficulty.

ETIOLOGY. Autosomal recessive.

References

Grebe, H.: Die Achondrogenesis. Ein einfach rezessives Erbmerkmal. Folia Hered. Pathol. (Milano), *2*:23, 1952.

Quelce-Salgado, A.: A new type of dwarfism with various bone aplasias and hypoplasia of the extremities. Acta Genet., *14*:63, 1964.

Scott, C. I.: Skeletal dysplasias. Birth Defects, *5*(3):14, 1969.

Garcio-Castro, J. M., and Pereze-Comas, A.: Nonlethal achondrogenesis in two Puerto Rican sibships. J. Pediatr., *87*:948, 1975.

Romeo, G., et al.: Heterogeneity of non-lethal severe short-limb dwarfism. J. Pediatr., *91*:918, 1977.

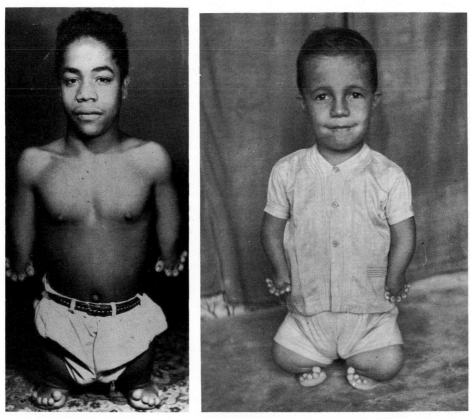

Grebe syndrome. (From Quelco-Salgado, A.: Acta Genet., *14*:63, 1964.)

POLAND ANOMALY

Unilateral Defect of
Pectoralis Muscle and Syndactyly of Hand

In 1841, Poland reported unilateral absence of the pectoralis minor and the sternal portion of the pectoralis major muscles in an individual who also had cutaneous syndactyly of the hand on the same side. This unique pattern of defects has subsequently been noted in numerous cases and has an incidence of about 1 in 20,000. It has been estimated that 10 per cent of patients with syndactyly of the hand have the Poland anomaly.

ABNORMALITIES. Variable *unilateral* features from among the following:
Thorax. Hypoplasia to absence of the pectoralis major muscle, nipple, and areola. Rib defects.
Upper Limbs. Hypoplasia distally with varying degrees of syndactyly, brachydactyly, oligodactyly, and occasionally, more severe reduction deficiency.
Other. Occasional hemivertebrae, renal anomaly, Sprengel's anomaly.

NATURAL HISTORY. Generally an otherwise normal individual.

ETIOLOGY. Unknown. It is three times as common in the male as in the female and is 75 per cent right-sided. Bouvet et al. have presented evidence of diminished blood flow to the affected side and have suggested that the primary defect may be in the development of the proximal subclavian artery, with early deficit of blood flow to the distal limb and the pectoral region, yielding partial loss of tissue in those regions. Bavinck and Weaver have proposed that interruption of the subclavian artery occurs proximal to the origin of the internal thoracic artery but distal to the origin of the vertebral artery. It is suspected that the defect occurs in all gradations, and the disorder is more common than has been appreciated. The author is aware of two sibships in which the propositus had the "full" Poland anomaly, whereas a sibling in one instance had only absence of the pectoral muscle and, in the other instance, only syndactyly of the hand.

References

Poland, A.: Deficiency of the pectoral muscles. Guy's Hosp. Rep., *6*:191, 1841.
Clarkson, P.: Poland's syndactyly. Guy's Hosp. Rep., *111*:335, 1962.
David, T. J.: Nature and etiology of the Poland anomaly. N. Engl. J. Med. *287*:487, 1972.
Mace, J. W., et al.: Poland's syndrome. Clin. Pediatr. (Phila.), *11*:98, 1972.
Bouvet, J., Maroteaux, P., and Briard-Guillemot, M.: Poland's syndrome: clinical and genetic studies—physiopathology. Nouv. Presse Med., *5*:185, 1976.
Bavinck, J. N. B., and Weaver, D. D: Subclavian artery supply disruption sequence: Hypothesis of a vascular etiology for Poland, Klippel-Feil and Möebius anomalies. Am. J. Med. Genet., *23*:903, 1986.

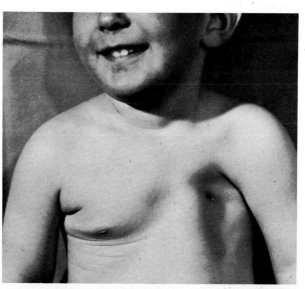

Poland anomaly. The absence of the pectoralis minor and the sternal portion of the pectoralis major plus the ipsilateral syndactyly of the hand are the more usual features of this complex anomaly. The bony thoracic anomaly and the hypoplasia of the hand, as noted in this otherwise normal boy, are more severe expressions of this defect.

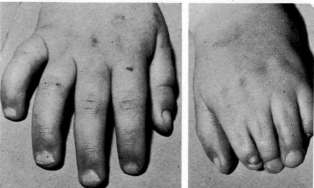

POPLITEAL PTERYGIUM SYNDROME

(Facio-Genito-Popliteal Syndrome)

Popliteal Web, Cleft Palate, Lower Lip Pits

This disorder was first reported by Trelat in 1869; about 47 cases have been recorded.

ABNORMALITIES
Oral. Cleft palate with or without cleft lip. Salivary lower lip pits.

Limbs. Popliteal web, in extreme form from heel to ischium. Toenail dysplasia, syndactyly of toes.

Genitalia. Hypoplastic labia majora, scrotal dysplasia, cryptorchidism.

OCCASIONAL ABNORMALITIES.
Oral frenula, cutaneous webs between eyelids, intercrural pterygium, syndactyly of fingers, hypoplasia or aplasia of digits, fusion of distal interphalangeal joints, valgus deformity of feet, pyramidal form to skin over hallux, hypoplasia of tibia, bifid or absent patella, posterior dislocation of fibulae, low acetabular angle, spina bifida occulta, other vertebral anomalies, scoliosis, ambiguous external genitalia, inguinal hernia, abnormal scalp hair, mental retardation (two cases).

NATURAL HISTORY.
There is usually a dense fibrous cord in the posterior portion of the popliteal pterygium, and extreme care must be exercised in the surgical repair because this cord may contain the sciatic nerve and popliteal artery.

There may be associated defects of muscle in the lower extremities, with limitation of function despite repair of the pterygium. Other webbing across the eyelids or in the mouth may require excision. The palate tends to be short, such that, even with repair of the cleft, function is impaired. Intelligence is usually normal, and these individuals are otherwise healthy. Cosmetic and orthopedic corrective procedures are merited.

ETIOLOGY. Autosomal dominant inheritance has been implied, with wide variability in severity.

References

Trelat, U.: Sur un vice conformation très-rare de la lèvre-inférieure. J. Med. Chir. Prat., *40*:442, 1869.

Hecht, F., and Jarvinen, J. M.: Heritable dysmorphic syndrome with normal intelligence. J. Pediatr., *70*:927, 1967.

Escobar, V., and Weaver, D.: The facio-genito-popliteal syndrome. Birth Defects Original Article Series, *14*:185, 1978.

Raithel, H., Schweckendiek, W., and Hillig, U.: The popliteal pterygium syndrome in three generations. Z. Kinderchir., *26*:56, 1979.

Hall, J. G., et al.: Limb pterygium syndromes: A review and report of eleven patients. Am. J. Med. Genet., *12*:377, 1982.

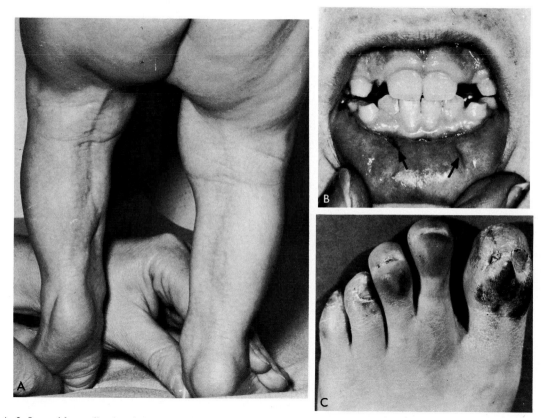

A, Infant with popliteal web. Note rod-like taut core. *B*, Boy with lower lip pits (*arrows*). *C*, Toenail dysplasia, a variable feature. (From Hecht, F., and Jarvinen, J. M.: J. Pediatr., *70*:927, 1967.)

ESCOBAR SYNDROME

(Multiple Pterygium Syndrome)

Multiple Pterygia, Camptodactyly, Syndactyly

Originally described by Bussiere in 1902, this disorder was fully delineated as a distinct entity by Escobar et al. in 1978. About 50 cases have been noted.

ABNORMALITIES
Growth. Small stature.
Facies. Ptosis of eyelids with antimongoloid slant of palpebral fissures, inner canthal folds, hypertelorism, micrognathia with downturning corners of mouth, cleft palate, sad, flat, emotionless face.
Pterygia. Pterygia of neck, axillae, antecubital, popliteal, and intercrural areas.
Limbs. Pterygia plus camptodactyly, syndactyly, equinovarus and/or rocker-bottom feet.
Genitalia. Cryptorchidism, absence of labia majora.

Other. Failure of posterior fusion of vertebrae, fusion of cervical vertebrae, rib anomalies.

OCCASIONAL ABNORMALITIES. Scoliosis, dislocation of hip, hypoplastic nipples.

NATURAL HISTORY. The majority of affected individuals become ambulatory. Intelligence is normal.

ETIOLOGY. Autosomal recessive.

References

Escobar, V., et al.: Multiple pterygium syndrome. Am. J. Dis. Child., *132*:609, 1978.
Hall, J. G., et al.: Limb pterygium syndromes: A review and report of eleven patients. Am. J. Med. Genet., *12*:377, 1982.

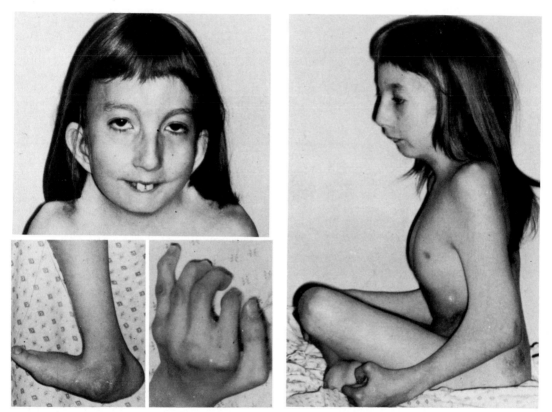

Twelve year old girl showing features of Escobar syndrome. (From Escobar, V., et al.: Am. J. Dis. Child., *132*:609, 1978.)

CHILD SYNDROME

*Unilateral Hypomelia and Skin Hypoplasia,
Cardiac Defect*

Falek et al. reported two female siblings with this unique pattern of malformation in 1968, and Shear noted a comparable case. At least 20 cases have now been reported. The term CHILD is an acronym for Congenital Hemidysplasia with Ichthyosiform erythroderma and Limb Defects.

ABNORMALITIES

Growth. Mild prenatal growth deficiency.

Limbs. Unilateral hypomelia varying from absence to hypoplasia of some metacarpals and phalanges. Webbing at elbows and knees. Joint contractures.

Skin. Unilateral erythema and scaling, with sharp midline demarcation anteriorly and posteriorly. Unilateral alopecia, hyperkeratosis, and nail destruction.

Other Skeletal. Unilateral hypoplasia of bones involving any part of the skeleton, including mandible, clavicle, scapula, ribs, and vertebrae. Punctate epiphyseal calcifications.

Other. Cardiac septal defects. Single coronary ostium. Single ventricle. Unilateral renal agenesis.

OCCASIONAL ABNORMALITIES. Ipsilateral hypoplasia of brain, cranial nerves, spinal cord, lung, thyroid, adrenal gland, ovary, and fallopian tube. Mild mental deficiency. Mild contralateral anomalies of skin, bone, and/or viscera. Cleft lip. Umbilical hernia. Hearing loss.

NATURAL HISTORY. The erythema and scaling usually present at birth may develop during the first few weeks of life. New areas of involvement may occur as late as nine years. The face is spared. The right side of the body has been involved in 14 cases, the left side in six. Treatment with etretinate, an aromatic retinoid, has been successful in management of the skin problems in some cases.

ETIOLOGY. Unknown. All but one affected individual has been a female, raising the possibility of X-linked dominant inheritance; lethal in the hemizygous male.

References

Falek, A., et al.: Unilateral limb and skin deformities with congenital heart disease in twin siblings. A lethal syndrome. J. Pediatr., *73*:910, 1968.

Shear, C. S., et al.: Syndrome of unilateral ectromelia, psoriasis, and central nervous system anomalies. Birth Defects, 7:197, 1971.

Happle, R., Koch, H., and Lenz, W.: The CHILD syndrome. Eur. J. Pediatr., *134*:27, 1980.

Christiansen, J. R., Petersen, H. O., and Søgaard, H.: The CHILD syndrome—congenital hemidysplasia with ichthyosiform erythroderma and limb defects. A case report. Acta Derm. Venereol. (Stockh.), *64*:165, 1984.

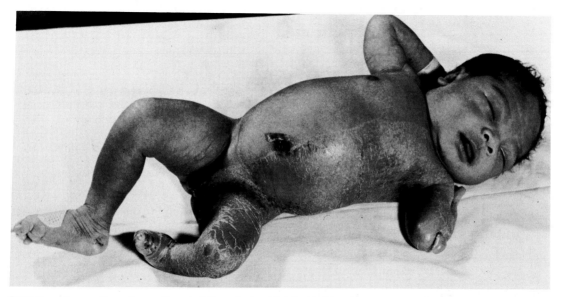

CHILD syndrome. One of two affected siblings, both with left-sided involvement. (From Falek, A., et al.: J. Pediatr., 73:910, 1968.)

FEMORAL HYPOPLASIA–
UNUSUAL FACIES SYNDROME

Femoral Hypoplasia, Short Nose, Cleft Palate

Following single case reports in 1961 and 1965 by Franz and O'Rahilly and by Kucera et al., Daentl et al. recognized four additional patients and set forth this unique syndrome in 1975.

ABNORMALITIES

Growth. Small stature, predominantly the result of short lower limbs.

Facial. Short nose with hypoplastic alae nasi, long philtrum, and thin upper lip. Micrognathia, cleft palate. Upslanting palpebral fissures.

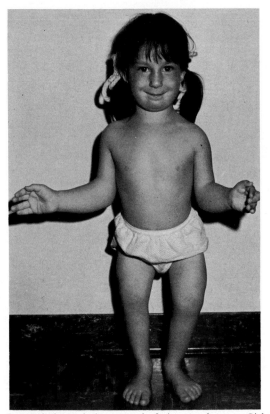

Femoral hypoplasia–unusual facies syndrome. Girl showing short humeri with synostosis at the elbow, in addition to femoral shortness.

Limbs. Hypoplastic to absent femora and fibulae. Variable hypoplasia of humeri with restricted elbow movement, including synostosis. Talipes.

Pelvis. Hypoplastic acetabulae, constricted iliac base with vertical ischial axis, and large obturator foramina.

Spine. Dysplastic sacrum. Missing vertebrae and/or hemivertebrae. Sacralization of lumbar vertebrae. Scoliosis.

Genitourinary. Cryptorchidism. Inguinal hernia. Small penis, testes, or labia majora. Polycystic kidneys, absent kidneys, abnormal collecting system.

OCCASIONAL ABNORMALITIES. Astigmatism; esotropia; short third, fourth, and fifth metatarsals; inguinal hernia; cryptorchidism.

NATURAL HISTORY. Though there may be problems in speech development, the patients have been of normal intelligence. Most of them have been ambulatory.

ETIOLOGY. Unknown. Although the vast majority of cases are sporadic, an affected male whose daughter is similarly affected raises the possibility of autosomal dominant inheritance. Maternal diabetes has been documented frequently.

References

Franz, C. H., and O'Rahilly, R.: Congenital skeletal limb deficiencies. J. Bone Joint Surg. [Am.], *43*:1202, 1961.

Kucera, V. J., Lenz, W., and Maier, W.: Missbildungen der Beine und der Kaudalen Wirbelsaeule bei Kindern diabetischer Muetter. Dtsch. Med. Wochenschr., *90*:901, 1965.

Daentl, D. L., et al.: Femoral hypoplasia–unusual facies syndrome. J. Pediatr., *86*:107, 1975.

Lampert, R. P.: Dominant inheritance of femoral hypoplasia–unusual facies syndrome. Clin. Genet., *17*:255, 1980.

Johnson, J. P., et al.: Femoral hypoplasia–unusual facies syndrome in infants of diabetic mothers. J. Pediatr., *102*:866, 1983.

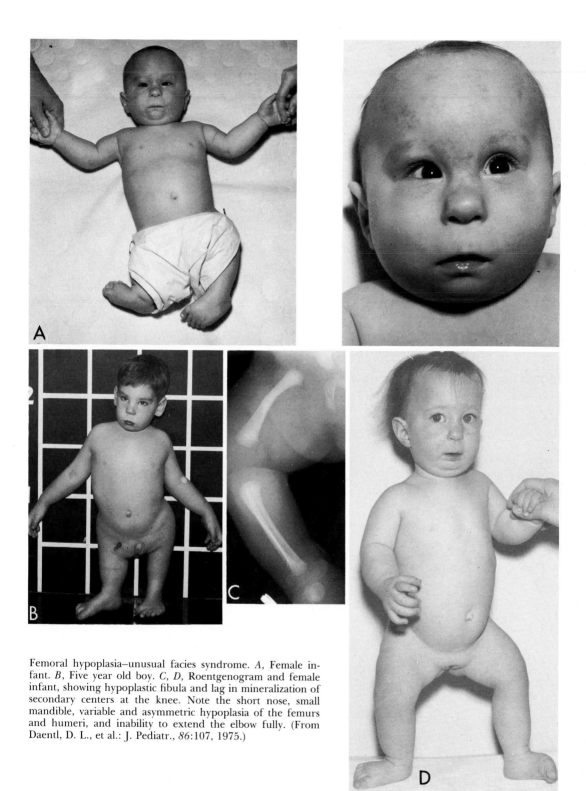

Femoral hypoplasia–unusual facies syndrome. *A*, Female infant. *B*, Five year old boy. *C, D*, Roentgenogram and female infant, showing hypoplastic fibula and lag in mineralization of secondary centers at the knee. Note the short nose, small mandible, variable and asymmetric hypoplasia of the femurs and humeri, and inability to extend the elbow fully. (From Daentl, D. L., et al.: J. Pediatr., *86*:107, 1975.)

ADAMS-OLIVER SYNDROME

Aplasia Cutis Congenita,
Terminal Transverse Defects of Limbs

Adams and Oliver described eight members of a family with this disorder in 1945. More than 40 affected individuals have been reported.

ABNORMALITIES

Growth. Mild growth deficiency (third to tenth percentile).

Scalp. Aplasia cutis congenita over posterior parietal region, with or without an underlying defect of bone. Tortuous veins over posterior scalp.

Limbs. Variable degrees of terminal transverse defects, including those of lower legs, feet, hands, fingers, toes, and/or distal phalanges. Short fingers. Small toenails.

Skin. Cutis marmorata.

OCCASIONAL ABNORMALITIES. Cryptorchidism. Esotropia. Accessory nipples. Microphthalmia. Duplicated collecting system. Cleft lip.

ETIOLOGY. Autosomal dominant with marked variability in expression. A careful physical examination and radiographs of hands and feet are indicated in first degree relatives of affected individuals.

References

Adams, F. H., and Oliver, C. P.: Hereditary deformities in man due to arrested development. J. Hered., *36*:3, 1945.

Scribanu, N., and Tamtamy, S. A.: The syndrome of aplasia cutis congenita with terminal transverse defects of limbs. *87*:79, 1975.

Bonafede, R. P., and Beighton, P.: Autosomal dominant inheritance of scalp defects with ectrodactyly. Am. J. Med. Genet., *3*:35, 1979.

Toriello, H. V., Stawiski, M., and Larsen, J.: Autosomal dominant skin and limb defects: Probable Adams-Oliver syndrome with unusual manifestations. David W. Smith Workshop on Malformations and Morphogenesis. University of Vermont, Burlington, 1986.

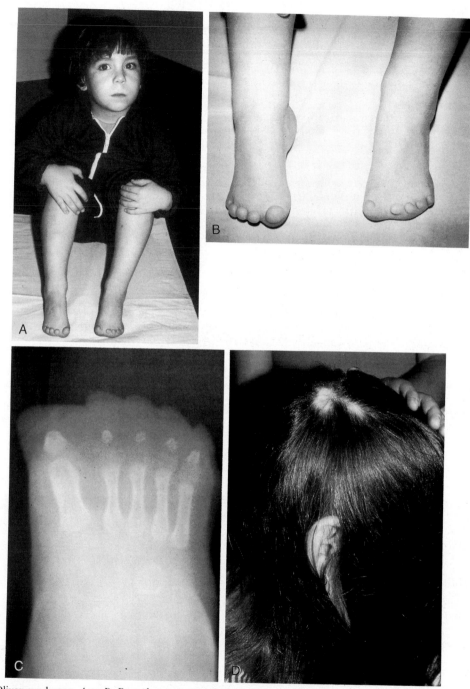

Adams-Oliver syndrome. *A* to *D*, Boy, three years and nine months old, and his mother's sister. Note the terminal transverse defects involving the toes (*A* to *C*) and the area of aplasia cutis congenita over his maternal aunt's posterior scalp (*D*). She was otherwise normal.

HOLT-ORAM SYNDROME

(Cardiac-Limb Syndrome)

*Upper Limb Defect, Cardiac Anomaly,
Narrow Shoulders*

This syndrome of skeletal and cardiovascular abnormalities was first described by Holt and Oram in 1960.

ABNORMALITIES

Skeletal. All gradations of defect in the upper limb and shoulder girdle, from thumb hypoplasia to phocomelia. Asymmetric involvement is frequently seen. There is no correlation between the severity of the limb defect and the cardiac defect. Finger-like hypoplastic to absent triphalangeal thumb with syndactyly. Hypoplasia to absence of first metacarpal and radius. Defects of ulna, humerus, clavicle, scapula, sternum.

Cardiovascular. Auricular septal defect, sometimes with arrhythmia, and ventricular septal defect have been the most common defects, and about one third of of the patients have had other types of congenital heart defects. Hypoplasia of distal blood vessels.

OCCASIONAL ABNORMALITIES. Hypertelorism.
Patent ductus arteriosus, pulmonic stenosis. Absent pectoralis major muscle. Pectus excavatum, thoracic scoliosis. Vertebral anomalies. Absence of one or more ossification centers in the wrist.

ETIOLOGY. Autosomal dominant with variable expression. Rarely only unilateral involvement of thumb. To insure diagnosis, at-risk individuals with a normal physical examination should have radiographs of wrists, arms, and hands and an echocardiogram.

References

Holt, M., and Oram, S.: Familial heart disease with skeletal malformations. Br. Heart J., *22*:236, 1960.

Lewis, K. B., et al.: The upper limb–cardiovascular syndrome. An autosomal dominant genetic effect on embryogenesis. J.A.M.A., *193*:1080, 1965.

Poznauski, A., et al.: Objective evaluation of the hand in the Holt-Oram syndrome. Birth Defects, *8*:125, 1972.

Kaufman, R. L., et al.: Variable expression of the Holt-Oram syndrome. Am. J. Dis. Child., *127*:21, 1974.

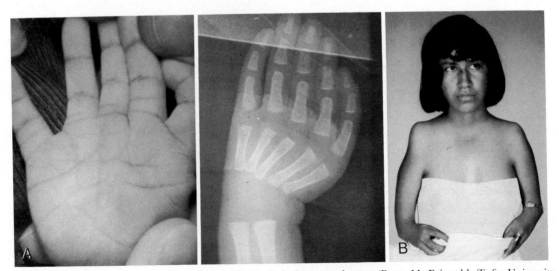

A, Finger-like thumb (to right) in an infant with the Holt-Oram syndrome. (From M. Feingold, Tufts University School of Medicine, Boston.) *B*, Fifteen year old with auricular septal defect. Note severe forearm hypoplasia, absence of thumbs, and altered shoulder girdle.

LEVY-HOLLISTER SYNDROME

(Lacrimo-Auriculo-Dento-Digital Syndrome)

Although Levy described the first affected patient in 1967, this disorder was first delineated by Hollister et al. in 1973. Fourteen cases have been reported.

ABNORMALITIES

Lacrimal Anomalies. Nasolacrimal duct obstruction; aplasia or hypoplasia of lacrimal puncta.

Ears. Simple, cup-shaped ears with short helix and underdeveloped antihelix.

Hearing. Mild to severe mixed conductive and sensorineural hearing loss.

Dental. Hypodontia, peg-shaped incisors, enamel hypoplasia of both deciduous and permanent teeth.

Limb. Variable abnormalities of upper limbs, including digitalization of thumb; deficiency of bone and soft tissue of thumb and index finger; shortening of radius and ulna; preaxial polydactyly; triphalangeal thumb; duplication of distal phalanx of thumb; thenar muscle hypoplasia; syndactyly between index and middle fingers; clinodactyly of third and fifth fingers; absent radius and thumb.

OCCASIONAL ABNORMALITIES. Absence of parotid glands and Stensen's ducts. Nasolacrimal fistulae. Renal agenesis; coronal hypospadius. Nephrosclerosis. 2-3 syndactyly of toes.

ETIOLOGY. Autosomal dominant.

References

Levy, W. J.: Mesoectodermal dysplasia. Am. J. Ophthalmol., *63*:978, 1967.

Hollister, D. W., et al.: The lacrimo-auriculo-dento-digital syndrome. J. Pediatr., *83*:438, 1973.

Shiang, E. L., and Holmes, L. B.: The lacrimo-auriculo-dento-digital syndrome. Pediatrics, *59*:927, 1977.

Thompson, E., Pembrey, M., and Graham, J. M.: Phenotypic variation in LADD syndrome. J. Med. Genet., *22*:382, 1985.

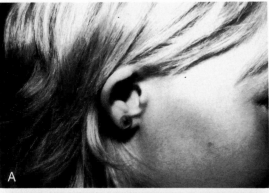
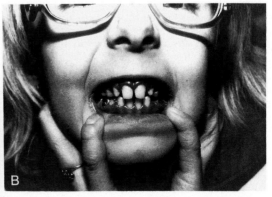

Levy-Hollister syndrome. Nine year old female showing small, cupped ears *(A)*, small, peg-shaped teeth with enamel dysplasia *(B)*, and *(C)* the digitalized thumb plus fifth finger clinodactyly on the hand at the right of the photograph and a long tapering thumb with absent creases and surgically removed index finger on the hand at the left of the photograph. (Courtesy of Dr. H. E. Hoyme, University of Arizona, Tucson.)

FANCONI PANCYTOPENIA SYNDROME

Radial Hypoplasia, Hyperpigmentation, Pancytopenia

Since Fanconi's original description of three affected siblings in 1927, over 160 cases have been reported. Recently, Glanz and Fraser have documented the marked variability of the clinical phenotype. Since 25 per cent of affected individuals are structurally normal, they have emphasized the importance of considering this diagnosis in any anemic child with chromosome breaks, even in the absence of dysmorphic features on the physical examination.

ABNORMALITIES

Growth. Short stature, frequently of prenatal onset.

Performance. Microcephaly (25 to 37 per cent). Mental deficiency in 25 per cent.

Skeletal. Hypoplasia to aplasia of thumb, with supernumerary thumbs in some cases. Hypoplastic or aplastic radii. Congenital hip dislocation.

Urogenital. Hypoplastic and/or malformed kidneys. Double ureters. Small penis, small testes, and/or cryptorchidism.

Hematologic. Pancytopenia manifested by poikilocytosis, anisocytosis, reticulocytopenia, thrombocytopenia, and leukopenia. Splenic hypoplasia is a frequent autopsy finding.

Skin. Brownish pigmentation.

OCCASIONAL ABNORMALITIES.
Ptosis of eyelid, strabismus, nystagmus, microphthalmos, auricular anomaly, deafness, osteoporosis, broad base of proximal phalanges, hypoplasia to aplasia of first metacarpal, diminished carpal centers, syndactyly, dislocation of hip, congenital heart defect, hypospadias, leukemia.

NATURAL HISTORY.
The majority of patients are relatively small at birth. Respiratory tract infections may be a frequent problem. The uneven brownish pigmentation of the skin tends to increase with age, being most evident in the anogenital area, groin, axillae, and trunk. Development of bleeding, pallor, and/or recurring infection usually appears between five and ten years of age,

although pancytopenia may occur in infancy or as late as the third decade. There are nests of hematopoiesis in the generally hypoplastic marrow. Some erythrocytes are macrocytic; there is a high percentage of fetal hemoglobin, and the red cell life span is shortened. The leukopenia is predominantly granulocytopenia. Previously, the survival following discovery of pancytopenia was seldom more than two years, although recently, combined therapy with testosterone and hydrocortisone analogue has extended the survival period.

ETIOLOGY.
Autosomal recessive. An occasional parent may have a malformation (one case), slight pancytopenia (one case), or neutropenia, and leukemia was found in an otherwise normal relative in 4 of 48 affected families; all possible heterozygote manifestions.

COMMENT.
Successful prenatal and postnatal diagnoses of this disorder can now be accomplished by demonstrating a high frequency of diepoxybutane-induced chromosomal breakage in peripheral blood lymphocytes as well as in cultured amniotic fluid cells.

References

Fanconi, G.: Familiäre infantile pernizosaaritige anämie. Z. Kinderheilkd. *117*:257, 1927.

Garriga, S., and Crosby, W. H.: The incidence of leukemia in families of patients with hypoplasia of the marrow. Blood, *14*:1008, 1959.

Nilsson, L. R.: Chronic pancytopenia with multiple congenital abnormalities (Fanconi's anaemia). Acta Paediatr., *49*:518, 1960.

Schmid, W. K., et al.: Chromosomenbrueihigkeit bei der familiären Panmyelopathie (Typus Fanconi). Schweiz. Med. Wochenschr., *95*:1461, 1965.

Glanz, A., and Fraser, F. C.: Spectrum of anomalies in Fanconi anemia. J. Med. Genet., *19*:412, 1982.

Auerbach, A. D., Sagi, M., and Adler, B.: Fanconi anemia: Prenatal diagnosis in 30 infants at risk. Pediatrics, *76*:794, 1985.

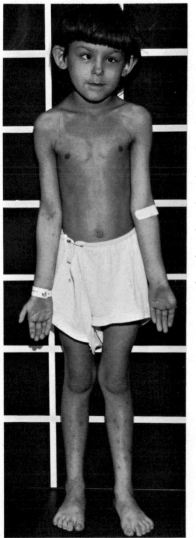

+ PIGMENTATION (BROWN) OF SKIN

+ SHORT STATURE

+ SMALL CRANIUM

+ MENTAL RETARDATION

+ STRABISMUS

+ ABNORMAL EARS

+ ABNORMAL THUMBS

+ RENAL ANOMALY

+ HYPOPLASIA OF MARROW, WITH TIME

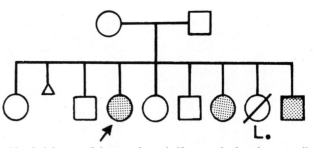

Fanconi pancytopenia syndrome. Seven year old with a height age of three and one-half years who has the anomalies listed above. The pedigree notes two affected siblings and one otherwise normal brother who died of leukemia during infancy. (From Smith, D. W.: J. Pediatr., *70*:479, 1967.)

RADIAL APLASIA–THROMBOCYTOPENIA SYNDROME

(TAR Syndrome)

Gross, Groh, and Weippl described this entity in siblings in 1956; subsequently, over 31 cases have been reported.

ABNORMALITIES

Hematologic. Most severe in early infancy. Thrombocytopenia with absence or hypoplasia of megakaryocytes (absent in 66 per cent, decreased in 12 per cent, inactive in 12 per cent). "Leukemoid" granulocytosis in 62 per cent of patients, especially during bleeding episodes. Eosinophilia in 53 per cent. Anemia, often out of proportion to apparent blood loss.

Limbs. Absence or hypoplasia of radius. Usually bilateral; often with associated ulnar hypoplasia and defects of the hands, legs, and/or feet. However, the thumbs are present.

OCCASIONAL ABNORMALITIES.

About 33 per cent have a congenital heart defect. Small stature, nevus flammeus of forehead, genu varum, renal anomaly, spina bifida, brachycephaly, strabismus, micrognathia, syndactyly, short humerus, hypoplastic shoulder girdle, dislocation of the hip, talipes foot deformity, severe reduction defect of legs, Meckel's diverticulum. Mental deficiency occurs in about 7 per cent of patients.

NATURAL HISTORY. About 40 per cent of the patients have died, usually as a result of hemorrhage during early infancy. With advancing age, the severity of the hematologic disorder usually becomes less profound, and therefore, vigorous early management is indicated. The babies are liable to have eosinophilia and seem more prone to developing cow milk allergy.

ETIOLOGY. Autosomal recessive. Of interest is the fact that an uncle of one patient died of leukemia. Prenatal diagnosis can be made by showing the defect of the upper limb on sonography.

References

Gross, H., Groh, C., and Weippl, G.: Congenitale hypoplastische Thrombopenie mit Radialaplasie. Neue Osterr. Z. Kinderheilkhd., *1*:574, 1956.

Shaw, S., and Oliver, R. A. M.: Congenital hypoplastic thrombocytopenia with skeletal deformities in siblings. Blood, *14*:374, 1956.

Hall, J. G., et al.: Thrombocytopenia with absent radius (TAR). Medicine, *48*:441, 1969.

Anyane-Yeboa, K., et al.: Brief clinical report: Tetraphocomelia in the syndrome of thrombocytopenic with absent radii (TAR syndrome). Am. J. Med. Genet., *20*:571, 1985.

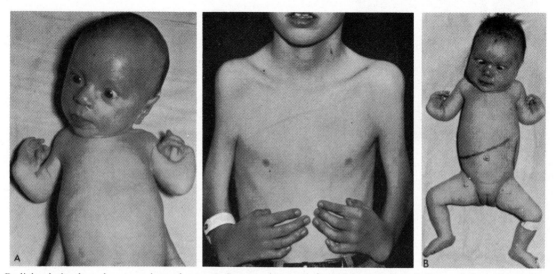

Radial aplasia–thrombocytopenia syndrome. *A,* Same patient, as infant and young boy. *B,* Young infant with serious bleeding and hepatosplenomegaly. Patient also had a cardiac defect. (Courtesy of J. M. Opitz, Helena, Montana, and R. Hunter, University of Washington, Seattle.)

AASE SYNDROME

Triphalangeal Thumb, Congenital Anemia

Aase and Smith described this disorder in two male siblings in 1969. At least six additional cases have been recognized.

ABNORMALITIES. Based on eight cases.
Growth. Mild growth deficiency, about third percentile.
Hematologic. Hypoplastic anemia that tends to improve with age. Variable leukopenia.
Skeletal. Triphalangeal thumbs, mild radial hypoplasia, narrow shoulders, late closure of fontanels.
Other. Cardiac defects, especially ventricular septal defect. Variable hepatosplenomegaly.

OCCASIONAL ABNORMALITIES. Found in one patient: cleft lip, cleft palate, retinopathy, webbed neck.

NATURAL HISTORY. The anemia, which has been responsive to prednisone therapy, tends to improve with age.

ETIOLOGY. Unknown. Occurrence in siblings and in both sexes makes autosomal recessive inheritance most likely.

References

Aase, J. M., and Smith, D. W.: Congenital anemia and triphalangeal thumbs: A new syndrome. J. Pediatr., 74:417, 1969.
Murphy, S., and Lubin, B.: Triphalangeal thumbs and congenital erythroid hypoplasia: Report of a case with unusual features. J. Pediatr., 81:987, 1972.
Jones, B., and Thompson, H.: Triphalangeal thumbs associated with hypoplastic anemia. Pediatrics, 52:609, 1973.
Van Weel-Sipman, M., van der Kamp, J. J. P., and deKoning, J.: A female patient with Aase syndrome. J. Pediatr., 91:753, 1977.
Higginbottom, M. C., et al.: Case report: The Aase syndrome in a female patient. J. Med. Genet., 15:484, 1978.

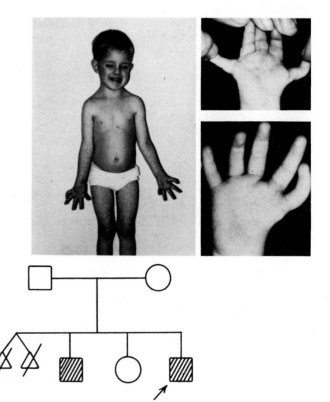

Aase syndrome. Affected boy who had been seriously anemic in infancy, during which time the anemia responded to prednisone therapy. He is now mildly anemic without therapy. His brother, whose hand is also shown, is similarly affected. (From Aase, J. M., and Smith, D. W.: J. Pediatr., 74:417, 1969.)

J. OSTEOCHONDRODYSPLASIAS

ACHONDROGENESIS, TYPES IA AND IB

Low Nasal Bridge, Very Short Limbs,
Incomplete Ossification of Lower Spine

This early lethal disorder was described in 1925 by Donath and Vogl and termed achondrogenesis by Fraccaro in 1952. More than 15 cases have been reported. Recent studies by Borochowitz et al. indicate that achondrogenesis type I (previously referred to as Parenti-Fraccaro type) represents two radiographically and histopathologically distinct disorders referred to as types IA and IB. In the classification set forth by Whitley and Gorlin, type I is synonymous with type IA and type II with type IB.

ABNORMALITIES

Growth. Extreme small stature, 22 to 30 cm.
Craniofacies. Cranium large for gestational age. Low nasal bridge, micrognathia.
Limbs. Severe micromelia.
Radiographs. In both types, the skull, vertebral bodies, fibula, talus, and calcaneus are poorly ossified, the ilia are crenated, the long bones are stellate, and the ribs are extremely short. In type IA, multiple rib fractures are present, and the proximal femurs have metaphyseal spikes. Conversely, in type IB, rib fractures do not occur, and the distal femurs have metaphyseal irregularities.

NATURAL HISTORY AND COMMENT. The defect in the development of cartilage and bone is severe. In type IA, normal-appearing but hypervascular cartilage matrix is present with increased cellular density. Large lacuna surround the chondrocytes, which contain round cytoplasmic inclusion bodies. In type IB, sparse interterritorial cartilaginous matrix is present, with a marked deficiency of collagen fibers. The chondrocytes are large, have a central round nucleus, and are surrounded by a dense collagenous ring.

Developmental pathology beyond the skeletal system is implied by the frequent findings of polyhydramnios, hydrops, and early lethality. Most infants are stillborn or die shortly after birth.

ETIOLOGY. Autosomal recessive.

References

Donath, J., and Vogl, A.: Untersuchungen über den chondrodystrophischen Zwergwuchs. Wien. Arch. Intern. Med., *10*:1, 1925.

Fraccaro, M.: Contributo allo studio delle malattie del mesenchima osteopoietico. L'achondrogenesi. Folia Hered. Pathol. (Milano), *1*:190, 1952.

Maroteaux, P., and Lamy, M.: Le diagnostic des nanismes chondrodystrophiques chez les nouveaunés. Arch. Fr. Pediatr., *25*:241, 1968.

Whitley, C. B., and Gorlin, R. J.: Achondrogenesis: New nosology with evidence of genetic heterogeneity. Radiology, *148*:693, 1983.

Borochowitz, Z., et al.: Achondrogenesis Type I—Further heterogeneity. J. Pediatr. (in press).

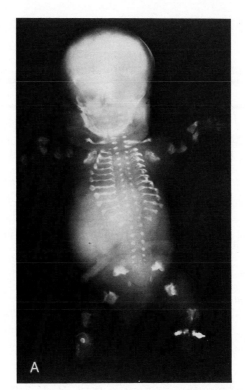

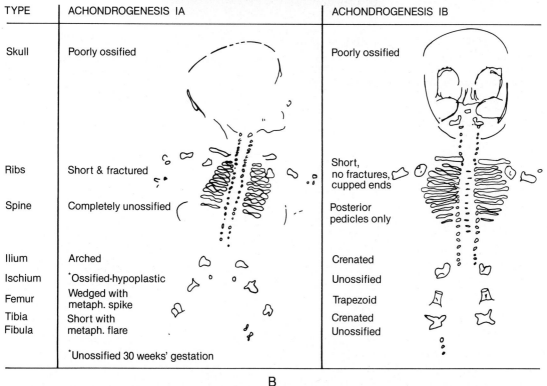

TYPE	ACHONDROGENESIS IA	ACHONDROGENESIS IB
Skull	Poorly ossified	Poorly ossified
Ribs	Short & fractured	Short, no fractures, cupped ends
Spine	Completely unossified	Posterior pedicles only
Ilium	Arched	Crenated
Ischium	*Ossified-hypoplastic	Unossified
Femur	Wedged with metaph. spike	Trapezoid
Tibia	Short with	Crenated
Fibula	metaph. flare	Unossified
	*Unossified 30 weeks' gestation	

B

A, Stillborn infant at 30 weeks' gestation with achrondrogenesis, type IA. *B,* Radiographic features that differentiate type IA from type IB are delineated on the drawings. (Courtesy of Dr. R. Lachman, Harbor–UCLA Medical Center, and Dr. D. Rimoin, Cedars-Sinai Medical Center, Los Angeles.)

ACHONDROGENESIS, TYPE II

(Langer-Saldino Achondrogenesis; Hypochondrogenesis)

Initially described by Langer et al. and Saldino, this early lethal disorder has recently been more completely delineated by Chen et al. and Borochowitz et al.

ABNORMALITIES
Growth. Extremely short stature (27 to 36 cm).
Craniofacies. Large calvarium with large anterior and posterior fontanels, flat nasal bridge, small anteverted nostrils, micrognathia.
Limbs. Short.
Radiographs. Normal cranial ossification. Short ribs without fractures. Short, broad long bones with disproportionately long fibula and metaphyseal irregularity of distal ulna. Variable degrees of failure of ossification of lumbar spine, cervical spine, sacrum, ischial and pubic bones, and calcaneus and talus.
Other. Polyhydramnios.

OCCASIONAL ABNORMALITIES. Cleft soft palate.

NATURAL HISTORY AND COMMENT. Although one child survived to 3 months, the majority are stillborn or die in the first few hours of life. Chondro-osseous histology has revealed hypervascularity and hypercellularity of cartilage, with multiple small, round dilated cysternae of rough endoplasmic reticulum.

ETIOLOGY. Autosomal recessive.

COMMENT. Recent data indicate that hypochondrogenesis previously thought to be a distinct disorder, and achondrogenesis type II represent a spectrum of the same disorder, with marked phenotypic variability.

References

Langer, L. O., et al.: Thanatophoric dwarfism: A condition confused with achondroplasia in the neonate, with brief comments on achondrogenesis and homozygous achondroplasia. Radiology, *92*:285, 1969.

Saldino, R. M.: Lethal short-limbed dwarfism: Achondrogenesis and thanatophoric dwarfism. Am. J. Roentgenol., *112*:185, 1971.

Chen, H., Lin, C. T., and Yang, S. S.: Achondrogenesis: a review with special consideration of achondrogenesis type II (Langer-Saldino). Am. J. Med. Genet., *10*:379, 1981.

Borochowitz, Z., et al.: Achondrogenesis II–hypochondrogenesis: Variability versus heterogeneity. Am. J. Med. Genet., *24*:273, 1986.

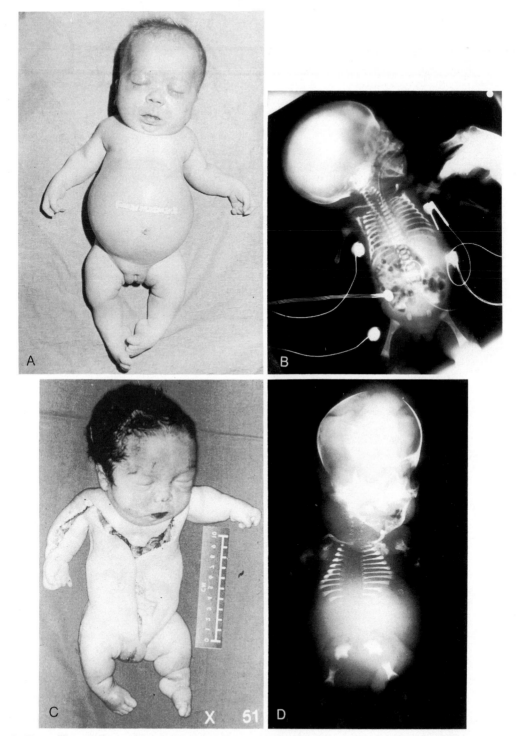

A to D, Two stillborn infants with achondrogenesis, type II, showing the variation in severity of the disorder. Note the relatively normal cranial ossification, short ribs, and variable degrees of failure of ossification of lumbar and cervical spines, sacrum, and ischial and pubic bones. (Courtesy of Dr. R. Lachman, Harbor–UCLA Medical Center, and Dr. D. Rimoin, Cedars-Sinai Medical Center, Los Angeles.)

FIBROCHONDROGENESIS

Lazzaroni-Fossati described a patient with this early lethal disorder in 1978. Subsequently, four additional patients have been reported. A distinctive fibrosis of the growth-plate cartilage led to the designation fibrochondrogenesis.

ABNORMALITIES
Growth. Short stature.
Craniofacies. Widely patent anterior fontanel, coronal and sagittal sutures. Protuberant eyes with large corneae. Flat nasal bridge and anteverted nares. Cleft palate. Short neck. Low-set, malformed ears.
Trunk. Flattened vertebrae with posterior vertebral hypoplasia and a sagittal midline cleft. Short, thin ribs with anterior and posterior cupping. Long, thin clavicles. Small chest.
Other. Omphalocele.
Limbs. Rhizomelic shortening. Camptodactyly. Fifth finger clinodactyly. Hypoplastic finger and toenails. Broad, irregular metaphyses of long bones, with peripheral spur formation. Short fibulae.

Pelvis. Small sacroscratic notch with medial spikes. Small iliac bones. Flattened acetabula. Short ischial and pubic bones. Broad ischii.

NATURAL HISTORY. Two patients have been stillborn; one died immediately after birth, a fourth died after three weeks of mechanical ventilation.

ETIOLOGY. Probably autosomal recessive.

References

Lazzaroni-Fossati, F., et al.: La fibrochondrogenese. Arch. Fr. Pediatr., *35*:1096, 1978.
Eteson, D. J., et al.: Fibrochondrogenesis:Radiologic and histologic studies. Am. J. Med. Genet., *19*:277, 1984.
Whitley, C. B., et al.: Fibrochondrogenesis: Lethal, autosomal recessive chondrodysplasia with distinctive cartilage histopathology. Am. J. Med. Genet., *19*:265, 1984.

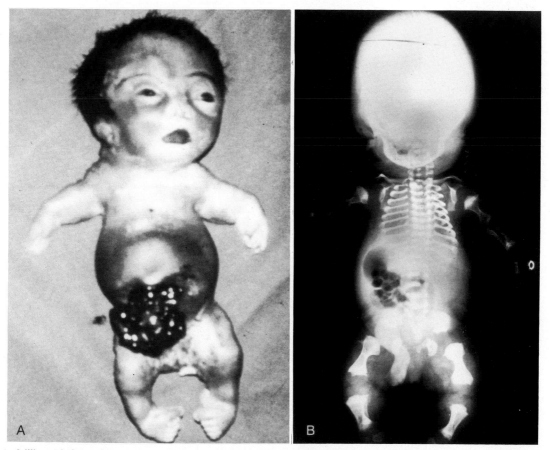

A, Stillborn infant with fibrochondrogenesis. Note the flat, wide nasal bridge, anteverted nares, short limbs, and equinovarus position of the feet. *B*, The radiograph reveals long, thin clavicles, short, thin ribs, flattened acetabula, narrow sacrosciatic notches, metaphyseal widening of the tibia and fibula, and dumbbell-shaped femora. (From Eteson, D. J., et al.: Am. J. Med. Genet., *19*:277, 1984.)

ATELOSTEOGENESIS

(Giant Cell Chondrodysplasia)

This early lethal short-limb dwarfing condition has recently been set forth by Maroteaux et al. and Sillence et al. Atelosteogenesis derives from the Greek word for incomplete and relates to the marked lack of complete ossification of certain bones.

ABNORMALITIES

Growth. Short stature with proximal shortness of limbs.

Radiographs. Short rounded to absent humerus. Absent fibula. Short femora with rounded proximal ends but square and tapered distal ends. Flattened, hypoplastic vertebrae, particularly in the cervicodorsal and lumbosacral regions, with multiple coronal clefts throughout. Markedly delayed ossification of proximal phalanges and middle phalanges with well-ossified distal phalanges.

Other. Polyhydramnios.

OCCASIONAL ABNORMALITIES. Depressed nasal bridge. Cleft palate.

NATURAL HISTORY. All affected infants have been stillborn or have died immediately after birth.

ETIOLOGY. Unknown. All cases have been sporadic.

COMMENT. Multinucleated "giant cells" are found scattered throughout resting cartilage.

References

Maroteaux, P., et al.: Atelosteogenesis. Am. J. Med. Genet., *13*:15, 1982.

Sillence, D. O., et al.: Spondylohumerofemoral hypoplasia (giant cell chondrodysplasia): A neonatally lethal short-limb skeletal dysplasia. Am. J. Med. Genet., *13*:7, 1982.

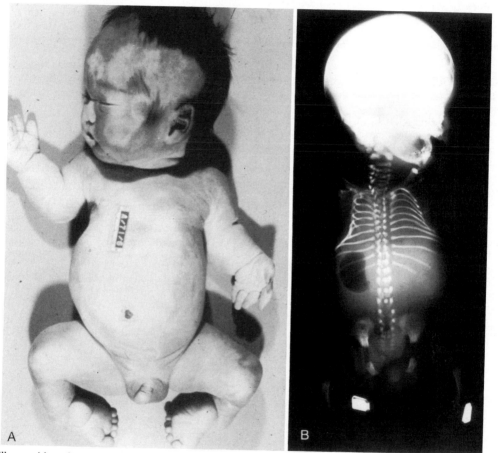

A, Stillborn with atelosteogenesis. Note the depressed nasal bridge, flexion contractures at knees, and equinovarus position of feet. *B*, The radiograph reveals lack of calcification of humerus and hypoplasia of much of the skeleton. (Courtesy of Dr. R. Lachman, Harbor–UCLA Medical Center, and Dr. D. Rimoin, Cedars-Sinai Medical Center, Los Angeles.)

SHORT RIB–POLYDACTYLY SYNDROME, MAJEWSKI TYPE

(Short Rib Syndrome [With or Without Polydactyly], Type II)

In 1971, Majewski et al. described four infants with this early lethal form of short-limb dwarfism. Spranger et al. differentiated it from other forms of short rib–polydactyly in 1974, and subsequently a number of additional cases have been described.

ABNORMALITIES

Growth. Short stature with disproportionate short limbs.

Craniofacies. Midline cleft lip. Cleft palate. Low-set, small, malformed ears.

Limbs. Both preaxial and postaxial polysyndactyly of hands and/or feet. Brachydactyly. Disproportionately short, oval-shaped tibiae. Short, rounded metacarpals and metatarsals. Premature ossification of proximal epiphyses of humeri, femora, and lateral cuboids. Underossified phalanges.

Trunk. Narrow thorax. Short, horizontal ribs. High clavicles.

Other. Ambiguous genitalia. Hypoplasia of epiglottis and larynx. Multiple glomerular cysts and focal dilatation of distal tubules of kidney.

OCCASIONAL ABNORMALITIES. Microglossia. Absent gallbladder. Brain anomalies, including pachygyria, a small vermis, and absence of olfactory bulbs. Persisting left superior vena cava. Hydrops. Polyhydramnios.

NATURAL HISTORY. Respiratory insufficiency secondary to pulmonary hypoplasia has led to death soon after birth in all cases.

ETIOLOGY. Autosomal recessive.

References

Majewski, F., et al.: Polysyndaktylie, verkürzte Gliedmassen und Genitalfehlbildungen: Kennzeichen eines selbaständigen Syndroms? Z. Kinderheilkd., *111*:118, 1971.

Spranger, J., et al.: Short rib–polydactyly (SRP) syndromes, types Majewski and Saldino-Noonan. Z. Kinderheilkd., *116*:73, 1974.

Motegi, T., et al.: Short rib–polydactyly syndrome, Majewski type, in two males. Hum. Genet., *49*:269, 1979.

Chen, H., et al.: Short rib–polydactyly syndrome, Majewski type. Am. J. Med. Genet., *7*:215, 1980.

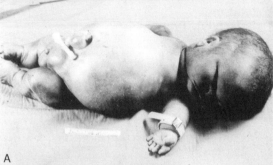

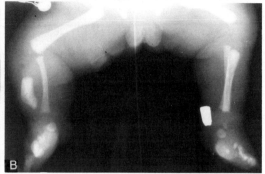

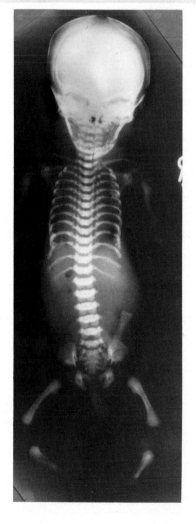

A to *C*, Neonate with short rib–polydactyly syndrome, Majewski type. Note the disproportionately short limbs, postaxial polydactyly, and, on the radiographs, the narrow thorax with short ribs and disproportionately short, abnormally shaped tibia. (Courtesy of Dr. R. Lachman, Harbor–UCLA Medical Center and Dr. D. Rimoin, Cedars-Sinai Medical Center, Los Angeles.)

SHORT RIB–POLYDACTYLY SYNDROME, NON-MAJEWSKI TYPE

(Short Rib Syndrome [With or Without Polydactyly], Type I)

This disorder was originally described by Saldino and Noonan in 1972. Although Naumoff et al. and Yang et al. have published cases suggesting that short rib–polydactyly syndrome, non-Majewski type, represents two separate disorders, clinical, radiographic, and morphologic studies set forth by Sillence suggest that only one disorder exists, with wide variability in expression. This issue remains to be completely resolved.

ABNORMALITIES

Growth. Short stature.

Limbs. Short. Postaxial polydactyly of hands and/or feet. Syndactyly. Metaphyseal irregularities of long bones, with spurs extending longitudinally from medial and lateral segments. Underossified phalanges.

Trunk. Short, horizontal ribs. Notch-like ossification defects around periphery of vertebral bodies.

Pelvis. Small iliac bones with horizontal acetabular roof. Triangular ossification defect above lateral aspect of acetabulum.

Other. Cardiac defects, including transposition of great vessels, double-outlet left ventricle, double-outlet right ventricle, endocardial cushion defect, and hypoplastic right heart. Polycystic kidneys. Hypoplasia of penis. Defects of cloacal development. Imperforate anus.

OCCASIONAL ABNORMALITIES. Natal teeth.

NATURAL HISTORY. Death from respiratory insufficiency secondary to pulmonary hypoplasia has occurred in all infants within the first few hours after birth.

ETIOLOGY. Autosomal recessive.

References

Saldino, R. M., and Noonan, C. D.: Severe thoracic dystrophy with striking micromelia, abnormal osseous development, including the spine, and multiple visceral anomalies. Am. J. Roentgenol., *114*:257, 1972.

Spranger, J., et al.: Short rib–polydactyly (SRP) syndromes, types Majewski and Saldino-Noonan. Z. Kinderheilkd., *116*:73, 1974.

Naumoff, P., et al.: Short rib–polydactyly syndrome type 3. Radiology, *122*:443, 1977.

Sillence, D. O.: Invited editorial comment: Non-Majewski short rib–polydactyly syndrome. Am. J. Med. Genet., 7:223, 1980.

Yang, S. S., et al.: Short rib–polydactyly syndrome, type 3 with chondrocytic inclusions: report of a case and review of the literature. Am. J. Med. Genet., 7:205, 1980.

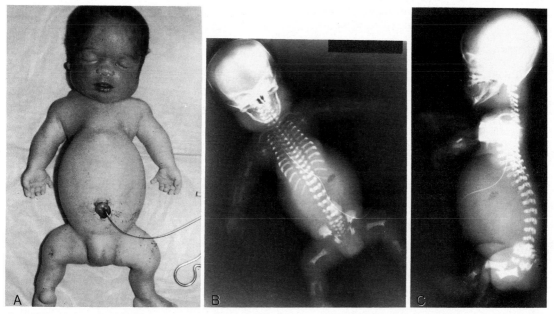

Short rib–polydactyly syndrome, non-Majewski type. *A,* Stillborn male infant. Note the narrow thorax, short limbs, postaxial polydactyly, and hypoplastic penis. *B, C,* Radiographs show short, horizontal ribs; metaphyseal irregularities of long bones, with spurs extending from medial and lateral segments; and triangular ossification defects above lateral aspect of acetabulum.

THANATOPHORIC DYSPLASIA

Short Limbs, Flat Vertebrae,
Large Cranium With Low Nasal Bridge

Maroteaux et al. set forth this disorder in 1967 and utilized the Greek term thanatophoric (death-bringing) to emphasize that such patients usually die shortly after birth. In the past, this disorder was often misdiagnosed as achondroplasia. For example, Harris and Patton considered ten of the 17 patients diagnosed as having achondroplasia among 64,000 births at St. Mary's Hospital in Manchester to be instances of thanatophoric dysplasia, an incidence of about one in 6400.

ABNORMALITIES
Performance. Hypotonia.
Growth. Severe growth deficiency; 36 to 46 cm tall, with an average height of 40 cm.
Craniofacial. Large cranium and fontanel; 36 to 47 cm, average of 37 cm. Small foramen magnum and short base of skull, with full forehead, low nasal bridge, and small facies.
Limbs. Short, with small sausage-like fingers, bowed long bones with cupped spur-like irregular flaring of metaphyses, and lack of ossification in secondary centers at knee. Disorganized chondrocytes and bony trabeculae, especially in central epiphyseal-metaphyseal region.
Thorax. Narrow with short ribs.
Spine. Short, flattened vertebrae with relatively wide intervertebral disc space. Lack of caudal widening of spinal canal.
Scapulae. Small and squarish.
Pelvis. Squarish and short, with small sciatic notch and medial spurs.

ABNORMALITIES OF UNCERTAIN INCIDENCE.
Brain anomalies, including microgyria, absent corpus callosum, and faulty organization, especially in temporal lobe and cerebellum. Extramedullary hematopoiesis.

OCCASIONAL ABNORMALITIES.
Hydrocephalus, patent ductus arteriosus, auricular septal defect, horseshoe kidney, hydronephrosis, imperforate anus, radioulnar synostosis. Craniostenosis, even to the degree of cloverleaf skull.

NATURAL HISTORY.
Feeble fetal activity and/or polyhydramnios is frequent in this disorder. Should such features lead to a prenatal ultrasonographic diagnosis, early induction of delivery has been recommended in order to avoid serious delivery problems at a later date (related to large head and/or breech presentation).

These patients usually die shortly after birth, at least partially owing to the small thoracic cage and respiratory insufficiency. The longest survival was 169 days. The author recommends no medical intervention toward survival for patients with this disorder.

ETIOLOGY.
Unknown. Although one instance of affected siblings has been reported, all other well-documented cases have been sporadic. Therefore, the vast majority of patients most likely represent a dominant new mutation. Recurrence risk is negligible. Documentation of monozygotic twins with thanatophoric dysplasia discordant for cloverleaf skull suggests that the skull anomaly is a variable manifestation of thanatophoric dysplasia.

COMMENT.
There is a striking resemblance between this disorder and an autosomal recessive early lethal type of achondroplasia in the rabbit. Studies in the rabbit homozygote have demonstrated a mitochondrial defect in energy generation.

References

Maroteaux, P., Lamy, M., and Robert, J. M.: Le nanisme thanatophore. Presse Med., 75:2519, 1967.

Giedion, A.: Thanatophoric dwarfism. Helv. Paediatr. Acta, 23:175, 1968.

Huguenin, M., et al.: Two different mutations within the same sibship: Thanatophoric dwarfism and Ulrich-Feichtiger syndrome. Helv. Paediatr. Acta, 24:239, 1969.

Goutières, F., Aicardi, J., and Farkas-Bargeton, E.: Une malformation cérébrale particulière associée au nanisme thanatophore. Presse Med., 79:960, 1971.

Harris, R., and Patton, J. R.: Achondroplasia and thanatophoric dwarfism in the newborn. Clin. Genet., 2:61, 1971.

Thompson, B. H., and Parmley, T. H.: Obstetric features of thanatophoric dwarfism. Am. J. Obstet. Gynecol., 109:396, 1971.

Horton, W. A., Harris, D. J., Collins, D. L.: Discordance for the Kleeblattschädel anomaly in monozygotic twins with thanatophoric dysplasia. Am. J. Med. Genet., 15:97, 1983.

Stensvold, K., Ek, J., and Havland, A. R.: An infant with thanatophoric dwarfism surviving 169 days. Clin. Genet., 29:157, 1986.

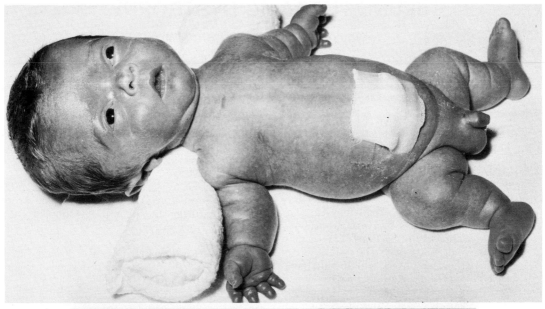

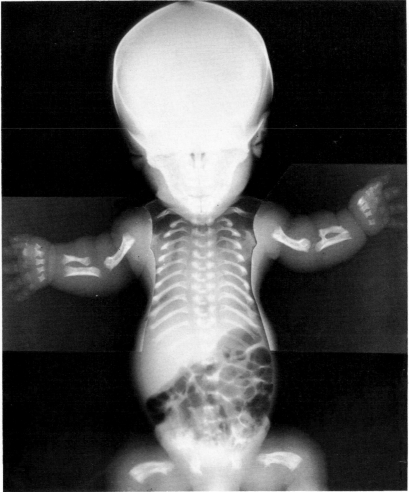

Thanatophoric dysplasia. Neonate. (From Giedion, A.: Helv. Paediatr. Acta, *23*:175, 1968.)

JEUNE THORACIC DYSTROPHY

(Asphyxiating Thoracic Dystrophy)

Small Thorax, Short Limbs, Hypoplastic Iliac Wings

First described by Jeune et al. in 1955, over 100 cases have now been reported.

ABNORMALITIES

Growth. Short stature.

Skeletal. Infancy: Short ribs with irregular costochondral junctions and small thoracic cage. Hypoplastic iliac wings. Horizontal acetabular roofs with spur-like projections at lower margins of sciatic notches. Early ossification of capital femoral epiphysis. Childhood: Irregular epiphyses and metaphyses with relatively short limbs, especially the hands. Ulnae and fibulae relatively short. Cone-shaped epiphyses and early fusion between epiphyses and metaphyses of distal and middle phalanges.

Respiratory. Lung hypoplasia, presumably secondary to the small thoracic cage, is the major cause of death in early infancy.

Renal. Cystic tubular dysplasia and/or glomerular sclerosis.

Hepatic. Variable proliferation of small duct radicals.

OCCASIONAL ABNORMALITIES.

Polydactyly, usually of hands and feet, notching of distal end of metacarpal and metatarsal bones; lacunar skull; pancreatic cysts; retinal degeneration with predominantly cone-type cells remaining.

NATURAL HISTORY.

Early death, usually the consequence of asphyxia with or without pneumonia, occurs in the majority of patients. Those who survive usually have progressive improvement in the relative growth of the thoracic cage and may have only slight to moderate shortness of stature. Chronic nephritis leading to renal failure is a serious potential feature of this disorder. Renal insufficiency may be evident by two years of age. However, survival to the fourth decade has occurred.

Autopsy has revealed disordered growth at the costochondral juncture with hyperplastic proliferating cartilage and poor progression of endochondral mineralization.

ETIOLOGY. Autosomal recessive. Prenatal diagnosis utilizing ultrasonography has been accomplished successfully at 18 weeks' gestation.

References

Jeune, M., Beraud, C., and Carron, R.: Dystrophie thoracique asphyxiante de caractère familial. Arch. Fr. Pediatr., *12*:886, 1955.

Pirnar, T., and Neuhauser, E. B. D.: Asphyxiating thoracic dystrophy of the newborn. Am. J. Roentgenol. Radium Ther. Nucl. Med., *98*:358, 1966.

Herdman, R. C., and Langer, L. O.: The thoracic asphyxiant dystrophy and renal disease. Am. J. Dis. Child., *116*:192, 1968.

Langer, L. O.: Thoracic-Pelvic-Phalangeal dystrophy. Radiology, *91*:447, 1968.

Friedman, J. M., Kaplan, H. G., and Hall, J. G.: The Jeune syndrome in an adult. Am. J. Med., *59*:857, 1975.

Okerklaid, F., et al.: Asphyxiating thoracic dystrophy. Arch. Dis. Child., *52*:758, 1977.

Allen, A. W., et al. Ocular findings in thoracic-pelvic-phalangeal dystrophy. Arch. Ophthalmol., *97*:489, 1979.

Shah, K. J.: Renal lesions in Jeune's syndrome. Br. J. Radiol., *53*:432, 1980.

Elejalde, B. R., Mercedes de Elejalde, M., and Pansch, D.: Prenatal diagnosis of Jeune syndrome. Am. J. Med. Genet., *21*:433, 1985.

Affected children with Jeune thoracic dystrophy. Note the small thoracic cage, short hands, and mild bowing of legs. (Courtesy of Dr. Jaime Frias, University of Nebraska Medical School, Omaha.)

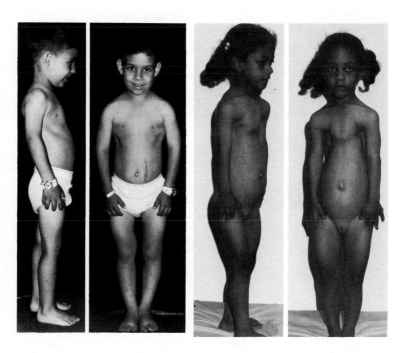

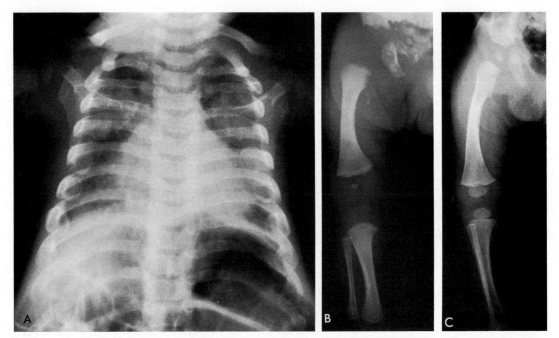

Jeune thoracic dystrophy. *A*, Four month old. Note short ribs, high position of clavicles. *B, C*, Right lower extremity at one month and ten months of age showing improvement in long bones and pelvis, though fibula remains relatively short. (From Hanissian, A. S., et al.: J. Pediatr., *71*:855, 1967.)

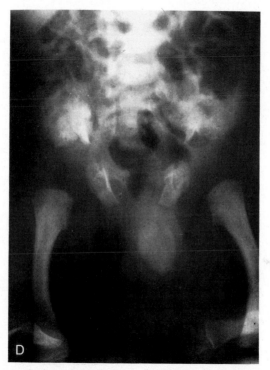

D, Horizontal acetabular roofs with spur-like projections at lower margins of sciatic notches.

CAMPTOMELIC DYSPLASIA

Bowed Tibiae, Hypoplastic Scapulae, Flat Facies

Though reports of this condition appeared in the 1950s by Bound et al. and Bain and Barrett, it was not until the 1970s that the syndrome became more broadly recognized by Spranger et al. and Maroteaux et al., who utilized the term "camptomelique," meaning bent limb, to epitomize the disorder. Three recent reports provide excellent summaries of large numbers of patients.

ABNORMALITIES

Growth. Prenatal onset growth deficiency with retarded osseous maturation and large head. Birth length, 35 to 49 cm. Average occipitofrontal circumference is 37 cm.

CNS. Tendency toward having large brain with gross cellular disorganization, most evident in cerebral cortex, thalamus, and caudate nucleus. Absence or hypoplasia of olfactory tract or bulbs. Hydrocephalus.

Facies. Flat-appearing small face with high forehead, anterior frontal upsweep, large anterior fontanel, low nasal bridge, micrognathia, cleft palate, short palpebral fissures, and malformed and/or low-set ears.

Limbs. Anterior bowing of tibiae with skin dimpling over convex area, short fibulae, mild bowing of femurs, and talipes equinovarus.

Radiographic. Short and somewhat flat vertebrae, particularly cervical. Hypoplastic scapulae, small thoracic cage with slender and/or decreased number of ribs, kyphoscoliosis, small iliac wings with relatively wide pelvic outlet. Absent mineralization of sternum. Lack of ossification of proximal tibial and distal femoral epiphysis and talus.

Tracheobronchial. Incomplete cartilaginous development with tracheobronchiomalacia.

Genitalia. Some of the affected XY individuals fail to develop masculine characteristics and have XY gonadal dysgenesis with ovarian, müllerian duct, and vaginal development.

OCCASIONAL ABNORMALITIES. Cardiac defects. Hydronephrosis. Polyhydramnios.

NATURAL HISTORY. The great majority of patients die in the neonatal period from respiratory insufficiency, and those surviving into early infancy have feeding problems, failure to thrive, and evidence of serious central nervous system deficiency, including apneic spells. The oldest survivors include a seven month old, a 19 month old, and a 17 year old boy with an I.Q. of 45.

ETIOLOGY. Autosomal recessive. Prenatal diagnosis utilizing ultrasonography has been accomplished successfully at 18 weeks' gestation.

References

Bound, J. P., Finlay, H. V. L., and Rose, F. C.: Congenital anterior angulation of the tibia. Arch. Dis. Child., *27*:179, 1952.

Bain, A. D., and Barrett, H. S.: Congenital bowing of the long bones: Report of a case. Arch. Dis. Child., *34*:516, 1959.

Spranger, J., Langer, L. O., and Maroteaux, P.: Increasing frequency of a syndrome of multiple osseous defects? Lancet, *2*:716, 1970.

Maroteaux, P., et al.: Le syndrome camptomélique. Presse Med., *79*:1157, 1971.

Hoefnagel, D., et al.: Camptomelic dwarfism. Lancet, *1*:1068, 1972.

Schmickel, R. D., Heidelberger, K. P., and Poznanski, A. K.: The campomelique syndrome. J. Pediatr., *82*:299, 1973.

Hall, B. D., and Spranger, J. W.: Camptomelic dysplasia. Am. J. Dis. Child., *134*:285, 1980.

Houston, C. S., et al.: The camptomelic syndrome: Review, report of 17 cases, and follow-up on the currently 17 year old boy first reported by Maroteaux et al in 1971. Am. J. Med. Genet., *15*:3, 1983.

Belluffi, G., and Fraccaro, M.: Genetical and clinical aspects of camptomelic dysplasia. *In* Papadatos, C. J., and Bartsocas, C. S. (eds.): Skeletal Dysplasias. New York, Alan R. Liss., 1982, pp. 53–65.

Winter, R., et al.: Prenatal diagnosis of camptomelic dysplasia by ultrasonography. Prenat. Diagn., *5*:1, 1985.

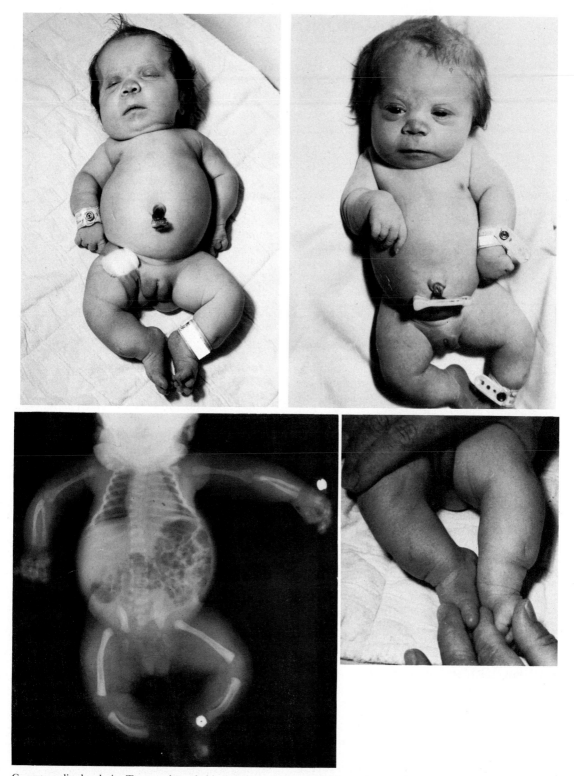

Camptomelic dysplasia. Two newborn babies, showing low nasal bridge, micrognathia, small thorax, aberrant hand positioning, and bowed tibiae with dimples at the maximal point of bowing. Roentgenogram shows the slim, poorly developed bones and osseous immaturity (knee and foot). (From D. Hoefnagel, et al.: Lancet, *1*:1068, 1972.)

ACHONDROPLASIA

Short Limbs, Low Nasal Bridge, Caudal Narrowing of Spinal Canal

The most common chondrodysplasia, true achondroplasia, occurs with a frequency of about 1:26,000.

ABNORMALITIES

Growth. Small stature. Mean adult height in males is 131 ± 5.6 cm and in females is 124 ± 5.9 cm.

Craniofacial. Megalocephaly, small foramen magnum. Short cranial base with early spheno-occipital closure. Low nasal bridge with prominent forehead. Mild midfacial hypoplasia with narrow nasal passages.

Skeletal. Small cuboid-shaped vertebral bodies with short pedicles and progressive narrowing of lumbar interpedicular distance. Lumbar lordosis, mild thoracolumbar kyphosis with anterior beaking of first and/or second lumbar vertebra. Small iliac wings with narrow greater sciatic notch. Short tubular bones, especially humeri; metaphyseal flare with ball and socket arrangement of epiphysis to metaphysis. Short trident hand, fingers being similar in length, with short proximal and midphalanges. Short femoral neck; incomplete extension of elbow.

Other. Mild hypotonia. Early motor progress is often slow, although eventual intelligence is usually normal. Relative glucose intolerance evident with an oral glucose tolerance test.

OCCASIONAL COMPLICATIONS.
Hydrocephalus secondary to a narrow foramen magnum may occur. Spinal cord and/or root compression can happen as a consequence of kyphosis, stenosis of the spinal canal, or disc lesions. About 46 per cent of patients have spinal complications, and therefore a cautious orthopedic-neurologic follow-up is merited.

NATURAL HISTORY.
Macrocephaly may represent mild hydrocephaly relating to a small foramen magnum. Because of the difficulty in clinically documenting hydrocephalus during the first year of life, Hall has suggested that ultrasonographic studies of the brain be done at birth, two, four, and six months to establish ventricular size and to rule out an intracranial bleed secondary to cephalopelvic disproportion. Todorov et al. have developed a screening test that establishes normal milestones for children with achondroplasia up to two years of age.

Respiratory problems secondary to a small chest, upper airway obstruction, and sleep-disordered breathing are common, whereas apnea secondary to cervical spinal cord and lower brain stem compression sometimes occurs.

The physician should be alert to detect any neurologic complications due to bone or disc compression. Osteoarthritis is not a usual feature in the adult. Osteotomies for severe bowlegs are usually deferred until full growth has occurred. Siebens et al. discourage early sitting, standing, and walking, since the large head produces a great load on the hypotonic spine, enhancing the lumbar lordosis. They recommend extending the hips while stabilizing the spine, by bracing if need be, in an effort to forestall lumbar lordosis and later crowding of the spinal cord. Exercises may also be utilized in an attempt to flatten the lumbosacral curve. Relative overgrowth of the fibula may accentuate bowing and require early stapling.

Short eustachian tubes may lead to middle ear infection, and tympanic tubes may be indicated. The mandibular teeth may become crowded, possibly requiring removal of one or more.

There is a tendency toward late childhood obesity, and females are more prone to have menorrhagia, fibroids, and large breasts.

ETIOLOGY.
Autosomal dominant, about 90 per cent of the cases representing a fresh mutation, yielding a mutation rate of 1.9×10^{-5} per generation. Older paternal age has been a contributing factor in fresh achondroplasia mutations.

COMMENT.
Histologic evaluation at the epiphyseal line discloses shorter cartilage columns that lack the usual linear arrangement, and some cartilage cells appear to be undergoing a mucinoid degeneration.

References

Maroteaux, P., and Lamy, M.: Achondroplasia in man and animals. Clin. Orthop., *33*:91, 1964.

Caffey, J.: Pediatric X-Ray Diagnosis, 5th ed. Chicago, Year Book Medical Publishers, 1967, p. 819.

Cohen, M. E., Rosenthal, A. D., and Matson, D. D.: Neurological abnormalities in achondroplastic children. J. Pediatr., *71*:367, 1967.

Shepard, T. H., and Graham, B.: The congenitally malformed. XIII. Achondroplastic dwarfism; diagnosis and management. Northwest Med., *66*:451, 1967.

Collipp, P. J., et al.: Abnormal glucose tolerance in children with achondroplasia. Am. J. Dis. Child., *124*:682, 1972.

Nelson, M. A.: Spinal stenosis in achondroplasia. Proc. R. Soc. Med., *65*:1028, 1972.

Horton, W. A., et al.: Standard growth curves for achondroplasia. J. Pediatr., *93*:435, 1978.

Siebens, A. A., Hungerford, A. S., and Kirby, N. A.: Curves of the achondroplastic spine: A new hypothesis. Johns Hopkins Med. J., *142*:205, 1978.

Oberklaid, F., et al.: Achondroplasia and hypochondroplasia. J. Med. Genet., *16*:140, 1979.

Todorov, A. B., et al.: Developmental screening tests in achondroplastic children. Am. J. Med. Genet., *9*:19, 1981.

Hall, J. G., et al.: Letter to the editor: Head growth in achondroplasia: Use of ultrasound studies. Amer. J. Med. Genet., *13*:105, 1982.

Stokes, D. C., et al.: Respiratory complications of achondroplasia. J. Pediatr., *102*:534, 1983.

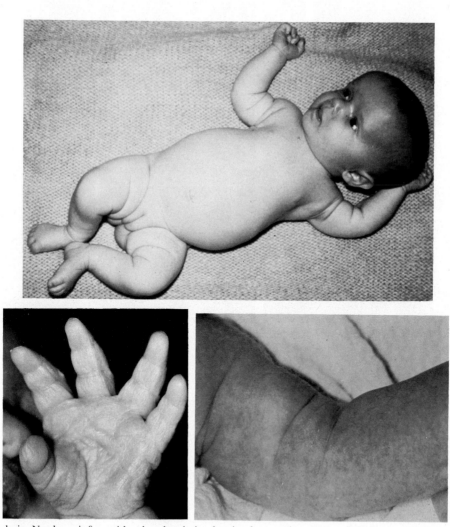

Achondroplasia. Newborn infant with achondroplasia, showing hypotonia, macrocephaly, low nasal bridge, relatively small thoracic cage, shortness of humeri and femurs (rhizomelia), "trident" position of the open, small hand, and inability to extend fully at the elbow.

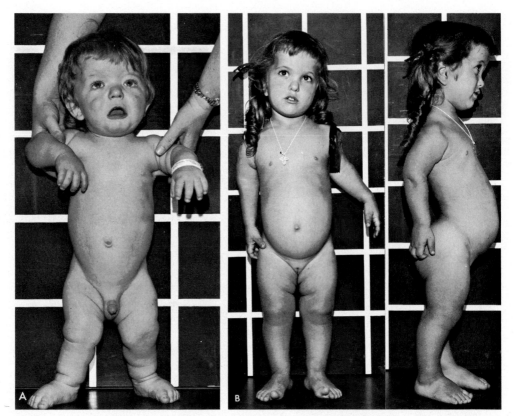

Achondroplasia. *A*, One year old with height age of four months. (From Smith, D. W.: J. Pediatr., *70*:504, 1967.) *B*, Four year old with height age of 20 months.

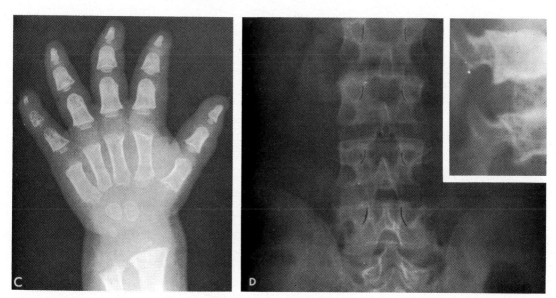

C, Short "trident" hand with short metacarpals and phalanges. *D*, Caudal narrowing of spinal canal (pedicles marked) with short pedicles (*upper right*).

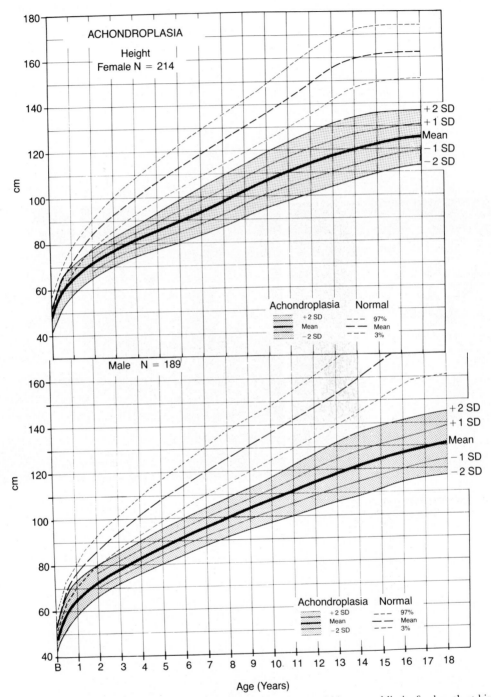

Note that about one half of the newborn babies with achondroplasia are within normal limits for length at birth, but there is a progressive deceleration of growth rate beginning in infancy. (From Horton, W. A., et al.: J. Pediatr., *93*:435, 1978.)

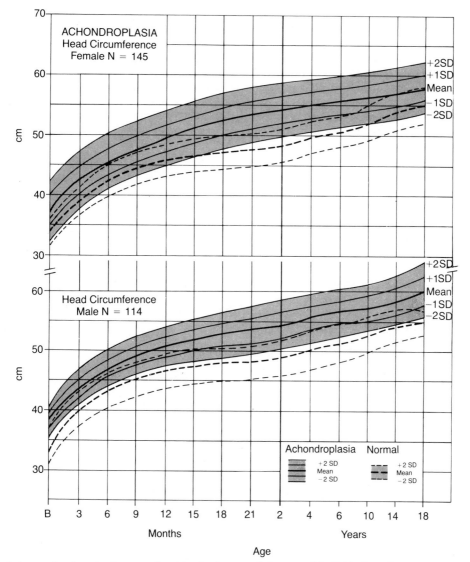

Macrocephaly, predominantly due to a large brain, is a usual feature of individuals with achondroplasia. (From Horton, W. A., et al.: J. Pediatr., *93*:435, 1978.)

HYPOCHONDROPLASIA

Short Limbs, Caudal Narrowing of Spine, Near-Normal Craniofacies

Though the features of this disorder were described by Ravenna in 1913, and its designation as hypochondroplasia and mode of inheritance were set forth in 1924, the majority of cases have been misdiagnosed as achondroplasia until recent times. Hypochondroplasia has an incidence of about one twelfth that of achondroplasia and can be distinguished from it by the relative lack of craniofacial involvement and milder features in the hands and spine.

ABNORMALITIES

Growth. Small stature, usually of postnatal onset. Mean birth length, 47.7 cm, and birth weight, 2.9 kg. Macrocephaly.

Limbs. Relatively short without rhizomelic, mesomelic, or acromelic predominance. Short tubular bones with mild metaphyseal flare. Short, broad femoral necks. Long distal fibulae, short distal ulnae, and long ulnar styloids. Brachydactyly. Bowing of legs. Stubby hands and feet. Mild limitation in elbow extension and supination.

Spine. Anteroposterior shortening of lumbar pedicles on anteroposterior view. Spinal canal narrowing or unchanged caudally, with or without lumbar lordosis.

Pelvis. Squared and short ilia.

OCCASIONAL ABNORMALITIES.
Mental deficiency, brachycephaly with short base of skull, mild frontal bossing, esotropia, cataract, ptosis, postaxial toe polydactyly, high vertebrae, flat vertebrae.

NATURAL HISTORY.
Slow growth, if not evident by birth, is usually obvious by three years of age. Final height attainment in adults ranged from 46.5 to 60 inches. Outward bowing of the lower limbs and genu varum may become pronounced with weight-bearing. Though this may improve in childhood, the condition may merit surgical straightening. The relatively long fibulae can result in inversion of the feet. Exercise may provoke mild aching in the knees, ankles, and/or elbows during childhood, and such discomfort is usually worse and may include the low back in the adult. Cesarean section is often required for delivery in pregnant women with this disorder.

Mental deficiency, a rare feature in achondroplasia, was noted in four of the 13 cases reported by Walker et al, with I.Q.s ranging from 50 to 80, and in 9 per cent of the patients reported by Hall and Spranger.

ETIOLOGY.
Autosomal dominant mutant gene etiology has been implicated by direct inheritance from affected individuals and by older paternal age among the presumed fresh mutation cases from unaffected parents, which represent the majority of cases.

References

Ravenna, F.: Achondroplasie et chondrohypoplasie: Contribution clinique. N. Iconog. Salpêtrière, *26*:157, 1913.

Léri, A., and Linossier (Mlle.): Hypochondroplasia héréditaire. Bull. Mem. Soc. Med. Hop. (Paris), *48*:1780, 1924.

Beals, R. K.: Hypochondroplasia. A report of five kindred. J. Bone Joint Surg. [Am.], *51*:728, 1969.

Walker, B. A., et al.: Hypochondroplasia. Am. J. Dis. Child., *122*:95, 1971.

Hall, B. D., and Spranger, J.: Hypochondroplasia: Clinical and radiological aspects in 39 cases. Radiology, *133*:95, 1979.

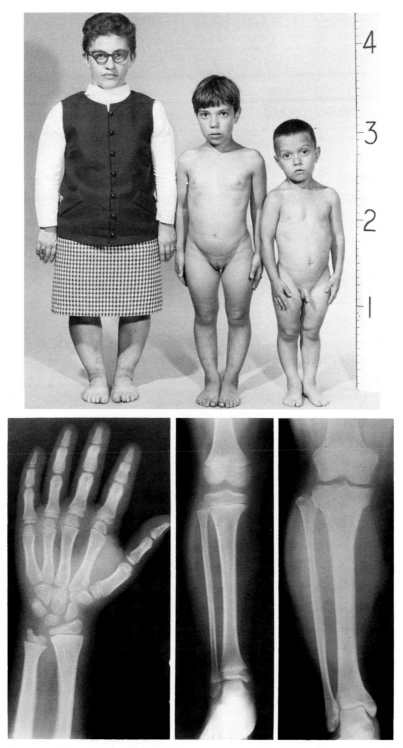

Hypochondroplasia. *Above,* Affected mother and children (seven and six years), showing short stature, most striking in the bowed lower limbs. *Lower left,* Note slight ulnar shortening, metaphyseal flaring with bulbous radial enlargement, and elongation of the styloid process (from a ten year old). *Lower middle,* Seven year old, showing elongation of distal fibula and slight "squaring off" of the proximal tibial epiphysis. *Lower right,* Adult, showing more striking squaring of proximal tibial epiphysis, with sharp flare of metaphysis and elongation of distal fibula with varus deformity of ankle mortise. (From Beals, R. K.: J. Bone Joint Surg. [Am.], *51*:728, 1969.)

PSEUDOACHONDROPLASTIC SPONDYLOEPIPHYSEAL DYSPLASIA (SED)

Small Irregular Epiphyses, Irregular Mushroomed Metaphyses, Flattening and/or Anterior Beaking of Vertebrae, With Normal Craniofacial Appearance

Maroteaux and Lamy described three individuals with this pattern of altered bone morphogenesis in 1959, and subsequently at least four additional cases have been published.

ABNORMALITIES

Growth. Apparently postnatal onset of short-limb growth deficiency by second year. Adult stature, 82 to 130 cm.

Metaphyses. Irregular, mushroomed.

Epiphyses. Small, irregular or "fragmented," especially the capital femoral epiphyses.

Diaphyses. Short, bowing, especially in lower extremities.

Vertebrae. Variable degrees of flattening, anterior, tongue-shaped short pedicles. Lumbar lordosis, kyphosis, scoliosis.

Ribs. Tend to be spatulate.

Joints. Hypermobility of major joints except elbows.

OCCASIONAL ABNORMALITIES. Pelvis: short sacroiliac notch, flaring of iliac crests.

NATURAL HISTORY. The patients have been described as "normal" at birth, with small size and waddling gait becoming evident between six months and four years of age. Bowed lower extremities with waddling gait and scoliosis are the principal orthopedic problems, and there may be some limitation in joint motility. Intelligence is normal.

ETIOLOGY. Autosomal dominant. Most of the cases have been sporadic and presumably represent fresh mutations. Rare cases of affected siblings born to unaffected parents are most likely the result of gonadal mosaicism.

COMMENT. The postnatal onset and normal craniofacial appearance readily differentiate this entity from true achondroplasia.

References

Maroteaux, P., and Lamy, M.: Les formes pseudo-achondroplastiques des dysplasies spondyloépiphysaires. Presse Med., *67*:383, 1959.

Ford, N., Silverman, F. N., and Kozlowski, K.: Spondylo-epiphyseal dysplasia (pseudoachondroplastic type). Am. J. Roentgenol. Radium Ther. Nucl. Med., *86*:462, 1961.

Rubin, P.: Achondroplasia versus pseudoachondroplasia. Radiol. Clin. North Am., *1*:621, 1963.

Lindseth, R. E., et al.: Spondylo-epiphyseal dysplasia (pseudoachondroplastic type). Case report with pathologic and metabolic investigations. Am. J. Dis. Child., *113*:721, 1967.

Hall, J. G., and Rotta, J.: Gonadal mosaicism of a new mutation leading to pseudoachondroplasia. Clin. Research, *35*:211A, 1987.

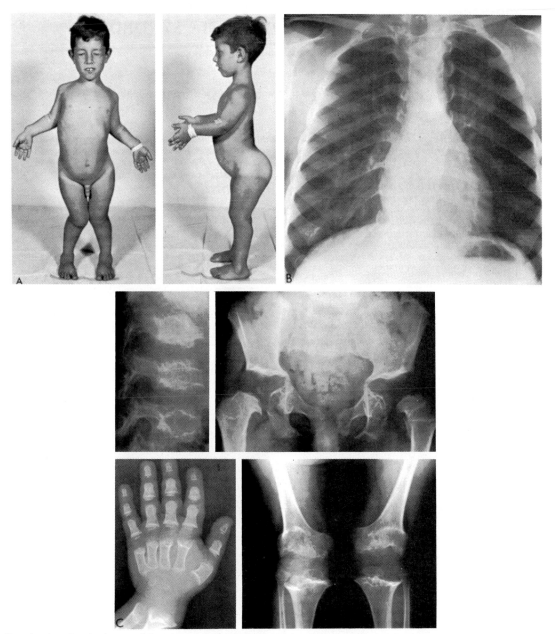

Pseudoachondroplastic spondyloepiphyseal dysplasia. *A*, Eight year old with height age of three years. *B*, Mildly spatulate ribs; scoliosis. *C*, Flattened irregular vertebral bodies, hypoplastic abnormal iliac wings, and short tubular bones with irregular "ball-in-socket" epiphyses in relation to metaphyses. (From Lindseth, R. E., et al.: Am. J. Dis. Child. *113*:721, 1967.)

ACROMESOMELIC DYSPLASIA

(Acromesomelic Dwarfism)

*Short Distal Limbs, Frontal Prominence, Low
Thoracic Kyphosis*

Maroteaux et al. recognized this disorder in 1971, and Langer et al. summarized the manifestations in 19 patients in 1977.

ABNORMALITIES. Seen in 19 patients.
Craniofacial. Relative frontal prominence, +/− relatively short nose.
Limbs. Short limbs, epecially distally, with dysplasia that may include coned epiphyses and limited elbow extension. Short fingers with redundant skin and short nails.
Spine. Development of lower thoracic kyphosis.

OCCASIONAL ABNORMALITIES. Relatively large great toe. Corneal clouding.

NATURAL HISTORY. Birth weight may be normal, and the linear growth deficiency becomes more evident during the first year. Lower thoracic kyphosis is liable to occur, and most joints tend to be relatively lax. There may be some lag in gross motor performance, but intelligence is normal. Final height in eight adults ranged from 38 to 49 inches.

ETIOLOGY. Autosomal recessive.

References

Maroteaux, P., Martinelli, B., and Campailla, E.: Le nanisme acromesomelique. Presse Med., *79*:1838, 1971.
Langer, L. O., et al.: Acromesomelic dwarfism: Manifestations in childhood. Am. J. Med. Genet., *1*:87, 1977.

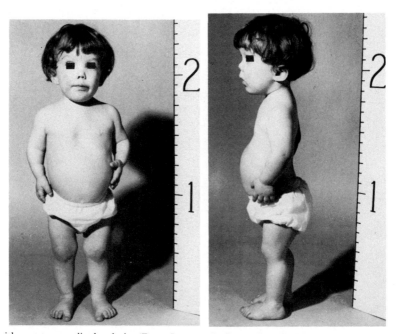

Infant with acromesomelic dysplasia. (From Langer, L. O., et al.: Am. J. Med. Genet., *1*:87, 1977.)

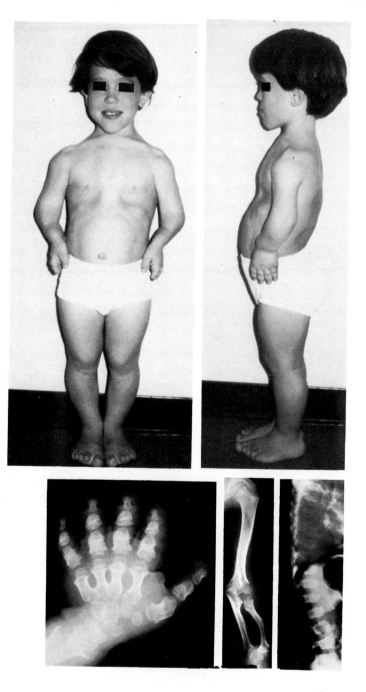

Child with acromesomelic dysplasia and roentgenographic findings. (From Langer, L. O., et al.: Am. J. Med. Genet., *1*:87, 1977.)

SPONDYLOEPIPHYSEAL DYSPLASIA CONGENITA

Short Trunk, Lag in Epiphyseal Mineralization, Myopia

Spranger and Wiedemann established this disorder in 1966 when they reported six new cases and summarized 14 from the past literature.

ABNORMALITIES. Onset at birth.

Growth. Prenatal onset growth deficiency, final height, 37 to 52 inches.

Facies. Variable flat facies, malar hypoplasia, cleft palate.

Eyes. Myopia, retinal detachment (50 per cent).

Spine. Short, including neck with ovoid flattened vertebrae with narrow intervertebral disc spaces, odontoid hypoplasia, kyphoscoliosis, lumbar lordosis.

Chest. Barrel chest with pectus carinatum.

Limbs. Lag in mineralization of epiphyses, which tend to be flat, with no os pubis, talus, calcaneus, or knee centers mineralized at birth. Coxa vara. Diminished joint mobility at elbows, knees, and hips.

Muscles. Weakness, easy fatigability, hypoplasia of abdominal muscles.

OCCASIONAL ABNORMALITIES. Talipes varus, dislocation of hip.

NATURAL HISTORY. The hypotonic weakness and orthopedic situation contribute to a late onset of walking, usually with a waddling gait. Myopia should be suspected, and frequent ophthalmologic evaluation is merited to guard against retinal detachment. Morning stiffness may be a feature, but there is usually no undue joint pain.

ETIOLOGY. Autosomal dominant in vast majority of cases. Documentation of three families in which affected siblings have been born to unaffected parents suggests genetic heterogeneity.

References

Spranger, J., and Wiedemann, H. R.: Dysplasia spondyloepiphysaria congenita. Helv. Paediatr. Acta, *21*: 598, 1966.

Spranger, J., and Langer, L. O.: Spondyloepiphyseal dysplasia congenita. Radiology, *94*:313, 1970.

Harrod, M. J. E., et al.: Genetic heterogeneity in spondyloepiphyseal dysplasia congenita. Am. J. Med. Genet., *18*:311, 1984.

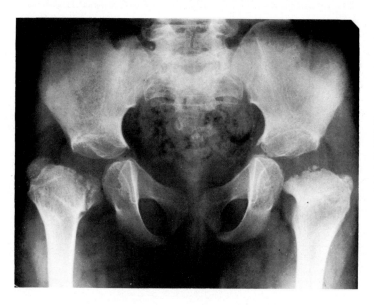

Spondyloepiphyseal dysplasia congenita. Pelvis at seven years, showing horizontal acetabula and lack of ossification of femoral heads and femoral necks, which are in severe varus position. (From Dr. Jurgen Spranger, Mainz, Germany.)

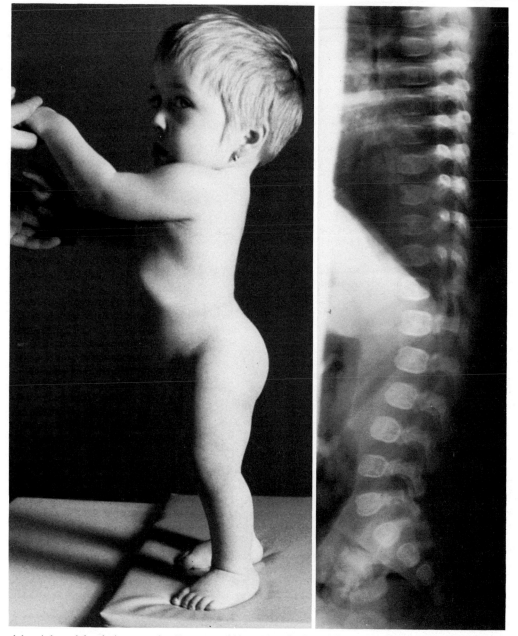

Spondyloepiphyseal dysplasia congenita. Four year old boy. Note the flat midface and lumbar lordosis. Roentgenogram of spine at nine months, showing mild dorsal flattening and minimal beaking at L2–L3. (From Dr. Jurgen Spranger, Mainz, Germany.)

KNIEST DYSPLASIA

Flat Facies, Thick Joints, Platyspondyly

Though Kniest described this disorder in 1952, it has been more generally recognized only in recent years.

ABNORMALITIES

Growth. Disproportionate short stature with short, barrel-shaped chest.

Craniofacies. Flat facies with prominent eyes, low nasal bridge, myopia that may progress to retinal detachment, cleft palate with frequent ear infections.

Limbs. Enlarged joints with limited joint mobility and variable pain and stiffness. Short limbs, often with bowing. Some irregularity of epiphyses with late ossification of femoral heads. Flexion contractures in hips. Inability to form fist secondary to bony enlargements at interphalangeal joints.

Spine. Lumbar kyphoscoliosis. Platyspondyly with vertical "cleft" in early infancy.

Other. Inguinal and umbilical hernias, small pelvis, short clavicles. Hearing loss. Tracheomalacia.

Radiographs. Platyspondyly, vertical cleft of vertebral bodies, low and broad ilia, shortened tubular bones, retarded ossification of proximal femora, flared metaphyses, and large epiphyses.

NATURAL HISTORY. Short extremities with stiff joints in neonatal period. Marked lumbar lordosis and kyphoscoliosis lead to disproportionate shortening of trunk in childhood. Late walking because of orthopedic disability with contracted hips. Chronic otitis media related to cleft palate. Normal intelligence. Final height, 106 to 145 cm.

ETIOLOGY. Generally sporadic. The occurrence in a parent and offspring suggests autosomal dominant inheritance, with most cases representing a fresh gene mutation.

References

Kniest, W.: Zur Abgrenzung der Dysostosis enchondralis von der Chondrodystrophie. Z. Kinderheilkd., *70*:633, 1952.

Kim, H. J., et al.: Kniest syndrome with dominant inheritance and mucopolysacchariduria. Am. J. Hum. Genet., *77*:755, 1975.

Rimoin, D. L., et al.: Metatropic dwarfism, the Kniest syndrome and the pseudoachondroplastic dysplasias. Clin. Orthop. Related Research, *114*:70, 1976.

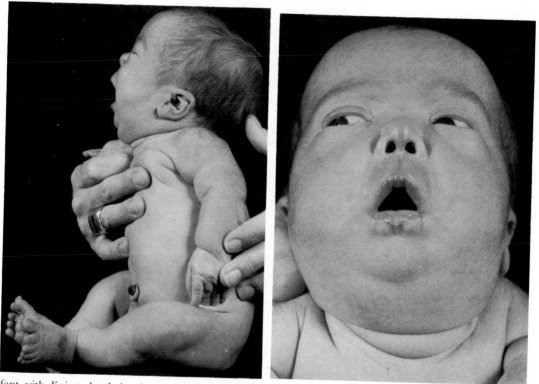

Infant with Kniest dysplasia, showing malproportionment and unusual facies. (Courtesy of Dr. John Graham, Dartmouth Medical School, Hanover, New Hampshire.)

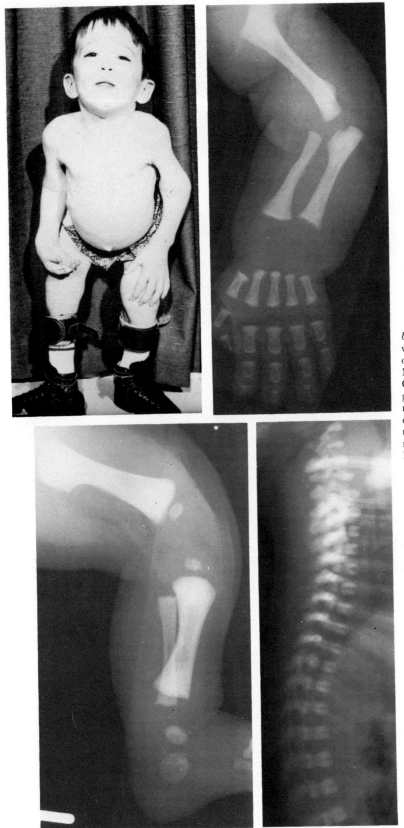

Upper left, Three year old boy with Kniest dysplasia. (Courtesy of Dr. D. L. Rimoin, Cedars-Sinai Medical Center, Los Angeles, CA.) *Upper right and lower*, Roentgenograms showing altered limb morphogenesis and platyspondyly with coronal clefting. (Courtesy of Dr. J. H. Graham, Dartmouth Medical School, Hanover, NH.)

DYGGVE-MELCHIOR-CLAUSEN SYNDROME

Initially described in 1962 by Dyggve et al., the clinical and radiographic features were set forth more completely in 1975 by Spranger et al.

ABNORMALITIES
Growth. Deficiency of postnatal onset, with short trunk dwarfism becoming evident before 18 months.
Performance. Mental deficiency. Microcephaly.
Spine. Flattened vertebrae with anterior pointing of the bodies and notch-like ossification defects of the superior and inferior end plates. Odontoid hypoplasia. Scoliosis. Kyphosis. Lordosis.
Thorax. Sternal protrusion. Barrel chest.
Pelvis. Small ilia with irregularly calcified (lace-like) iliac crests. Lateral displacement of capital femoral epiphyses.
Limbs. Restricted joint mobility. Waddling gait. Genu valga and vera. Short long bones with irregular metaphyses and epiphyses, short metacarpals, particularly the first, and short notched phalanges. Cone-shaped epiphyses. Small carpals.

NATURAL HISTORY. Manifestations become evident between one and 18 months. Feeding problems frequently occur during infancy. Restriction of joint mobility primarily affects the elbows and hips. Spinal cord compression due to atlantoaxial instability is a preventable complication. The degree of mental retardation has varied from moderate to severe. Three known adults measured 128 cm., 127 cm., and 119 cm., respectively.

ETIOLOGY. Autosomal recessive.

References

Dyggve, H. V., Melchior, J. C., and Clausen, J.: Morquio-Ullrich's disease. An inborn error of metabolism? Arch. Dis. Child., *37*:525, 1962.

Spranger, J., Maroteaux, P., Der Kaloustian, V. M.: The Dyggve-Melchior-Clausen syndrome. Radiology, *114*:415, 1975.

Naffah, J.: The Dyggve-Melchior-Clausen syndrome. Am. J. Hum. Genet., *28*:607, 1976

Spranger, J., Bierbaum, B., and Herrmann, J.: Heterogeneity of Dyggve-Melchior-Clausen dwarfism. Hum. Genet., *33*:279, 1976.

Bonafede, R. P., and Beighton, P.: The Dyggve-Melchior-Clausen syndrome in adult siblings. Clin. Genet., *14*:24, 1978.

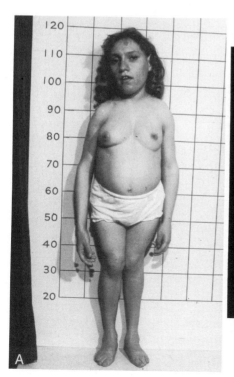
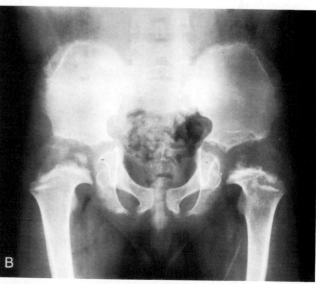

A, B, Adolescent with Dyggve-Melchior-Clausen syndrome. Note the irregularly calcified iliac crests. (Courtesy of Dr. R. Lachman, Harbor–UCLA Medical Center, and Dr. D. Rimoin, Cedars-Sinai Medical Center, Los Angeles.)

KOZLOWSKI SPONDYLOMETAPHYSEAL DYSPLASIA
(Kozlowski Spondylometaphyseal Chondrodysplasia)

Early Childhood Onset Short Spine, Irregular Metaphyses, Pectus Carinatum

Kozlowski et al. established this disorder in 1967, and several additional cases have been recognized. Spondylometaphyseal dysplasia comprises a group of disorders in which the spine and metaphyses of the tubular bones are affected. The different types can be distinguished both radiographically and genetically. The Kozlowski type is the most well known and the most common.

ABNORMALITIES
Growth. Growth deficiency, especially of trunk, from one to four years of age. Adult height, 4 feet 3 inches to 5 feet.
Spine. Short neck and trunk with dorsal kyphosis. Platyspondyly with anterior narrowing in lumbar region. Odontoid hypoplasia.
Thorax. Pectus carinatum.
Pelvis. Squarish, short iliac wings; flat, irregular acetabula.
Limbs. Irregular rachitic-like metaphyses, especially the proximal femur with very short femoral necks. Hypoplastic carpal bones with late ossification.

NATURAL HISTORY. Waddling gait with limitation of joint mobility and early degenerative joint changes leading to discomfort.

ETIOLOGY. Autosomal dominant, with most cases representing fresh mutation.

References

Kozlowski, K., Maroteaux, P., and Spranger, J.: La dysostose spondylo-métaphysaire. Presse Med., 75:2769, 1967.

Riggs, W., Jr., and Summitt, R. L.: Spondylometaphyseal dysplasia (Kozlowski). Report of affected mother and son. Radiology, *101*:375, 1971.

Le Quesne, G. W., and Kozlowski, K.: Spondylometaphyseal dysplasia. Br. J. Radiol., *46*:685, 1973.

Kozlowski, K., et al.: Spondylo-metaphyseal dysplasia. (Report of 7 cases and essay of classification). *In* Papadatos, C. J., and Bartsocas, C. S. (eds.): Skeletal Dysplasias. New York, Alan R. Liss, 1982, pp. 89–101.

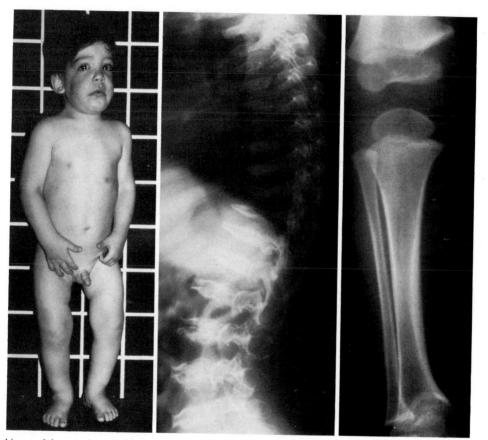

Kozlowski spondylometaphyseal dysplasia. Young boy. Note bowed legs, flattened vertebrae, and metaphyseal flare. (From Riggs, W., Jr., and Summitt, R. L.: Radiology, *101*:375, 1971.)

METATROPIC DYSPLASIA

(Metatropic Dwarfism Syndrome)

*Small Thorax, Thoracic Kyphoscoliosis, Metaphyseal
Flaring*

Maroteaux et al. set forth this entity with five cases of their own and 12 unrecognized cases from the literature. The striking early findings, shown on the following three pages, include huge epiphyses.

ABNORMALITIES

Skeletal. Small stature, severe. Early platyspondyly with progressive kyphosis and scoliosis in infancy to early childhood. Narrow thorax with short ribs. Short limbs with metaphyseal flaring and epiphyseal irregularity with hyperplastic trochanters. Prominent joints with restricted mobility at knee and hip but increased extensibility of finger joints. Hypoplasia of basilar pelvis with horizontal acetabula, short deep sacroiliac notch, and squared iliac wings.

NATURAL HISTORY. Often evident at birth, the vertebral changes are severe during infancy. The trunk, originally long, becomes extremely short secondary to rapidly progressing kyphoscoliosis.

ETIOLOGY. Genetic heterogeneity suggested by three different presentations; a nonlethal autosomal recessive form, a nonlethal autosomal dominant form with less severe spinal and pelvic changes, and a lethal autosomal recessive form with severe mushrooming and shortening of tubular bones and severe underossification of vertebral bodies.

References

Fleury, J., de Menibus, C. H., and Hazard, E.: Un cas singulier de dystrophie ostéo-chondrale congénitale (nanisme métatropique de Maroteaux). Ann. Pediatr. (Paris), *13*:453, 1966.

Maroteaux, P., Spranger, J., and Wiedemann, H. R.: Der metatropische Zwergwuchs. Arch. Kinderheilkd., *173*:211, 1966.

Larose, J., H., and Gay, B. G.: Metatropic dwarfism. Am. J. Roentgenol. Radium Ther. Nucl. Med., *106*:156, 1969.

Beck, M., et al.: Heterogeneity of metatropic dysplasia. Eur. J. Pediatr., *140*:231, 1983.

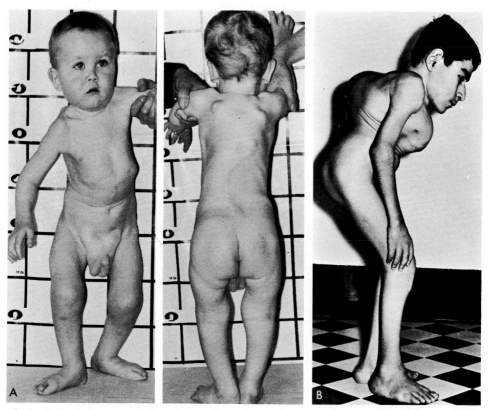

Metatropic dysplasia. *A*, A two year old. *B*, A 16 year old. (Courtesy of P. Maroteaux, Hospital des Enfants-Malades, Paris.)

Illustration continued on following page

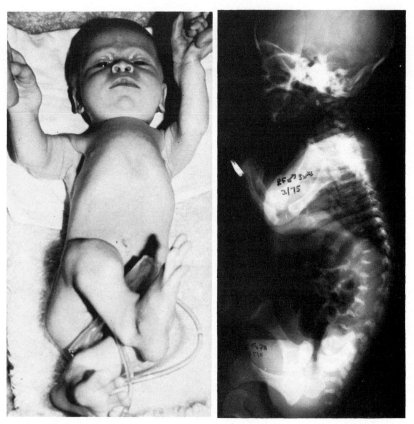

Above, One week old with metatropic dwarfism and the platyspondyly at three weeks.

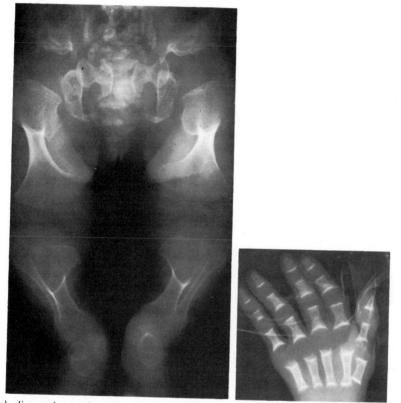

Above, The grossly distorted metaphyses at six months and the hand at two months. (Courtesy of Dr. Paul S. Bergeson, Good Samaritan Hospital, Phoenix, Arizona.)

GELEOPHYSIC DYSPLASIA

Initially described by Spranger et al. in 1971, a total of six cases have now been reported. The term geleophysic (geleos, meaning happy, and physis, meaning nature) refers to the happy-natured facial appearance typical of this disorder.

ABNORMALITIES

Growth. Short stature predominantly of postnatal onset. However, the two patients whose birth length was reported were 46 cm. and "very short."

Performance. Delayed speech development may be related to chronic otitis media. Seizures (one case).

Craniofacies. Round, full face. Short nose. Up-slanting palpebral fissures; long, smooth philtrum with thin, inverted vermilion. Thickened helix of normally formed ear. "Pleasant, happy-natured" appearance.

Limbs. Short hands and feet. Markedly short tubular bones of hands. Wide shafts of first and fifth metacarpals and proximal and middle phalanges. Progressive contractures of multiple joints. Small, irregular capital femoral epiphyses (after four years).

Cardiac. Progressive thickening of heart valves, with incompetence.

Other. Hepatomegaly. Developmental delay (one patient). Thickened, tight skin.

NATURAL HISTORY. Recognizable at birth because of typical face and small hands and feet, growth deficiency and the characteristic facies become more obvious with time. Prognosis is poor owing to progressive cardiac failure. One patient was stillborn. Two others died of heart failure at four years and five years of age, respectively.

ETIOLOGY. Autosomal recessive. Evidence suggests a primary defect of glycoprotein metabolism with lysosomal storage in fibroblasts of cardiac valve leaflets and hepatocytes.

References

Spranger, J. W., et al.: Geleophysic dwarfism—A "focal" mucopolysaccharidosis? Lancet, 2:97, 1971.

Koiffmann, C. P., et al.: Brief clinical report: Familial recurrence of geleophysic dysplasia. Amer. J. Med. Genet., *19*:483, 1984.

Spranger, J., et al.: Geleophysic dysplasia. Amer. J. Med. Genet., *19*:487, 1984.

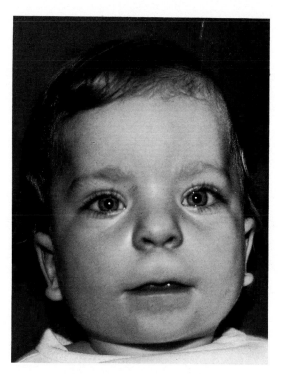

Geleophysic dysplasia. Two year old boy. (From Spranger, J. W., et al.: Lancet, 2:97, 1971.)

CHONDROECTODERMAL DYSPLASIA

(Ellis-van Creveld Syndrome)

*Short Distal Extremities,
Polydactyly, Nail Hypoplasia*

Ellis and van Creveld set forth this entity in 1940. About 40 cases were reported by 1964 when McKusick et al. added 52 cases from an inbred Amish population.

ABNORMALITIES

Growth. Small stature of prenatal onset.

Skeletal. Disproportionate, irregularly short extremities. Polydactyly of fingers, occasionally of toes. Extra carpal bone, malformed carpals, fusion of capitate, hemata, and extra carpal bones. Small thorax. Hypoplasia of upper lateral tibia, with knock-knee.

Nails. Hypoplastic.

Teeth. Neonatal teeth, partial anodontia, small teeth, and/or delayed eruption.

Mouth. Short upper lip bound by frenula to alveolar ridge; defects in alveolar ridge with accessory frenula.

Cardiac. About one half of the patients have a cardiac defect, most commonly an atrial septal defect.

OCCASIONAL ABNORMALITIES. Mental retardation, heterotopic masses of gray matter, scant or fine hair, cryptorchidism, epispadias, talipes equinovarus, renal agenesis.

NATURAL HISTORY. About one half of the patients die in early infancy as a consequence of cardiorespiratory problems. The majority of survivors are of normal intelligence. Eventual stature is in the range of 43 to 60 inches. There is usually some limitation in hand function, such as inability to form a clenched fist. Dental problems are frequent.

ETIOLOGY. Autosomal recessive.

References

Ellis, R. W. B., and van Creveld, S.: A syndrome characterized by ectodermal dysplasia, polydactyly, chondro-dysplasia and congenital morbus cordis. Report of three cases. Arch. Dis. Child., *15*:65, 1940.

McKusick, V. A., et al.: Dwarfism in the Amish. The Ellis–van Creveld syndrome. Bull. Hopkins Hosp., *115*:306, 1964.

Feingold, M., et al.: Ellis-van Creveld syndrome. Clin. Pediatr. (Phila.), *5*:431, 1966.

Rosemberg, S., et al.: Brief clinical report: Chondroectodermal dysplasia (Ellis–van Creveld) with anomalies of CNS and urinary tract. Am. J. Med. Genet., *15*:291, 1983.

Taylor, G. A., et al.: Polycarpaly and other abnormalities of the wrist in chondroectodermal dysplasia: The Ellis–van Creveld syndrome. Radiology, *151*:393, 1984.

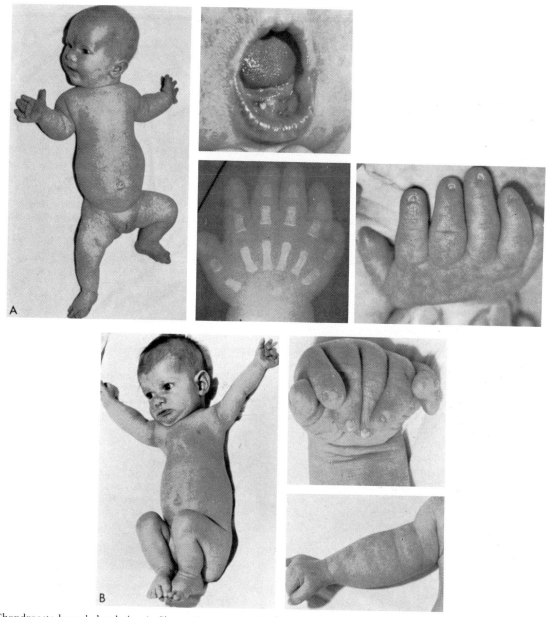

Chondroectodermal dysplasia. *A,* Six week old. Note the hypoplasia of the alveolar ridge, with frenula and an aberrant tooth. The patient is now doing well at several years of age. *B,* Five month old. Note the small thorax. The patient expired as a consequence of a congenital heart defect plus the small thorax. (*B* Courtesy of Professor H. Willi, Kantonsspital, Zurich.)

DIASTROPHIC* DYSPLASIA

(Diastrophic Nanism Syndrome)

*Short Tubular Bones (Especially First Metacarpal),
Joint Limitation with Talipes, Hypertrophied
Auricular Cartilage*

The 1960 report of Lamy and Maroteaux concerning three cases of their own and 11 similar cases from the literature established this pattern of malformation as a distinct entity. It is now recognized with frequency.

ABNORMALITIES
Growth. Short stature of prenatal onset. Mean birth length, 42 cm.
Limbs. Talipes varus plus limitation of flexion at proximal phalangeal joints and of extension at elbow, with or without dislocation of hip or knee with weight-bearing. Short and thick tubular bones with development of broad metaphyses and flattened irregular epiphyses that are late in mineralizing. Carpal bones may be accelerated in ossification in contrast with the remainder of the hand. First metacarpal unduly small, with proximal thumb. Variable symphalangism of proximal interphalangeal joints. Variable webbing at joints. Talipes equinovarus.
Spine. Development of scoliosis with or without kyphosis. Interpedicular narrowing.
Pinnae. Soft cystic masses in auricle develop into hypertrophic cartilage in early infancy in 84 per cent of patients.

OCCASIONAL ABNORMALITIES. Thick pectinate strands at root of iris, cleft palate (25 per cent), micrognathia, lateral displacement of patellae, subluxation of cervical vertebrae, elbow dislocation of head of radius, hyperelasticity of skin, cryptorchidism. Early mineralization of ribs, intracranial calcification. Deafness secondary to fusion or lack of ossicles, stenosis of the external auditory canal. Laryngotracheal stenosis. Midfacial capillary hemangiomata.

NATURAL HISTORY. Two affected infants with cleft palate and micrognathia, similar in this respect to those with the Robin sequence, died of respiratory obstruction. The mortality rate related to respiratory obstruction, including laryngeal stenosis, can be as high as 25 per cent in early infancy. For the survivors, general health is usually good, and the patients have normal intelligence, although there exists a risk for development of neurologic complications due to cervical spine anomalies. Unfortunately, the talipes varus and the scoliosis that develop have been rather resistant to corrective orthopedic measures, and the functional problem is aggravated by the limitation in joint motility. Spinal cord compression may occur as a consequence of severe kyphoscoliosis. When present, the unusual defect of hypertrophied auricular cartilage may eventually give way to ossification.

Linear growth is persistently slow; adult stature varies from 100 to 140 cm, with a mean of 125 cm.

ETIOLOGY. Autosomal recessive.

COMMENT. Diastrophic dysplasia can readily be distinguished from other chondrodystrophies and from arthrogryposis multiplex congenita by physical examination alone.

References

Lamy, M., and Maroteaux, P.: Le nanisme diastrophique. Presse Med., *68*:1977, 1960.
Langer, L. O.: Diastrophic dwarfism in early infancy. Am. J. Roentgenol. Radium Ther. Nucl. Med., *93*:399, 1965.
Walker, B. A., et al.: Diastrophic dwarfism. Medicine, *51*:41, 1972.
Horton, W. A., et al.: The phenotypic variability of diastrophic dysplasia. J. Pediatr., *93*:608, 1978.
Bethern, D., Winter, R. B., and Luther, L.: Disorders of the spine in diastrophic dwarfism. J. Bone Joint Surg., *62A*:529, 1980.

---

*Diastrophic = crooked.

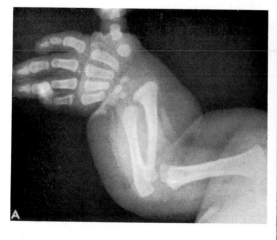

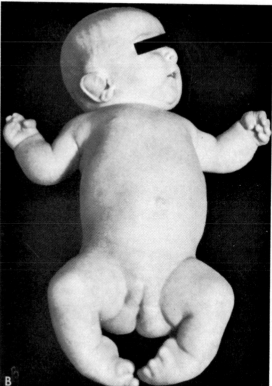

A, Diastrophic dwarfism in four month old. Note small first metacarpal. *B*, One month old. Note cystic swelling of ear. (From Langer, L. O.: Am. J. Roentgenol. Radium Ther. Nucl. Med., *93*:399, 1965.) *C*, Twenty-one month old. Note hypertrophy of ear and position of thumbs. (From Smith, D. W.: J. Pediatr., *70*:502, 1967.)

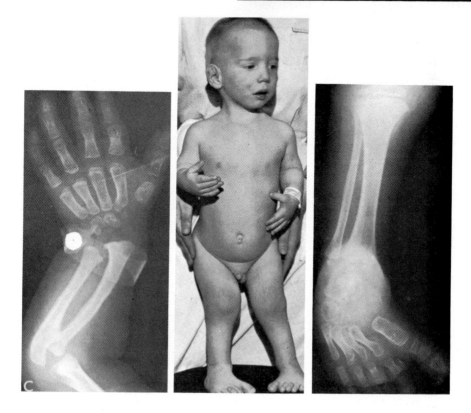

SPONDYLOEPIPHYSEAL DYSPLASIA TARDA

(X-Linked Spondyloepiphyseal Dysplasia)

Flattened Vertebrae of Midchildhood, Small Iliac Wings, Short Femoral Neck

This disorder was recognized in 1939 by Jacobsen.

ABNORMALITIES. Onset between five and ten years of age.
Growth. Short stature; final height, 52 to 62 inches.
Spine. Flattened vertebrae with central hump. Kyphosis, mild scoliosis, short neck.
Pelvis. Small iliac wings.
Limbs. Short femoral neck. Mild epiphyseal irregularity with flattening of femoral head.
Joints. Eventual hip pain and stiffness, back pain.

NATURAL HISTORY. Shortening of trunk. Back, knee, and especially hip pain due to osteoarthritis by 40 years of age; often disabling by 60 years.

ETIOLOGY. X-linked recessive in the vast majority of cases. However, both autosomal dominant and autosomal recessive late-onset spondyloepiphyseal dysplasia, clinically indistinguishable from the X-linked type, have been reported.

References

Jacobsen, A. W.: Hereditary osteochondrodystrophia deformans. A family with twenty members affected in five generations. J.A.M.A., *113*:121, 1939.

Maroteaux, P., Lamy, M., and Bernard, J.: La dysplasie spondylo-epiphysaire tardive. Description clinique et radiologique. Presse Med., *65*:1205, 1957.

Langer, L. O.: Spondyloepiphyseal dysplasia tarda. Hereditary chondrodysplasia with characteristic vertebral configuration in the adult. Radiology, *82*:833, 1964.

Bannerman, R. M., Ingall, G. B., and Mohn, J. F.: X-linked spondyloepiphyseal dysplasia tarda. J. Med. Genet., *8*:291, 1971.

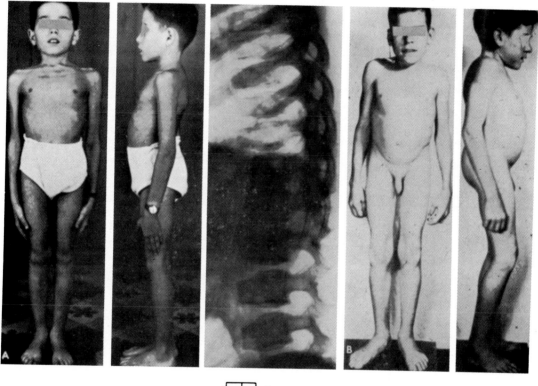

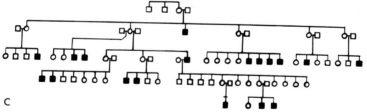

Spondyloepiphyseal dysplasia tarda. *A*, Twelve year old. Note shortening of trunk due to flattened vertebrae, each of which has a central "hump" in the area of its epiphyses. (Courtesy of P. Maroteaux, Hospital for Sick Infants, Paris.) *B*, Fifteen year old. (From Jacobsen, A. W.: J.A.M.A., *113*:121, 1939.) *C*, Pedigree, of which patient shown in *B* is a member, showing evidence of X-linked recessive inheritance. (Courtesy of R. Bannaman, Buffalo General Hospital, Buffalo, New York.)

MULTIPLE EPIPHYSEAL DYSPLASIA

Small Irregular Epiphyses,
Pain and Stiffness in Hips, Short Stature

This condition was described by Ribbing in 1937 and by Fairbank in 1947. It is frequently misdiagnosed as bilateral Legg-Perthes disease.

ABNORMALITIES

Growth. Slight to moderate shortness of stature. Adult stature, 145 to 170 cm.

Limbs. Late ossifying, small, irregular, mottled epiphyses with eventual osteoarthritis due to loss of articular cartilage in many large joints, especially in hips and knees. Short femoral neck. Mild metaphyseal flare. Shortness of metacarpals and phalanges.

Spine. Blunted, slightly ovoid, sometimes flattened vertebral bodies.

NATURAL HISTORY. Evident by two to ten years because of waddling gait and slow growth. Back pain is common. Slowly progressive pain and stiffness in joints, particularly in the hips, may be a complaint as early as five years, but usually not until 30 to 35 years.

ETIOLOGY. Autosomal dominant with wide variability in expression. More severely affected individuals are generally referred to as having the Fairbank type, whereas the Ribbing type is used to designate more mildly affected individuals. The two types do not overlap within families.

References

Ribbings, S.: Studien über hereditäre multiple ëpiphysenstörungen. Acta. Radiol. [Suppl.], 34, 1937.

Fairbank, T.: Dysplasia epiphysealis multiplex. Br. J. Surg., *34*:225, 1947.

Maudsley, R. H.: Dysplasia epiphysialis multiplex. A report of fourteen cases in three families. J. Bone Joint Surg., *37B*:228, 1955.

Hoefnagel, D., et al.: Hereditary multiple epiphyseal dysplasia. Ann. Hum. Genet., *30*:201, 1967.

Spranger, J.: The epiphyseal dysplasias. Clin. Orthop. Rel. Res., *114*:46, 1976.

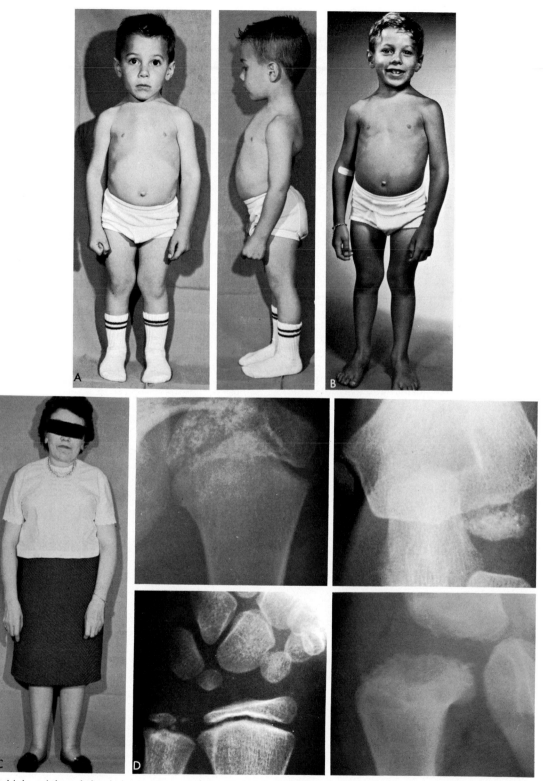

Multiple epiphyseal dysplasia. *A*, Five year old with height age of two and one-half years. Patient had occasional aching in legs. *B*, Same patient at eight and one-half years; height age, four and one-half years. He now has ankle and hip discomfort. *C*, Affected mother of patient shown in *A* and *B*. She is short of stature and has hip discomfort. *D*, Late and irregular mineralization of epiphyses, which may be small or aberrant in shape, or both.

METAPHYSEAL CHONDRODYSPLASIA, SCHMID TYPE

(Metaphyseal Dysplasia, Schmid Type)

Since the initial description by Schmid in 1949, several large pedigrees of affected individuals have been reported.

ABNORMALITIES

Growth. Mild to moderate shortness of stature. Adult height, 130 to 160 cm.

Skeletal. Splaying of broad irregular metaphyses. Relatively short tubular bones. Tibial bowing, especially at ankle. Waddling gait with coxa vara and genu varum. Flare to lower rib cage. Mild limitation in full extension of fingers.

NATURAL HISTORY. Short stature and bowed legs usually evident in second year. Pain in legs during childhood. Symptomatic and radiographic improvement beginning as early as three years of age, with orthopedic measures indicated only for unusual degrees of deformity and usually not until growth is complete. Since the epiphyses are not affected, there are usually no osteoarthritic symptoms.

ETIOLOGY. Autosomal dominant with variable expression. Biopsy discloses cartilage hypoplasia.

References

Schmid, F.: Beitrag zur Dysostosis Enchondralis Metaphysaria. Monatsschr. Kinderheilkd., *97*:393, 1949.

Stickler, G. B., et al.: Familial bone disease resembling rickets (hereditary metaphysial dysostosis). Pediatrics, *29*:996, 1962.

Rosenbloom, A. L., and Smith, D. W.: The natural history of metaphyseal dysostosis. J. Pediatr., *66*:857, 1965.

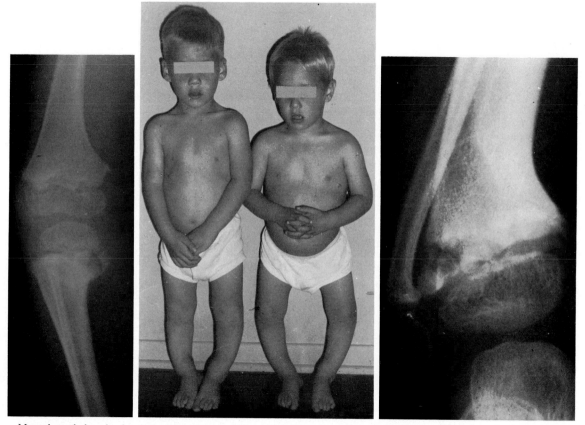

Metaphyseal chondrodysplasia, Schmid type. Affected brothers showing bowing of legs, mild changes in thorax, and metaphyseal alterations. (From Rosenbloom, A. L., and Smith, D. W.: J. Pediatr., *66*:857, 1965.)

METAPHYSEAL CHONDRODYSPLASIA, McKUSICK TYPE

(Cartilage-Hair Hypoplasia Syndrome)

Mild Bowing of Legs, Wide Irregular Metaphyses, Fine Sparse Hair

Discovered by McKusick et al. among an inbred Amish population, this condition has subsequently been detected in non-Amish individuals.

ABNORMALITIES

Growth. Small stature: adult height, 107 to 147 cm.

Skeletal. Irregular scalloped metaphyses. Relatively short limbs, mild bowing of legs. Short tibia in relation to fibula. Prominent heel. Flat feet. Short hands, fingernails, toenails. Decreased height of vertebrae. Incomplete extension of elbow. Mild flaring of lower rib cage with prominent sternum. Lumbar lordosis, small pelvic inlet.

Hair. Fine, sparse, light, relatively fragile.

Other. Loose-jointed "limp" hands and feet.

OCCASIONAL ABNORMALITIES.

Brachycephaly. Severe or fatal response to varicella with lymphopenia and diminished cellular immune response. Intestinal malabsorption in infancy. Altered T-cell responses. Congenital hypoplastic anemia.

NATURAL HISTORY. The early history is often indicative of an intestinal malabsorption problem, which tends to improve with time. Biopsy of the metaphyseal area reveals diminished cartilage cells forming poorly organized columns.

ETIOLOGY. Autosomal recessive.

References

McKusick, V. A., et al.: Dwarfism in the Amish. II. Cartilage-hair hypoplasia. Bull. Hopkins Hosp., *116*:285, 1965.

Lux, S. E., et al.: Chronic neutropenia and abnormal cellular immunity in cartilage-hair hypoplasia. New Engl. J. Med., *282*:231, 1970.

Harris, R. E., et al.: Cartilage hair hypoplasia, defective T-cell function, and Diamond-Blackfan anemia in an Amish child. Am. J. Med. Genet., *8*:291, 1981.

Metaphyseal chondrodysplasia, McKusick type. Five and one-half year old; height age, 18 months. (From McKusick, V. A., et al.: Bull. Hopkins Hosp., *116*:285, 1965.)

METAPHYSEAL CHONDRODYSPLASIA, JANSEN TYPE

(Metaphyseal Dysostosis, Jansen Type)

Wide Irregular Metaphyses, Flexion Joint Deformity, Small Thorax

Since Jansen described this severe type of metaphyseal dysostosis, at least 12 cases have been reported.

ABNORMALITIES

Growth. Severe short stature of postnatal onset. Adult stature about 125 cm.

Facies. Small, immature in appearance, with prominent eyes. Mild supraorbital and frontonasal hyperplasia in the adult. Micrognathia.

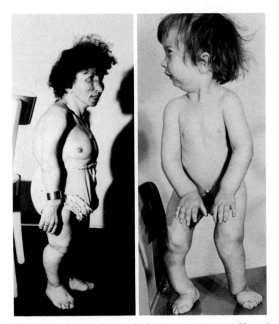

Metaphyseal chondrodysplasia, Jansen type. Affected mother and daughter. (Courtesy of W. Lenz, Münster, Germany.)

Skeletal and Joint. Gross irregular cyst-like areas due to lack of metaphyseal ossification. Pelvis similarly affected. Small thoracic cage. Flexion deformities of joints, especially at knee and hip, yielding a squatting stance with symmetric para-articular widening.

Other. Waddling gait. Clinodactyly. Short clubbed fingers. Hyperostosis of calvarium with thick dense base of skull. Hypercalcemia. Variable deafness.

NATURAL HISTORY. Skeletal changes have been noted at birth or in early infancy. The defective growth and joint dysfunction are severe.

ETIOLOGY. Autosomal dominant, with most cases being fresh mutations.

COMMENT. Radiographic features change with age. At birth, diffuse radiolucency and irregularity of metaphyses of long bones. Wide growth plates of tubular bones. In childhood, cupping of metaphyses with a wide zone of irregular calcification. In adult, the large calcified masses in the metaphyses turn into bone, resulting in bulbous deformities at the ends of short, bowed long bones.

References

Jansen, M. Über atypische Chondrodystrophie (Achondroplasia) und über eine noch nicht beschriebene angeborene Wachstumsstörung des Knochensystems: Metaphysäre Dysostosis. 2. Orthop. Chir., *61*:253, 1934.

Charrow, J., and Poznanski, A. K.: The Jansen type of metaphyseal chondrodysplasia: confirmation of dominant inheritance and review of radiographic manifestations in the newborn and adult. Am. J. Med. Genet., *18*:321, 1984.

SHWACHMAN SYNDROME

(Metaphyseal Chondrodysplasia With Pancreatic Insufficiency and Neutropenia)

Metaphyseal Chondrodysplasia, Neutropenia, Pancreatic Insufficiency

In 1963, Shwachman et al. described five children with evidence of pancreatic insufficiency and leukopenia, none of whom had cystic fibrosis of the pancreas. Burke et al. subsequently documented the association of metaphyseal chondrodysplasia with this syndrome. A total of at least 39 cases have been documented.

ABNORMALITIES. Lack of exocrine pancreas, which is replaced by adipose tissue. Pancreatic trypsin, lipase, and amylase are absent. Leukopenia, variable in degree. Skeletal changes, including short ribs with widely flared costochondral junctions, ovoid vertebral bodies, widening and irregularity of metaphyses of long bones, and focal lack of mineralization in epiphyses. Narrow sacroiliac notch.

OCCASIONAL ABNORMALITIES. Anemia, thrombocytopenia, eczema, immunoglobulin deficiency, leukemia.

NATURAL HISTORY. Failure to thrive with diarrhea is the most common presenting situation at two to ten months of age. Of interest is the observation that there is no steatorrhea; presumably the intestinal lipases are adequate in the absence of pancreatic lipase. The viscosity of duodenal secretions is also normal in contrast with cystic fibrosis of the pancreas, which can be readily excluded by sweat electrolyte studies. The diarrhea tends to improve with age even without pancreatic enzyme replacement therapy. The therapy is followed by dramatic response in some

patients but not in others. The leukopenia can occur intermittently and may be accompanied by a high frequency of bacterial infections.

ETIOLOGY. Presumed autosomal recessive.

COMMENT. The exocrine pancreas is replaced by adipose tissue, whereas the islet cells of Langerhans are intact. Both are derived from a common endodermal outpouching from the foregut, and therefore, it is assumed that the exocrine pancreatic cells are lost early in life and replaced by fat. One possibility is a defect in the integrity of the lysozymes in these cells, allowing the cells to be destroyed by the very enzymes they produce.

References

Shwachman, H., et al.: Pancreatic insufficiency and bone marrow dysfunction. A new clinical entity. J. Pediatr., *63*:835, 1963.

Burke, V., et al.: Association of pancreatic insufficiency and chronic neutropenia in childhood. Arch. Dis. Child., *42*:147, 1967.

McLennan, T. W., and Steinbach, H. L.: Schwachman's syndrome: The broad spectrum of bony abnormalities. Radiology, *112*:167, 1974.

Danks, D. M., et al.: Metaphyseal chondrodysplasia, neutropenia, and pancreatic insufficiency presenting with respiratory distress in the neonatal period. Arch. Dis. Child., *51*:697, 1976.

Woods, W. G., et al.: The occurrence of leukemia in patients with the Shwachman syndrome. J. Pediatr., *99*:425, 1981.

CHONDRODYSPLASIA PUNCTATA, CONRADI-HÜNERMANN TYPE

(Conradi-Hünermann Syndrome)

Asymmetric Limb Shortness, Early Punctate Mineralization, Large Skin Pores

Initially described by Conradi and later by Hünermann, this disorder was clearly distinguished from the autosomal recessive type of chondrodysplasia punctata by Spranger et al.

ABNORMALITIES
Growth. Mild to moderate growth deficiency.
Facies. Variable low nasal bridge with flat facies; hypoplasia of malar eminences with downslanting palpebral fissures.
Limbs. Asymmetric shortening related to areas of punctate mineralization in epiphyses. Variable joint contractures.
Spine. Frequent scoliosis, even in infancy, related to areas of punctate mineralization.
Skin. Variable follicular atrophoderma with large pores resembling "orange peel." Sparse hair that tends to be coarse.

OCCASIONAL ABNORMALITIES. Cataracts (17 per cent), ichthyosiform skin (27 per cent), short neck. Hydramnios, hydrops. Mild to moderate mental deficiency. Tracheal calcifications with associated tracheal stenosis.

NATURAL HISTORY. Failure to thrive and/or infection may occur in early infancy. If the patient survives the first few months, the prognosis for survival is good. Orthopedic problems including scoliosis are frequent, and there is an enhanced risk of cataract formation.

ETIOLOGY. Both X-linked dominant and autosomal dominant inheritance have been documented. The former, lethal in males, is characterized by asymmetric skeletal and eye involvement, patchy distribution of the scalp and skin manifestations, usually normal intelligence, and a good prognosis.

References

Conradi, E.: Vorzeitiges Auftreten von Knochen und eigenartigen Verkalkungskernen bei Chondrodystrophia foetalis hypoplastica. Jahrb. Kinderheilkd., *80*:86, 1914.

Hünermann, C.: Chondrodystrophia calcificans congenita als abortive Form der Chondrodystrophie. Z. Kinderheilkd., *51*:1, 1931.

Spranger, J., Opitz, J. M., and Bidder, U.: Heterogeneity of chondrodysplasia punctate. Humangenetik, *11*:190, 1971.

Happle, R.: X-linked dominant chondrodysplasia punctata. Review of literature and report of a case. Human Genet., *53*:65, 1979.

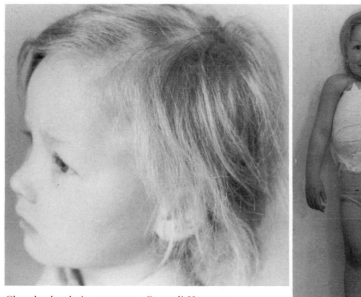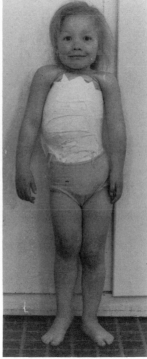

Chondrodysplasia punctata, Conradi-Hünermann type. Four and one-half year old girl, showing asymmetry (note shorter right leg), relatively short neck, scoliosis (casted), and coarse and somewhat sparse hair. She had large skin pores, most notably on the lower arms. Intelligence is normal. (From P. MacLeod, Kingston, Ontario.)

RHIZOMELIC CHONDRODYSPLASIA PUNCTATA SYNDROME

(Chondrodysplasia Punctata, Rhizomelic Type)

Short Humeri and Femora, Coronal Cleft in Vertebrae, Punctate Epiphyseal Mineralization

Spranger et al. clearly distinguished the rhizomelic (short proximal limb) type of chondrodysplasia punctata as a separate entity from the Conradi-Hünermann type of chondrodysplasia punctata. Besides the nine personal cases, Spranger et al. were able to find 33 additional cases from the past literature.

ABNORMALITIES
Growth. Slow.
CNS. Mental deficiency, with or without spasticity, microcephaly.
Craniofacies. Low nasal bridge and flat facies with or without upward slanting palpebral fissures. Cataracts (72 per cent).
Limbs. Symmetric proximal shortening of humeri and femora. Metaphyseal splaying and cupping, especially at the knee, with sparse and irregular trabeculae. Epiphyseal and extraepiphyseal foci of calcification in early infancy with later epiphyseal irregularity. Multiple joint contractures.
Spine. Coronal cleft noted on lateral roentgenogram with dysplasia and irregularity of vertebrae.
Pelvis. Trapeziform dysplasia of upper ilium.

OCCASIONAL ABNORMALITIES. Ichthyosiform skin dysplasia (28 per cent).

NATURAL HISTORY. These patients usually have a severe problem in growth and mental development and die prior to one to two years of age. The majority die in the neonatal period of respiratory insufficiency. Only one patient is known to have survived to the age of five years. Effective management of the disorder has not been determined. Punctate epiphyseal and nonepiphyseal mineralization, which is not specific to this disorder, may not be found in all cases, especially when the diagnosis is not made in early infancy.

ETIOLOGY. Autosomal recessive. Recent evidence suggests that this condition is associated with impairment of peroxisomes (subcellular organelles that play an important role in several metabolic processes).

References

Spranger, J. W., Bidder, U., and Voelz, C.: Chondrodysplasia punctata (Chondrodystrophia calcificans). II. Der rhizomele Type. Fortschr. Geb. Roentgenstr. Nuklearmed., *114*:327, 1971.

Spranger, J. W., Optiz, J. M., and Bidder, U.: Heterogeneity of chondrodysplasia punctata. Humangenetik, *11*:190, 1970.

Gilbert, E. F., et al.: Chondrodysplasia punctata: Rhizomelic form. Eur. J. Pediatr., *123*:89, 1976.

Heselson, N. G., Cremin, B. J., and Beighton, P.: Lethal chondrodysplasia punctata. Clin. Radiol., *29*:679, 1978.

Schutgens, R. B. H., et al.: Peroxisomal disorders: A newly recognized group of genetic diseases. Eur. J. Pediatr., *144*:430, 1986.

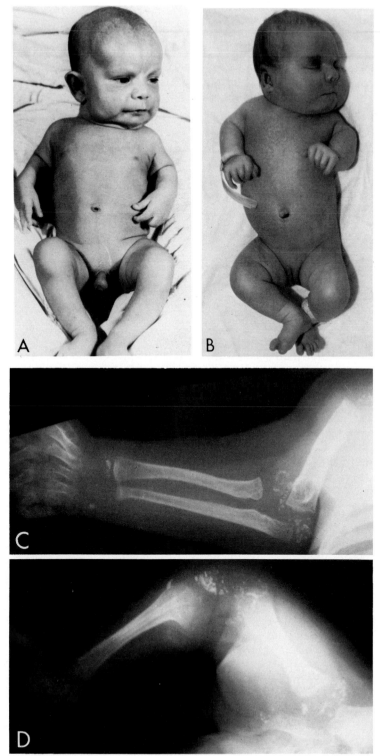

Rhizomelic chondrodysplasia punctata syndrome. *A*, Seven week old male. (From Ford, G. D., et al.: Pediatrics, *8*:380, 1951.) *B*, Young infant. Note the short upper arms. (Courtesy of J. M. Opitz, Helena, Montana, and J. Spranger, Mainz, Germany.) *C, D*, Roentgenograms of the arm and leg of an infant, showing proximal shortening with aberrant form and punctate mineralization. (Courtesy of R. A. Hadley and G. Gibbs, University of Nebraska, Omaha.)

X-LINKED HYPOPHOSPHATEMIC RICKETS

(Vitamin D–Resistant Rickets)

*Hypophosphatemia and Rickets,
Unresponsive to Usual Dosage of Vitamin D*

ABNORMALITIES

Growth. Mild to moderate growth deficiency. Adult stature, 130 to 160 cm.

Metabolic. Hypophosphatemia with diminished renal tubular reabsorption of phosphorus, questionably diminished absorption of phosphorus and calcium from the gastrointestinal tract, and diminished rate of new bone formation. Roentgenographic evidence of rickets, unresponsive to physiologic amounts of vitamin D.

Skeletal. Rickets. Bowing of lower limbs with weight-bearing, slow growth, shortness of stature, waddling gait, coxa vara.

OCCASIONAL ABNORMALITIES

Dental. Large pulp chamber with enamel hypoplasia. Gingival and periapical infection. Delayed eruption of dentition.

Skeletal. Craniosynostosis, dolichocephaly, scoliosis, pseudofractures, bony protuberances at the site of major muscle attachments in the adult.

NATURAL HISTORY. Harrison et al. have emphasized that growth is normal in early infancy until the serum phosphorus level falls to low values at about six months of age. Although large amounts of vitamin D can improve the roentgenographic appearance of the bone and limit the amount of deformity, the serum phosphorus level usually remains subnormal, and the patients continue to grow at a slow pace. Vitamin D taken in large dosage is potentially more harmful than the untreated disease, and therefore, such therapy should be utilized only when the serum calcium level can be monitored every two to four weeks; normal growth should not be anticipated as a response. Combined treatment with 1-alpha-hydroxyvitamin D_3 and oral phosphate has been successful based on healing of rickets, change in growth rate, decrease in alkaline phosphatase ac-

tivity, and symptomatic improvement. Deformities may progress into adult life; these include exostoses at the sites of muscle attachment, spinal fusion, and scoliosis.

ETIOLOGY. X-linked dominant in terms of hypophosphatemia with lesser severity in affected females. DeLuca et al. administered tritiated vitamin D_3 to two patients and two controls and found a longer half-life of the tritiated D_3 in the hypophosphatemic rickets patients, who had a twentyfold greater amount of aqueous soluble metabolites of D_3 in the serum than did the controls. These data, although inconclusive, suggest an abnormality in degradation of vitamin D in this disorder.

It is important in the differential diagnosis to note that there is a severe autosomal recessive form of hypophosphatemic rickets that has been rather intractable to therapy.

References

Winters, R. W., et al.: A genetic study of familial hypophosphatemia and vitamin D resistant rickets with a review of the literature. Medicine, *37*:97, 1958.

Archad, H. O., and Witkop, C. J.: Hereditary hypophosphatemia (vitamin D–resistant rickets) presenting primary dental manifestations. Oral Surg., *22*:184, 1966.

Harrison, H. E., et al.: Growth disturbance in hereditary hypophosphatemia. Am. J. Dis. Child., *112*:290, 1966.

DeLuca, H. F., et al.: Metabolism of tritiated vitamin D_3 in familial vitamin D–resistant rickets with hypophosphatemia. J. Pediatr., *70*:828, 1967.

Glorieux, F. H., et al.: Use of phosphate and vitamin D to prevent dwarfism and rickets in X-linked hypophosphatemia. N. Engl. J. Med., *287*:481, 1972.

Stamp, T. C. B., and Baker, L. R. L.: Recessive hypophosphatemic rickets. Arch. Dis. Child., *51*:360, 1976.

Rasmussen, H., et al.: Long-term treatment of familial hypophosphatemic rickets with oral phosphate and 1-α-hydroxyvitamin D_3. J. Pediatr., *99*:16, 1981.

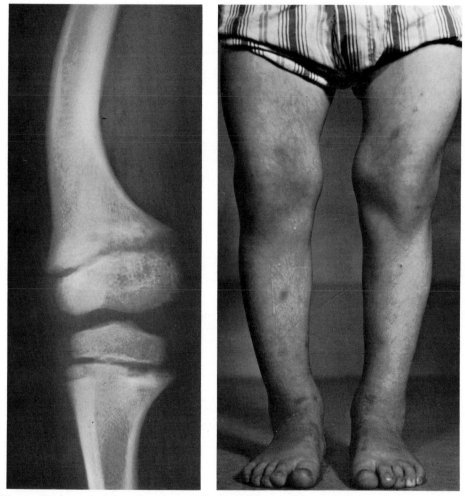

X-linked hypophosphatemic rickets. Seven year old, with height age of four and one-half years. Serum phosphorus, 2.2 mg per 100 ml.

PSEUDO-VITAMIN D DEFICIENCY RICKETS

Rickets, Hypotonia, Hypocalcemia,
Unresponsive to Usual Dosage of Vitamin

Prader et al. described this disorder in 1961, and increasing recognition has resulted in about 40 cases being reported.

ABNORMALITIES

General. Growth deficiency, hypotonia, slow motor progress, +/−seizures (tetany).
Skeletal. Rickets, +/−fractures, large fontanels.
Dental. Enamel hypoplasia of postnatal onset.
Metabolic. Hypocalcemia, elevated serum alkaline phosphatase, +/− mild to moderate hypophosphatemia, hyperaminoaciduria, mild renal tubular acidosis.

NATURAL HISTORY AND THERAPY. The natural history is highly comparable to that of severe early infantile vitamin D deficiency rickets, with onset of hypotonia, growth deficiency, skeletal evidences of rickets, with or without signs of hypocalcemia, such as seizures, in the first six to nine months. These patients are not responsive to vitamin D in the usual dosage, but large amounts of the vitamin will bring about a complete return to normal, including catch-up growth. The initial dosage of vitamin D has been 50,000 to 300,000 units per day, and the maintenance dosage has varied from 20,000 to 150,000 units, most commonly being 30,000 to 40,000 units per day.

This disorder differs from X-linked hypophosphatemic rickets by virtue of having an earlier onset with hypotonia, more severe hypocalcemia, less severe hypophosphatemia, and complete clinical and laboratory restitution on a relatively high dosage of vitamin D.

ETIOLOGY. Autosomal recessive, with a question of autosomal dominant inheritance in some families. These findings suggest possible genetic heterogeneity for this clinical disorder.

Impaired intestinal absorption of calcium has been noted in one case, and the question has been raised of there being a metabolic problem in the hydroxylation of 25-hydroxycholecalciferol to the biologically active form, 1α,25-dihydroxycholecalciferol in the kidney.

References

Prader, A., Illig, R., and Heierli, E.: Eine besondere Form der primären vitamin-D-resistenten Rachitis mit Hypocalcämie und autosomal-dominantem Erbgana: die hereditäre Pseudomangelrachitis. Helv. Paediatr. Acta, *16*:452, 1961.

Stoop, J. W., Schraagen, M. J. C., and Tiddens, H. A. W. M.: Pseudo vitamin D deficiency rickets. Report of four new cases. Acta Paediatr. Scand., *56*:607, 1967.

Hamilton, R., et al.: The small intestine in Vitamin D dependent rickets. Pediatrics, *45*:364, 1970.

Fraser, D., et al.: Pathogenesis of hereditary vitamin D–dependent rickets, an inborn error of vitamin D metabolism involving defective conversion of 25-hydroxyvitamin D to 1α,25-dihydroxy-vitamin D. New Engl. J. Med., *289*:817, 1973.

KENNY SYNDROME

Short Stature, Slim Medullary Cavity,
Transient Hypocalcemia, Myopia

Kenny and Linarelli described this entity in a mother and her son. Lee et al. have summarized the characteristic features in 15 patients.

ABNORMALITIES

Growth. Short stature usually of postnatal onset. However, three of 11 affected individuals were small for gestational age. Adult heights ranged from 48 to 59 inches.

Skeleton. Inner cortical thickening of bone with slim medullary cavities. Variable calvarial abnormalities including thickness or thinness of calvarium with or without diploic spaces and sclerosis. Delayed closure of anterior fontanel and widely separated metopic sutures.

Eye. Myopia. Hyperopia. Microphthalmia.

Metabolic. Transient hypocalcemia secondary to hypoparathyroidism leading to tetany.

Other. Anemia. Delayed bone age.

ETIOLOGY. Presumed autosomal dominant.

References

Kenny, F. M., and Linarelli, L.: Dwarfism and cortical thickening of tubular bones. Am. J. Dis. Child., *111*:201, 1966.

Caffey, J.: Congenital stenosis of medullary spaces in tubular bones and calvaria in two proportionate dwarfs, mother and son, coupled with transitory hypocalcemic tetany. Am. J. Roentgenol. Radium Ther. Nucl. Med., *100*:1, 1967.

Lee, W. K., et al.: The Kenny-Caffey syndrome: Growth retardation and hypocalcemia in a young boy. Am. J. Med. Genet., *14*:773, 1983.

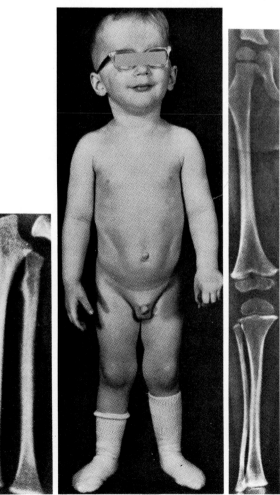

Kenny syndrome. Three and one-half year old, with height age of 16 months. (Courtesy of F. M. Kenny, Children's Hospital of Pittsburgh.)

HYPOPHOSPHATASIA

Poorly Mineralized Cranium, Short Ribs,
Hypoplastic Fragile Bones

Rathbun recognized this disease in 1948, and numerous cases of this autosomal recessive, invariably lethal condition have been documented subsequently.

ABNORMALITIES
Growth. Small stature.
Cranium. Poorly mineralized globular cranium.
Other Skeletal. Hypoplastic fragile bone of varying density with irregular lack of metaphyseal mineralization, bowed lower extremities with overlying cutaneous dimpling, and short ribs with rachitic rosary and small thoracic cage.

NATURAL HISTORY. Death secondary to respiratory insufficiency during early infancy is usual. Of those who survive, early failure to thrive, hypotonia, irritability and occasionally seizures, anemia and/or hypercalcemia, and nephrocalcinosis are common. The hypercalcemia may be responsive to hydrocortisone analogue therapy.

ETIOLOGY. Autosomal recessive. The homozygote has a severe deficiency of tissue and serum alkaline phosphatase and an excessive urinary excretion of phosphoethanolamine. The heterozygote may have a low value for serum alkaline phosphatase and mildly elevated phosphoethanolamine excretion. Prenatal diagnosis has been accomplished successfully with mid-trimester ultrasonography and recently by alkaline phosphatase assay on chorionic villus sample taken in the first trimester.

COMMENT. A much milder autosomal dominant form of hypophosphatasia, characterized by decreased serum alkaline phosphatase, elevated urinary phosphoethanolamine, premature deciduous tooth loss, and later onset, has been described. Affected individuals have late closure of wide fontanels and irregular, rachitic-appearing, incomplete metaphyseal mineralization, with bowing of the lower extremities and awkward gait. Bone pain, dental problems, and occasionally fractures occur, but the osseous abnormalities tend to improve with time.

References

Rathbun, J. C.: "Hypophosphatasia." A new developmental anomaly. Am. J. Dis. Child., 75:822, 1948.

Rathbun, J. C., et al.: Hypophosphatasia: a genetic study. Arch. Dis. Child., 36:540, 1961.

Kellsey, D. C.: Hypophosphatasia and congenital bowing of the long bones. J.A.M.A., 179:187, 1962.

MacPherson, R. I., Kroeker, M., and Houston, C. S.: Hypophosphatasia. J. Can. Assoc. Radiol., 23:16, 1972.

Rasmussen, H.: Hypophosphatasia. In: Stanbury, J. B., et al. (eds.): The Metabolic Basis of Inherited Disease, 5th ed. New York, McGraw-Hill, 1983, pp. 1497–1507.

Warren, R. C., McKenzie, C. F., Rodeck, C. H.: First trimester diagnosis of hypophosphatasia with a monoclonal antibody to the liver/bone/kidney isoenzyme of alkaline phosphatase. Lancet, 2:856, 1985.

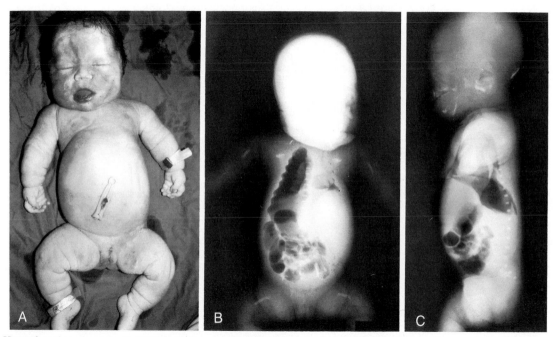

Hypophosphatasia. *A* to *C*, Stillborn infant with almost complete lack of mineralization of bony skeleton. Serum alkaline phosphatase was low, and there was an increased urinary phosphoethanolamine.

HAJDU-CHENEY SYNDROME

(Cheney Syndrome, Acro-osteolysis Syndrome, Arthro-Dento-Osteo Dysplasia)

Early Loss of Teeth, Acro-osteolysis, Lax Joints

Originally described by Hajdu and Kauntze in 1948, and more extensively reported by Cheney, the features of this disorder in 13 patients were summarized by Herrmann et al. The basic defect appears to be one of connective tissue, most strikingly affecting the development and persistence of skeletal tissues. There are several other osteolytic disorders that are not set forth in this text.

ABNORMALITIES

Growth. Small stature, aggravated by osseous compression.

Cranium. Wormian bones, failure of ossification of sutures, absence of frontal sinus, elongated sella turcica; development of basilar impression and bathrocephaly.

Facies. Thick straight hair with prominent eyebrows and eyelashes. Low-set ears with prominent lobes. Broad nose.

Mandible. Small, with diminished ramus.

Dentition. Resorption of alveolar process with early loss of teeth.

Spine. Biconcave vertebrae, kyphoscoliosis.

Limbs. Short distal digits and nails with acro-osteolysis and pseudoclubbing. Crowded carpal bones. Joint laxity.

NATURAL HISTORY. Though the diagnosis is seldom made in childhood, the onset of the disorder usually occurs during that time, as indicated by the hand changes. Pain is a frequent manifestation, especially in the hands. The patients are often weak, and pathologic fractures are liable to occur. Osseous compression may actually result in a decrease in stature, and the basilar compression can be life-threatening.

ETIOLOGY. Autosomal dominant, with sporadic cases presumably representing fresh gene mutation.

References

Hajdu, N., and Kauntze, R.: Cranio-skeletal dysplasia. Br. J. Radiol., *21*:42, 1948.

Cheney, W. D.: Acro-osteolysis. Amer. J. Roentgenol. Radium Ther. Nucl. Med., *94*:595, 1965.

Herrmann, J., et al.: Arthro-Dento-Osteo-Dysplasia (Hajdu-Cheney syndrome). Review of a genetic "Acro-Osteolysis" syndrome. Z. Kinderheilkd., *114*:93, 1973.

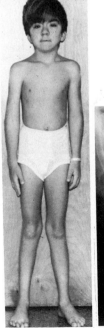
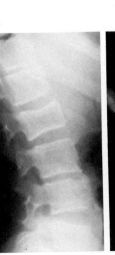
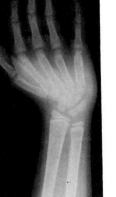

Hajdu-Cheney syndrome. Note the knock-knees, biconcave vertebra, diminished distal phalanges, crowded carpal bones, and relative lack of metaphyseal flare in the long bones. (From Hermann, J., et al.: Z. Kinderheilkd., *114*:93, 1973.)

CRANIOMETAPHYSEAL DYSPLASIA

*Bony Wedge Over Bridge of Nose,
Mild Splaying of Metaphyses*

Often confused with the Pyle metaphyseal dysplasia syndrome, this disorder has more profound craniofacial hyperostosis and less metaphyseal broadening than in Pyle disease.

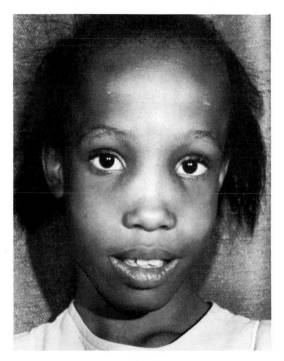

Craniometaphyseal dysplasia. Eleven year old girl with the autosomal dominant type. The hyperostosis is already causing the fullness noted in the area of the nasal bridge. Hearing loss began at age nine years. The long bones show the Erlenmeyer-flask shape at the metaphyseal area. (Courtesy of D. L. Rimoin, Cedars-Sinai Medical Center, Los Angeles, California.)

ABNORMALITIES

Craniofacial. Thick, with dense base, cranial vault, facial bones, and mandible. Variable absence of pneumatization. Unusual thick bony wedge over bridge of nose and supraorbital area with hypertelorism and relatively small nose. Variable proptosis of eyes. Compression of foramina with cranial nerve deficits, headache, and narrow nasal passages with rhinitis.

Limbs. Mild to moderate metaphyseal broadening with diaphyseal sclerosis.

NATURAL HISTORY. The disease is evident from infancy, and these individuals may have serious problems from compression of the brain and cranial nerves and from deafness. They are of normal intelligence. The autosomal recessive type is more severe and may result in facial paralysis and loss of vision.

ETIOLOGY. Both an autosomal dominant type and a presumed autosomal recessive type have been delineated, the latter being more severe in degree. The problem in bone morphogenesis is thought to be one of osteoclasis, with defective reabsorption and remodeling of secondary substantia spongiosa.

References

Spranger, J., Paulsen, K., and Lehmann, W.: Die kraniometaphysare Dysplasie. Z. Kinderheilkhd., *93*:64, 1965.

Millard, D. R., Jr., et al.: Craniofacial surgery in craniometaphyseal dysplasia. Am. J. Surg., *113*:615, 1967.

Gorlin, R. J., Spranger, J., and Koszalka, M.: Genetic craniotubular bone dysplasias and hyperostoses. A critical analysis. Birth Defects, *5*:79, 1969.

Penchaszadeh, V. B., Gutierrez, E. R., Figuero, P.: Autosomal recessive craniometaphyseal dysplasia. Am. J. Med. Genet., *5*:43, 1980.

FRONTOMETAPHYSEAL DYSPLASIA

*Prominent Supraorbital Ridges,
Joint Limitations, Splayed Metaphyses*

More than 20 cases of this disorder have been recognized since Gorlin and Cohen's initial report in 1969.

ABNORMALITIES

Craniofacial. Coarse facies with wide nasal bridge and prominent supraorbital ridges. Incomplete sinus development. Partial anodontia, delayed eruption, and retained deciduous teeth. High palate. Small mandible with decreased angle and prominent antigonial notch.

Limbs. Flexion defects of fingers, wrists, elbows, knees, and ankles. Arachnodactyly with disproportionately wide and elongated phalanges. Increased density in diaphyseal region with lack of modeling in metaphyseal region, giving Erlenmeyer-flask appearance to femur and tibia. Partial fusion of carpal and of tarsal bones.

Other Skeletal. Wide foramen magnum with various cervical vertebral anomalies and wide interpedicular distance of vertebrae. Flared pelvis with constriction of supra-acetabular area; chest cage deformities; winged scapulae; scoliosis.

Other. Mixed conductive and sensorineural hearing loss, which progresses. Wasting of muscles of arms and legs, especially hypothenar and interosseous muscles of hands.

OCCASIONAL ABNORMALITIES. Mental retardation. Ocular hypertelorism with downslanting palpebral fissures. Obstructive uropathy. Cardiac murmur, cause unknown. Subglottic tracheal narrowing.

ETIOLOGY. X-linked with severe manifestations in males and variable but more mildly affected females.

References

Gorlin, R. J., and Cohen, M. M.: Frontometaphyseal dysplasia: a new syndrome. Am. J. Dis. Child., *118*:487, 1969.

Danks, D. M., et al.: Fronto-metaphyseal dysplasia. A progressive disease of bone and connective tissue. Am. J. Dis. Child., *123*:254, 1972.

Gorlin, R. J., and Winter, R. B.: Frontometaphyseal dysplasia—Evidence for X-linked inheritance. Am. J. Med. Genet., *5*:81, 1980.

Fitzsimmons, J. S., et al.: Frontometaphyseal dysplasia. Further delineation of the clinical syndrome. Clin. Genet., *22*:195, 1982.

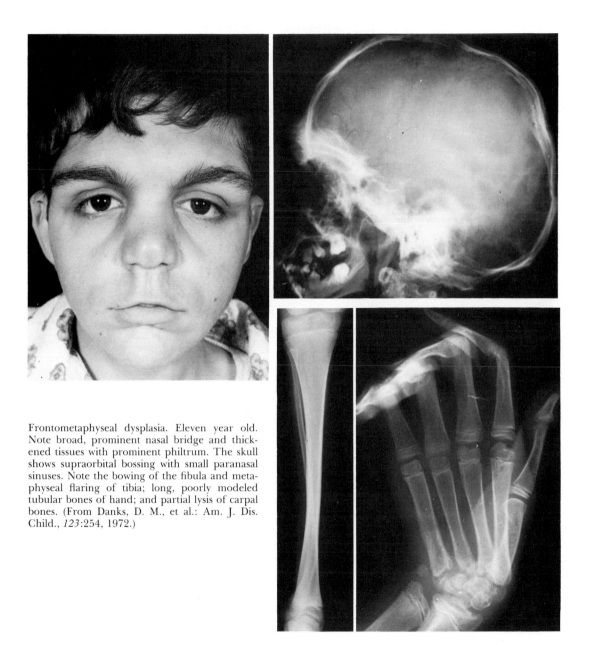

Frontometaphyseal dysplasia. Eleven year old. Note broad, prominent nasal bridge and thickened tissues with prominent philtrum. The skull shows supraorbital bossing with small paranasal sinuses. Note the bowing of the fibula and metaphyseal flaring of tibia; long, poorly modeled tubular bones of hand; and partial lysis of carpal bones. (From Danks, D. M., et al.: Am. J. Dis. Child., *123*:254, 1972.)

PYLE METAPHYSEAL DYSPLASIA

(Pyle Disease)

Marked Splaying Metaphyses,
Mild Supraorbital Hyperplasia

Described in 1931 by Pyle, this disorder was more fully characterized and distinguished from craniometaphyseal dysplasia by Gorlin et al. in 1970. More than 20 cases have been recognized.

ABNORMALITIES

Craniofacial. Mild supraorbital hyperplasia and thickening of calvarium.

Limbs. Marked Erlenmeyer flask–like flare of distal femur and proximal tibia, with cortical thinning and osteoporosis. Similar but less striking changes in other distal long bones plus distal metacarpals and proximal phalanges. Genu valgum. Limited elbow extension.

Other Skeletal. Thickening of ribs, pubic and ischial bones, and proximal clavicle.

OCCASIONAL ABNORMALITIES. Muscle weakness, joint pain, scoliosis, platyspondyly, fractures, carious and misplaced teeth, elongated big toe.

ETIOLOGY. Autosomal recessive.

References

Pyle, E.: A case of unusual bone development. J. Bone Joint Surg. [Am.], *13*:874, 1931.

Gorlin, R. J., Koszalka, M. F., and Spranger, J.: Pyle's disease (familial metaphyseal dysplasia). J. Bone Joint Surg. [Am.], *52*:347, 1970.

Heselson, N. G., et al.: The radiological manifestations of metaphyseal dysplasia (Pyle disease). Br. J. Radiol., *52*:431, 1979.

K. OSTEOCHONDRODYSPLASIA WITH OSTEOPETROSIS

OSTEOPETROSIS: AUTOSOMAL RECESSIVE— LETHAL
(Severe Osteopetrosis)

Dense, Thick, Fragile Bone,
Secondary Pancytopenia, Cranial Nerve Compression

More than 50 cases of this lethal disorder have been reported since its initial description.

ABNORMALITIES
Skeletal. Thick, dense, fragile bone with modeling alterations such as obtuse mandibular angle, partial aplasia of distal phalanges, straight femora, blocky "bone within a bone" metacarpals, and macrocephaly with frontal bossing. Marrow compression leads to pancytopenia, and compression of cranial foramina may lead to cranial nerve palsies, blindness, and/or hydrocephalus. Primary molars and permanent dentition tend to be distorted. Periodontal attachment is poor, allowing for exfoliation.
Metabolic. Serum calcium level may be low and serum phosphorus level elevated. Increased alkaline phosphatase.

NATURAL HISTORY. Usually evident at birth, with subsequent severe complications and death from anemia, bleeding, or overwhelming infection in infancy or childhood. No affected person has survived adolescence. Problems of dentition and dental infection may become serious.

ETIOLOGY. Autosomal recessive. There appears to be defective reabsorption of immature bone.

The question has been raised as to whether this disease may represent an abnormality in thyrocalcitonin metabolism, a possibility that merits close study.

A relatively common mild form of osteopetrosis with delayed manifestations and autosomal dominant inheritance is referred to as Albers-Schönberg syndrome. Diagnosis is often made by chance when radiographs are taken for other reasons. Facial palsy and deafness, as well as involvement of the optic and trigeminal nerves, only rarely occur. Mild skeletal changes become apparent in childhood. Life span is normal.

References

Albers-Schönberg, H.: Eine bisher nicht beschriebene Allgemeinekrankung des Skelettes im Röntgenbilde. Fortschr. Geb. Roentgenstr. Nuklearmed., *11*:261, 1907.
Tips, R. L., and Lynch, H. T.: Malignant congenital osteopetrosis resulting from a consanguineous marriage. Acta Paediatr. Scand., *51*:585, 1962.
Beighton, P., Horan, F., and Hamersma, H.: A review of the osteopetroses. Postgrad. Med. J., *53*:507, 1977.
Bjorvatn, K., Gilhuos-Moe, O., and Aarskog, D.: Oral aspects of osteopetrosis. Scand. J. Dent. Res., *87*:245, 1979.

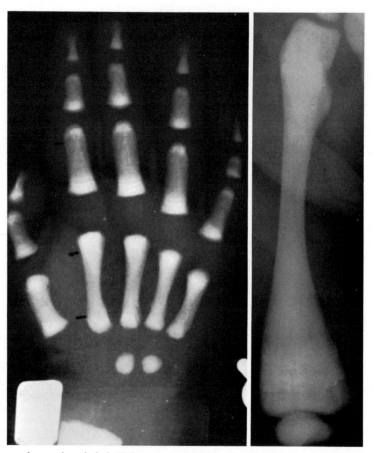

Osteopetrosis: autosomal recessive—lethal. Eight month old. The sclerotic skeleton shows the "bone within a bone" (endobone) appearance, vertical striations at the metaphyseal-diaphyseal juncture, and broad metaphyses.

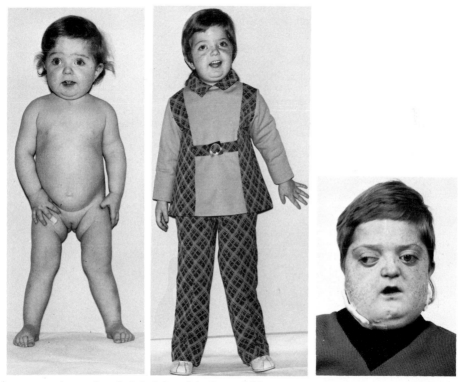

Osteopetrosis: autosomal recessive—lethal. *Left to right,* Same child at *(A)* two years, with length at third percentile and beginning genu valgum; at *(B)* three years and nine months, with lost vision, despite attempted decompression of optic nerve; and at *(C)* ten and one-half years, with proptosis and mandibular osteitis. Her death at 11 years resulted from carotid artery compression. (Courtesy of Dr. Dag Aarskog, Bergen, Norway.)

SCLEROSTEOSIS

Syndactyly, Thickening and Overgrowth of Bone

Hansen described the disorder in 1967, and Beighton et al. set forth the findings in 25 individuals in 1976.

ABNORMALITIES. Progressive thickening and overgrowth of bone.

Growth. Overgrowth leading to mild or moderate gigantism becomes evident in midchildhood.

Craniofacies. Development of prominent, sometimes asymmetric mandible. Occlusion of cranial foramina leads to deafness and facial palsy in later childhood. Proptosis of eyes occurs in adulthood, and blindness may be a consequence.

Limbs. Syndactyly of second to third fingers (not 100 per cent), nail dysplasia, thickening of bones with some irregularity of fingers.

NATURAL HISTORY. The progression of the dense thickening of bone not only leads to occlusion of multiple cranial foramina but may lead to increased intracranial pressure. The latter may cause headaches and may even be fatal.

ETIOLOGY. Autosomal recessive. The 25 cases have occurred in 15 kindreds of Afrikaner Dutch in South Africa. Similar clinical and radiographic manifestations have led Beighton et al. to suggest that sclerosteosis and Van Buchem disease are the same disorder. The only significant difference between the two is greater severity and syndactyly in the majority of patients with sclerosteosis.

References

Hansen, H. G.: Sklerosteose. *In* Opitz, J., and Schmid, F. (eds.): Handbuch der Kinderheilkunde, Vol. 6. New York, Berlin, 1967, pp. 351–355.

Beighton, P., Durr, L., and Hamersma, H.: The clinical features of sclerosteosis. Ann. Intern. Med., *84*:393, 1976.

Beighton, P., et al.: The syndrome status of sclerosteosis and Van Buchem disease. Clin. Genet., *25*:175, 1984.

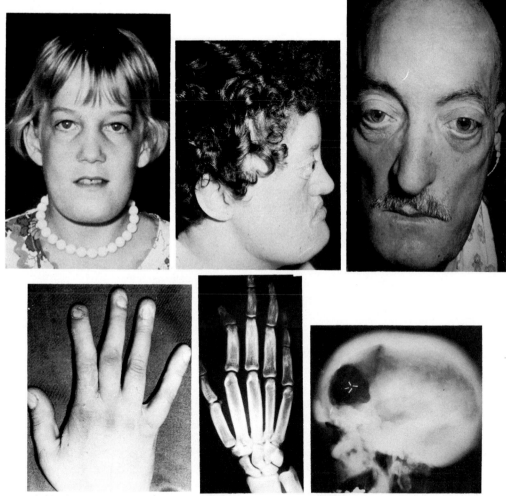

Sclerosteosis. Facies showing mandibular overgrowth, asymmetry, and proptosis; hand showing nail hypoplasia, irregular fingers, diaphyseal thickening with dense bone; and skull showing dense thickening. A piece of calvarium was removed to reduce the increased intracranial pressure. (From Beighton, P., et al.: Ann. Intern. Med., *84*:393, 1976.)

LENZ-MAJEWSKI HYPEROSTOSIS SYNDROME

Dense, Thick Bone; Symphalangism;
Hypotrophic Skin

Since 1974, when Lenz and Majewski first proposed this condition as a distinct syndrome, only five patient reports have appeared in the literature. However, at least three other isolated cases have been published as "unknown" multiple malformation syndromes. The features in infancy differ greatly from those in older childhood, producing difficulties in early diagnosis.

ABNORMALITIES
Growth. Early failure to thrive, postnatal short stature. Eventual severe emaciation.
Performance. Moderate to severe mental deficiency.
Craniofacial. Disproportionately large cranium with broad and prominent forehead, late closure of large fontanels. Hypertelorism with protuberant eyes. Frequent choanal stenosis or atresia, nasolacrimal duct stenosis.
Skin. Cutis laxa in infancy. Later, skin becomes hypotrophic and thin with prominent subcutaneous veins, especially over the scalp. Cutaneous syndactyly of the digits. Absence of elastic fibers on skin biopsy.
Hair. Sparse in infancy.
Teeth. Dysplastic enamel.
Skeletal. Proximal symphalangism, delayed ossification of ulnar rays, short or absent middle phalanges and dorsiflexion of fingers. Broad, thick ribs and clavicles. Widespread cortical sclerosis and thickening of bone in diaphyses, calvarium, and skull base. Shallow and distorted orbits. Long, flared, and radiolucent metaphyses, osteopenic epiphyses. Delayed bone age.
Genitalia. Cryptorchidism and inguinal hernia in boys.

OCCASIONAL ABNORMALITIES. Large, floppy ears, small tongue, micrognathia, cerebral atrophy, flexion-contractures at elbows and knees, hypospadias/chordee, dislocated hips (one case), early death.

NATURAL HISTORY. At birth, cutis laxa, large fontanels, and syndactyly are the most prominent features. Progressive hyperostosis becomes evident only after the first six months of life, often leading to erroneous diagnosis in infancy. Choanal stenosis may cause respiratory insufficiency and repeated episodes of pneumonia. Later, this problem may be aggravated by relative thoracic immobility due to rib widening. Poor weight gain and slow statural growth persist even after resolution of infantile feeding difficulties. No affected patient has yet survived to adulthood.

ETIOLOGY. Unknown. All cases have been sporadic. New mutation for a dominant gene has been suggested because of a tendency toward increased paternal age.

References

Kaye, C. I., Fischer, D. E., and Esterly, B. E.: Cutis laxa, skeletal anomalies and ambiguous genitalia. Am. J. Dis. Child., *127*:115, 1974.
Lenz, W. D., and Majewski, F.: A generalized disorder of the connective tissues with progeria, choanal atresia, symphalangism, hypoplasia of dentine and craniodiaphyseal hyperostosis. Birth Defects Original Article Series, X(12):133, 1974.
Robinow, M., Johanson, A. J., and Smith, T. H.: The Lenz-Majewski hyperostotic dwarfism: a syndrome of multiple congenital anomalies, mental retardation and progressive skeletal sclerosis. J. Pediatr., *91*:417, 1977.
Gorlin, R. J., and Whitley, C. B.: Lenz-Majewski syndrome. Radiology, *149*:129, 1983.

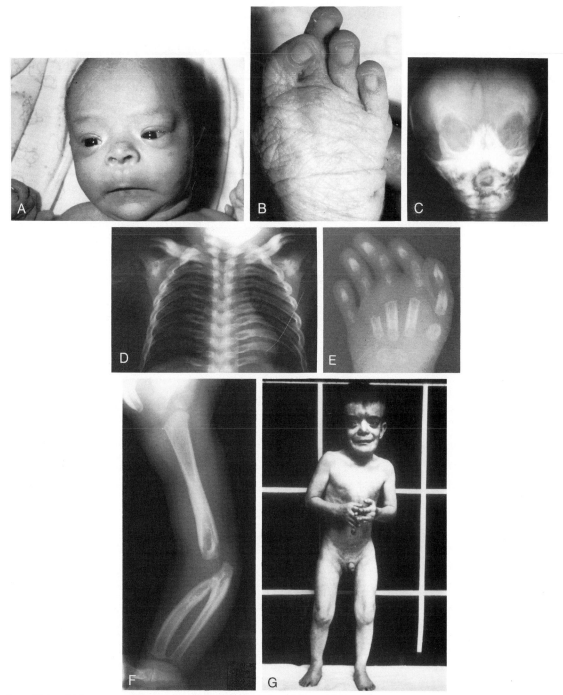

Lenz-Majewski hyperostosis syndrome. *A, B,* Two month old boy with broad, prominent forehead, ocular hyperte-lorism, cutaneous syndactyly with dorsiflexed fingers, and cutis laxa. Radiographs of the same patient at one year reveal sclerosis of skull base *(C),* broad ribs and clavicles *(D),* symphalangism and hypoplasia of middle phalanges *(E),* and diaphyseal undermodeling and cortical thickening with radiolucent metaphyses and epiphyses *(F).* (*A* to *F* Courtesy of Dr. Jon Aase, University of New Mexico, Albuquerque.) *G,* The changing phenotype is demonstrated by a boy, four years and seven months old, who has a square forehead with bifrontal bossing, ocular hypertelorism, and flexion contractures at elbows and knees. (*G* Courtesy of Dr. Meinhard Robinow, Children's Medical Center, Dayton, Ohio.)

PYKNODYSOSTOSIS

*Osteosclerosis, Short Distal Phalanges, Delayed
Closure of Fontanels*

Though cleidocranial dysostosis associated with osteosclerosis and bone fragility had been recognized prior to 1962, this condition was not well clarified until Maroteaux and Lamy described it as pyknodysostosis (pyknos = dense).

ABNORMALITIES

Growth. Small stature.

Skeletal. Osteosclerosis with tendency toward transverse fracture.

Craniofacial. Frontal and occipital prominence, delayed closure of sutures, persistence of anterior fontanel, wormian bones, lack of frontal sinus. Facial hypoplasia with prominent nose and narrow grooved palate. Obtuse angle to mandible, which may be small.

Dentition. Irregular permanent teeth with or without partial anodontia, delayed eruption, caries.

Clavicle. Dysplasia to loss of acromion end.

Digits. Acro-osteolytic dysplasia of distal phalanges, especially of index finger. Wrinkled skin over dorsa of distal fingers. Flattened and grooved nails.

OCCASIONAL ABNORMALITIES. Mental retardation (six of 32). Scoliosis.

NATURAL HISTORY. About two thirds of the patients have had fractures, most commonly in the mandible, clavicle, and lower extremities, including the metatarsals. There may be a progressive degeneration of the distal phalanges and outer clavicle and persistent open fontanels, especially posteriorly. Special dental care is often indicated.

ETIOLOGY. Consanguinity in seven of 32 families and sibship occurrence from unaffected parents are indicative of an autosomal recessive determination. However, Shuler discovered the syndrome in a maternal uncle of an affected male and therefore raised the question of X-linked recessive inheritance in that family.

COMMENT. The artist Toulouse-Lautrec is considered to have had pyknodysostosis.

References

Thomsen, G., and Guttadauro, M.: Cleidocranial dysostosis associated with osteosclerosis and bone fragility. Acta Radiol., *37*:559, 1952.

Maroteaux, P., and Lamy, M.: La pycnodysostose. Presse Med., *70*:999, 1962.

Shuler, S. E.: Pycnodysostosis. Arch. Dis. Child., *38*:620, 1963.

Elmore, S. M.: Pycnodysostosis: a review. J. Bone Joint Surg. [Am.], *49A*:153, 1967.

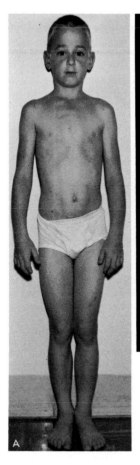

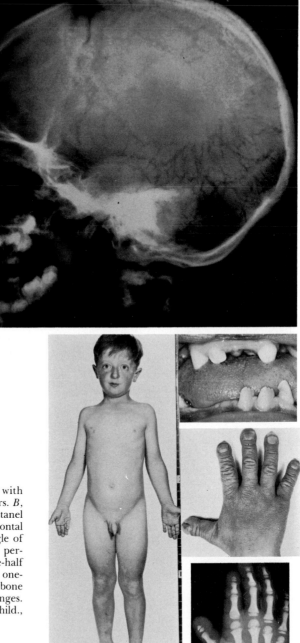

Pyknodysostosis. *A*, Ten year old with height age of eight and one-half years. *B*, Patient shown in *A*. Note the open fontanel and lambdoid suture, absence of frontal sinus or mastoid air cells, obtuse angle of mandible, and delay in eruption of permanent dentition. *C*, Seven and one-half years old with height age of four and one-half years. Note the generally dense bone and partial loss of several distal phalanges. (*C* From Shuler, S. E.: Arch. Dis. Child., *38*:620,1963.)

CLEIDOCRANIAL DYSOSTOSIS

*Defect of Clavicle, Late Ossification of Cranial
Sutures, Delayed Eruption of Teeth*

A possible example of this rather generalized dysplasia of osseous and dental tissues was detected in the skull of a Neanderthal man. The more obvious features of the defect in the clavicle and cranium prompted Marie and Sainton to utilize the term cleidocranial dysostosis for this condition. However, the more generalized dysplasia of bone and teeth has been emphasized, and the term cleidocranial dysostosis depicts only a portion of the abnormal development. Well over 500 cases have been reported.

ABNORMALITIES. The following are frequent but not constant features:

Growth. Slight to moderate shortness of stature.

Craniofacial. Brachycephaly with bossing of frontal, parietal, and occipital bones; late closure of fontanels and mineralization of sutures; late or incomplete development of accessory sinuses and mastoid air cells; wormian bones; small sphenoid bones. Calvarial thickening. Midfacial hypoplasia with low nasal bridge, narrow high-arched palate. Hypertelorism.

Dentition. Late eruption, especially the permanent teeth, which are often abnormal with aplasia, malformed roots, retention cysts, enamel hypoplasia, enhanced caries, supernumerary teeth.

Clavicle and Chest. Partial to complete aplasia of clavicle with associated muscle defects, small thorax with short oblique ribs.

Hands. Hand anomalies including asymmetric length of fingers with long second metacarpal, short middle phalanges of second and fifth fingers, short and tapering distal phalanges with or without downcurving nails, cone-shaped phalangeal epiphyses in childhood, accessory proximal metacarpal epiphyses that fuse in childhood, and slow rate of carpal ossification.

Other Skeletal. Delayed mineralization of pubic bone, with wide symphysis pubis, narrow pelvis, broad femoral head with short femoral neck, with or without coxa vara. Lateral notching of proximal femoral ossification centers. Spondylolysis. Spondylolisthesis.

OCCASIONAL ABNORMALITIES. Cervical rib, small scapulae, scoliosis, kyphosis, flat acetabula, osteosclerosis, increased bone fragility, deafness, cleft palate.

ETIOLOGY. Autosomal dominant with wide variability in expression, but usually showing penetrance. About one third of the cases represent fresh mutations. A rare autosomal recessive form of this disorder has been described in three individuals from two consanguineous families.

NATURAL HISTORY. Though stature is often reduced, mentality is usually normal. Hearing should be assessed, and dental problems should be anticipated. Removal of deciduous teeth does not seem to hasten the eruption of permanent teeth, and the permanent teeth may be difficult to extract because of malformed roots. A narrow pelvis may necessitate cesarean section in the pregnant female with this condition. A narrow thorax may lead to respiratory distress in early infancy.

COMMENT. The degree of variance in expression includes a lack of defective clavicular development. Many of the radiologic signs, such as metacarpal pseudoepiphyses and late mineralization of the pubic ramus, depend on the age of the patient.

References

Marie, P., and Sainton, P.: Observation d'hydrocephalie héréditaire (père et fils) par vice de développement du crane et du cerveau. Bull. Mem. Soc. Med. Hôp. (Paris), *14*:706, 1897.

Grieg, D. M.: Neanderthal skull presenting features of cleidocranial dysostosis and other peculiarities. Edinburgh Med. J., *40*:407, 1933.

Lasker, G. W.: The inheritance of cleidocranial dysostosis. Hum. Biol., *18*:103, 1946.

Jackson, W. P. U.: Osteo-dental dysplasia (Cleidocranial dysostosis). The "Arnold head." Acta Med. Scand., *139*:292, 1951.

Forland, M.: Cleidocranial dysostosis. A review of the syndrome and report of a sporadic case, with hereditary transmission. Am. J. Med., *33*:792, 1962.

Fauré, C., and Maroteaux, P.: Cleidocranial dysplasia. *In* Kaufman, H. J. (ed.): Progress in Pediatric Radiology, Vol. 4. Basel, Karger, 1973, pp. 211–238.

Jarvis, J. L., and Keats, T. E.: Cleidocranial dysostosis. A review of 40 new cases. Am. J. Roentgenol., *121*:5, 1974.

Goodman, R. M., et al.: Evidence for an autosomal recessive form of cleidocranial dysostosis. Clin. Genet., *8*:20, 1975.

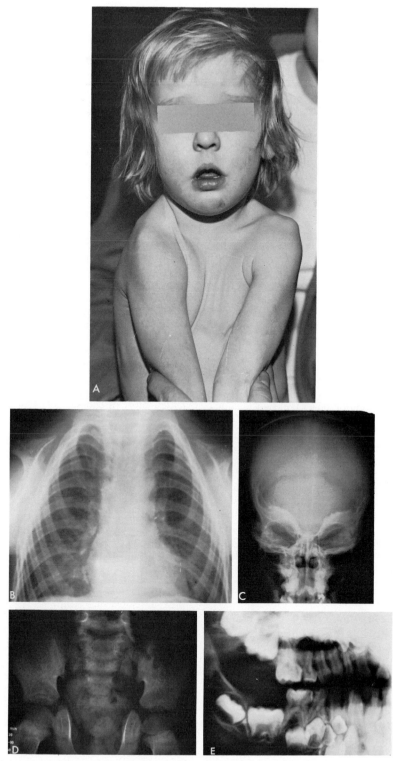

Cleidocranial dysostosis. *A*, Three and one-half year old; height age, two and one-half years. (From Smith, D. W.: J. Pediatr. *70*:500, 1967.) *B*, Absent clavicles. *C*, Poorly mineralized cranial sutures. *D*, Hypoplasia of ilia, wide-spread pubic rami. *E*, Mandible showing delay in eruption of permanent teeth in a seven year old. (*C* and *E* Courtesy of R. Scherz, Madigan General Hospital, Tacoma, Washington.)

L. CRANIOSYNOSTOSIS SYNDROMES

SAETHRE-CHOTZEN SYNDROME

*Brachycephaly with Maxillary Hypoplasia, Prominent
Ear Crus, Syndactyly*

Originally described by Saethre and by Chotzen in the early 1930s, this disorder has only more recently been appreciated as a distinct entity. The syndrome has frequently been undiagnosed in past reports. In the experience of the author, this has been the most common heritable disorder in which coronal craniostenosis may be an associated feature.

ABNORMALITIES. Variability of almost all features.
Craniofacial. Brachycephaly with high forehead, presumably due to synostosis of coronal suture. Maxillary hypoplasia with narrow palate. Facial asymmetry with deviation of nasal septum. Shallow orbits. Hypertelorism. Ptosis of eyelid. Prominent ear crus extending from the root of the helix across the concha. Small ears. Large fontanels, late in closing.
Limbs. Cutaneous syndactyly, usually partial, most commonly of second and third fingers and/or third and fourth toes. Mild to moderate brachydactyly with small distal phalanges and clinodactyly of fifth finger. Single upper palmar crease. Broad thumbs and great toes. Finger-like thumbs. Hallux valgus. Limited elbow extension.
Other. Short clavicles with distal hypoplasia.

OCCASIONAL ABNORMALITIES. Craniosynostosis to the point of increased intracranial pressure. Mental deficiency, small stature, cleft palate, deafness, strabismus, vertebral anomalies, short fourth metacarpals, presumed cardiac anomaly (murmur), cryptorchidism, renal anomaly. Parietal foramina.

NATURAL HISTORY. Though most patients are apparently of normal intelligence, mental deficiency of mild to moderate degree has been a feature. Whether this is secondary to craniosynostosis remains to be clarified. Facial appearance tends to improve during childhood.

ETIOLOGY. Autosomal dominant with rather wide variance in expression. The author has evaluated one family in which the child had coronal craniostenosis requiring early surgical intervention but did not have limb defects. The father, who had no craniosynostosis, had syndactyly of the hands and feet and broad thumbs and toes. Combining the findings in the father and son yielded most of the variable features of Saethre-Chotzen syndrome.

References

Saethre, H.: Ein Beitrag zum Turmschaedelproblem (Pathogenese, Erblichkeit und Symptomatologie). Z. Nervenheilkd., *117*:533, 1931.
Chotzen, F.: Eine eigenartige familiare Entwicklungsstörung. (Akrocephalosyndaktylie, Dysostosis craniofacialis und Hypertelorismus). Monatsschr. Kinderheilkd., *55*:97, 1932.
Aase, J. M., and Smith, D. W.: Facial asymmetry and abnormalities of palms and ears: A dominantly inherited developmental syndrome. J. Pediatr., *76*:928, 1970.
Bartsocas, C. S., Weber, A. L., and Crawford, J. D.: Acrocephalosyndactyly type III: Chotzen's syndrome. J. Pediatr., *77*:267, 1970.
Kreiborg, S., Pruzansky, S., and Pashayan, H.: The Saethre-Chotzen syndrome. Teratology, *6*:287, 1972.
Pantke, O. A., et al.: The Saethre-Chotzen syndrome. Birth Defects Original Article Series, *XI*(2):190, 1975.
Friedman, J. M., et al.: Saethre-Chotzen syndrome: a broad and variable pattern of skeletal malformations. J. Pediatr., *91*:929, 1977.

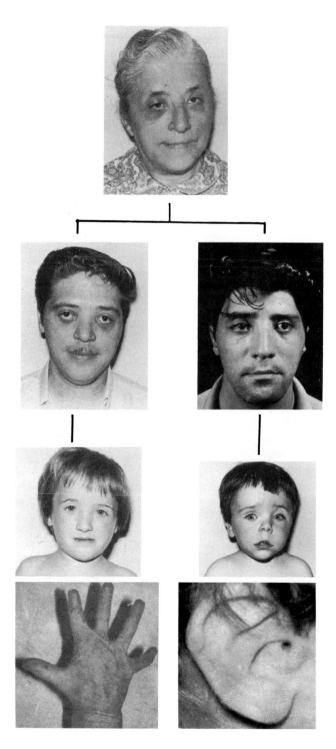

Saethre-Chotzen syndrome. Five affected family members. Note the variable ptosis, facial asymmetry, and strabismus. The hand of the girl shows a simian crease, clinodactyly, and mild webbing between the second and third fingers (the only individual with syndactyly *noted* in this family). The ear of the boy shows the unusually prominent crus across the concha, found in all affected individuals in this family. (From Aase, J. M., and Smith, D. W.: J. Pediatr., 76:928, 1970.)

Illustration continued on following page

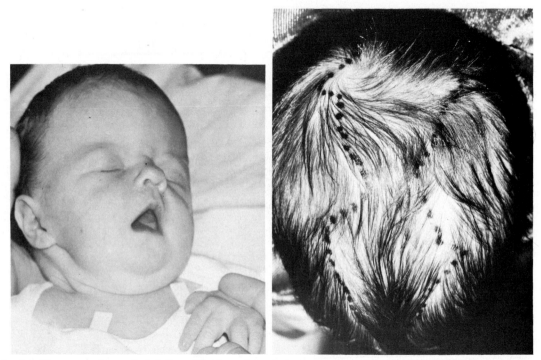

Saethre-Chotzen syndrome. *Left*, Infant with bilateral craniosynostosis and third and fourth finger syndactyly. *Right*, Infant with huge anterior and posterior fontanels (outlined). (Courtesy of Dr. J. M. Friedman, University of British Columbia, Vancouver.)

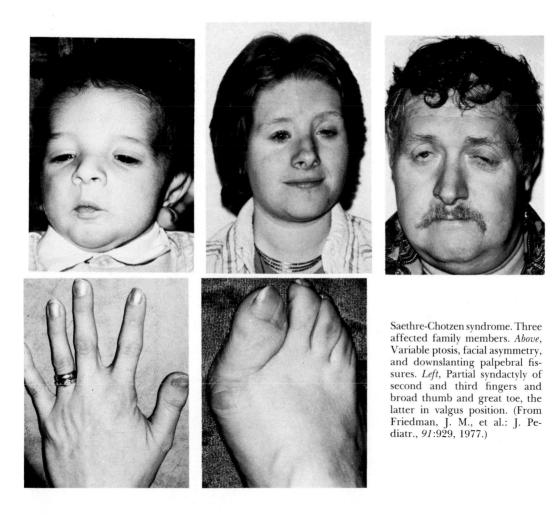

Saethre-Chotzen syndrome. Three affected family members. *Above*, Variable ptosis, facial asymmetry, and downslanting palpebral fissures. *Left*, Partial syndactyly of second and third fingers and broad thumb and great toe, the latter in valgus position. (From Friedman, J. M., et al.: J. Pediatr., *91*:929, 1977.)

PFEIFFER SYNDROME
(Pfeiffer-type Acrocephalosyndactyly)

Brachycephaly, Mild Syndactyly,
Broad Thumbs and Toes

Only a few cases of this disorder have been recognized, and they were reported by Pfeiffer in 1964. The major unresolved question is whether Pfeiffer syndrome is a separate entity or simply represents a part of the variable expression of Saethre-Chotzen syndrome.

ABNORMALITIES

Craniofacial. Brachycephaly with craniosynostosis of coronal, +/− sagittal sutures with full high forehead, ocular hypertelorism, antimongoloid upslanting palpebral fissures, small nose with low nasal bridge, narrow maxilla.

Hands and Feet. Broad distal phalanges of thumb and big toe, +/− small middle phalanges of fingers, +/− partial syndactyly of second and third fingers and second, third, and fourth toes.

OCCASIONAL ABNORMALITIES. Choanal atresia. Kleeblattschädel anomaly. Radiohumeral synostosis of elbow. Mental retardation. Hydrocephalus. Arnold-Chiari malformation. Seizures. Fifth finger clinodactyly.

NATURAL HISTORY. The craniofacial appearance tends to improve with age, depending on severity of the craniosynostosis. Intelligence has usually been within normal limits.

ETIOLOGY. Autosomal dominant with many cases representing fresh mutations.

References

Pfeiffer, R. A.: Dominant erbliche Akrocephalosyndactylie. Z. Kinderheilkd., *90*:301, 1964.
Martsolf, J. T., et al.: Pfeiffer syndrome. An unusual type of acrocephalosyndactyly with broad thumbs and great toes. Am. J. Dis. Child., *121*:257, 1971.

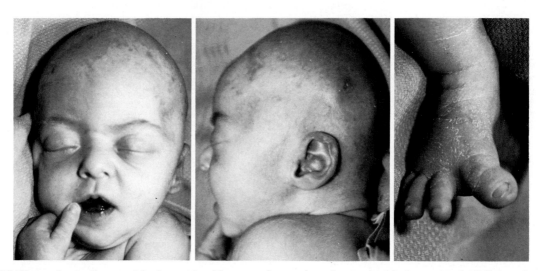

Pfeiffer syndrome. Presumed fresh mutational instance of coronal craniostenosis with aberrant and mildly broad toe and questionable mildly altered thumbs.

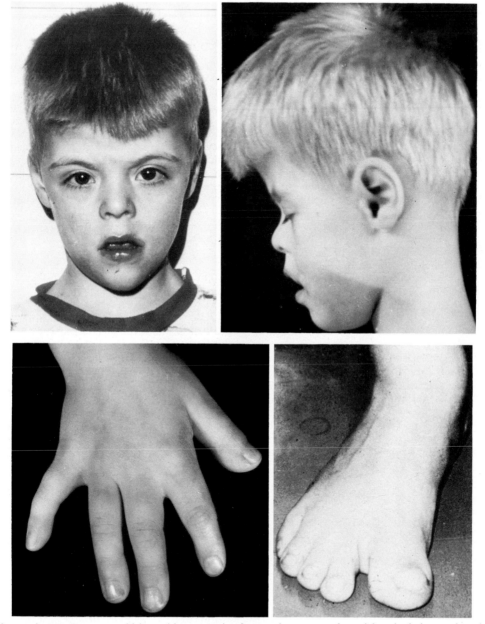

Pfeiffer syndrome. Four year old boy with synostosis of coronal sutures and partial sagittal closure, broad thumbs and great toes, and partial syndactyly between second and third fingers and second through fourth toes. (From Martsolf, J. T., et al.: Am. J. Dis. Child., *121*:257, 1971.)

CARPENTER SYNDROME

*Acrocephaly, Polydactyly and Syndactyly of Feet,
Lateral Displacement of Inner Canthi*

Although Carpenter described this condition in 1901, it was not firmly established as an entity until Temtamy's report in 1966. Some of the cases reported in the literature had been mistakenly identified as Apert syndrome or the Lawrence-Moon-Biedl syndrome.

ABNORMALITIES

Growth. Obesity.

Performance. Variable delay in intellectual performance. I.Q.s have ranged from 60 to 104.

Craniofacial. Brachycephaly with variable synostosis of coronal, sagittal, and lambdoid sutures. Shallow supraorbital ridges. Lateral displacement of the inner canthi with or without inner canthal folds.

Limbs. Brachydactyly of hands with clinodactyly, partial syndactyly, and camptodactyly. Single flexion crease. Subluxation at distal interphalangeal joints. Angulation deformities at knees. Preaxial polydactyly of the feet with partial syndactyly.

Other. Hypogenitalism.

OCCASIONAL ABNORMALITIES. Postaxial polydactyly, low-set auricles, preauricular pits, congenital heart defects (patent ductus arteriosus, ventricular septal defect, pulmonic stenosis, transposition of great vessels), duplication of second phalanx of thumb, metatarsus varus, flat acetabulum, flare to pelvis, coxa valga, genu valgum, lateral displacement of patellae, pilonidal dimple, accessory spleen, abdominal hernias, short stature, renal anomalies, conductive and neurosensory hearing loss.

NATURAL HISTORY. Recent reports indicate that mental retardation is not an obligate feature of this condition and probably does not relate to the timing of craniofacial surgery. Fine motor dysfunction secondary to the digital anomalies is a continuing problem. Articulation errors attributed to inability to perform rapidly alternating movements of the lips and tongue can lead to speech problems. Eustachian tube dysfunction is secondary to the short cranial base.

ETIOLOGY. Presumed autosomal recessive.

References

Carpenter, G.: Two sisters showing malformations of the skull and other congenital abnormalities. Rep. Soc. Study Dis. Child Lond., *1*:110, 1901.

Temtamy, S. A.: Carpenter's syndrome: Acrocephalopolysyndactyly, an autosomal recessive syndrome. J. Pediatr., *69*:111, 1966.

Frias, J. L., et al.: Normal intelligence in two children with Carpenter syndrome. Am. J. Med. Genet., *2*:191, 1978.

Robinson, L. K., et al.: Carpenter syndrome: Natural history and clinical spectrum. Am. J. Med. Genet., *20*:461, 1985.

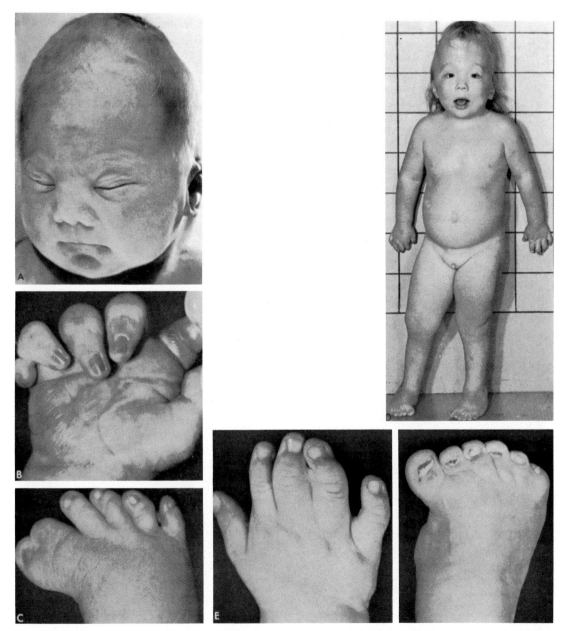

Carpenter syndrome. *A* to *C*, Neonate, necropsy photos. (Courtesy of A. W. Bauer, Group Health Cooperative, Seattle.) *D, E*, Three year old. (From Temtamy, S. A.: J. Pediatr., *69*:111, 1966.)

APERT SYNDROME

(Acrocephalosyndactyly)

Irregular Craniosynostosis, Midfacial Hypoplasia,
Syndactyly, Broad Distal Phalanx of Thumb
and Big Toe

The condition was reported by Wheaton in 1894. In 1906, Apert summarized nine cases, and in 1920, Park and Powers published an exceptional essay on this entity. By 1960, Blank noted the recording of 150 cases.

ABNORMALITIES

Performance. Mental deficiency may be present, but normal intelligence has been observed, and the incidence of mental defect is not known.

Craniofacial. Short anteroposterior diameter with high, full forehead and flat occiput. Irregular craniosynostosis, especially of coronal suture. Fontanels may be large and late in closure. Flat facies, supraorbital horizontal groove, shallow orbits, hypertelorism, strabismus, downslanting of palpebral fissures, small nose, maxillary hypoplasia. Narrow palate with median groove, with or without cleft palate or bifid uvula.

Limbs. Osseous and/or cutaneous syndactyly, varying from total fusion to partial fusion, most commonly with complete fusion of second, third, and fourth fingers. Distal phalanges of the thumbs are often broad and in valgus position. Fingers may be short. Cutaneous syndactyly of all toes with or without osseous syndactyly. Distal hallux may be broad and malformed.

Skin. Moderate to severe acne, including the forearms, at adolescence.

OCCASIONAL ABNORMALITIES.
Short humerus, synostosis of radius and humerus, limitation of joint mobility.

Pyloric stenosis, ectopic anus, pulmonary aplasia, atrophy of pulmonary arteries, anomalous tracheal cartilage, pulmonic stenosis overriding aorta, ventricular septal defect, endocardial fibroelastosis, polycystic kidney, hydronephrosis, bicornuate uterus.

NATURAL HISTORY.
There are no adequate data on the long-term follow-up of patients. Early surgery for craniosynostosis, however, would seem indicated when the condition is of sufficient magnitude to give rise to increased intracranial pressure. Though there can be mental deficiency in patients who have no evidence of increased intracranial pressure, it is an irregular occurrence. There should be vigorous early management of the syndrome. When the thumb is immobilized, early surgery to allow for a pincer grasp is indicated, with later attempts at further improvement of hand function. Newer techniques allow for vastly improved facial cosmetic reconstruction.

ETIOLOGY.
Autosomal dominant, with the vast majority of cases representing a fresh mutation. One factor in the sporadic cases is older paternal age.

The recurrence risk for the unaffected parents of a child with Apert syndrome is negligible, whereas the recurrence risk for the offspring of the affected individual is 50 per cent.

COMMENT.
The osseous developmental pathology appears to be irregular bridging between the early islands of mesenchymal blastema that will become bone, especially in the distal extremities and cranium. Indications of hypoplasia and abnormal shape of bone are also evident, and the mutant gene may adversely affect the organization of other tissues. This is evident in the irregular occurrence of mental deficiency and the greater than expected concurrence of a number of nonskeletal malformations. Therefore, every neonate suspected of having Apert syndrome deserves a complete evaluation for other malformations.

References

Wheaton, S. W.: Two specimens of congenital cranial deformity in infants associated with fusion of the fingers and toes. Trans. Path. Soc. London, *45*:238, 1894.

Apert, E.: De l'Acrocephalosyndactylie. Bull. Soc. Med., *23*:1310, 1906.

Park, E. A., and Powers, G. F.: Acrocephaly and scaphocephaly with symmetrically distributed malformations of the extremities. A study of the so-called "Acrocephalosyndactylism." Am. J. Dis. Child., *20*:235, 1920.

Blank, C. E.: Apert's syndrome (a type of acrocephalosyndactyly). Observations on British series of thirty-nine cases. Ann. Hum. Genet., *24*:151, 1960.

Cohen, M. M.: An etiologic and nosologic overview of craniosynostosis syndromes. Birth Defects Original Article Series, *11*:137, 1975.

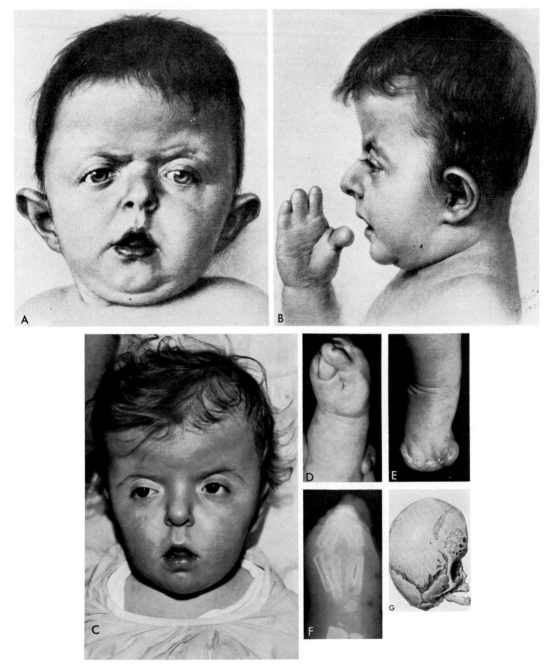

Apert syndrome. *A, B,* A boy, drawn by the late M. Brödel. *C,* Two year old girl, her hand *(D)*, foot *(E)*, and x-ray film of the hand *(F)*. *G,* The cranium of an infant with Apert syndrome, showing the irregular synostosis of the coronal suture and the aberrant development in the frontal bone. *(A, B,* and *G* from Park, E. A., and Powers, G. F.: Am. J. Dis. Child., *20:*235, 1920.)

CROUZON SYNDROME
(Craniofacial Dysostosis)

Shallow Orbits, Premature Craniosynostosis,
Maxillary Hypoplasia

Originally described in 1912 by Crouzon in a mother and her daughter, this condition usually has an adverse effect on craniofacial development alone. With complete examination, including the hands and feet, many of the patients who have been diagnosed as having Crouzon syndrome in the past have been recognized as having Saethre-Chotzen syndrome. Furthermore, others represent the coronal stenosis sequence due to fetal head constraint in utero, a nongenetic type of disorder.

ABNORMALITIES

Craniofacial. Ocular proptosis due to shallow orbits with or without divergent strabismus, hypertelorism. Frontal bossing. Exposure conjunctivitis or keratitis. Hypoplasia of maxilla with or without curved parrot-like nose, inverted V shape to palate. Conductive hearing loss. Craniosynostosis, especially of coronal, lambdoid, and sagittal sutures with palpable ridging. Short anteroposterior and wide lateral dimensions of the cranium may occur.

OCCASIONAL ABNORMALITIES. Mental retardation. Seizures. Agenesis of corpus callosum. Poor vision. Optic atrophy. Iris coloboma. Atresia of auditory meatus. Cleft lip with or without cleft palate. Bifid uvula. Subluxation of radial heads.

NATURAL HISTORY. The degree of craniosynostosis, as well as the age of onset, is variable. One infant is described who showed no roentgenographic evidence of craniosynostosis at four months but complete sutural closure by 11 months of age. Surgical morcellation procedures to allow for more normal brain development are indicated when there is increased intracranial pressure. Otherwise, the indications are usually cosmetic, and the decision toward surgery is usually mitigated by the severity of the aberrant shape plus the competency of the surgeon who will perform the procedure. Newer techniques allow for cosmetic reconstruction of the facial bones. Obstruction of the upper airway frequently results in obligatory mouth breathing and rarely leads to acute respiratory distress.

Although craniosynostosis limits the growth of the brain, the cranium can undergo some further enlargement even when all sutures are fused at an early age.

ETIOLOGY. Autosomal dominant with variable expression, shallow orbits being the most consistent feature. About one quarter of the reported cases have had a negative family history and presumably represent fresh mutations.

References

Bertelsen, T. I.: The premature synostosis of the cranial sutures. Acta Ophthalmol. [Suppl. 51] (Kbh.), *1*:176, 1958.

Crouzon, O.: Dysostose cranio-faciale héréditaire. Bull. Mem. Soc. Med. Hop. (Paris), *33*:545, 1912.

Dodge, H. W., Jr., Wood, M. W., and Kennedy, R. L. J.: Craniofacial dysostosis: Crouzon's disease. Pediatrics, *23*:98, 1959.

Gorlin, R. J., and Pindborg, J. J.: Syndromes of the Head and Neck. New York, McGraw-Hill Book Co., 1964, p. 172.

Vulliamy, D. G., and Normandale, P. A.: Craniofacial dysostosis in a Dorset family. Arch. Dis. Child., *41*:375, 1966.

Kreiborg, S.: Crouzon syndrome: A clinical and roentgencephalometric study. Scand. J. Plast. Reconstr. Surg., Suppl. 18, 1981.

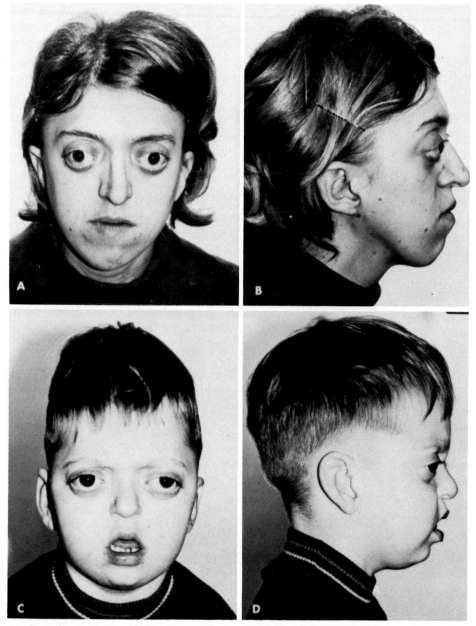

Mother *(A, B)* and son *(C, D)* with Crouzon syndrome. (Courtesy of Dr., Michael Cohen, Dalhousie University, Halifax, Nova Scotia.)

GREIG CEPHALOPOLYSYNDACTYLY SYNDROME

Preaxial and Postaxial Polydactyly, Syndactyly, Frontal Bossing

Initially described by Greig in 1926, additional cases were reported by Temtamy and McKusick, Marshall and Smith, and Hootnick and Holmes. Subsequently, at least 36 cases have been published.

ABNORMALITIES
Craniofacies. High forehead with frontal bossing. Macrocephaly. Hypertelorism. Broad nasal root.
Hands. Postaxial polydactyly. Broad thumbs. Syndactyly.
Feet. Preaxial polydactyly. Broad halluces. Syndactyly.

OCCASIONAL ABNORMALITIES. Broad, late-closing cranial sutures. Advanced bone age. Downslanting palpebral fissures. Mild mental deficiency. Agenesis of corpus callosum (one patient). Mild degrees of hydrocephaly. Craniosynostosis. Camptodactyly.

ETIOLOGY. Autosomal dominant. An affected family with concordance between the phenotype and the occurrence of a reciprocal translocation between the short arm of chromosome 3 and the short arm of chromosome 7 suggests that the gene for this condition resides on one of the translocation chromosomes.

References

Greig, D. M.: Oxycephaly. Edinburgh Med. J., *33*:189, 1926.

Temtamy, S., and McKusick, V. A.: Synopsis of hand malformation with particular emphasis on genetic factors. Birth Defects Original Article Series, *V*(3):125, 1969.

Marshall, R. E., and Smith, D. W.: Frontodigital syndrome: A dominant inherited disorder with normal intelligence. J. Pediatr., *77*:129, 1970.

Hootnick, D., and Holmes, L. B.: Family polysyndactyly and craniofacial anomalies. Clin. Genet., *3*:128, 1972.

Tommerup, N., and Nielsen, F.: A familial translocation t(3;7) (p21.1;p13) associated with the Greig polysyndactyly-craniofacial anomalies syndrome. Am. J. Med. Genet., *16*:313, 1983.

Gollop, T. R., and Fontes, L. R.: The Greig cephalopolysyndactyly syndrome: report of a family and review of the literature. Am. J. Med. Genet., *22*:59, 1985.

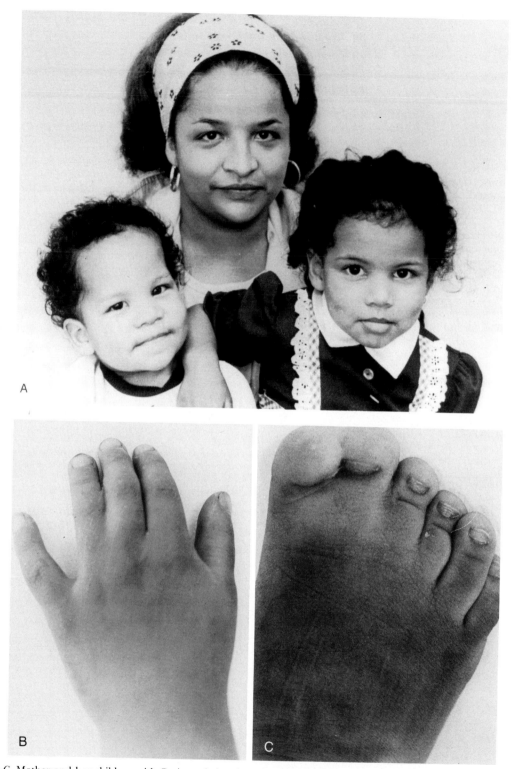

A

B

C

A to *C*, Mother and her children with Greig cephalopolysyndactyly syndrome. Note the high forehead, syndactyly of fingers 3 and 4, and preaxial polydactyly of foot. (From Duncan, P. A., et al.: Am. J. Dis. Child., *133*:818, 1979.)

ANTLEY-BIXLER SYNDROME

(Multisynostotic Osteodysgenesis, Trapezoidcephaly/Multiple Synostosis)

Craniosynostosis, Choanal Atresia, Radiohumeral Synostosis

First described by Antley and Bixler in 1975, subsequent cases have been reported by DeLozier et al. and Robinson et al. Schinzel et al. documented the first instance of affected siblings.

ABNORMALITIES

Craniofacial. Brachycephaly. Frontal bossing. Large anterior fontanel. Craniosynostosis. Midfacial hypoplasia. Depressed nasal bridge. Proptosis. Choanal stenosis and/or atresia. Dysplastic ears.

Limbs. Radiohumeral synostosis. Joint contractures, including inability to extend fingers and decreased range of motion at wrists, hips, knees, and ankles. Arachnodactyly associated with enlarged interphalangeal joints, increased numbers of flexion creases, and distal tapering with narrow nails. Femoral bowing. Femoral fractures.

OCCASIONAL ABNORMALITIES.
Hydrocephalus. Preauricular tags. Vaginal atresia. Atrial septal defects. Renal defect. Multiple hemangiomata.

NATURAL HISTORY.
Respiratory compromise secondary to upper airway obstruction has varied from severe nasal congestion to multiple apneic episodes leading to death. Although gross and fine motor function have been difficult to assess because of joint contractures, psychosocial development has been normal in two patients greater than 1 year of age. Joint contractures have improved with age and passive range of motion exercises. Resection of the radiohumeral synostosis was attempted in one child at six months of age. However, recurrence of the bony fusion recurred within three months. There has been no propensity to fracture postnatally.

ETIOLOGY. Probable autosomal recessive inheritance based on one example of affected sisters born to unaffected parents.

References

Antley, R. M., and Bixler, D.: Trapezoidcephaly, midface hypoplasia, and cartilage abnormalities with multiple synostoses and skeletal fractures. Birth Defects Original Article Series, *XI* (2):397, 1975.

DeLozier, C. D., et al. The syndrome of multisynostotic osteodysgenesis with long-bone fractures. Am. J. Med. Genet., 7:391, 1980.

Robinson, L. K., et al.: The Antley-Bixler syndrome. J. Pediatr., *101*:201, 1982.

Schinzel, A., et al.: Antley-Bixler syndrome in sisters: A term newborn and a prenatally diagnosed fetus. Am. J. Med. Genet., *14*:139, 1983.

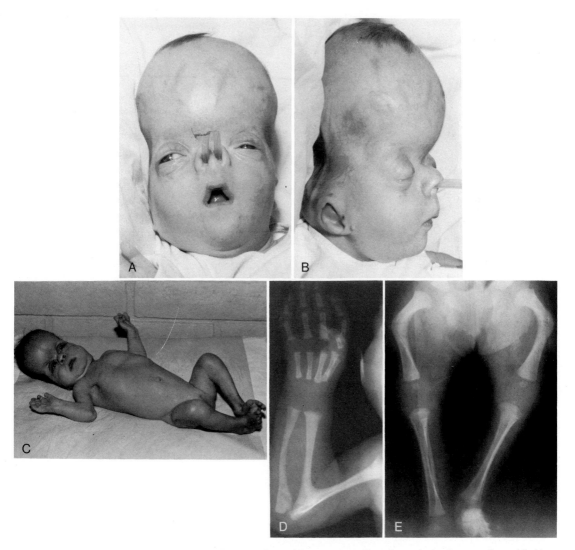

Antley-Bixler syndrome. *A* to *E*, Newborn female infant with severe maxillary hypoplasia, depressed nasal bridge, proptosis, and dysplastic ears. Note the multiple joint contractures, radiohumeral synostosis, and femoral bowing. (From Robinson, L. K., et al.: J. Pediatr., *101*:201, 1982.)

BALLER-GEROLD SYNDROME

(Craniosynostosis–Radial Aplasia Syndrome)

Baller described a 26 year old woman in 1950, and Gerold subsequently reported affected siblings.

ABNORMALITIES. Based on eight patients.
Performance. Fifty per cent of those followed beyond infancy have been mentally deficient.
Growth. Prenatal and postnatal growth deficiencies.
Craniofacies. Craniosynostosis. Dysplastic ears.
Limbs. Radial aplasia/hypoplasia. Short curved ulna. Missing carpals, metacarpals, and phalanges. Fused carpals. Absent or hypoplastic thumbs.
Anal. Imperforate anus. Anteriorly placed anus.

OCCASIONAL ABNORMALITIES. Epicanthal folds. Strabismus. Optic atrophy. Conductive hearing loss. Prominent nasal bridge. Capillary hemangiomata over nose and philtrum. Vertebral defects. Scoliosis. Hypoplastic humerus. Hypoplastic patellae. Coxa valga. Spina bifida occulta.

Subaortic valvular hypertrophy. Ventricular septal defect. Pelvic kidney.

ETIOLOGY. Autosomal recessive inheritance.

References

Baller, F.: Radiusaplasie und Inzucht. Z. Menschl. Vererb.-Konstit.-Lehre, *29*:782, 1950.
Gerold, M.: Frakturheilung bei einem seltenen Fall kongenitaler Anomalie der oberen Gliedmassen. Zentralbl. Chir., *84*:831, 1959.
Greitzer, L. J., et al.: Craniosynostosis–radial aplasia syndrome. J. Pediatr., *84*:723, 1974.
Sklower, S. L., et al.: Clinical memoranda: Craniosynostosis–radial aplasia: Baller-Gerold syndrome. Am. J. Dis. Child., *133*:1279, 1979.
Pelias, M. Z., Superneau, D. W., and Thurmon, T. F.: A sixth report (eighth case) of craniosynostosis–radial aplasia (Baller-Gerold) syndrome. Am. J. Med. Genet., *10*:133, 1981.

Baller-Gerold syndrome. *A, B,* Newborn infant with metopic craniosynostosis, mildly dysplastic ears, and radial dysplasia with absent thumbs. (From Greitzer, L. J.: J. Pediatr., *84*:723, 1974.)

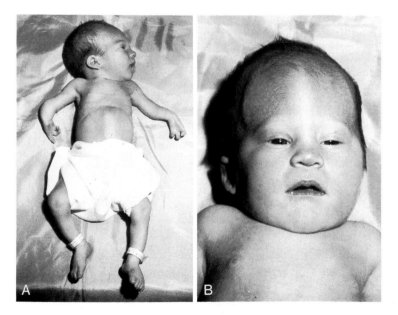

M. OTHER SKELETAL DYSPLASIAS

MULTIPLE SYNOSTOSIS SYNDROME
(Symphalangism Syndrome)

Symphalangism, Hypoplasia of Alae Nasi

In the past, this disorder was generally termed symphalangism (synostosis of finger joints), a nonspecific anomaly. The multiple synostosis character of the disorder herein set forth was emphasized by Maroteaux et al.

ABNORMALITIES
Facies. Narrow, with hypoplasia of alae nasi, hypoplastic nasal septum, fusion of the nasal bone and the frontal process of the maxilla, short philtrum, occasional strabismus.
Limbs. Multiple fusion of midphalangeal joints, elbows, and carpal and tarsal bones (especially navicular to talus). Variable clinodactyly, brachydactyly, and distal bone hypoplasia or aplasia in phalanges. Limited forearm pronation/supination, rotation of hips, and abduction of shoulders.
Spine. Vertebral anomalies.
Middle Ear. Variable fusion of middle ear ossicles, with conductive deafness, most commonly fusion of stapes to the round window.

OCCASIONAL ABNORMALITIES. Moderate
mental deficiency.

ETIOLOGY. Autosomal dominant with appreciable variance in expression.

COMMENT. Potential for significant partial or complete restoration of hearing by otologic surgery is excellent. Symphalangism is progressive and is not always present in childhood.

References

Vesell, E. S.: Symphalangism, strabismus and hearing loss in mother and daughter. N. Engl. J. Med., *263*:839, 1960.
Fuhrmann, W., et al.: Dominant erbliche Brachydaktylie mit Gelenksaplasien. Humangenetik, *1*:337, 1965.
Strasburger, A. K., et al.: Symphalangism: Genetic and clinical aspects. Bull. Johns Hopkins Hosp., *117*:108, 1965.
Elkington, S. G., and Huntsman, R. G.: The Talbot fingers. A study in symphalangism. Br. Med. J., *1*:407, 1967.
Maroteaux, P., Bouvet, J. P., and Briard, M. L.: La maladie des synostoses multiples. Nouv. Presse Med., *1*:3041, 1972.
Herrmann, J.: Symphalangism and brachydactyly syndrome. Birth Defects, *10*(5):23, 1974.
da-Silva, E. O., Filho, S. M., and de Albuquerque, S. C.: Multiple synostosis syndrome: study of a large Brazilian kindred. Am. J. Med. Genet., *18*:237, 1984.

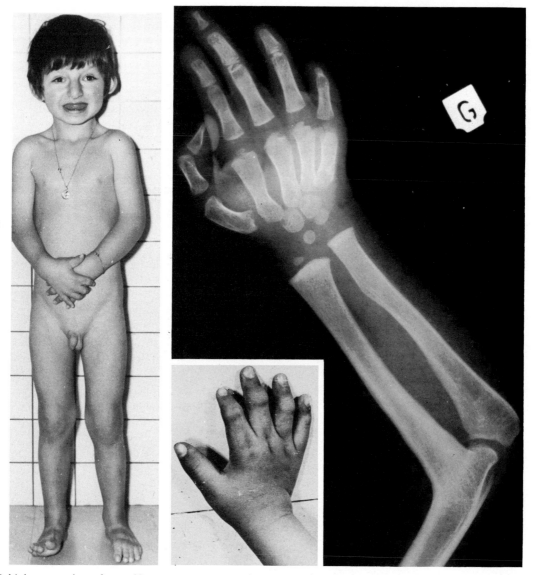

Multiple synostosis syndrome. Note narrow nose, prominent external ear, and variable brachydactyly, aplasia of distal phalanges, and synostoses. (From Maroteaux, P., et al.: Nouv. Presse Med., *1*:3041, 1972.)

MULTIPLE EXOSTOSES SYNDROME

(Diaphyseal Aclasis, External Chondromatosis Syndrome)

Diaphyseal Outgrowths Leading to Limb Deformity, With or Without Short Metacarpals

More than 1000 cases have been reported.

ABNORMALITIES

Skeletal. Diaphyseal juxtaepiphyseal outgrowths develop, capped by hyaline cartilage, and tend to grow away from the joint, leading to deformity. Though often present at birth, they are usually not appreciated until early childhood. There is a slowing in their growth at adolescence, and no further growth occurs in the adult. They are most prominent at the ends of long bones, especially at the knees, with variable involvement of the pelvis, scapulae, and ribs. Involved bone may be relatively short, especially the ulna, with consequent bowing of the forearm. Shortness of stature is a variable feature, with the mean male adult height being 169 cm and that of the female being 159 cm.

OCCASIONAL ABNORMALITIES.   Enchondromata. Short metacarpal (fourth and fifth) bones.

NATURAL HISTORY. New outgrowths and enlargement of old exostoses may occur through adolescence. Thereafter, no further growth takes place, although there is a 2 to 10 per cent incidence of sarcoma from such lesions in the adult, a risk that does not pertain to childhood. In a retrospective review of 32 affected patients, Shapiro et al. documented that an average of 2.7 operative procedures were performed per patient, that the most severe bony deformities involved the forearm and leg, and that the leg-length discrepancies were great enough to warrant epiphyseal arrest in approximately one half of cases.

ETIOLOGY. Autosomal dominant, with 62 per cent of cases being familial.

References

Rubin, P.: Dynamic Classification of Bone Dysplasias. Chicago, Year Book Medical Publishers, 1964, p. 297.

Solomon, L.: Hereditary multiple exostosis. Am. J. Hum. Genet., 16:351, 1964.

Shapiro, F., Simon, S., and Glimcher, M. J.: Hereditary multiple exostosis. J. Bone Joint Surg., 61A:815, 1979.

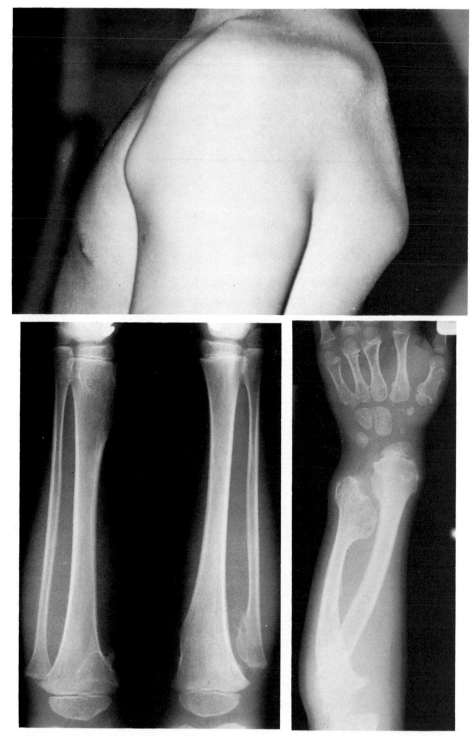

Multiple exostoses syndrome. *Upper*, Grossly evident exostoses in upper humerus and in scapula. *Lower*, Metaphyseal distribution of exostoses, which may be deforming, as seen in the wrist in this example.

NAIL-PATELLA SYNDROME
(Hereditary Osteo-onychodysplasia)

Nail Dysplasia, Patella Hypoplasia, Iliac Spurs

Little's report in 1897, limited to a presentation of patellar defect, is usually credited as the initial description of this syndrome, whereas this pattern includes multiple other dysplasias of osseous as well as nonosseous mesenchymal tissues. More than 200 cases have been reported.

ABNORMALITIES. Relative frequency of expression given in percentages.

Nails

Hypoplasia, splitting, most commonly of thumbnail; discoloration, longitudinal ridging, poorly formed lunulae and triangular lunulae	98%

Knees

Hypoplastic to absent patella, hypoplasia of lateral femoral condyle and small head of fibula	92%

Elbows

Hypoplastic capitellum, small head of radius	90%

Ilia

Spur in midposterior ilium, 71 per cent palpable	81%

Scapulae

Hypoplasia, convex thick outer border	44%

Irides

Dark, "cloverleaf" pigmentation at inner margin	46%

Renal

Proteinuria with or without hematuria, casts, renal insufficiency	30%

Other Frequent Features
Absence of dorsal distal phalangeal joints, delayed ossification of secondary centers of ossification, valgus deformity of femoral neck, talipes.

OCCASIONAL ABNORMALITIES
Skeletal. Prominent outer clavicle, malformed sternum, spina bifida, scoliosis, enlarged ulnar styloid process, clinodactyly of fifth finger, dislocation of head of radius.
Eyes. Keratoconus, microcornea, microphakia, cataract, ptosis.
Muscles. Aplasia of pectoralis minor, biceps, triceps, quadriceps.
CNS. Occasional mental deficiency, psychosis.

NATURAL HISTORY. Patients may have problems due to limitation of joint mobility, dislocation, or both, especially at the elbow and knee, where osteoarthritis may eventually limit function. Children should be closely followed for scoliosis. Albuminuria is the most common early indication of a renal problem. Studies show hyaline thickening of the glomerular basement membrane, cause unknown. Renal failure is apparently rare prior to the fourth decade.

ETIOLOGY. Autosomal dominant, always showing some expression. Close linkage with the genetic determinants of ABO blood group substances. A closer correlation for the extent of nail dysplasia has been found among affected siblings than between affected parent and offspring. This evidence implies a strong effect of the normal allele (always derived from the unaffected parent) on the expression of the mutant allele for the nail-patella syndrome.

COMMENT. The osseous abnormality consists of specific regions of hypoplasia, such as the lateral knee and elbow, and other specific regions of hyperplasia, such as the iliac spurs. The latter defect, as yet unknown in any other species or in other diseases of man, appears to be pathognomonic as an expression of this mutant gene.

References

Little, E. M.: Congenital absence or delayed development of the patella. Lancet, *2*:781, 1897.
Carbonara, P., and Alpert, M.: Hereditary osteoonychodysplasia (Hood). Am. J. Med. Sci., *248*:139, 1964.
Lucas, G. L., and Opitz, J. M.: The nail-patella syndrome. Clinical and genetic aspects of 5 kindreds with 38 affected family members. J. Pediatr., *68*:273, 1966.
Darlington, D., and Hawkins, C. F.: Nail-patella syndrome with iliac horns and hereditary nephropathy. Necropsy report and anatomical dissection. J. Bone Joint Surg. [Br.], *49-B*:164, 1967.
Beals, R. K., and Eckardt, A. L.: Hereditary onychoosteodysplasia. A report of nine kindreds. J. Bone Joint Surg. [Am.], *51*:505, 1969.
Daniel, C. R., Osment, L. S., Noojin, R. O.: Triangular lunulae. Arch. Dermatol., *116*:448, 1980.

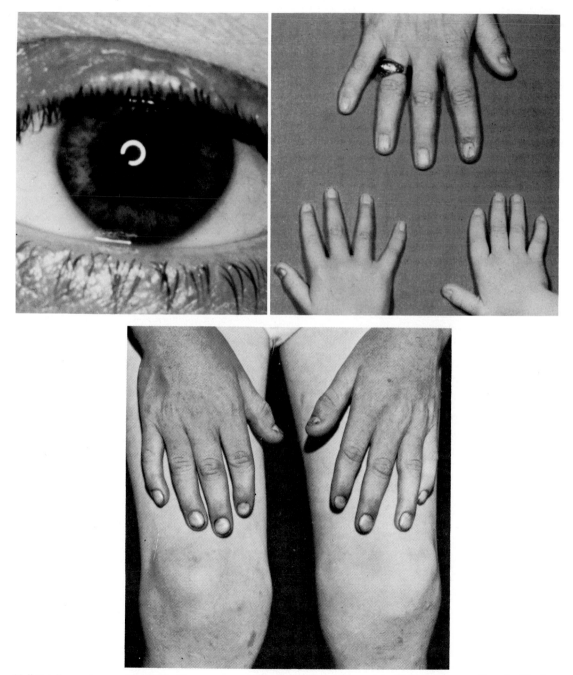

Nail-Patella syndrome. *Upper left*, Aberrant patterning of inner iris. *Upper right*, Father and two affected offspring showing nail hypoplasia, most striking for the thumbnails. *Below*, Adolescent showing nail hypoplasia, especially of thumbs, and displacement of small patellae. (Bottom photo courtesy of J. Opitz, Helena, Montana.)

LERI-WEILL DYSCHONDROSTEOSIS

Short Forearms with Madelung Deformity,
With or Without Short Lower Leg

Leri and Weill described this condition in 1929, and more than 30 cases have been reported subsequently. Most patients previously categorized as having Madelung deformity have Leri-Weill dyschondrosteosis.

ABNORMALITIES

Growth. Variable small stature, adult height from 135 cm to normal.

Extremities. Short forearm with bowing of radius, widened gap between radius and ulna, and altered osseous alignment at wrist. May have partial dislocation of ulna at wrist, elbow, or both, with limitation of movement. Short lower leg.

OCCASIONAL ABNORMALITIES. Short hands and feet with metaphyseal flaring in metacarpal and metatarsal bones, short fourth metacarpal and/or metatarsal bones, curvature of tibia, exostoses from proximal tibia and/or fibula, abnormal femoral neck, coxa valga, abnormal tuberosity of humerus.

NATURAL HISTORY. Associated paramyotonia has been noted in affected individuals in one family; whether this is a frequent feature remains to be determined. Otherwise, the only usual problems are moderate shortness of stature and limitation of joint mobility at the wrist, elbow, or both.

ETIOLOGY. Autosomal dominant, with an excess of affected females in the recorded cases.

References

Leri, A., and Weill, J.: Une affectation congenitale et symétrique du développement osseus: la dyschondrosteose. Bull. Mem. Soc. Med. Hop. (Paris), *45*:1491, 1929.

Langer, L. O.: Dyschondrosteosis, a hereditary bone dysplasia with characteristic roentgenographic features. Am. J. Roentgenol. Radium Ther. Nucl. Med., *45*:178, 1965.

Herdman, R. C., Langer, L. O., and Good, R. A.: Dyschondrosteosis. The most common cause of Madelung's deformity. J. Pediatr., *68*:432, 1966.

Felman, A. H., and Kirkpatrick, J. A.: Dyschondrosteoses. Am. J. Dis. Child., *120*:329, 1970.

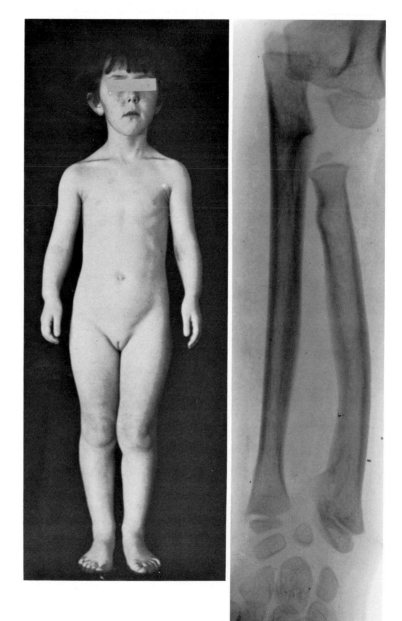

Leri-Weill dyschondrosteosis. Age, seven years and five months; height age, five and one-half years. (From Lamy and Maroteaux: Les chondrodystrophies génotypiques. Paris, L'expansion Scientifique Française, 1960.)

LANGER MESOMELIC DYSPLASIA

(Homozygous Leri-Weill Dyschondrosteosis Syndrome)

Mesomelic Dwarfism,
Rudimentary Fibula, Micrognathia

Langer summarized this disorder as a distinctive entity in 1967, citing numerous cases from past literature. The original report was presented by Brailsford.

ABNORMALITIES

Facies. Small mandible.

Limbs. Short, especially forearms and lower legs (mesomelia). The fibula is rudimentary, the ulna is reduced distally, and the radius is dorsolaterally bowed and short.

NATURAL HISTORY. One adult male was 130 cm tall. Normal intelligence with surprisingly good function.

ETIOLOGY. The homozygous state for the autosomal dominant gene for Leri-Weill dyschondrosteosis syndrome. Heterozygote individuals with the latter disorder have mild to moderate shortness of stature and relatively short forearms with the Madelung deformity. The homozygous state is a much more severe shortness of stature with striking smallness of the forearms and lower legs (mesomelia) plus the additional feature of micrognathia.

References

Brailsford, J. F.: Dystrophies of the skeleton. Br. J. Radiol., *8*:533, 1935.

Blockey, N. J., and Lawrie, J. H.: An unusual symmetrical distal limb deformity in siblings. J. Bone Joint Surg. [Br.], *45*:745, 1963.

Langer, L. O.: Mesomelic dwarfism of the hypoplastic ulna, fibula, mandible type. Radiology, *89*:654, 1967.

Espiritu, C., Chen, H., and Woolley, P. V., Jr.: Probable homozygosity for the dyschondrosteosis genes. Am. J. Dis. Child., *129*:375, 1975.

Kunze, J., and Klemm, T.: Mesomelic dysplasia, type Langer—A homozygous state for dyschondrosteosis. Eur. J. Pediatr., *134*:269, 1980.

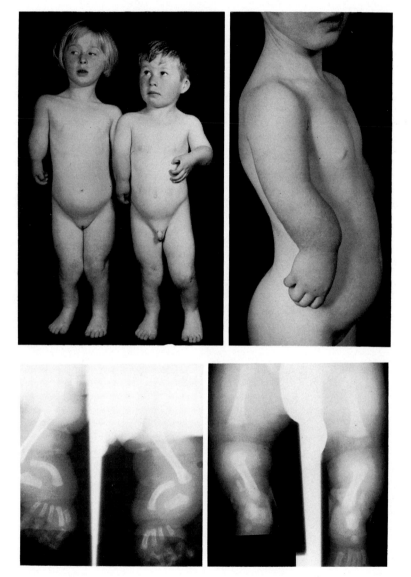

Langer mesomelic dysplasia. Siblings with unusual shortness of stature with disproportionate smallness of forearms and lower legs, especially the ulnae and fibulae. (From Blockley, N. J., and Lawrie, J. H.: J. Bone Joint Surg. [Br.], *45*:745, 1963.)

ACRODYSOSTOSIS

*Short Hands with Peripheral Dysostosis,
Small Nose, Mental Deficiency*

Maroteaux and Malamut first described this disorder in three patients in 1968, and there are now over 20 published cases.

ABNORMALITIES
Growth. Mild to moderate prenatal onset growth deficiency.
Performance. Mental deficiency in about 90 per cent.
Craniofacial. Brachycephaly, low nasal bridge, broad and small upturned nose, tendency to hold mouth open, hypoplastic maxilla with prognathism.
Limbs. Short, especially distally, with progressive deformity in distal humerus, radius, and ulna, and cone-shaped epiphyses that fuse prematurely in hands and feet. Hands appear short and broad, with wrinkling of dorsal skin.

OCCASIONAL ABNORMALITIES. Epicanthal folds, hypertelorism, optic atrophy, dimpled nasal tip, malocclusion of teeth, calvarial hyperostosis, hydrocephalus, recurrent ear infections with occasional hearing loss, pigmented nevi, hypogenitalism, hypogonadism, dislocated radial heads, small vertebrae that may collapse, spinal curvatures.

NATURAL HISTORY. Most patients do relatively well except for the problems of mental deficiency and arthritic complaints. Progressive restriction of movement of the hands, elbows, and spine may occur.

ETIOLOGY. Unknown, sporadic occurrence. Older paternal age suggests autosomal dominant fresh mutation.

COMMENT. It has been suggested that individuals felt to have this disorder in fact have Albright hereditary osteodystrophy. Complete resolution of this issue awaits further study.

References

Maroteaux, P., and Malamut, G. L.: L'acrodysostose. Presse Med., 76:2189, 1968.

Robinow, M., et al.: Acrodysostosis. A syndrome of peripheral dysostosis, nasal hypoplasia, and mental retardation. Am. J. Dis. Child., 121:195, 1971.

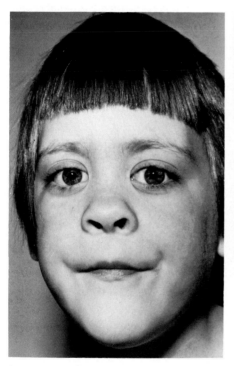

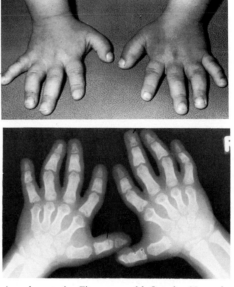

Acrodysostosis. Five year old female. Note the low nasal bridge, epicanthal folds, prominent mandible, short, broad fingers with skin wrinkling, and the broad and short metacarpals and phalanges with cone-shaped epiphyses.

ALBRIGHT HEREDITARY OSTEODYSTROPHY

(Pseudohypoparathyroidism, Pseudopseudohypoparathyroidism)

Short Metacarpals, Rounded Facies, With or Without Hypocalcemia and/or Vicarious Mineralization

Albright described this condition in 1942 and referred to it as pseudohypoparathyroidism because of hypocalcemia and hyperphosphatemia that were unresponsive to parathormone. Subsequently, patients were detected with a comparable phenotype but with normocalcemia, even in the same family as a patient with hypocalcemia. The term pseudopseudohypoparathyroidism was utilized to designate such instances. Because it is now obvious that hypocalcemia is a variable expression in this heritable disease, the term Albright hereditary osteodystrophy seems preferable. Phenotypic variation is marked.

ABNORMALITIES

Growth. Small stature; final height, 54 inches to 5 feet; occasionally normal. Moderate obesity. Span decreased for height.

Performance. Mental deficiency, I.Q.s of 20 to 99, mean I.Q. of approximately 60; occasionally normal.

Face and Neck. Rounded, low nasal bridge. Short neck. Cataracts.

Dentition. Delayed dental eruption, aplasia, and/or enamel hypoplasia.

Limbs. Short metacarpals and metatarsals, especially the fourth and fifth. Short distal phalanx of thumb. Cone-shaped epiphyses. Osteoporosis.

Extraskeletal Calcification. Areas of mineralization in subcutaneous tissues, basal ganglia.

Calcium and Phosphorus. Variable hypocalcemia and hyperphosphatemia.

OCCASIONAL ABNORMALITIES.

Distal palmar axial triradii, osteochondromata, thick calvarium, short ulna, short phalanges, epiphyseal dysplasia, genu valgum, hypothyroidism, hypogonadism with or without gonadal dysgenesis, peripheral lenticular opacities, nystagmus, unequal size of pupils, blurring of disc margins, tortuosity of vessels, diplopia, microphthalmia, optic atrophy, macular degeneration, hypertelorism, fibrous dysplasia, exostosis, osteitis fibrosa cystica, advanced bone age, clavicular abnormalities.

NATURAL HISTORY.

The shortened metacarpal and/or phalangeal bones represent early epiphyseal fusion and may not be evident until several years of age. Hypocalcemia, when present, usually becomes evident in childhood, seizures being the most common presenting symptom. Hypocalcemia may become manifest during periods of increased calcium utilization, as in adolescence or in pregnancy. Cautious vitamin D therapy in a dosage of 25,000 to 100,000 units per day may be necessary; however, the therapy should be discontinued every few years to reassess the situation, because spontaneous amelioration of the hypocalcemia may occur with time.

ETIOLOGY.

The family data are indicative of a single mutant gene giving rise to this syndrome. The findings of a 2:1 female to male sex incidence have favored an X-linked dominant mode of determination. However, documentation of both male to male transmission and unaffected females born to affected men, as well as the presence of equal numbers of severely affected males and females, makes autosomal dominant inheritance equally likely. An abnormally low urinary excretion of cyclic adenosine monophosphate following parathormone administration has been documented, suggesting that there exists an abnormality in the parathormone receptor adenylate cyclase complex of the renal cell plasma membrane.

References

Albright, F., et al.: Pseudohypoparathyroidism—an example of "Seabright-bantam syndrome." Report of three cases. Endocrinology, *30*:922, 1942.

Christiaen, L., et al.: Le pseudohypoparathyroidisme chronique. A propos de trois cas familiaux. Acta Paediatr. Belg., *21*:5, 1967.

Spranger, J. W.: Skeletal dysplasia and the eye: Albright's hereditary osteodystrophy. Birth Defects Original Article Series, 5:122, 1969.

Mann, E., et al.: Pseudohypoparathyroidism, a difficult diagnosis in early childhood. Acta Paediatr. Scand., *65*:487, 1976.

Poznanski, A. K., Werder, E. A., and Giedion, A.: The patterning of shortening of the bones of the hand in PHP and PPHP. Pediatr. Radiol., *123*:707, 1977.

Fitch, N.: Albright's hereditary osteodystrophy: A review. Am. J. Med. Genet., *11*:11, 1982.

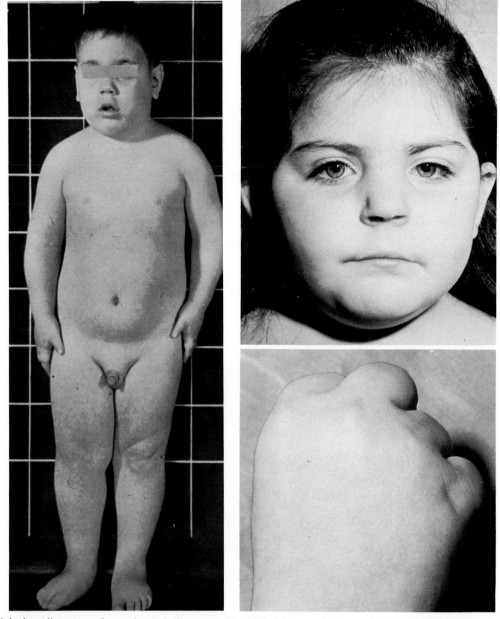

Albright hereditary osteodystrophy. *Left*, Five year old with height age of three and one-half years and bone age of five years. Hypocalcemia and hyperphosphatemia were first detected at one year of age. *Right*, Moderately retarded girl showing rounded facies and indications of short fourth and fifth metacarpal bones in fisted hand.

BRACHYDACTYLY SYNDROME, TYPE E

*Short Metacarpals, Brachydactyly,
Mild to Moderate Short Stature*

In 1951, Bell classified genetic forms of brachydactyly into five types, A to E. Riccardi and Holmes have recently summarized the findings in type E.

ABNORMALITIES
Growth. Mild to moderate shortness of stature with relatively short limbs.
Limbs. Short hands and feet with short metacarpals and metatarsals, especially the fourth and fifth; short phalanges, especially the terminal phalanx of thumb and big toe and the middle phalanx of the fifth finger. Variable cone-shaped epiphyses in hand.

NATURAL HISTORY. Small size is usually evident by birth, with a consistently slow pace of postnatal growth.

ETIOLOGY. Autosomal dominant.

References

Bell, J.: On brachydactyly and symphalangism. *In* Penrose, L. S. (ed.): Treasury of Human Inheritance, Vol. V. London, Cambridge University Press, 1951, pp. 1–31.

Riccardi, V. M., and Holmes, L. B.: Brachydactyly, type E. J. Pediatr., *84*:251, 1974.

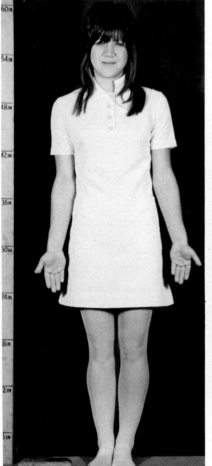

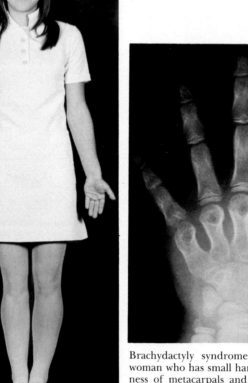

Brachydactyly syndrome, type E. Mildly short young woman who has small hands with disproportionate shortness of metacarpals and some phalanges and indented epiphyses (cone-shaped) in some phalanges. (From Riccardi, V. M., and Holmes, L. B.: J. Pediatr., *84*:251, 1974.)

WEILL-MARCHESANI SYNDROME

(Brachydactyly-Spherophakia Syndrome)

Brachydactyly, Small Spherical Lens, Short Stature

More than 18 instances of this condition have been described since the initial recognition by Weill in 1932 and the broader description by Marchesani in 1939.

ABNORMALITIES

Growth. Small stature.

Craniofacial. Broad skull, small shallow orbits, mild maxillary hypoplasia with narrow palate.

Eyes. Small spherical lens, myopia with or without glaucoma, ectopia lentis in half of cases, blindness in one third.

Teeth. Malformed and malaligned.

Limbs. Brachydactyly with broad metacarpals and phalanges, with or without late ossification of epiphyses. Stiff joints, particularly of hands.

OCCASIONAL ABNORMALITY. Cardiac anomaly.

NATURAL HISTORY. The mean age of recognition of an ocular problem in this disorder is 7.5 years, the youngest recorded age being nine months. Dilatation of the pupil is often necessary to appreciate the lens defect. Intelligence is usually not affected. There is the occasional development of carpal tunnel nerve compression at adolescence or later.

ETIOLOGY. Autosomal recessive inheritance with partial expression in the heterozygote, manifested by short stature. Gorlin et al. reported a family in which a father and two of his three children were affected, suggesting genetic heterogeneity or the possibility of pseudodominance (the phenotypic expression of a recessive allele on one chromosome due to deletion of the dominant allele from the homologue).

References

Weill, G.: Ectopie du cristallin et malformations générales. Ann. Ocul. (Paris), *169*:21, 1932.

Marchesani, O.: Brachydaktylie und angeborene Kugellinse als Systemerkrankung. Klin. Monatsbl. Augenheilkd., *103*:392, 1939.

Zabriskie, J., and Reisman, M.: Marchesani syndrome. J. Pediatr., *52*:158, 1958.

Feinberg, S. B.: Congenital mesodermal dysmorphodystrophy (brachymorphic type). Radiology, *74*:218, 1960.

Gorlin, R. J., L'Heureux, P. R., Shapiro, I.: Weill-Marchesani syndrome in two generations: Genetic heterogeneity or pseudodominance. J. Pediatr. Ophthalmol. *11*:139, 1974.

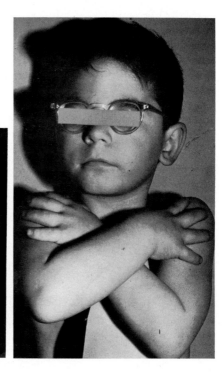

Weill-Marchesani syndrome. Nine year old with height age of five and one-half years. Small lens and myopia. (From Zabriskie, J., and Reisman, M.: J. Pediatr., *52*:158, 1958.)

BEALS AURICULO-OSTEODYSPLASIA SYNDROME

*Hypoplasia of Capitellum,
Attached Ear Lobule, Short Stature*

Beals described this disorder in 29 affected individuals in two families in 1967.

ABNORMALITIES

Growth. Mild to moderate short stature.

Ears. Elongated attached lobules with small, posteriorly placed lobule at point of attachment.

Elbows. Hypoplasia of capitellum with or without dislocation of radius.

Shoulders. Broad shoulders with wide base of neck and horizontal alignment of clavicles.

OCCASIONAL ABNORMALITIES. Dislocation of hip in one third of affected females. Short carpal area of wrist with ulnar slope to distal radius.

NATURAL HISTORY. Patients tend to be below the fiftieth percentile for stature. Other than variable dislocation of the hip and arthritic manifestations of the elbow, affected individuals are in good health.

ETIOLOGY. Autosomal dominant inheritance.

Reference

Beals, R. K.: Auriculo-osteodysplasia: A syndrome of multiple osseous dysplasia, ear anomaly, and short stature. J. Bone Joint Surg. [Am.], *49A*:1541, 1967.

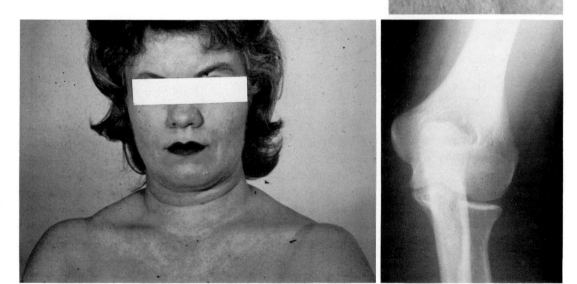

Beals auriculo-osteodysplasia syndrome. Note the horizontal clavicles, bulge of the upper portion of the scapulae lateral to the neck, dislocated radial head with hypoplasia of capitellum, and anomalous ear lobule in this adult female. (Courtesy of R. K. Beals, University of Oregon Medical School, Portland.)

N. STORAGE DISORDERS

GENERALIZED GANGLIOSIDOSIS SYNDROME, TYPE I (SEVERE INFANTILE TYPE)
(Caffey Pseudo-Hurler Syndrome, Familial Neurovisceral Lipidosis)

Coarse Facies, Joint Limitation, Kyphosis in Early Infancy

In 1951, Caffey described two neonates who had many of the features of Hurler syndrome, but of prenatal onset. Landing et al. reported pathologic studies in similar cases showing foamy histiocytes in the liver and spleen, swollen neurons, and vacuoles in the glomerular epithelium. They interpreted the storage material as a glycolipid and set forth the name "familial neurovisceral lipidosis," which was changed to "generalized gangliosidosis" by Okada and O'Brien on the basis of finding elevated levels of ganglioside GM_1 in the liver, spleen, and brain tissue from a patient. The molecular defect has been shown to be a deficiency of ganglioside GM_1 β-galactosidase.

ABNORMALITIES
Growth. Deficiency, with relatively low birth weight and severe postnatal growth deficit.
Performance. Severe early defect in developmental performance with hypotonia, poor coordination, and later, spasticity.
Orofacial. Coarse features with low nasal bridge, broad nose, flaring alae nasi, frontal bossing, long philtrum, hypertrophied alveolar ridges with prominent maxilla and mild macroglossia. Hirsutism.
Eyes. Cherry-red macular spot in about one half of the patients.
Skeletal. Moderate joint limitation with thick wrists, contractures at the elbows and knees, and development of clawhand. Early roentgenograms show poorly mineralized, coarsely trabeculated long bones with medullary midshaft broadening and a "cloak" of subperiosteal new bone formation, especially evident in the humerus. Some metaphyseal cupping and epiphyseal irregularity are usually present. With time, the bones appear more like those of the Hurler syndrome, including kyphosis

with anterior bullet wedging of vertebrae. Ribs are thick, legs may be bowed, and talipes may be present. Short broad hands. Kyphoscoliosis.
Viscera. Variable hepatomegaly with some foamy histiocytes. Vacuolation in glomerular epithelial cells containing swollen lysosomes.
Leukocytes. Vacuolation within cytoplasm of leukocytes and foam cells in marrow.
Urinary Excretion. Mucopolysaccharides occasionally may be increased with the excretion of keratan sulfate–like materials.
Other. Facial and peripheral edema in early infancy.

NATURAL HISTORY. Severe developmental lag with hypotonia, feeding problems with failure to thrive, and frequent infections usually culminate in death during early infancy. Deterioration of cerebral function is rapid if the patient survives the first year, leading to a decerebrate status with seizures and death prior to two years of age. The mean age of survival for 17 patients was 13.5 months, with a range from 3.5 to 25 months. No form of therapy other than life-supportive tube feeding and antibiotic management of infections has been effective. Considering the natural history of this disorder, the author favors discussion with the parents followed by the withholding of life-supportive medical treatment, if this course of management is acceptable to the parents.

ETIOLOGY. Autosomal recessive. Okada and O'Brien detected a deficit (one twentieth of normal) of the lysosomal enzyme β-galactosidase in the liver from these patients. The presumed developmental pathology of the disease is as follows: (1) inability to cleave the terminal galactose from ganglioside and mucopolysaccharide, (2) accumulation of these products within lysosomes where they would normally be degraded, and (3) the storage disease.

The diagnosis can be confirmed by the assay of β-galactosidase in the peripheral leukocytes or in cultured skin fibroblasts. Prenatal diagnosis has been established on the basis of cultured amniotic fluid cells.

References

Caffey, J.: Gargoylism (Hunter-Hurler disease, dysostosis multiplex, lipochondrodystrophy); prenatal and neonatal bone lesions and their early postnatal evolution. Bull. Hosp. Joint Dis., *12*:38, 1951.

Landing, B. H., et al.: Familial neurovisceral lipidosis. An analysis of eight cases of a syndrome previously reported as "Hurler-variant," "Pseudo-Hurler disease," and "Tay-Sachs disease with visceral involvement." Am. J. Dis. Child., *108*:503, 1964.

Okada, S., and O'Brien, J. S.: Generalized gangliosidosis: Beta-galactosidase deficiency. Science, *160*:1002, 1968.

Kaback, M. M., et al.: Gangliosidosis type I: In-utero detection and fetal manifestations. J. Pediatr., *82*:1037, 1973.

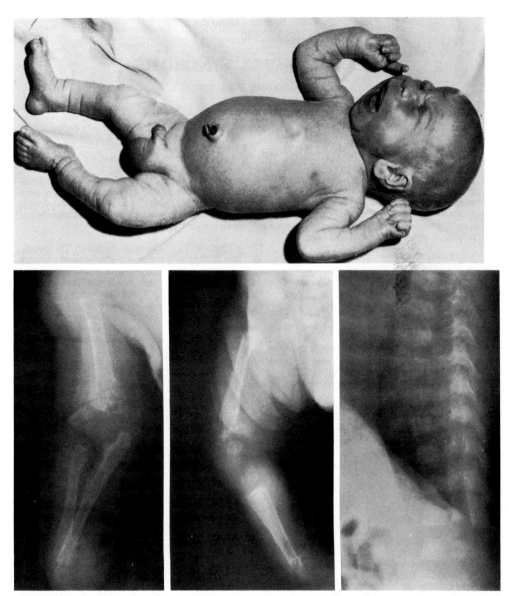

Generalized gangliosidosis syndrome, type I. Two week old with x-ray films of the arm, leg, and thoracolumbar vertebrae. Note the coarse facies, hypertrophied alveolar ridges, broad wrists, periosteal cloaking with thin cortices, altered shape of head of humerus and femur, and hypoplastic vertebrae. (From Scott, C. R., et al.: J. Pediatr., *71*:357, 1967.)

LEROY I-CELL SYNDROME

(Mucolipidosis II)

Early Alveolar Ridge Hypertrophy,
Joint Limitation, Thick Tight Skin in Early Infancy

This disorder was recognized by Leroy and DeMars when they noted unusual cytoplasmic inclusions in the cultured fibroblasts of a girl who had been considered to have the Hurler syndrome despite the fact that she did not have cloudy corneas or excessive acid mucopolysaccharide in the urine.

ABNORMALITIES

Growth. Birth weight less than 5½ pounds. Marked growth deficiency with lack of linear growth after infancy.

Performance. Slow progress from early infancy, reaching a plateau at approximately 18 months with no apparent deterioration subsequently.

Craniofacial. High, narrow forehead. Thin eyebrows, puffy eyelids, inner epicanthal folds, clear or faintly hazy corneas. Low nasal bridge, anteverted nostrils. Long philtrum.

Mouth. Progressive hypertrophy of alveolar ridges.

Skeletal and Joints. Moderate joint limitation in flexion, especially of hips. Dorsolumbar kyphosis. Broadening of wrists and fingers. Roentgenographic findings in the later phases similar to those seen in children with the Hurler syndrome. In early infancy, periosteal new bone formation leading to a "cloaking" of the long tubular bones is best seen in femora and humeri.

Skin. Thick, relatively tight skin during early infancy that becomes less tight as the patients become older. Cavernous hemangiomata.

Other. Minimal hepatomegaly. Diastasis recti. Inguinal hernia (one case). Systolic murmurs after one year of age.

Note. No metachromatic granules noted in leukocytes. Urinary mucopolysaccharides normal to mildly increased.

NATURAL HISTORY.

By 18 months of age, most patients can sit with support, and some stand with support. However, severe progressive retardation of growth and development occur. Recurrent bouts of bronchitis, pneumonia, and otitis media have been frequent during early childhood. Death, which usually occurs by five years of age, is often associated with congestive heart failure.

ETIOLOGY. Autosomal recessive. The consistent finding is a deficiency of lysosomal enzymes within cultured skin fibroblasts and an increase in lysosomal enzymes in plasma, cerebrospinal fluid, and urine. Cultured fibroblasts contain an abundance of mucopolysaccharide and glycolipid material within lysosomal structures. It is currently believed that in I-cell disease the lysosomal enzymes are missing a common recognition marker that directs them into lysosomes. This recognition marker is believed to be 6-phosphomannose. A marked increase in serum activity of beta-hexosaminidase, iduronate sulfatase, and arylsulfatase A is seen in this disorder as well as in mucolipidosis III (pseudo-Hurler polydystrophy).

Heterozygotes cannot be detected. Prenatal diagnosis can be established on the basis of cultured amniotic fluid cells.

References

Leroy, J. G., and DeMars, R. I.: Mutant enzymatic and cytological phenotypes in cultured human fibroblasts. Science, *157*:804, 1967.

Matalon, R., et al.: Lipid abnormalities in a variant of the Hurler syndrome. Proc. Natl. Acad. Sci. U.S.A., *59*:1097, 1968.

Leroy, J. G., DeMars, R. I., and Opitz, J. M.: "I-cell" disease. *In* Bergsma, D. S. (ed.): The First Conference on the Clinical Delineation of Birth Defects, Part IV. Baltimore, Williams and Wilkins, 1969.

Leroy, J. G., et al.: I-cell disease, a clinical picture. J. Pediatr., *79*:360, 1971.

Hickman, S., and Neufeld, E. F.: A hypothesis for I-cell disease: defective hydrolases that do not enter lysosomes. Biochem. Biophys. Res. Commun., *49*:992, 1972.

Kaplan, A., Achord, D. T., and Sly, W. S.: Phosphohexosyl components of a lysosomal enzyme are recognized by pinocytosis receptors on human fibroblasts. Proc. Natl. Acad. Sci., U.S.A., *74*:2026, 1977.

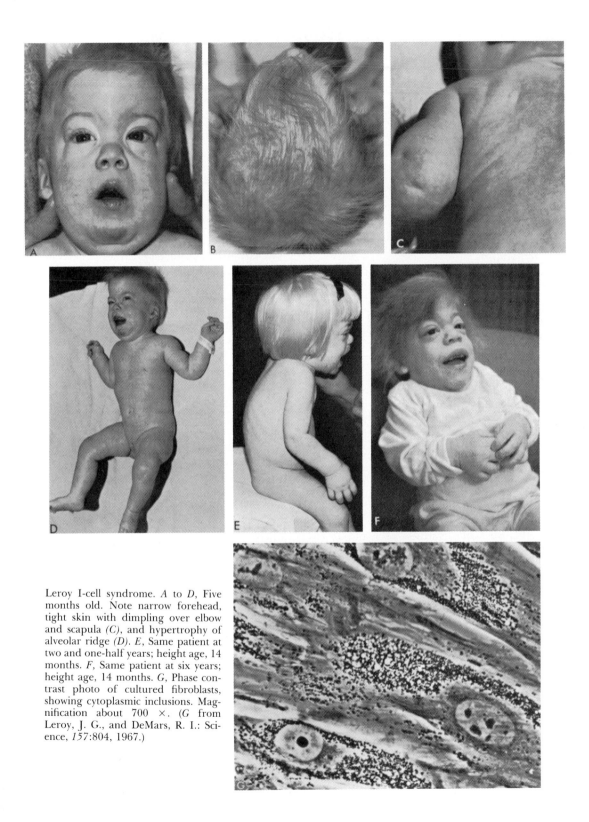

Leroy I-cell syndrome. *A* to *D,* Five months old. Note narrow forehead, tight skin with dimpling over elbow and scapula *(C),* and hypertrophy of alveolar ridge *(D). E,* Same patient at two and one-half years; height age, 14 months. *F,* Same patient at six years; height age, 14 months. *G,* Phase contrast photo of cultured fibroblasts, showing cytoplasmic inclusions. Magnification about 700 ×. (*G* from Leroy, J. G., and DeMars, R. I.: Science, *157*:804, 1967.)

PSEUDO-HURLER POLYDYSTROPHY SYNDROME

(Mucolipidosis III)

*Coarse Facies, Stiff Joints by
Two to Four Years, No Mucopolysacchariduria*

Recognized by Maroteaux and Lamy in 1966, more than 15 cases have been reported subsequently. Clinically, the disorder is of milder degree than the Hurler syndrome and is similar to the Scheie syndrome, but the patients do not have hepatosplenomegaly, cloudy corneas, or mucopolysacchariduria.

ABNORMALITIES. Onset usually appreciated at four to five years.
Growth. Decreasing growth rate in early childhood.
Performance. Mild mental deficiency, I.Q.s of 64 to 85.
Facies. Development of mildly coarse facies by six years.
Eyes. Mild corneal opacities, evident by slit lamp, by six to eight years.
Joints. Stiffness, especially in hands, elbows, shoulders, and knees.
Skeletal. Mild platyspondyly, flaring iliac wings, flattening of femoral epiphyses, changes in hands.
Cardiac. Aortic valve disease, often with regurgitation.
Other. Inguinal hernia. Acne.

NATURAL HISTORY. Stiffness of joints usually becomes evident by four to five years of age. Carpal tunnel compression is a potential complication. Mild to moderate deterioration of central nervous system function. Some patients have lived into their 20's.

ETIOLOGY. Autosomal recessive inheritance. Marrow plasma cells show vacuolated plasma cells with swollen lysosomes, but there is no mucopolysacchariduria. Lysosomal enzymes are elevated in the serum and decreased in cultured fibroblasts. The disorder is considered similar to I-cell disease, but is of a milder nature. As with mucolipidosis II, there is a marked increase in serum beta-hexosaminidase, iduronate sulfatase, and arylsulfatase A. These two disorders are best differentiated by their clinical courses.

References

Maroteaux, P., and Lamy, M.: La pseudopolydystrophie de Hurler. Presse Med., *74*:2889, 1966.

Scott, C. I., Jr., and Grossman, M. S.: Pseudo-Hurler polydystrophy. Birth Defects, *4*(5):349, 1969.

McKusick, V. A.: Heritable Disorders of Connective Tissue, 4th ed. St. Louis, C. V. Mosby Co., 1972, p. 652.

Melhem, R., et al.: Roentgen findings in mucolipidosis III (pseudo-Hurler polydystrophy). Radiology, *106*:153, 1973.

Thomas, G. H., et al.: Mucolipidosis III (pseudo-Hurler polydystrophy): Multiple lysosomal enzyme abnormalities in serum and cultured fibroblast cells. Pediatr. Res., 7:751, 1973.

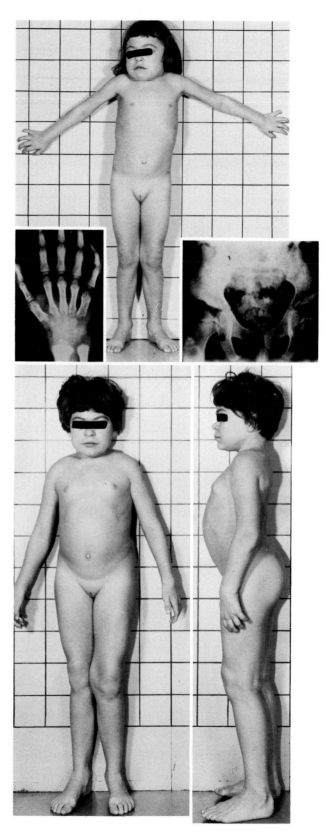

Pseudo-Hurler polydystrophy syndrome. *Above,* Six year old girl with roentgenograms of hand and pelvis. *Below,* Early adolescent girl showing mild facial coarsening, joint contractures, and lumbar lordosis. (From Scott, C. I., Jr., and Grossman, M. S.: Birth Defects., *4*:349, 1969.)

HURLER SYNDROME

(Mucopolysaccharidosis I H)

*Coarse Facies, Stiff Joints, Mental
Deficiency, Cloudy Corneas by One to Two Years*

Hurler set forth this entity in 1919, two years after the Hunter syndrome was described.

ABNORMALITIES

Growth. Deceleration of growth between six and 18 months; maximal stature, 110 cm.

Performance. Grossly retarded progress at six to 12 months, with failure of advancement by two to five years.

Craniofacial and Eyes. Scaphocephalic macrocephaly with frontal prominence, coarse facies with full lips, flared nostrils, low nasal bridge, and tendency toward hypertelorism. Inner epicanthal folds. Hazy corneas, retinal pigmentation.

Mouth. Hypertrophied alveolar ridge and gums with small malaligned teeth. Enlarged tongue.

Skeletal and Joints. Diaphyseal broadening of short misshapen bones and joint limitation result in the clawhand and other joint deformities, with more limitation of extension than flexion. Flaring of the rib cage. Kyphosis and thoracolumbar gibbus secondary to anterior vertebral wedging, short neck. J-shaped sella turcica. Widening of medial end of clavicle.

Cardiac. Murmurs; cardiac failure may be due to intimal thickening in the coronary vessels or the cardiac valves.

Other. Hirsutism, hepatosplenomegaly, inguinal hernia, umbilical hernia, dislocation of hip, mucoid rhinitis, deafness.

Urinary Excretion. Dermatan sulfate and heparan sulfate.

OCCASIONAL ABNORMALITIES. Hydrocephalus, presumably a result of meningeal involvement. Hydrocele. Arachnoid cysts.

NATURAL HISTORY. Growth during the first year actually may be more rapid than usual, with subsequent deterioration. Subtle changes in the facies, macrocephaly, hernias, limited hip motility, noisy breathing, and frequent respiratory tract infections may be evident during the first six months. Deceleration of developmental and mental progress is evident during the latter half of the first year. These patients are usually placid, easily manageable, and often loveable. Death usually occurs in childhood secondary to respiratory tract or cardiac complications, and survival past ten years of age is unusual.

ETIOLOGY. Autosomal recessive. The primary defect is an absence of lysosomal α-L-iduronidase in all tissues. The pathologic consequence is an accumulation of mucopolysaccharides in parenchymal and mesenchymal tissues and the storage of lipids within neuronal tissues.

Diagnosis is confirmed by the physical appearance, the excretion of dermatan sulfate and heparan sulfate in the urine, and the absence of α-L-iduronidase in cultured fibroblasts. Heterozygote detection is not readily available. Prenatal diagnosis is possible by measuring α-L-iduronidase in cultured amniotic fluid cells.

References

Hurler, G.: Ueber einen Typ multipler Abartungen, vorwiegend am Skelettsystem. Z. Kinderheilkd., *24*:220, 1919.

Leroy, J. G., and Crocker, A. C.: Clinical definition of the Hurler-Hunter phenotypes. A review of 50 patients. Am. J. Dis. Child., *112*:518, 1966.

Matalon, R., and Dorfman, A.: Hurler's syndrome, and α-L-iduronidase deficiency. Biochem. Biophys. Res. Commun., *47*:959, 1972.

McKusick, V.: Heritable Disorders of Connective Tissue, 4th ed. St. Louis, C. V. Mosby Co., 1972.

Spranger, J.: The systemic mucopolysaccharidoses. *In* Ergebnisse delr Inneren Medizin und Kinderheilkunde. New York, Springer-Verlag, 1972.

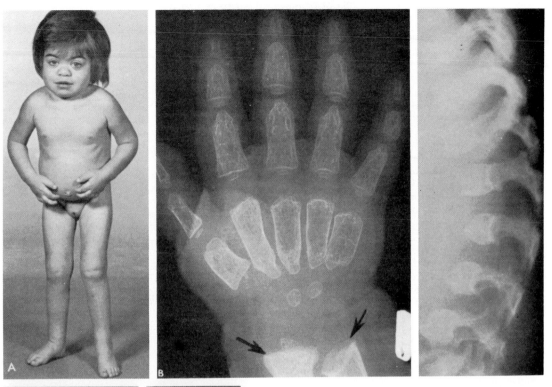

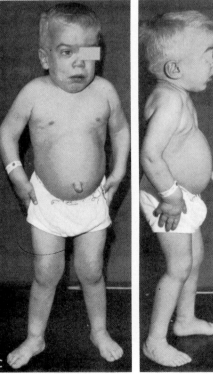

Hurler syndrome. *A*, Two year old who sat at one year and walked at 21 months. Height age at six months was ten months; at one year, 16 months; and at two years, two years. *B*, Broad, irregular bone, especially at metaphyses. Thoracic and lumbar vertebrae are short with anterior wedging. *C*, Five year old with height age of three years.

SCHEIE SYNDROME

(Mucopolysaccharidosis I S)

Broad Mouth With Full Lips,
Early Corneal Opacity, Normal Mentality

This disorder was originally described by Scheie et al. in 1962.

ABNORMALITIES

General. Little, if any, impairment of intelligence.

Facies. Broad mouth with full lips by five to eight years of age. Mandibular prognathism.

Corneas. Early clouding of cornea, becoming most dense in periphery.

Limbs. Joint limitation leading to clawhand, small carpal bones, femoral head dysplasia. Broad and short hands and feet.

Cardiac. Aortic valvular defect.

Other. Body hirsutism. Retinal pigmentation. Inguinal and umbilical hernias. Short neck.

Urinary Excretion. Proportionately more dermatan sulfate than usual.

OCCASIONAL ABNORMALITIES. Carpal tunnel narrowing may cause median nerve compression. Bone cysts. Psychosis and possible mental deterioration may occur. Mild impairment of growth. Hearing loss. Hepatomegaly. Macroglossia. Glaucoma, myopia. Sleep apnea.

ETIOLOGY. Autosomal recessive, with excess urinary excretion of dermatan sulfate and absence of α-L-iduronidase in cultured fibroblasts. Differentiation between this and mucopolysaccharidosis I H can be made only on the basis of the clinical course and phenotype.

References

Scheie, H. G., Hambrick, G. W., Jr., and Barness, L. A.: A newly recognized forme fruste of Hurler's disease (gargoylism). Am. J. Ophthalmol., 53:753, 1962.

Emerit, I., Maroteaux, P., and Vernant, P.: Deux observations de mucopolysaccharidose avec atteinte cardiovasculaire. Arch. Fr. Pediatr., 23:1075, 1966.

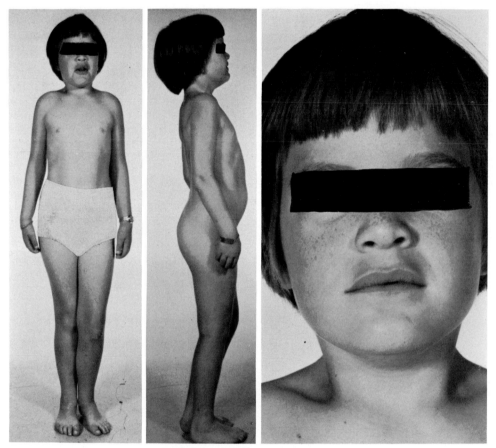

Scheie syndrome. Child, nine years and nine months old, with height age of nine years and I.Q. of 102. Mild to moderate limitation of shoulder, elbow, and hand movement. Mild corneal opacity. (Courtesy of R. Scott, University of Washington, Seattle.)

HURLER-SCHEIE COMPOUND SYNDROME

(Mucopolysaccharidosis I H/S)

Stevenson et al. set forth the genetic compound of the Hurler syndrome and the Scheie syndrome in 1976. They estimated that the frequency of occurrence of the compound would be intermediate between that of the Hurler syndrome and that of the Scheie syndrome. The phenotype is a strikingly intermediate compounding of the effects of these two allelic mutant genes.

ABNORMALITIES. Gradual development of signs and symptoms during the first few years, especially at one to two years of age.
Performance. Mild mental deficiency to normal.
Growth. During the first year, growth may be accelerated; thereafter, it decelerates to growth deficiency.
Craniofacial. Development of scaphocephaly with macrocephaly, low nasal bridge, prominent lips, corneal clouding. Micrognathia.
Skin. Thickened, with fine hirsutism.
Skeletal. Moderate joint limitation. Mild to moderate dysostosis multiplex changes with broadening of bone but without gibbus.
Other. Chronic rhinorrhea, middle ear fluid, inguinal hernia, +/− umbilical hernia, hepato-splenomegaly, +/− cardiac valvular changes. Deafness. Arachnoid cyst.

NATURAL HISTORY. The progression is intermediate between that of Hurler syndrome and that of Scheie syndrome, with a very gradual progression toward mild to moderate disabilities.

ETIOLOGY. Both Hurler syndrome and Scheie syndrome represent apparently allelic mutations affecting the enzyme protein α-L-iduronidase. The Hurler-Scheie compound represents the double heterozygote state for these allelic genes, yielding an intermediary problem in the enzyme function and hence in the child. It is a situation similar to the hemoglobin S-C compound disorder. The recurrence risk for the parents (25 per cent) is the same as for those with an autosomal recessive disorder, but there is no excess of consanguinity as for a homozygous autosomal recessive disorder.

Reference

Stevenson, R. E., et al.: The iduronidase-deficient mucopolysaccharidoses; clinical and roentgenographic features. Pediatrics, 57:111, 1976.

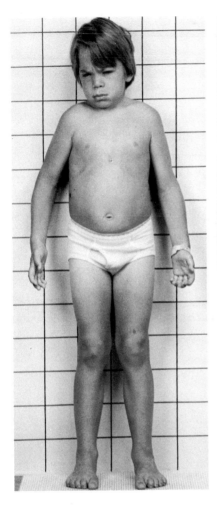

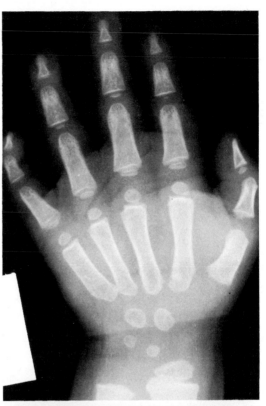

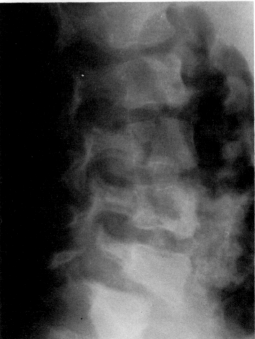

Hurler-Scheie compound syndrome. *Left*, Young boy showing mildly altered facies and joint limitations that are most evident at elbow and in the fingers. *Right*, Subtle dysostosis multiplex type of changes in hand and in lumbar spine. (From Stevenson, R. E., et al.: Pediatrics, *57*:111, 1976.)

HUNTER SYNDROME

(Mucopolysaccharidosis II)

Coarse Facies, Growth Deficiency,
Stiff Joints by Two to Four Years, Clear Corneas

Hunter described this condition found in two brothers in 1917. The clinical phenotype may vary from mild to severe, even in the same sibship.

ABNORMALITIES. Onset at about two to four years.
Growth. Deficiency, onset at one to four years. Adult height, 120 to 150 cm.
Performance. Juvenile type: Mental and neurologic deterioration at approximately two to five years of age to the point of severe mental deficiency with aggressive hyperactive behavior and spasticity. Late type: Mild mental deficiency to normal intelligence.
Craniofacial. Coarsening of facial features, full lips. Macrocephaly.
Joints and Skeletal. Stiff partial contracture of joints, clawhand. Broadening of bone.

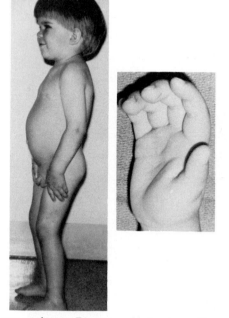

Hunter syndrome. Four year old showing evidence of tight joints, especially fingers. Presumably the "late type," as his intelligence seemed within normal limits at four years of age.

Other. Hepatosplenomegaly, hypertrichosis, inguinal hernias, mucoid nasal discharge, progressive deafness. Delayed tooth eruption. Dentigerous cysts. Hoarse voice.
Urinary Excretion. Dermatan sulfate and heparan sulfate.

OCCASIONAL ABNORMALITIES. Diarrhea, nodular skin lesions over scapular area and on arms, kyphosis, pes cavus, osteoarthritis of head of femur, retinal pigmentation, congestive heart failure, coronary occlusion. Papilledema. Hydrocephalus. Airway obstruction.

IMPORTANT DIFFERENCES IN CONTRAST WITH THE HURLER SYNDROME. (1) Clear corneas. (2) Less severe gibbus. (3) No affected females. (4) More gradual onset of features.

NATURAL HISTORY. Gradual decline in growth rate from two to six years. Deafness frequently is evident by two to three years. Cardiac complications not uncommonly lead to death prior to 20 years; however, survival to 60 years has been recorded. The more severe juvenile-type patients tend to die earlier, between four and 14 years of age.

ETIOLOGY. X-linked, with no overt expression in the heterozygous female, who may be recognized by the fact that cultured fibroblasts show cytoplasmic accumulation of mucopolysaccharide, though to a lesser extent than those of the hemizygous male. The primary defect is a deficiency of iduronate sulfatase. Excess dermatan sulfate and heparan sulfate are found in urine.

References

Hunter, C.: A rare disease in two brothers. Proc. R. Soc. Med., *10*:104, 1917.

Leroy, J. G., and Crocker, A. C.: Clinical definition of the Hurler-Hunter phenotypes. A review of 50 patients. Am. J. Dis. Child., *112*:518, 1966.

McKusick, V.: Heritable Disorders of Connective Tissue, 4th ed. St. Louis, C. V. Mosby Co., 1972, p. 346.

Yatziv, S., Erickson, R. P., and Epstein, C. J.: Mild and severe Hunter syndrome (MPS II) within the same sibships. Clin. Genet., *11*:119, 1977.

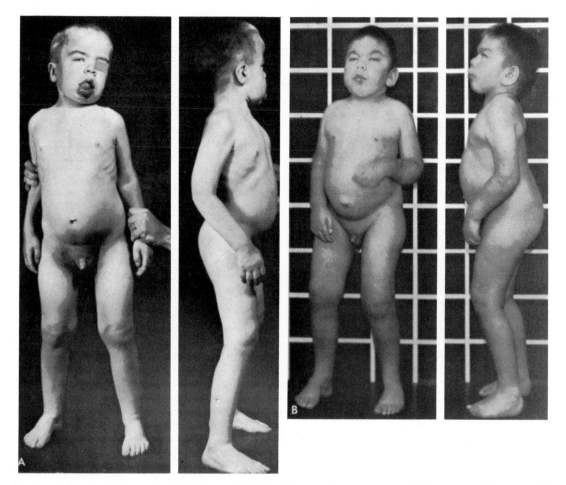

Hunter syndrome. *A*, Nine and one-half year old with height age of seven years and eight months. (Courtesy of A. C. Crocker, Boston Children's Hospital.) *B*, Thirteen and one-half year old with height age of seven years.

SANFILIPPO SYNDROME

(Mucopolysaccharidosis III, Types A, B, C, and D)

Mild Coarse Facies,
Mild Stiff Joints, Mental Deficiency

This clinical disorder was recognized by San-filippo et al. in 1963 and appears to be the most common mucopolysaccharidosis disorder. The excess urinary excretion of mucopolysaccharide is heparan sulfate alone. These individuals usually have clear corneas.

ABNORMALITIES. Onset in early childhood.
Growth. Normal to accelerated growth for one to three years, followed by slow growth.
Performance. Slowing mental development by one and one-half to three years, followed by deterioration, including gait, speech, and behavior.
Craniofacies. Dense calvarium. Mildly coarse facies with synophrys.
Other. Variable hepatomegaly. Obliteration of pulp chambers of teeth by irregular secondary dentin. Ovoid dysplasia of vertebrae. Mild cardiac involvement.

NATURAL HISTORY. Sleep disturbances and frequent upper respiratory tract infections may be early evidence of the disorder prior to the slowing of growth and mental deterioration. Unfortunately, the usual result is severe mental deficiency in a strong, often difficult to manage, individual. The syndrome may be compatible with long survival, but many die of pneumonia by 10 to 20 years.

ETIOLOGY. Autosomal recessive. Sanfilippo A is a defect of heparan N-sulfatase; Sanfilippo B, a deficiency of N-acetyl-α-D-glucosaminidase; Sanfilippo C, a deficiency of acetyl-CoA:α-glucosaminide-N-acetyltransferase; and Sanfilippo D, a deficiency of N-acetyl-α-D-glucosaminide-6-sulfatase. Excess heparan sulfate is excreted in the urine in all four types, and the clinical phenotype is identical in each.

References

Sanfilippo, S. J., et al.: Mental retardation associated with acid mucopolysacchariduria (heparitin sulfate type). J. Pediatr., *63*:837, 1963.

McKusick, V.: Heritable Disorders of Connective Tissue, 3rd ed. St. Louis, C. V. Mosby Co., 1966, p. 357.

Spranger, J., et al.: Die HS-Mucopolysaccharidose von Sanfilippo (Polydystrophe Oligophrenie). Bericht über 10 Patienten. Z. Kinderheilkd., *101*:71, 1967.

Kriel, R. L., et al.: Neuroanatomical and EEG correlations in Sanfilippo syndrome, type A. Arch. Neurol., *35*:838, 1978.

Andria, G., et al.: Sanfilippo B syndrome. Clin. Genet., *15*:500, 1979.

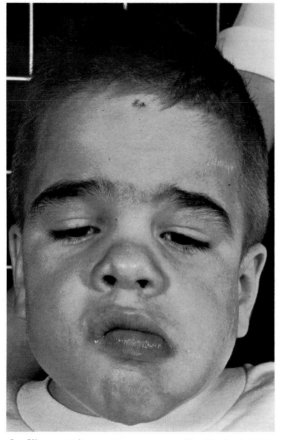

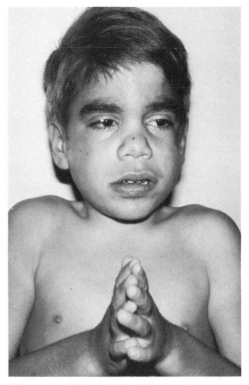

Sanfilippo syndrome. A seven year old with the height age of five years and nine months. His capabilities have been regressing, and his present intelligence quotient is about 50. A sibling is similarly affected. (Courtesy of R. Scott, University of Washington School of Medicine, Seattle.)

Nine year old boy with Sanfilippo syndrome, type B, whose I.Q. was about 20. (Courtesy of Dr. Robert Summitt, University of Tennessee College of Medicine, Memphis.)

MORQUIO SYNDROME

(Mucopolysaccharidosis IV, Types A and B)

Onset at One to Three Years of Age,
Mild Coarse Facies,
Severe Kyphosis and Knock-knees, Cloudy Corneas

Mistakenly interpreted by Osler in 1898, this condition was described by Morquio in 1929; it was recognized as a mucopolysaccharidosis in 1963. Deficiencies of two different enzymes leading to a severe form, mucopolysaccharidosis IV A, and a mild form, mucopolysaccharidosis IV B, are now recognized.

ABNORMALITIES. Onset between one and three years.

Growth. Severe limitation with cessation by later childhood. Adult stature 82 to 115 cm.

Craniofacial. Mild coarsening of facial features, with broad mouth and short anteverted nose.

Eyes. Cloudy cornea evident by slit lamp examination, usually after five to ten years of age.

Skeletal and Joints. Marked platyspondyly, with vertebrae changing to ovoid, ovoid with anterior projection, to flattened form with short neck and trunk plus kyphoscoliosis. Odontoid hypoplasia. Early flaring of rib cage progressing to bulging sternum. Short, curved long bones with irregular tubulation, widened metaphyses, abnormal femoral neck, flattening of femoral head, knock-knee with medial spur of tibial metaphysis, conical bases of widened metacarpals, irregular epiphyseal form, osteoporosis. Short, stubby hands. Joint laxity, most evident at wrists and small joints, and joint restriction in some of the larger joints, especially the hips.

Mouth. Widely spaced teeth with thin enamel that tends to become grayish in color.

Cardiac. Late onset of aortic regurgitation.

Other. Hearing loss. Inguinal hernia. Hepatomegaly.

Urinary Excretion. Keratan sulfate.

OCCASIONAL ABNORMALITIES. Macrocephaly, mental deficiency.

NATURAL HISTORY. The earliest recognized indications of the disease have been flaring of the lower rib cage, prominent sternum, frequent upper respiratory tract infections (including otitis media), hernias, and growth deficiency, all becoming evident by 18 months to two years of age. Severe defects of vertebrae may result in cord compression or respiratory insufficiency. These and cardiac complications may result in death prior to 20 years. In the milder form, longer survival is the rule, dental enamel is normal, and C2–C3 subluxation has been documented in addition to C1–C2 subluxation. Mentality is usually normal in both the severe and the mild forms.

ETIOLOGY. Autosomal recessive. The basic defect in type IVA is a deficiency of N-acetylgalactosamine-6-sulfatase, whereas in type IVB there is a deficiency of β-galactosidase.

Confirmation of the diagnosis is dependent upon the identification of an excessive excretion of keratan sulfate in the urine and/or the deficiency of the enzyme in cultured skin fibroblasts or leukocytes. Both assays are difficult and not readily available.

Heterozygote detection is not reliable. Prenatal diagnosis may be possible in selected laboratories.

References

Osler, W.: Sporadic cretinism in America. Trans. Cong. Am. Phys., *4*:169, 1898.

Morquio, L.: Sur une forme de dystrophie osseuse familiale. Arch. Med. Enf., *32*:129, 1929.

Robins, M. M., Stevens, H. F., and Linker, A.: Morquio's disease: an abnormality of mucopolysaccharide metabolism. J. Pediatr., *62*:881, 1963.

Langer, L. O., and Carey, L. S.: The roentgenographic features of the ks mucopolysaccharidosis of Morquio (Morquio-Brailsford's disease). Am. J. Roentgenol. Radium Ther. Nucl. Med., *97*:1, 1966.

Linker, A., Evans, L. R., and Langer, L. O.: Morquio's disease and mucopolysaccharide excretion. J. Pediatr., *77*:1039, 1970.

Matalon, R., et al.: Morquio's syndrome: deficiency of a chondroitin sulfate N-acetylhexosamine sulfatase. Biochem. Biophys. Res. Commun., *61*:759, 1974.

McKusick, V. A., and Neufeld, E. F.: Mucopolysaccharidosis IV (MPS IV, Morquio syndrome, keratansulfaturia), type A and B. *In* Stanbury, J. B., et al. (eds.): The Metabolic Basis of Inherited Disease. New York, McGraw-Hill Book Co., 1982, pp. 766–768.

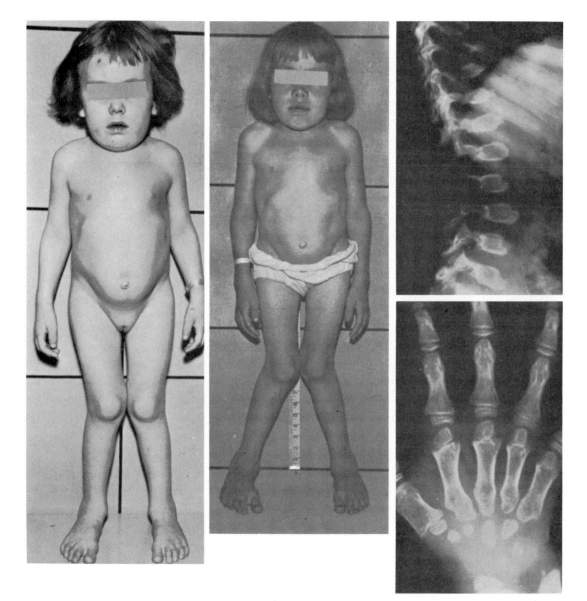

Morquio syndrome. *Left*, Patient at three and one-half years; height age, two years and nine months. *Center*, Same patient at seven years; height age, two years and nine months. *Right*, X-ray films of patient at seven years. (From Robins, M. M., et al.: J. Pediatr., *62*:881, 1963.)

MAROTEAUX-LAMY MUCOPOLYSACCHARIDOSIS SYNDROME (MILD AND SEVERE TYPES)

(Mucopolysaccharidosis VI)

Coarse Facies, Stiff Joints,
Cloudy Corneas in Infancy, No Mental Deterioration

Maroteaux et al. recognized this disorder as being distinct from Hurler syndrome in that mental deterioration did *not* occur during early childhood. Two clinical subtypes have been indicated, one with a slow and milder course and the other with a rapid and more severe course.

ABNORMALITIES. Onset by one to three years of age.

Growth. Deficiency, usually evident between two and three years.

Craniofacial. Coarse facies with large nose and thick lips. Low nasal bridge.

Eyes. Fine corneal opacity. Cornea may be thick and/or large.

Skeletal and Joints. Mild stiffness of joints. Metaphyses, slightly broad and irregular. Epiphyseal irregularity, especially femoral epiphysis. Vertebrae flattened with anterior wedging of T-12 and L-1. Prominent sternum. Broad ribs. Elongated sella turcica. Odontoid hypoplasia. Lumbar kyphosis, genu valgum.

Other. Umbilical and inguinal hernias. Skin, thick and tight. Small, widely spaced teeth with late eruption. Hepatosplenomegaly. Varying degrees of deafness. Cytoplasmic granules in leukocytes.

OCCASIONAL ABNORMALITIES. Macroglossia. Macrocephaly. Hydrocephalus. Involvement of heart valves.

NATURAL HISTORY. Macrocephaly, frequent upper respiratory tract infections, diarrhea, hernias, and limitation of knee, hip, and elbow movement may be present in infancy. Thereafter, the two clinical subtypes diverge. Those with the mild, slow course usually survive until the second to third decade and succumb to cardiac complications. Those with the severe type rapidly deteriorate physically and by three to six years have serious deformity. The age of onset of growth deficiency is usually a little later than in the Hurler syndrome; the extent of skeletal broadening, joint limitation, hepatosplenomegaly, and corneal opacification is generally less than with Hurler syndrome; and mental deficiency has not been noted during childhood. The data on prognosis after ten years of age are currently inadequate.

ETIOLOGY. Autosomal recessive. The molecular defect is a deficiency of *N*-acetylgalactosamine-4-sulfatase (arylsulfatase B). The enzyme is missing in all tissues, including cultured fibroblasts. There is an increased urinary excretion of mucopolysaccharides consisting predominantly of dermatan sulfate.

Heterozygote detection and prenatal diagnosis may be feasible in selected laboratories.

References

Maroteaux, P., et al.: Une nouvelle dysostose avec élimination urinaire de chondroitine-sulfate B. Presse Med., *71*:1849, 1963.

Maroteaux, P., and Lamy, M.: Hurler's disease, Morquio's disease, and related mucopolysaccharidoses. J. Pediatr., *67*:312, 1965.

Fallis, N., Barnes, F. L., II, and di Ferrante, N.: A case of polydystrophic dwarfism with urinary excretion of dermatan sulfate and heparan sulfate. J. Clin. Endocrinol. Metab., *28*:26, 1968.

Stumpf, D. A., et al.: Mucopolysaccharidosis type VI. I. Sulfatase B deficiency in tissues. Am. J. Dis. Child., *126*:747, 1973.

O'Brien, J. F., Cantz, M., and Spranger, J.: Maroteaux-Lamy disease, subtype A: deficiency of an *N*-acetylgalactosamine-4-sulfatase. Biochem. Biophys. Res. Commun., *60*:1170, 1974.

McKusick, V. A., and Neufield, E. F.: The mucopolysaccharide storage diseases. *In* Stanbury, J. B., et al. (eds.): The Metabolic Basis of Inherited Disease. New York, McGraw-Hill Book Co., 1982, pp 751–777.

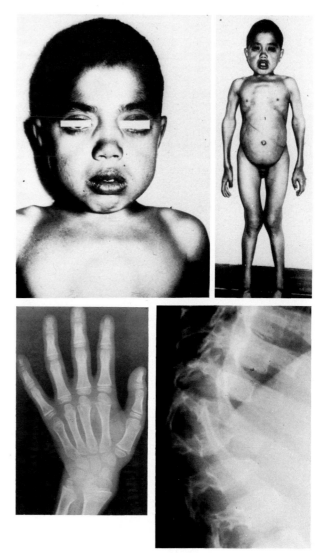

Maroteaux-Lamy mucopolysaccharidosis syndrome. Older boy, short of stature, with normal intelligence. (Courtesy of P. Maroteaux, Hôpital des Enfants-Malades, Paris.)

MUCOPOLYSACCHARIDOSIS VII

(Sly Syndrome; β-Glucuronidase Deficiency)

Initially described by Sly et al. in an infant with short stature, skeletal deformities, hepatosplenomegaly and mental deficiency, 12 cases have been reported subsequently. A widely variable clinical phenotype has been noted.

ABNORMALITIES
Growth. Postnatal growth deficiency.
Performance. Moderately severe mental deficiency.
Craniofacies. Macrocephaly. Coarsened facies.
Eyes. Corneal clouding.
Skeletal. Thoracolumbar gibbus. Metatarsus adductus. Flaring of lower ribs. Prominent sternum. J-shaped sella turcica. Acetabular dysplasia, narrow sciatic notches and hypoplastic basilar portions of ilia. Widening of ribs. Pointed proximal metacarpals.
Other. Inguinal hernia. Hepatosplenomegaly.

OCCASIONAL ABNORMALITIES.
Joint contractures. Hydrocephalus. Involvement of heart valves. Odontoid hypoplasia. Shortening and anterior irregularities of vertebral bodies, wedge deformities of lumbar vertebrae. Anterior, inferior beaking of lower thoracic and lumbar vertebrae. Hip dysplasia.

NATURAL HISTORY.
Unlike the other known mucopolysaccharidoses, MPS VII is frequently recognizable in the neonatal period. Onset of corneal clouding varies from seven months to eight years. Moderate mental deficiency is the rule.

ETIOLOGY. Autosomal recessive. The basic defect is a deficiency of β-glucuronidase, which can be documented in fibroblasts and leukocytes.

COMMENT. The existence of multiple allelic forms of this disorder most likely explains the wide variability in the clinical phenotype. There exists at least one form of β-glucuronidase deficiency that presents during the second decade of life and is characterized by mild skeletal abnormalities and normal intelligence.

References

Sly, W. S., et al.: Beta glucuronidase deficiency. Report of clinical, radiologic, and biochemical features of a new mucopolysaccharidosis. J. Pediatr., *82*:249, 1973.

Daves, B. S., and Degnan, M.: Different clinical and biochemical phenotype associated with beta glucuronidase deficiency. *In* Bergsma, D. (ed.): Skeletal Dysplasias. New York, National Foundation March of Dimes, 1974, p. 251.

Hoyme, H. E., et al.: Presentation of mucopolysaccharidosis VII (β-glucuronidase deficiency) in infancy. J. Med. Genet., *18*:237, 1981.

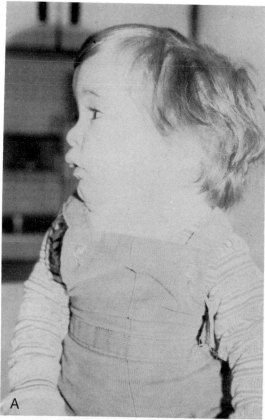

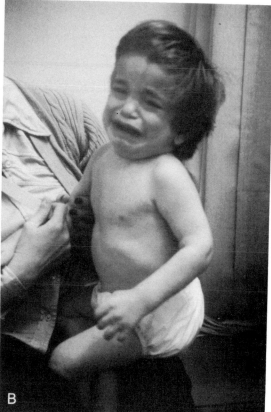

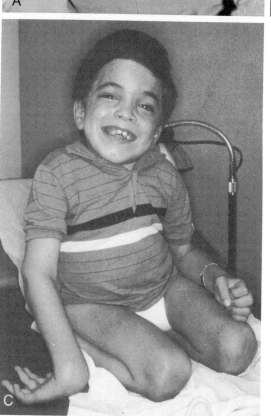

Mucopolysaccharidosis VII. Same child at one year *(A)*, two years *(B)*, and eight years *(C)* of age. Note the coarse facies and joint contractures.

O. CONNECTIVE TISSUE DISORDERS

MARFAN SYNDROME

Arachnodactyly with Hyperextensibility,
Lens Subluxation, Aortic Dilatation

Described as dolichostenomelia in the initial report by Marfan, this disorder has been extensively studied and recognized as a connective tissue disorder by McKusick.

ABNORMALITIES

Skeletal. Tendency toward tall stature with long slim limbs, little subcutaneous fat, and muscle hypotonia. Arachnodactyly. Decreased upper to lower segment ratio. Joint laxity with scoliosis (60 per cent) and kyphosis. Pectus excavatum or carinatum. Narrow facies with narrow palate.

Eyes. Lens subluxation, usually upward, with defect in suspensory ligament. Increased axial globe length. Myopia. Retinal detachment.

Cardiovascular. Dilatation with or without dissecting aneurysm of ascending aorta, less commonly of thoracic or abdominal aorta or pulmonary artery. Secondary aortic regurgitation. Mitral valve prolapse.

Other. Inguinal and/or femoral hernias.

OCCASIONAL ABNORMALITIES. Large ears, retinal detachment, striae in pectoral or deltoid area, diaphragmatic hernia, pulmonary malformation contributing to spontaneous pneumothorax and/or emphysema with an increased susceptibility to respiratory tract infection. Hemivertebrae, colobomata of iris, cleft palate, incomplete rotation of colon. Ventricular dysrhythmias. Neuropsychologic impairment, including learning disability and attention deficit disorder, in 42 per cent of 19 individuals (five to 18 years of age) despite normal I.Q.

NATURAL HISTORY. During childhood and adolescence, special care should be directed toward prevention of scoliosis. The serious vascular complications may develop at any time from fetal life through old age and are the chief cause of death. Pyeritz has documented a significantly reduced rate of aortic dilatation and its associated complications in both children and adults chronically treated with propranolol. In addition, based on a follow-up study of 50 consecutive patients (age range, nine to 52 years) who received a graft for the complete replacement of the ascending aortic aneurysm and aortic valve, Gott et al. recommend prophylactic repair for any patient with Marfan syndrome who has an ascending aorta with a diameter of 6 cm or more, regardless of symptoms or the presence of aortic regurgitation. Secondary glaucoma may occur, especially when the lens dislocates into the anterior chamber of the eye. The mean age of survival is 43 for men and 46 for women. These individuals are of normal intelligence. Estrogen therapy in early adolescence may merit consideration for the relatively tall girl with Marfan syndrome, in order to limit her statural growth.

ETIOLOGY. Autosomal dominant, with sufficiently wide variability in expression that the diagnosis is often tenuous in sporadic nonfamilial cases. The disorder can occur without ectopia lentis and without pronounced arachnodactyly. The basic defect in connective tissue has not been determined; however, accumulation of mucopolysaccharide has been noted within cells of the aorta from an affected individual, and the cultured fibroblast cells from individuals with the Marfan syndrome show cytoplasmic metachromatic inclusion.

References

Marfan, A. B.: Un cas de déformation congénitale des quatre membres plus prononcée aux extrémities charactérisée par l'allongement des os avec un certain degré d'amincissement. Bull. Mem. Soc. Med. Hop. (Paris), *13*:220, 1896.

McKusick, V.: Heritable Disorders of Connective Tissue, 3rd ed. St. Louis, C.V. Mosby Co., 1966, p. 38.

Skorby, F., and McKusick, V. A.: Estrogen treatment of tall stature in girls with Marfan syndrome. Birth Defects Original Article Series, *13*:155, 1977.

Pyeritz, R. E., and McKusick, V. A.: The Marfan syndrome: Diagnosis and management. N. Engl. J. Med., *300*:772, 1979.

Hofman, K. J., Bernhardt, B. A., and Pyeritz, R. E.: Increased incidence of neuropsychologic impairment in the Marfan syndrome. Am. J. Hum. Genet., 37:4A, 1985.

Gott, V. L., et al.: Surgical treatment of aneurysms of the ascending aorta in the Marfan syndrome. Results of composite-graft repair in 50 patients. N. Engl. J. Med., 314:1070, 1986.

Pyeritz, R. E.: Protection of the aortic root by propranolol in Marfan syndrome. J. Med. Genet., 23:469, 1986.

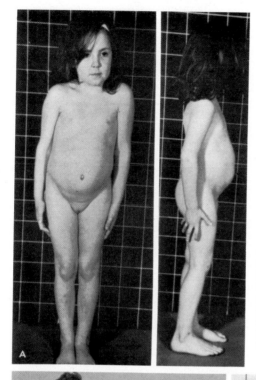

Marfan syndrome. *A*, Three and one-half year old, with height age of five years, who has lens dislocation, mild arachnodactyly of the hands and feet, unusually soft skin, and narrow palate. The family history of the Marfan syndrome in the mother and grandfather tends to confirm the diagnosis in this case. *B*, Girl, nine years and three months old, with height age of 12 years and three months, and her mother. Both have arachnodactyly, but only the mother has dislocation of the lenses. *C*, Sixteen year old with arachnodactyly, hyperextensible hands and knees, limitation of extension at elbow, scoliosis, systolic and diastolic murmurs, superiorly dislocated lenses, glaucoma, and retinal detachments, despite numerous surgical procedures. She represents a fresh mutation in that no other family members are affected. (*C* courtesy of Dr. Victor McKusick, Johns Hopkins Hospital, Baltimore, Maryland, and Dr. Judith Hall, University of British Columbia, Vancouver.)

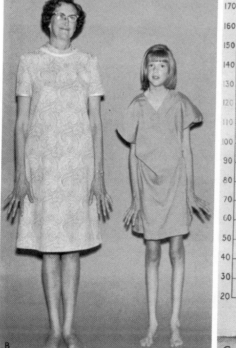

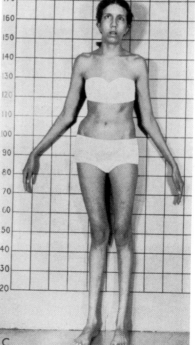

BEALS SYNDROME
(Beals Contractural Arachnodactyly Syndrome)

Joint Contractures,
Arachnodactyly, "Crumpled" Ear

Beals and Hecht described this syndrome in 1971. They found 11 probable past reports of the same entity, including the original Marfan report.

ABNORMALITIES

Limbs. Long slim limbs (dolichostenomelia) with arachnodactyly. Camptodactyly and ulnar deviation of fingers. Joint contractures, especially of knees, elbows, and hands.

Other Skeletal. Kyphoscoliosis, relatively short neck. Metatarsus varus. Hypoplasia of calf muscles.

Ears. "Crumpled" appearance with poorly defined conchas and prominent crura from the root of the helix.

Other. Mitral valve prolapse.

OCCASIONAL ABNORMALITIES.
Micrognathia. Iris coloboma. Subluxation of patella. Atrial septal defect, ventricular septal defect, hypoplasia of aorta.

NATURAL HISTORY. There tends to be gradual improvement in the joint limitations, but the scoliosis may be progressive.

ETIOLOGY. Autosomal dominant inheritance.

References

Beals, R. K., and Hecht, F.: Delineation of another heritable disorder of connective tissue. J. Bone Joint Surg. [Am.], *53*:987, 1971.

Hecht, F., and Beals, R. K.: "New" syndrome of congenital contractural arachnodactyly originally described by Marfan in 1896. Pediatrics, *49*:574, 1972.

Anderson, R. A., Koch, S., and Camerini-Otero, R. D.: Cardiovascular findings in congenital contractural arachnodactyly: Report of an affected kindred. Am. J. Med. Genet., *18*:265, 1984.

Ramos Arroyo, M. A., Weaver, D. D., and Beals, R. K.: Congenital contractural arachnodactyly. Report of four additional families and review of literature. Clin. Genet., *27*:570, 1985.

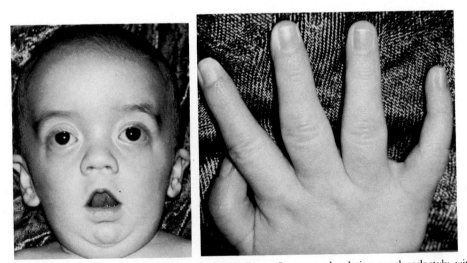

Beals syndrome. Young infant showing facies, folded helixes of ears, and relative arachnodactyly with minor camptodactyly. He developed severe scoliosis by two years of age.

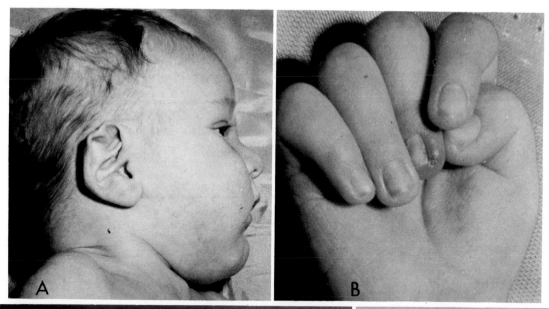

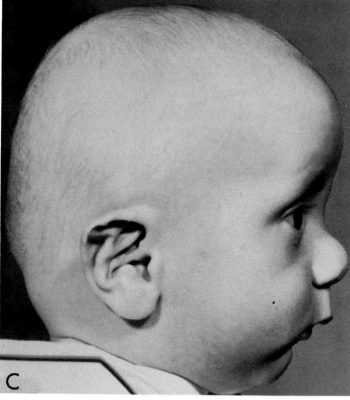

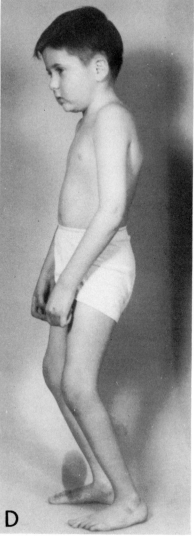

Beals syndrome. *A, B,* Infant showing "crumpled" ear and aberrant position of contracted fingers. *C,* Note similar appearance of ear to that in *A. D,* Six year old sibling of infant in *C.* (*C* and *D* from Beals, R. K., and Hecht, F.: J. Bone Joint Surg. [Am.], *53*:987, 1971.)

HOMOCYSTINURIA SYNDROME

Subluxation of Lens, Malar Flush, Osteoporosis

Urinary amino acid screening of mentally defective patients resulted in the independent discovery of this entity by Carson et al. and Gerritsen and Waisman in 1963. Finkelstein et al. found a lack of cystathionine synthetase activity in the liver of affected individuals, and this enzyme defect apparently leads to the accumulation of homocystine and methionine with a deficiency of cystathionine and cystine. Vitamin B_6–responsive and vitamin B_6–nonresponsive forms of this disorder have been delineated.

ABNORMALITIES

General. Mental defect in 58 per cent of 38 patients.

Eye. Subluxation, usually downward, of the lens by the age of ten years, the earliest instance noted being two years. Myopia.

Skeletal. Slim skeletal build, arachnodactyly, pectus excavatum or carinatum, genu valgum, pes cavus, everted feet with or without kyphoscoliosis. Osteoporosis.

Vasculature. Medial degeneration of aorta and elastic arteries with intimal hyperplasia and fibrosis leading to pads and ridges within the vessels. Both arterial and venous thromboses are frequent.

Skin. Malar flush with tendency toward patchy erythematous blotches elsewhere.

Hair. Tends to be fine, sparse, dry, and light in color.

OCCASIONAL ABNORMALITIES. Cataracts, glaucoma, optic atrophy, cystic retinal degeneration or detachment, irregular crowded teeth, high arched palate, hernias, hepatomegaly with fatty liver.

NATURAL HISTORY. Seizures, with onset from six months to five years of age, have been noted, and the electroencephalographic pattern is usually abnormal. Excessive nervousness may be a feature, occasionally with schizophrenic behavior. Neurologic defect, especially spasticity, may be present and is often asymmetric—presumably the consequence of vascular thrombosis that can be arterial or venous and not infrequently involves the coronary artery. Venipuncture or surgical procedures may be followed by excessive vascular thrombosis and should be avoided when possible. Thromboembolic phenomena constitute the most life-threatening feature of this disease. Another problem, osteoporosis, frequently leads to partial collapse of vertebrae, and there is an increased likelihood of fractures.

Failure to thrive has been a feature of some cases, with severe mental defect. However, normal to tall stature is the more usual growth pattern.

A long-term follow-up evaluation of 629 affected patients has recently been reported. Lens dislocation at ten years of age, initial clinically detected thromboembolic events at 15 years, spinal osteoporosis at 15 years, and mortality at age 30 occurred less frequently in untreated B_6–responsive patients than in untreated B_6–nonresponsive patients.

ETIOLOGY. Autosomal recessive. Decreased cystathionine synthetase activity has been found in the liver of the parents of homocystinuric individuals, supporting the contention that they are heterozygotes. Interference with collagen cross-linking by sulfhydryl groups of homocystine causes ectopia lentis and skeletal changes. Sulfation factor–like effects contribute to the disruption of vascular endothelium, leading to platelet thrombosis and then to arterial and venous occlusions. Pyridoxine therapy may be beneficial in some cases when begun in infancy.

COMMENT. The urinary cyanide nitroprusside test may not always yield a positive result in patients with homocystinuria, and specific amino acid studies therefore constitute the most important diagnostic measure. A completely successful mode of therapy has not yet been demonstrated. A low methionine, high cystine diet is beneficial in preventing mental retardation in B_6–nonresponsive patients if begun in the neonatal period.

References

Carson, N. A. J., et al.: Homocystinuria: a new inborn error of metabolism associated with mental deficiency. Arch. Dis. Child., *38*:425, 1963.

Gerritsen, T., and Waisman, H. A.: Homocystinuria, an error in the metabolism of methionine. Pediatrics, *33*:413, 1964.

Finkelstein, J. D., et al.: Homocystinuria due to cystathionine synthetase deficiency: the mode of inheritance. Science, *146*:785, 1964.

White, H. H., et al.: Homocystinuria. Trans. Am. Neurol. Assoc., *89*:24, 1964.

Grieco, H. J.: Homocystinuria; pathogenetic mechanisms. Am. J. Med. Sci., *273*:120, 1977.

Mudd, S. H., et al.: The natural history of homocystinuria cystathionine β-sulfatase deficiency. Am. J. Hum. Genet., *37*:1, 1985.

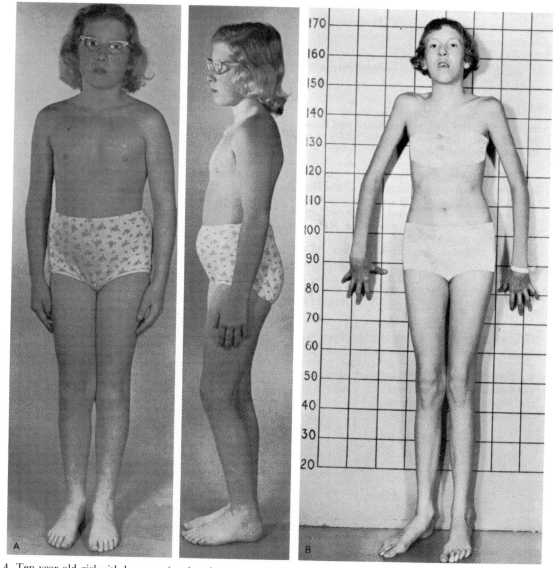

A, Ten year old girl with homocystinuria, who presented with lens subluxation that was first noted at four years of age. Her early developmental progress was within normal limits, but she has been receiving special schooling and her intelligence quotient is 67. *B*, Twelve year old girl with arachnodactyly, "tight" joints, and inferiorly and nasally dislocated lenses. She is of low normal intelligence with a "schizoid personality" and has had two episodes of gastrointestinal bleeding, one documented as being secondary to a gastric infarct. (*B* courtesy of Dr. Victor McKusick, Johns Hopkins Hospital, Baltimore, Maryland, and Dr. Judith Hall, University of British Columbia, Vancouver.)

CAMURATI-ENGELMANN SYNDROME

(Progressive Diaphyseal Dysplasia)

Diaphyseal Dysplasia, Weakness, Leg Pain

Originally described by Cockayne in 1920, this disorder was further delineated by Camurati and then Engelmann in the 1920s. About 70 cases have been reported.

ABNORMALITIES

Skeletal. Progressive diaphyseal broadening with thickened cortices and an abrupt transition toward more normal metaphyseal bone, most evident in femora and tibiae. May have sclerosis in base of skull.

Muscles. Relative weakness, most severe around pelvic girdle. Muscle biopsy may show atrophic fibers with degeneration.

Function. Waddling gait, leg pains, weakness.

Other. Elevated serum alkaline phosphatase level.

OCCASIONAL ABNORMALITIES. Deafness, headaches, scoliosis, late adolescence.

NATURAL HISTORY. Severely affected patients may have feeding problems, waddling gait, and leg pains even in infancy and often have an asthenic "malnourished" appearance. Mild cases may only be evident by roentgenogram. Hyperostosis may progress to optic nerve compression, for which surgical intervention is merited.

ETIOLOGY. Autosomal dominant with wide variance in expression.

References

Cockayne, E. A.: Case for diagnosis. Proc. R. Soc. Med., *13*:132, 1920.

Camurati, M.: Di un raro caso di osteite simmetrica erediatria degli arti inferiori. Chir. Organi. Mov., *6*:662, 1922.

Engelmann, G.: Ein Fall von Osteopathic hyperostotica (sclerotans) multiplex infantilis: Fortschr. Roentgenstr., *39*:1101, 1929.

Sparkes, R. S., and Graham, C. B.: Camurati Engelmann disease. Genetics and clinical manifestations with a review of the literature. J. Med. Genet., *9*:73, 1972.

Yen, J. K., et al.: Camurati-Engelmann disease. J. Neurosurg., *48*:138, 1978.

Yoshioka, H., et al.: Muscular changes in Engelmann's disease. Arch. Dis. Child., *55*:716, 1980.

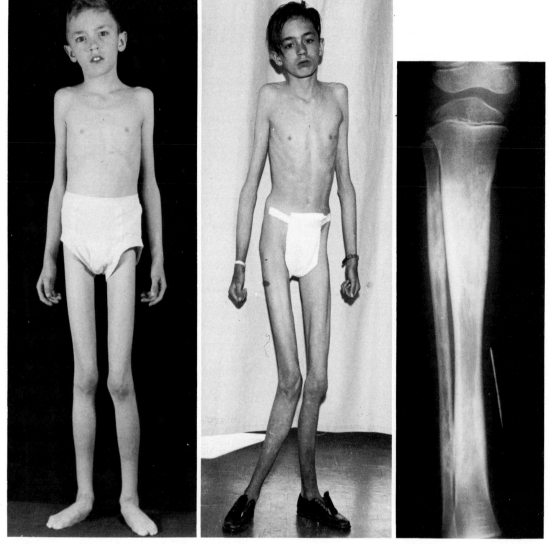

Camurati-Engelmann syndrome. Ten and 18 year old patients showing slim habitus, with bowing and angulation at the knees, and flat feet. Roentgenogram shows irregular cortical thickening with diaphyseal broadening. (From Clawson, D. K., and Loop, J. W.: J. Bone Joint Surg. [Am.], 46:143, 1964.)

EHLERS-DANLOS SYNDROME

Hyperextensibility of Joints, Hyperextensibility of Skin, Poor Wound Healing with Thin Scar

Originally described by Van Meekeren in 1682, this condition was further clarified by Ehlers in 1901 and Danlos in 1908. More than 100 cases have been described, the most complete review being that of McKusick. The possibility has been raised that the celebrated violinist Paganini may have had Ehlers-Danlos syndrome, thus accounting for his unusual dexterity and reach.

Eight distinct forms of the Ehler-Danlos syndrome have now been delineated. Only type I has been set forth in detail in this text.

ABNORMALITIES. The most consistent features are provided here.

Face. Narrow maxilla.

Auricles. Hypermobile, with tendency toward "lop ears."

Skin. Velvety, hyperextensible, and fragile, with poor wound healing leaving parchment-thin scars. Small, movable subcutaneous spherules contain either mucinous material or adipose.

Joints. Hyperextensibility with liability toward dislocation at hip, shoulder, elbow, knee, or clavicle. Pes planus.

Blood Vessels. Easy bruisability.

Cardiac. Mitral valve prolapse +/− tricuspid valve prolapse. Aortic root and/or sinus of Valsalva dilatation.

OCCASIONAL ABNORMALITIES

Eyes and Facies. Wide nasal bridge. Epicanthal folds, blue sclerae, myopia, microcornea, keratoconus, glaucoma, ectopia lentis, retinal detachment.

Skeletal. Small stature, kyphoscoliosis (27 per cent), long neck, slim skeletal build, downsloping ribs, talipes deformity, overlapping toes. Talipes equinovarus.

Dentition. Small; irregular placement; partial anodontia.

Cardiovascular. Dissecting aneurysm, intracranial aneurysm, hemorrhage. Atrial septal defect, abnormal aortic arch, other heart defects, anomalies of mitral valve.

Gastrointestinal. Inguinal hernia, diaphragmatic hernia, ectasia of intestine, intestinal diverticuli.

Renal. Ureteropelvic anomaly, renal tubular acidosis.

Other. Mental deficiency.

NATURAL HISTORY. Barabas discovered that most patients with Ehlers-Danlos syndrome are born prematurely following premature rupture of the membranes, possibly the first obvious indication of relative friability of tissues in these individuals. The integrity of tissues is easily disturbed, as evidenced by the fragility of skin and blood vessels. Wound healing is delayed, with relatively inadequate scar tissue, and prolonged hemorrhage may occur following trauma. Both of these factors, plus the tendency of sutures to tear out, rule out unnecessary surgical procedures. These patients should be cautioned to avoid traumatic situations. Gastrointestinal hemorrhage or hemoptysis may be a problem. The poor integrity of vessels occasionally may lead to a dissecting aneurysm, and affected women are liable to have postpartum hemorrhage. Whether or not the tendency to have chilblains and acrocyanosis is secondary to vascular alterations is undetermined.

The peculiar fat- or mucinoid-containing subcutaneous spherules, most commonly found in areas of frequent mild trauma, may mineralize and thereby be evident on roentgenograms.

ETIOLOGY. Autosomal dominant with wide variance in expression.

COMMENT. Major features of types II through VIII are summarized here.

Type II. A similar but much milder clinical picture and autosomal dominant inheritance.

Type III. Striking joint hypermobility, frequent joint dislocation, soft but otherwise normal skin, and autosomal dominant inheritance.

Type IV. The vascular or ecchymotic type. Thin or translucent skin with easily visible underlying veins, easy bruising, normal joint mobility with the exception of the small joints of the hands, bowel and/or arterial rupture leading to death, and autosomal dominant inheritance in the majority of cases. A defect in type III collagen has been documented.

Type V. A clinical picture similar to that of type II but with X-linked recessive inheritance.

Type VI. Soft, hyperextensible skin with moderate scarring and easy bruising, joint laxity, scoliosis, ocular fragility and keratoconus, lysyl hydroxylase deficiency resulting in hydroxylysine deficient collagen, and autosomal recessive inheritance.

Type VII. Soft but otherwise normal skin, marked joint hyperextensibility, congenital hip dislocation, and autosomal dominant inheritance.

Type VIII. Periodontitis, marked bruising, joint hypermobility, skin hyperextensibility, and autosomal dominant inheritance.

References

Van Meekeren, J. A.: De dilatabilitate extraordinaria cutis. Chapter 32 in Observations Medicochirogicae. Amsterdam, 1682.

Ehlers, E.: Cutis laxa, Neigung zu Harmorrhagien in der Haut, Lockerung mehrer Artikulationen. Dermat. Ztschr., *8*:173, 1901.

Danlos, H.: Un cas de cutis laxa avec tumeurs par contusion chronique des coudes et des genoux (santhome juvenile pseudodiabetique de MM. Hallopeau et Mace de Lepinay). Bull. Soc. Fr., Dermat. Syph., *19*:70, 1908.

Wechsler, H. L., and Fisher, E. R.: Ehlers-Danlos syndrome. Pathologic, histochemical, and electron microscopic observations. Arch. Pathol., *77*:613, 1964.

Barabas, A. P.: Ehlers-Danlos syndrome: associated with prematurity and premature rupture of foetal membranes; possible increase in incidence. Br. Med. J., 2:682, 1966.

McKusick, V. A., Heritable Disorders of Connective Tissue, 4th ed. St. Louis, C. V. Mosby Co., 1972, p. 292.

Leier, C. V., et al.: The spectrum of cardiac defects in Ehlers-Danlos syndrome, types I and III. Ann. Intern. Med., *92*:171, 1980.

Byers, P. H., Hollbrook, K. A., and Barsh, G. S.: Ehlers-Danlos syndrome. *In* Emery, A. E. H., and Rimoin, D. L.: Principles and Practice of Medical Genetics. Edinburgh, Churchill Livingstone, 1983.

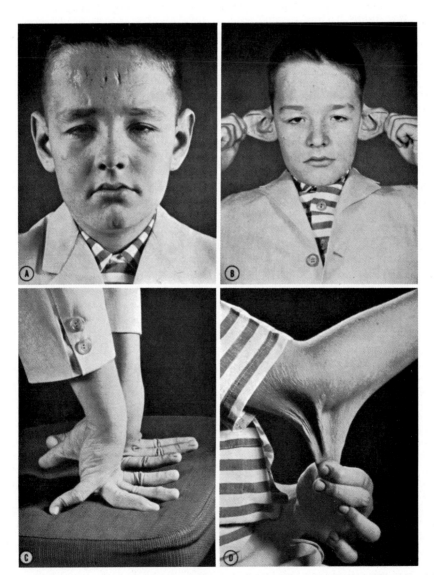

Ehlers-Danlos syndrome. Twelve year old boy showing thin persisting scars on forehead *(A)*, hyperelasticity of auricles and skin *(B and D)*, and hyperextensibility of joints *(C)*. (From Rees, T. D., et al.: Plast. Reconstr. Surg., *32*:39, 1963.)

OSTEOGENESIS IMPERFECTA SYNDROME, TYPE I

(Autosomal Dominant Osteogenesis Imperfecta, Lobstein Disease)

Fragile Bone, Blue Sclerae, Hyperextensibility, and/or Odontogenesis Imperfecta

At least four types of osteogenesis imperfecta exist. Only type I and type II are discussed in this text. Osteogenesis imperfecta Types III and IV are rare. Osteogenesis imperfecta type III, an autosomal recessive disorder, is associated with shortness, bowing, and angulation of the limbs; multiple fractures present in 47 per cent of cases; and normal sclerae and kyphoscoliosis occur in the majority of children who pass puberty. Osteogenesis imperfecta type IV, an autosomal dominant disorder, is associated with osteoporosis leading to fractures, variable but much milder deformity of long bones, and normal sclerae. Type IV osteogenesis imperfecta has been subdivided into A and B subtypes, depending on the presence or absence of dentinogenesis imperfecta.

The defects set forth below occur in roughly 25 to 60 per cent of patients with osteogenesis imperfecta type I, with no single alteration being a consistent feature.

ABNORMALITIES

Growth. Small stature in severe cases, sometimes with unduly short limbs.

Bones. Thin cortices and sparse trabeculae with fragility leading to bowing of leg bones in severe cases. Occasionally, soft, thin, calvarium with wide fontanels and wormian bones, with bulging in temporal and frontal regions and platybasia at base of skull; biconcave flattening of vertebrae; pectus carinatum or excavatum. Small facial bones.

Joints and Ligaments. Hyperextensible, sometimes leading to kyphoscoliosis, flat feet, and in extreme cases, joint dislocation.

Dentition. Hypoplasia of dentin and pulp with translucency of teeth, which have a yellowish or bluish-gray coloration, and susceptibility to caries, irregular placement, and late eruption.

Sclerae and Skin. The skin and sclerae tend to be thin and translucent; partial visualization of the choroid gives the sclerae a blue appearance.

Hearing. Deafness is usually secondary to otosclerosis and is seldom present until adult life.

Other. Inguinal and/or umbilical hernia. Poor muscle development. Increased bleeding tendency secondary to capillary fragility and/or abnormal thrombocyte function.

OCCASIONAL ABNORMALITIES

Eyes. Embryotoxon (opacity in the peripheral cornea), keratoconus, megalocornea.

Other. Syndactyly. Floppy mitral valve.

NATURAL HISTORY. There is wide individual variability with early mortality among severely affected infants, chiefly related to bronchopneumonia. Beyond infancy, the outlook for survival is good, and the chief problems are orthopedic deformity and otosclerosis. The long leg bones are the most frequent sites of breakage, with the peak ages for fractures being two to three years and ten to 15 years. After adolescence, the likelihood of fracture diminishes, although inactivity, pregnancy, or lactation can apparently enhance the likelihood of fracture. Intramedullary support by metal rods should be considered for treatment of the serious multiple fracture cases, and optimal orthopedic management is merited because many of these patients make a surprisingly good life adaptation. By 30 to 39 years of age, 35 per cent of patients are deaf; it occurs in 50 per cent by 60 years of age. Recently there has been some evidence that long-term calcitonin (salmon) may be beneficial in reducing the frequency of fractures. Also, fluoride, by yielding a stronger calcium apatite crystal, may be beneficial. With production of sex hormones at adolescence, there is usually partial improvement.

ETIOLOGY. Autosomal dominant. The majority of severe cases represent a sporadic occurrence within the family, presumably a fresh gene mutation, for which the parents need have little concern for recurrence. The disorder can be divided into A and B subtypes, depending on the presence or absence of dentinogenesis imperfecta.

From the molecular standpoint, in osteogenesis imperfecta type I, a quantitative defect in the production of type I procollagen appears to exist, the result (in most cases studied) of decreased synthesis of one of the constituent chains, pro-α 1 (I).

References

Freda, V. J., Vosburgh, G. J., and Di Liberti, C.: Osteogenesis imperfecta congenita. A presentation of 16 cases and review of the literature. Obstet. Gynecol., *18*:535, 1961.

Smars, G.: Osteogenesis Imperfecta in Sweden. Clinical, Genetic, Epidemiological, and Socio-Medical Aspects. Stockholm, Scandinavian University Books, 1961.

McKusick, V. A.: Heritable Disorders of Connective Tissue, 3rd ed. St. Louis, C. V. Mosby Co., 1966.

Sillence, D. O., Senn, A., and Danks, D. H.: Genetic heterogeneity in osteogenesis imperfecta. J. Med. Genet., *16*:101, 1979.

Byers, P. H., Bonadio, J. F., and Steinmann, B.: Invited editorial comment: Osteogenesis Imperfecta: Update and Perspective. Am. J. Med. Genet., *17*:429, 1984.

Sillence, D. O., et al.: Osteogenesis imperfecta Type III. Delineation of the phenotype with reference to genetic heterogeneity. Am. J. Med. Genet., *23*:821, 1986.

Illustrations on following page

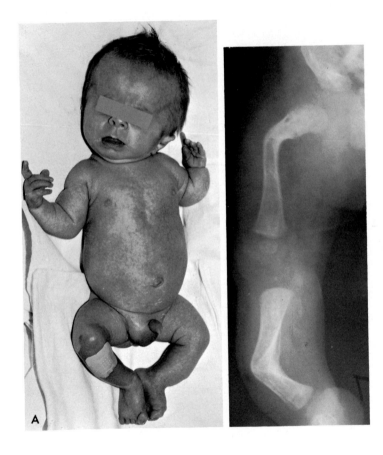

Osteogenesis imperfecta syndrome, type I. *A*, Two month old. Length, 19 inches; blue sclerae, inguinal hernia, hepatosplenomegaly.

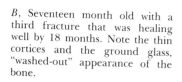

B, Seventeen month old with a third fracture that was healing well by 18 months. Note the thin cortices and the ground glass, "washed-out" appearance of the bone.

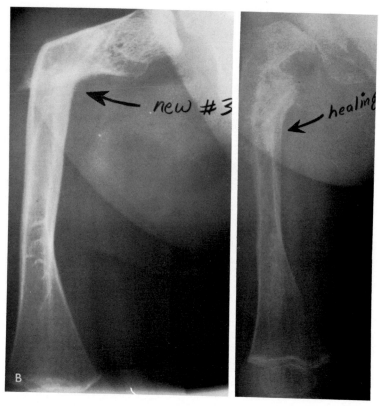

OSTEOGENESIS IMPERFECTA SYNDROME, TYPE II

(Osteogenesis Imperfecta Congenita, Vrolik Disease)

*Short Broad Long Bones,
Multiple Fractures, Blue Sclerae*

A perinatally lethal variety of osteogenesis imperfecta, this disorder is characterized by short limbs, short, broad long bones, radiologic evidence of severe osseous fragility and defective ossification. Based on subtle differences in radiographic features, Sillence et al. recently have subdivided this disorder into three groups. Group A is characterized by short, broad crumpled femora and continuously beaded ribs; group B by short, broad crumpled femora but normal ribs or ribs with incomplete beading; and group C by long, thin, inadequately modeled, rectangular long bones with multiple fractures and thin beaded ribs.

ABNORMALITIES
Growth. Prenatal short-limbed growth deficiency.
Craniofacial. Poorly mineralized, soft calvarium with large fontanels and multiple wormian bones. Deep blue sclerae, shallow orbits, small nose, low nasal bridge.
Limbs. Short, thick, ribbon-like, poorly mineralized long bones with multiple fractures and callus formation, especially in lower limbs.
Other. Flattened vertebrae, hypotonia, inguinal hernias, variable hydrocephalus. Hydrops.

NATURAL HISTORY. These patients usually are stillborn or die in early infancy of respiratory failure.

ETIOLOGY. Recent biochemical studies by Dr. Peter Byers at the University of Washington have now documented synthesis of both normal and abnormal type I collagen molecules in approximately 90 per cent of affected infants studied. This suggests that the majority of cases of type II osteogenesis imperfecta are the result of sporadic mutation of an autosomal dominant gene as opposed to autosomal recessive inheritance as had previously been suggested. For these cases, a recurrence risk of about 6 per cent has been observed and is felt to be the result of a parental germ cell mutation. However, biochemical evidence of autosomal recessive inheritance has been documented in a small number of affected infants. In those few cases, recurrence risk is 25 per cent.

References

Sillence, D. O., et al.: Osteogenesis imperfecta, type II. Delineation of the phenotype with reference to genetic heterogeneity. Am. J. Med. Genet., *17*:407, 1984.

Spranger, J.: Invited editorial comment: Osteogenesis imperfecta: A pasture for splitters and lumpers. Am. J. Med. Genet., *17*:425, 1984.

Byers, P. H., Bonadio, J. F., and Steinmann, B.: Invited editorial comment: Osteogenesis imperfecta. Update and perspective. Am. J. Med. Genet., *17*:429, 1984.

Horwitz, A. L., Lazda, V., and Byers, P. H.: Recurrent type II (lethal) osteogenesis imperfecta: Apparent dominant inheritance. Am. J. Hum. Genet., *37*:A59, 1985.

Tsipouras, P., et al.: Osteogenesis imperfecta type II is usually due to new dominant gene. Am. J. Hum. Genet., *37*:A79, 1985.

Peter Byers, M.D., University of Washington, Personal communication, 1987.

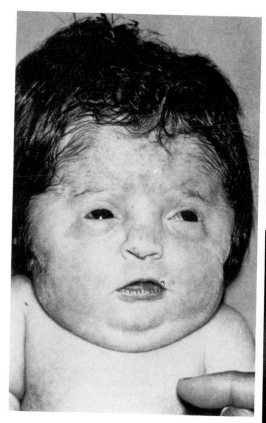
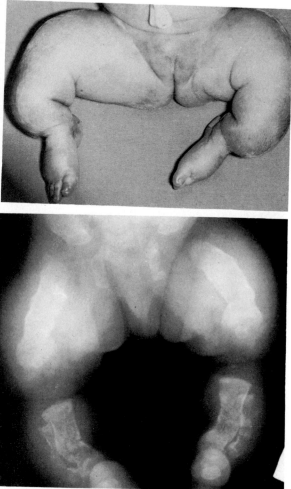

Osteogenesis imperfecta syndrome, type II. Young infant of normal parents. (Courtesy of P. Baird, University of British Columbia, Vancouver.)

FIBRODYSPLASIA OSSIFICANS PROGRESSIVA SYNDROME

Short Hallux, Fibrous Dysplasia Leading to Ossification in Muscles and Subcutaneous Tissues

This condition, described in a letter by Guy Patin in 1692, was extensively reviewed by Rosenstirn in 1918. Fibrodysplasia ossificans congenita is the terminology utilized by McKusick because myositis ossificans congenita is basically a misnomer. More than 350 cases have been reported.

ABNORMALITIES
Digits. Short hallux, often with synostosis. Less frequently, short thumb.
Fibrous Tissues. Swellings, sometimes with pain and fever, in aponeuroses, fasciae, and tendons, leading to ossification in muscles and fibrous tissues; most prominent in neck, dorsal trunk, and proximal limbs, with sternocleidomastoid frequently involved.

OCCASIONAL ABNORMALITIES.
Short phalanges other than hallux or thumb, clinodactyly of fifth finger, short femoral neck, hernia. Widely spaced teeth. Hypogenitalism and/or delayed sexual development. Easy bruising. Hearing loss.

NATURAL HISTORY.
The unusual fibrodysplasia leading to ossification may become evident during fetal life or as late as 25 years, with most patients experiencing onset in early childhood. Ossification is usually evident within two to eight months of the time swelling occurs. Although some affected individuals never express the fibrodysplasia, and others survive to late adult life with severe disability, the majority who have fibrodysplasia within the first five years succumb to the consequences of severe immobilization prior to 15 years of age. No effective treatment has been discovered, although symptomatic relief of pain may be achieved by salicylates or hydrocortisone analogue therapy. The natural history tends toward exacerbation and remission, and therefore, the results of therapy should be interpreted with caution. Another matter for caution is the interpretation of biopsies from affected tissues. The pathologic interpretation may be osteogenic sarcoma, although such a malignant growth is not a feature of this disease. Furthermore, any kind of trauma, including biopsy, surgery, and/or intramuscular injection, can be a focus for an area of ectopic ossification.

ETIOLOGY.
Autosomal dominant with almost full penetrance for short hallux and varying expression for the fibrodysplasia. About 90 per cent of patients represent fresh mutations, for which older paternal age has been noted as a factor.

COMMENT.
Although the fundamental defect in fibrous tissue is unknown, it is obvious that it allows for ossification to normal-appearing bone in tissues in which ossification normally would not occur.

References

Rosenstirn, J.: A contribution to the study of myositis ossificans progressiva. Ann. Surg., *68*:485, 1918.

McKusick, V.: Heritable Disorders of Connective Tissue, 3rd ed. St. Louis, C. V. Mosby Co., 1966, p. 400.

Tünte, W., Becker, P. E., and v. Knorr, G.: Zur Genetik der Myositis ossificans progressiva. Humangenetik, *4*:320, 1967.

Rogers, I. G., and Geho, W. B.: Fibrodysplasia ossificans progressiva. J. Bone Joint Surg. [Am.], *61*:909, 1979.

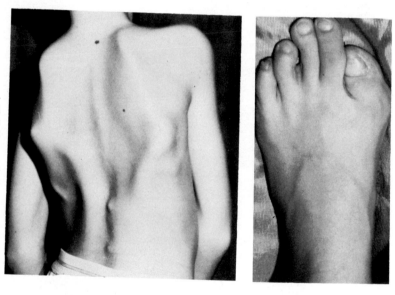

Fibrodysplasia ossificans progressiva syndrome. Thirteen year old showing progressive ossification in back musculature and short valgus hallux.

Illustration continued on following page

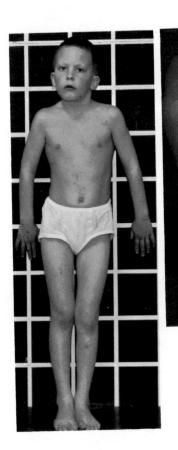

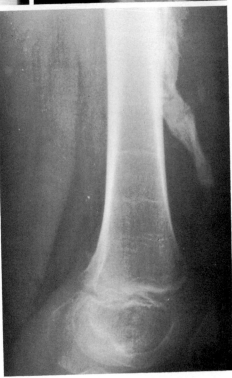

Fibrodysplasia ossificans progressiva syndrome. Seven year old with secondary torticollis, scoliosis, and partial contractures at elbow, hip, and knee joints. Note the short and deformed first metatarsal, hallux, and first metacarpal. Aberrant ossification is evident in the lower thigh. (From Herrmann, J., et al.: Birth Defects. Original Article Series, Vol. V, No. 5, 1969. Courtesy of Dr. John M. Opitz, Helena, Montana.)

P

P. HAMARTOSES

DISORDERS IN WHICH HAMARTOMATA ARE A PROMINENT FEATURE

Hamartosis implies an organizational defect leading to an abnormal admixture of tissues, often with a tumor-like excess of one or more components of the tissue. Included in this category are such features as hemangiomata, melanomata, irregular skin pigmentation, fibromata, lipomata, osteomata, dental tumors, and adenomata. There are also some strange tissue admixtures that create nosologic confusion because the histology of the lesions does not conform to a pathologic standard. For example, the "adenoma sebaceum" lesions in tuberous sclerosis are not adenomata of sebaceous glands. The very name tuberous sclerosis—potato-like lesions with sclerosis in the brain—emphasizes the nosologic problems.

The aberrant growth of particular tissues, a feature of many hamartomata, may allow for local growth toward a tumor or even metastasis beyond the local site. One advantage in recognizing some of the following patterns of malformation is the enhanced capability of anticipating future problems by knowing the natural history of the disorder. For example, malignant change of a colonic polyp in the Gardner syndrome is sufficiently frequent to justify resection of the colon by the age of 12 in a child who is recognized as having this syndrome with colonic polyps. However, in another syndrome with intestinal polyposis—the Peutz-Jeghers syndrome—the natural history indicates that intestinal malignancy is a rare occurrence, an important fact because the intestinal polyps excised from patients with the Peutz-Jeghers syndrome may be interpreted by the pathologist as potentially malignant.

The "occasional abnormalities" in some of the following syndromes may be "occasional tumors." The physician should be on guard for the occasional rhabdomyoma in tuberous sclerosis, the ovarian tumor in the Gardner syndrome, and the medulloblastoma in the basal cell nevus syndrome.

Hamartomatous lesions are a feature of many syndromes other than those that follow. For example, multiple exostoses represent a hamartomatous process in the diaphyseal portion of the bone, and this condition carries a small but distinct risk toward the development of osteosarcoma. Melanomata are a frequent feature in the XO (Turner) syndrome. Adrenal carcinoma and Wilms tumor are occasional complications for individuals with the Beckwith-Wiedemann syndrome. A looser association, in terms of being a distinct syndrome, has been noted in the occurrence of Wilms tumor in individuals with hemihypertrophy, aniridia, or both. These types of cases emphasize the close relationship that may exist between malformation and neoplasia. The same mutant gene that gives rise to an altered facies in the basal cell nevus syndrome also affects the growth stability of certain cells, allowing for nevi as a usual feature and basal cell carcinoma from such lesions as an occasional feature.

Finally, there would appear to be little value in persisting with the use of the term "phakomatoses" for some of the following conditions. The original "phakomatoses"—Sturge-Weber sequence, tuberous sclerosis, and neurofibromatosis—may now be viewed as separate entities, clinically distinct from each other, with no apparent etiologic relationship.

STURGE-WEBER SEQUENCE

*Flat Facial Hemangiomata,
Meningeal Hemangiomata with Seizures*

The association and localization of aberrant vasculature in the facial skin, eyes, and meninges are compatible with a defect arising in a limited part of the cephalic neural crest, cells of which migrate to the supraocular dermis, choroid, and pia mater.

ABNORMALITIES

Facial. Pink to purplish-red nonelevated cutaneous hemangiomata, most commonly in a trigeminal facial distribution, sometimes involving the choroid of the eye with secondary buphthalmos and/or glaucoma.

Meninges and CNS. Hemangiomata of arachnoid and pia mater, especially in occipital and temporal areas with secondary cerebral cortical atrophy, sclerosis, and "double contour" convolutional calcification. Seizures, paresis, mental deficiency.

OCCASIONAL ABNORMALITIES.

Hemangiomatosis in nonfacial areas, central nervous system, and other tissues. Macrocephaly. Cavernous hemangiomata. Colobomata of iris, coarctation of aorta, abnormal external ears.

NATURAL HISTORY.

The surface cutaneous hemangiomata are usually present at birth and seldom progress. Seizures most commonly begin between two and seven months of age and are grand mal in type, often asymmetric. The degree of central nervous system involvement is variable, with 30 per cent having paresis and 56 per cent having seizures; not all patients are mentally deficient. Cerebral calcification is usually not evident by x-ray until later infancy, the earliest occurring in a patient 13 months of age, first being noted in the occipital region.

Medical anticonvulsant treatment is of limited value, and occasionally, partial extirpation of affected meninges, brain tissue, or both may be merited in unilateral cases as a measure to control the seizures.

ETIOLOGY. Unknown. Sporadic, with rare exceptions. Occasionally, other family members may have hemangiomata of a lesser degree.

COMMENT. Only patients with lesions involving the ophthalmic distribution of the trigeminal nerve are at risk for neuro-ocular complications.

References

Chao, D. H.-C.: Congenital neurocutaneous syndromes of childhood. III. Sturge-Weber disease. J. Pediatr., 55:635, 1959.

Butterworth, T., and Strean, L. P.: Clinical Genodermatology. Baltimore, Williams and Wilkins Co., 1962.

Enrolras, O., Riche, M. C., and Merland, J. J.: Facial port-wine stains and Sturge-Weber syndrome. Pediatrics, 76:48, 1985.

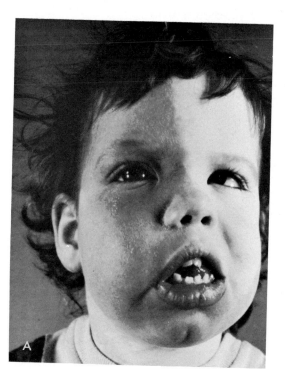

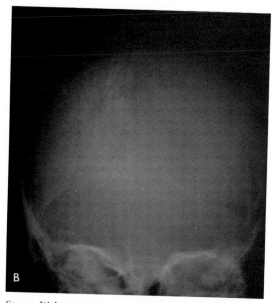

Sturge-Weber sequence. *A*, Affected child who has had grand mal seizures. *B*, Note the fine mineralization (left), which tends to reflect the convolutional pattern of the brain.

NEUROCUTANEOUS MELANOSIS SEQUENCE

Melanosis of Skin and Pia-arachnoid,
CNS Deterioration

This melanocytic hamartomatosis of the skin and pia-arachnoid was first described in 1861. More than 40 cases have been reported.

ABNORMALITIES

Skin. Blackish, thickened, sometimes hairy multiple nevi, most extensive in a "bathing trunk" distribution over the lower trunk, abdomen, and upper thighs.

Pia-arachnoid. Thick and pigmented with nests and sheets of melanoblasts, most striking at base of brain.

CNS. Liable to development of seizures and deterioration of central nervous system function. Communicating hydrocephalus secondary to blockage of cisternal pathways or obliteration of arachnoid villi by the tumor.

NATURAL HISTORY. The cutaneous melanosis is grossly evident at birth. Central nervous system function may be normal initially, but seizures and mental deterioration may begin before one year of age, apparently related to progression of the melanoblastic involvement of the pia-arachnoid, with diffuse or localized malignancy being implied in 12 of 18 patients.

The CNS consequences of the disorder often result in early demise. Three of the recognized patients were stillborn; the majority died before two years of age, and only one sixth of the patients are known to have survived past the age of 25 years. Although the frequency of leptomeningeal involvement in children with giant hairy nevi is unknown, involvement of the head and scalp is more likely to be associated with neurologic complications.

The risk of malignant melanoma degeneration is said to be 10 to 13 per cent, with half becoming evident by five years of age.

ETIOLOGY. Sporadic, cause unknown. Presumed to be an aberration in growth of early melanoblasts of neural crest origin, which contribute to the skin and pia-arachnoid. The sex incidence has been equal, and a family history of melanomata was noted in only one case.

References

Rokitansky, J.: Ein ausgezeichneter Fall von Pigment-mal mit ausgebreiteter Pigmentirung der inneren Hirn- und Rückenmarkshäute. Allg. Wien Med. Ztg., *6*:113, 1861.

Van Bogaert, L.: La mélanose neurocutanée diffuse hérédofamiale. Bull. Acad. R. Med. Belg. (6th Series), *13*:397, 1948.

Fox, H., et al.: Neurocutaneous melanosis. Arch. Dis. Child., *39*:508, 1964.

Hoffman, H. J., and Freeman, A.: Primary malignant leptomeningeal melanoma in association with giant hairy nevus. J. Neurosurg., *26*:62, 1967.

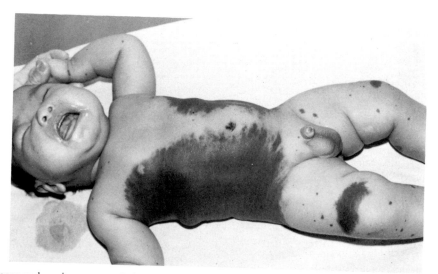

Neurocutaneous melanosis sequence. Infant who as yet shows no signs of CNS involvement. (Courtesy of S. Bintliff, Kauikeolani Children's Hospital, Honolulu.)

LINEAR SEBACEOUS NEVUS SEQUENCE

(Nevus Sebaceus of Jadassohn)

Midfacial Nevus Sebaceus, Seizures, Mental Deficiency

Nevus sebaceus of Jadassohn is most commonly found in an otherwise normal individual. However, the association of this type of lesion in the midfacial area with seizures and mental deficiency has been reported in at least 35 cases.

ABNORMALITIES

Skin. Nevus sebaceus with hyperpigmentation and hyperkeratosis. Lesions most commonly in the midfacial area, from the forehead down into the nasal area, tending to be linear in distribution. May also affect trunk and limbs.

CNS. Seizures of major motor, focal, or minor motor types. Mental deficiency.

OCCASIONAL ABNORMALITIES

Eyes. Esotropia, lipodermoid of conjunctiva, cloudy cornea, colobomata of eyelid, coloboma of iris and choroid.

CNS. Asymmetric "cortical atrophy," hydrocephalus.

Other. Pigmented nevi, spotty alopecia, coarctation of aorta, ventricular septal defect, hypoplastic teeth. Renal hamartomata, nephroblastoma.

NATURAL HISTORY. The nevus sebaceus is usually present at birth as a slightly yellow to orange to tan waxy-appearing lesion containing deficiencies and/or papillomatous excesses of epidermal elements, especially sebaceous glands and immature hair follicles. With time, the lesions tend to become verrucous and unsightly. Early surgical removal should be considered, since there is a 15 to 20 per cent risk of tumor, especially basal cell epithelioma. Furthermore, there may be unpredictable periods of rapid growth of the lesions. In the cases with associated central nervous system features, the onset of seizures has been from two months to two years, and they are difficult to control. The mental deficiency has been moderate to severe, though an occasional patient may have normal intelligence.

ETIOLOGY. Unknown. Whether this constitutes a single etiologic entity remains to be determined. Bianchine noted seizures and/or mental deficiency without skin lesions in several first degree relatives of one patient. Hence, a cautious family evaluation is indicated in cases of this clinical disorder.

References

Mehregan, A. H., and Pinkus, H.: Life history of organoid nevi. Special reference to nevus sebaceus of Jadassohn. Arch. Dermatol., *91*:574, 1965.

Marden, P. M., and Venters, H. D.: A new neurocutaneous syndrome. Am. J. Dis. Child., *112*:79, 1966.

Bianchine, J. W.: The nevus sebaceus of Jadassohn. A neurocutaneous syndrome and a potentially premalignant lesion. Am. J. Dis. Child., *120*:223, 1970.

Lansky, L. L., et al.: Linear sebaceous nevus syndrome. Am. J. Dis. Child., *123*:587, 1972.

Leonidas, J. C., et al.: Radiographic features of the linear sebaceous syndrome. Am. J. Roentgenol., *132*:277, 1979.

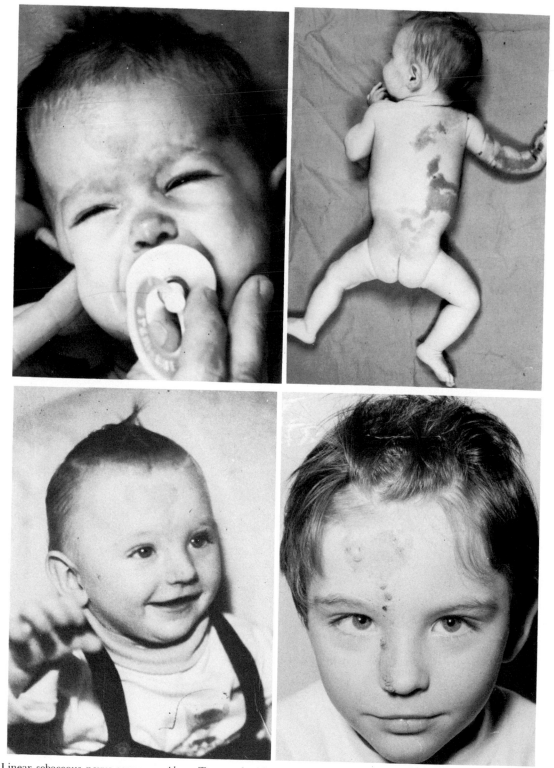

Linear sebaceous nevus sequence. *Above,* Two week old with facial and extensive body sebaceous nevi. Intractable seizures began at five months, and the patient died at nine months with pneumonia. Necropsy revealed renal nodular nephronoblastomatosis. (From Lansky, L. L., et al.: Am. J. Dis. Child., *123:*587, 1972.) *Below,* Verrucous change in sebaceous nevus from infancy to older childhood. (From Bianchine, J. W.: Am. J. Dis. Child., *120:*223, 1970.)

INCONTINENTIA PIGMENTI SYNDROME

(Bloch-Sulzberger Syndrome)

*Irregular Pigmented Skin Lesions
With or Without Dental Anomaly, Patchy Alopecia*

Bardach originally described the condition in twin sisters in 1925, and soon thereafter Bloch set forth the term incontinentia pigmenti to depict the unusual skin lesions. A major review of 635 cases by Carney includes only 16 affected males.

ABNORMALITIES

Skin. Most consistent feature. Vesiculation; verrucous changes; atrophy; irregular gray-brown pigmentation in fleck, whorl, or spidery form, especially on trunk and extremities.

Dentition. Thirty per cent have hypodontia, delayed eruption, and/or conical form.

Hair. Twenty per cent have atrophic patchy alopecia, especially on the posterior scalp.

CNS. About one third have mental deficiency, microcephaly, spasticity, and/or seizures.

Eyes. About 30 per cent have strabismus, retinal dysplasia, retinal detachment, uveitis, keratitis, cataract, retrolental dysplasia, and/or blue sclerae.

Osseous. About 20 per cent have hemivertebrae, kyphoscoliosis, extra rib, syndactyly, hemiatrophy, and/or short arms and legs.

OCCASIONAL ABNORMALITIES. Nail dystrophy, breast hypoplasia, dacryostenosis, eczema, short stature, hydrocephalus.

NATURAL HISTORY. Bullous skin lesions are generally present in early infancy and tend to progress from inflammatory or vesicular to pigmented and may fade in childhood. General eosinophilia is often present in infancy and the vesicles contain eosinophils. Verrucous lichenoid lesions develop during infancy in about one third of cases, especially over the dorsum of the hands and feet. The development of the irregular marble cake–like pigmentation may or may not coincide with the sites of bullous or verrucous lesions. The pigmented areas gradually fade in the second to third decades, and the adult may show only slightly atrophic depigmented "achromic stains," especially over the lower legs. About one half of the patients show other features, the most serious being the central nervous system abnormalities.

ETIOLOGY. Family studies indicate the effect of a single mutant gene, most likely lethal in affected males because the ratio of females to males in affected sibships is 2:1, with one half of the females affected. Whether the gene is autosomal or X-linked remains to be determined. Fifty-five per cent of the cases are familial, the remainder representing fresh mutational cases. The parents, especially the mother, should be closely examined for residual skin lesions, including achromatic spots, before genetic counseling is rendered.

References

Bardach, M.: Systematisierte Naevusbildungen bei einem cineiigen Zwillingspaar. Ein Beitrag zur Naevusätiologie. Z. Kinderheilkd., *39*:542, 1925.

Bloch, B.: Eigentümliche bisher nicht beschriebene Pigmentaffektion (Incontinentia pigmenti). Schweiz. Med. Wochenschr., *56*:404, 1926.

Carney, R. G.: Incontinentia pigmenti. A report of five cases and review of the literature. Arch. Dermatol. Syph., *64*:126, 1951.

Morgan, J. D.: Incontinentia pigmenti. Am. J. Dis. Child., *122*:294, 1971.

Carney, R. G.: Incontinentia pigmenti, a world statistical analysis. Arch. Dermatol., *112*:535, 1976.

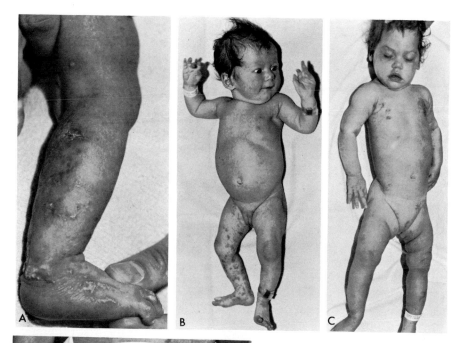

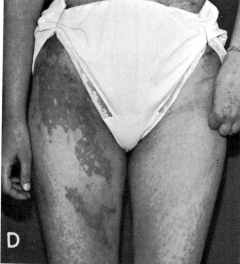

Incontinentia pigmenti syndromes. *A*, Early lesions in the young infant shown in *B*. *C*, Older mentally deficient infant with reticular pigmentation. *D*, Mentally deficient woman with spasticity and pseudogliomatous retinal detachment, showing advanced skin pigmentary change. *E*, Minor abnormalities of dentition in an affected girl. *F*, Reticular pigmentation in a three year old mentally deficient girl. (*A* to *E* courtesy of J. M. Opitz, Helena, Montana.)

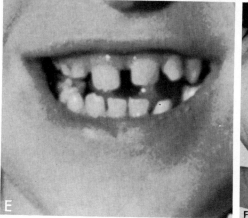

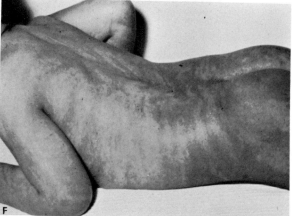

TUBEROUS SCLEROSIS SYNDROME

(Adenoma Sebaceum)

Hamartomatous Skin Nodules, Seizures, Phakomata, Bone Lesions

Von Recklinghausen is said to have described this disease over 100 years ago, but Bourneville is usually given credit for its recognition in 1880. Hamartomatous lesions develop in many tissues, especially the skin and brain. About 0.5 per cent of severely mentally defective individuals have this condition.

ABNORMALITIES
Brain and Eyes. Glioma-angioma lesions in cortex and white matter, with seizures (93 per cent) and mental deficiency (62 per cent) as apparent consequences. Roentgenographic evidence of intracranial mineralization (51 per cent), most commonly in basal ganglia or periventricular region. However, the periventricular lesions may be noted early in the clinical course by computed tomography scan as one of the most consistent features. Phakomata and similar retinal lesions in 53 per cent.

Skin. Fibrous-angiomatous lesions (83 per cent), varying in color from flesh to pink to yellow to brown, develop in the nasolabial fold, cheeks, and elsewhere. Ovoid "white nevi" from 0.5 to 8 cm in size that contain melanocytes without melanin are even more common. Café au lait spots. Fibromatous plaques and nodules.

Bone. Cyst-like areas in phalanges (66 per cent) and elsewhere, with areas of periosteal thickening yielding roentgenographic evidence of "sclerosis," palpable irregularity, or both.

Renal. Angiomyolipomata in 45 to 81 per cent, usually multiple and benign. Tubular enlargement and cyst formation with hyperplasia of tubular cells.

Dentition. Pit-shaped enamel defects, most evident by close inspection of labial premolar surfaces.

OCCASIONAL ABNORMALITIES.
Other hamartomata: fibromata (especially subungual), lipomata, angiomata, nevi, shagreen patches (goose flesh–like). Rhabdomyomata and angiomata of heart, cystic changes in lung, hamartomata of liver and pancreas. Hypothyroidism, thyroid adenomata. Sexual precocity. Astrocytoma.

NATURAL HISTORY. Hamartomata usually become evident in early childhood and may increase at adolescence. Facial nodular lesions are present in 50 per cent of children by five years, whereas 82 per cent have white nevi in childhood. Malignant transformation may occur, and about 6 per cent of patients develop a brain tumor. However, malignant transformation of the periventricular nodules is rare. The seizures, which tend to develop in early childhood, may initially be myoclonic and later grand mal in type and are difficult to control. EEG abnormality is found in 87 per cent of patients and may be of the grossly disorganized hypsarrhythmic pattern. The seizures and mental defect seem to be related to the extent of hamartomatous change in the brain. For those with mental deficiency, 100 per cent have seizures, 88 per cent by five years of age, whereas of those without serious mental deficiency, 69 per cent have seizures, 44 per cent by five years of age. Mental deterioration is unusual, except in relation to frequent seizures of status epilepticus.

An unknown percentage of patients die prior to 20 years of age as the consequence of status epilepticus, general debility, pneumonia, or tumor. However, it should be appreciated that there is wide variability in expression of the disease; all patients with skin lesions do not develop seizures, mental deficiency, or both, and the earlier noted pattern of abnormality is biased toward the more severe cases. One general survey showed a 69 per cent incidence of mental deficiency. However, of the nine patients diagnosed at a hospital for skin diseases, none were mentally deficient, whereas 93 per cent of those admitted to a children's hospital were mentally deficient.

ETIOLOGY. Autosomal dominant, with about 86 per cent representing fresh mutations from unaffected parents. Affected individuals usually show some manifestations of the disorder by adulthood. A search for depigmented spots and/

or hairs and CT scan for periventricular lesions appear to be the best methods for early detection of an affected individual. Older paternal age has not been a factor in fresh mutational cases of tuberous sclerosis from past studies.

COMMENT. The reader will note that the term "adenoma sebaceum" is not utilized, and this is because the skin lesions do not directly involve the sebaceous glands. The skin lesions are telangiectatic fibromata or angiofibromata. Actually, the term tuberous sclerosis (potato-like sclerotic lesions) pertains only to the brain lesions and is a poor descriptive term for this disease. Such terms are indicative of the difficulty in applying descriptive names to these admixed hamartomatous areas of faulty tissue morphogenesis.

References

Bourneville, D.: Sclereuse tubereuse des circonvolutions cerebrales. Idiote et epilepsie hemiplegique. Arch. Neurol. (Paris), *1*:81, 1880.

Lagos, J. C., and Gomez, M. R.: Tuberous sclerosis: reappraisal of a clinical entity. Mayo Clin. Proc., *42*:26, 1967.

Bundey, S., and Evans, K.: Tuberous sclerosis: A genetic study. J. Neurol. Neurosurg. Psychiatry, *32*:591, 1969.

Hoff, M., et al.: Enamel defects associated with tuberous sclerosis. Oral Surg., *40*:261, 1976.

Kenishi, Y., et al.: Tuberous sclerosis. Early neurologic manifestations and CT features in 18 patients. Brain Dev., *1*:31, 1979.

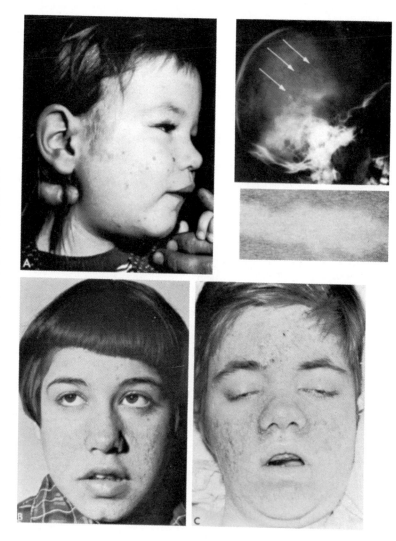

Tuberous sclerosis syndrome. *A*, Two year old with early pink to red nodular and flat skin lesions and seizures. *B*, Girl with mental deficiency and seizures. *C*, Young woman with mental deficiency and seizures, on Dilantin (phenytoin) therapy. (*B* and *C* courtesy of L. Dobbs, Rainier State Training School, Buckley, Washington.) *Upper right,* Skull roentgenogram showing periventricular calcification and skin showing depigmented "ash leaf" lesion. (Courtesy of Michael M. Cohen, Jr., D.D.S., Dalhousie University, Halifax, Nova Scotia.)

NEUROFIBROMATOSIS SYNDROME

Multiple Neurofibromata,
Café au Lait Spots, +/− Bone Lesions

Von Recklinghausen described this disease in 1882. Crowe et al. estimated the incidence at one in 3000 individuals.

ABNORMALITIES

Skin. Areas of hyper- or hypopigmentation with café au lait spots in 94 per cent, roughly three fourths of affected individuals having six or more spots measuring 1.5 cm or greater in size, most commonly on trunk. Axillary "freckling" may occur.

Subcutaneous. Dysplastic tumors consisting of connective tissue, neurilemma cells, and/or mast cells; occurring along nerves, in subcutaneous tissues, and sometimes in eyes and/or meninges.

Other. Lisch nodules or pigmented iris hamartomata (94 per cent after six months). Macrocephaly of postnatal onset. Mild short stature.

OCCASIONAL ABNORMALITIES

Central Nervous System. Tumors, including optic gliomas and other astrocytomas, acoustic neuromas, neurilemmomas, meningiomas, and neurofibromas, occurring in 5 to 10 per cent. Seizures and/or EEG abnormalities in about 20 per cent. Mental deficiency in 2 to 5 per cent, with learning disability, hyperactivity, and/or speech problems in an additional significant percentage. Cerebral vascular compromise. Headaches.

Skeletal. Scoliosis. Hypoplastic bowing of lower legs, with pseudoarthrosis at birth. Osseous lesions with localized osteosclerosis, rib fusion, spina bifida, absence of patella, dislocation of radius and ulna, local overgrowth, and scalloping of vertebral bodies with deformed pedicles.

Hamartomata. Cutaneous nevi, lipomata, angiomata, neurofibroma in kidney, stomach, heart, tongue, and bladder.

Other. Syndactyly. Glaucoma. Corneal opacity. Potentially malignant melanoma of iris. Verrucous nevus. Pheochromocytoma. Pulmonic stenosis. Vascular hyperplasia of the intima and media. Pruritus. Ptosis.

NATURAL HISTORY. Often evident in early childhood; 47 per cent of patients develop some neurologic impairment, sometimes secondary to nerve compression, as with blindness due to optic nerve pressure. Malignant change occurs in 5 to 10 per cent of patients, most commonly in males.

The complications of neurofibromatosis can be divided into those that are structural (macrocephaly, segmental hypertrophy, scoliosis, pseudoarthrosis, cardiac defects), those that are functional (seizures, speech disorders, hypertension, intellectual deficits), and those that relate to neoplasia. Screening for structural and functional complications can be done effectively through comprehensive physical evaluation every six months. The author believes that routine radiologic screening for central nervous system and visceral tumors is not warranted in the majority of cases. Rather, clinicians following affected individuals should maintain a high index of suspicion and evaluate specific signs and symptoms as they develop.

ETIOLOGY. Autosomal dominant with high penetrance but wide variability in expression. About 50 per cent of patients have a fresh gene mutation, and Crowe et al. calculated the mutation rate per gamete per generation to be 1×10^{-4}, the highest known for the human.

COMMENT. In addition to the classic form of neurofibromatosis, a second disorder exists, referred to as central or acoustic neurofibromatosis. Also autosomal dominant, it is characterized by a later age of onset, the presence of bilateral acoustic neuromas, which generally develop over the second and third decades, and other CNS tumors, such as meningiomas and neuromas of the dorsal spinal roots. Usually only a few café au lait spots and cutaneous neurofibromas are present. Finally, there exists a segmental form of neurofibromatosis characterized by café au lait spots, cutaneous neurofibromas, and intrathoracic and/or intra-abdominal neurofibromas limited to a circumscribed body segment. Because this disorder is most likely due to a somatic mutation, recurrence risk is negligible.

References

Von Recklinghausen, F.: Ueber die multiplen Fibroma der Haut und ihre Beziehung zu den multiplen Neuromen. Berlin, A. Hirschwald, 1882.

Crowe, F. W., Schull, W. J., and Neel, J. V.: Multiple Neurofibromatosis. American Lecture Series No. 281. Springfield, Ill., Charles C Thomas, 1952.

Canale, D., Bebin, J., and Knighton, R. S.: Neurologic manifestations of von Recklinghausen's disease of the nervous system. Confin. Neurol., *24*:359, 1964.

Fienman, N. L., and Yakovac, W. C.: Neurofibromatosis in childhood. J. Pediatr., *76*:339, 1970.

Mena, E., et al.: Neurofibromatosis and renovascular hypertension in children. Am. J. Roentgenol. Radium Ther. Nucl. Med., *118*:39, 1973.

Holt, J. F., and Kuhns, L. R.: Macrocranium and macroencephaly in neurofibromatosis. Skeletal Radiol., *1*:25, 1976.

Miller, R. M., and Sparkes, R. S.: Segmental neurofibromatosis. Arch. Dermatol., *113*:837, 1977.

Eldridge, R.: Central neurofibromatosis with bilateral acoustic neuromas. Adv. Neurol., *29*:57, 1981.

Riccardi, V. M.: Von Recklinghausen neurofibromatosis. N. Engl. J. Med., *305*:1617, 1981.

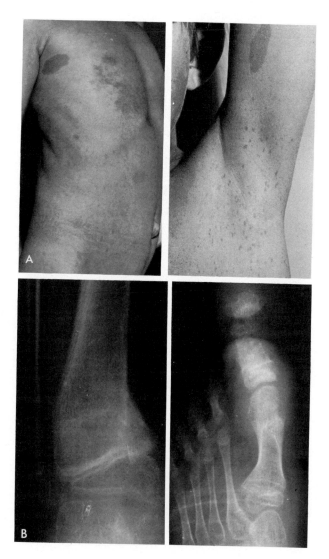

Neurofibromatosis syndrome. *A,* Café au lait, ovaloid, irregular, and minute pigmentary spots on the trunk of one child and in the axilla—axillary "freckling"—in another child. *B,* Pseudofracture of distal tibia and fibula. Hypertrophy of toe in relation to the hamartomatous process in that area.

McCUNE-ALBRIGHT SYNDROME

(Osteitis Fibrosa Cystica)

Polyostotic Fibrous Dysplasia,
Irregular Skin Pigmentation, Sexual Precocity

McCune and Albright et al. described this condition in 1936 and 1937, respectively. More than 100 cases have been reported. The relative frequency of diagnosis in females vs. males is 3:2.

ABNORMALITIES

Bone. Multiple areas of fibrous dysplasia, most commonly in long bones and pelvis; may also include facial bones, causing facial asymmetry. May result in deformity, increased thickness of bone, or both.

Skin. Irregular brown pigmentation, most commonly over sacrum, buttocks, upper spine; unilateral in about 50 per cent of patients.

Endocrine. Precocious puberty. Hyperthyroidism, hyperparathyroidism. Acromegaly. Cushing's syndrome. Hyperprolactinemia.

NATURAL HISTORY. The pigmentation is usually evident in infancy, and the bone dysplasia may progress during childhood, resulting in deformity, fracture, or both, most commonly in the upper femur. Thickening of bone in the calvarium can lead to cranial nerve compression with such serious consequences as blindness or deafness. The sexual precocity in the female is often unusual in character, with menstruation prior to development of breasts or pubic hair. The accelerated maturation coincident with sexual precocity may result in early attainment of full stature, so that adult height can be relatively short.

ETIOLOGY. The cases have been sporadic occurrences in the families, and the etiology is undetermined.

COMMENT. Recent evidence suggests that the endocrinologic abnormalities are the result of autonomous hyperfunction of several endocrine glands rather than being centrally mediated.

References

McCune, D. J.: Osteitis fibrosa cystica. Am. J. Dis. Child., *52*:745, 1936.

Albright, F., et al.: Syndrome characterized by osteitis fibrosa disseminata, areas of pigmentation and endocrine dysfunction, with precocious puberty in females. Report of five cases. N. Engl. J. Med., *216*:727, 1937.

Arlien-Soborg, U., and Iversen, T.: Albright's syndrome. A brief survey and report of a case in a seven year old girl. Acta Paediatr., *45*:558, 1956.

DiGeorge, A. M.: Albright syndrome: Is it coming of age? J. Pediatr., *87*:1018, 1975.

D'Armiento, M., et al.: McCune-Albright syndrome: Evidence for autonomous multiendocrine hyperfunction. J. Pediatr., *102*:584, 1983.

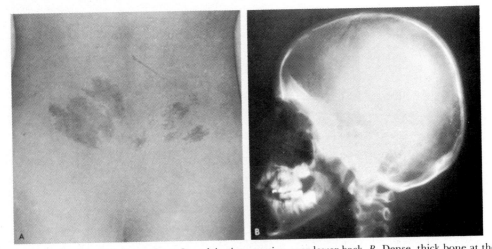

McCune-Albright syndrome. *A,* Irregular café au lait pigmentation over lower back. *B,* Dense, thick bone at the base of the skull.

VON HIPPEL-LINDAU SYNDROME

Retinal Angiomata, Cerebellar Hemangioblastoma

Lindau, in 1926, recognized this association of angiomatous retina (von Hippel disease) and angiomatous tumors of the cerebellum and other parts of the central nervous system.

ABNORMALITIES

Eyes. Angioma, often peripheral, with "beaded" artery leading into it and tortuous dilated vein from it.

Cerebellum. Hemangioblastoma, sometimes with cyst, most commonly in cortical area of cerebellum, occasionally in spinal cord or elsewhere in brain. May calcify.

OCCASIONAL ABNORMALITIES. Hemangiomata of face, adrenal, lung, and liver; multiple cysts of pancreas, kidney, and epididymis; hypernephromata; pheochromocytoma; pancreatic cancer; adenocarcinoma of ampulla of Vater; paragangliomas; polycythemia.

NATURAL HISTORY. Retinal lesions usually not apparent until approximately 25 years of age, with subsequent visual impairment. Cerebellar signs may appear in third decade. Light coagulation or cryotherapy may be effective in treating the retinal angiomata and avoiding retinal detachment. There is about a 25 per cent risk of renal cancer, not uncommonly bilateral, for which renal transplantation merits consideration.

ETIOLOGY. Autosomal dominant with varying expression.

References

Lindau, A.: Studien über Kleinhirnsystem. Bon Pathogenese und Beziehungen zur Angiomatosis retinae. Acta Path. Microbiol. Scand. [Suppl.], *1*:1, 1926.

Christoferson, L. A., Gustafson, M. B., and Petersen, A. G.: Von Hippel–Lindau's disease. J.A.M.A., *178*:280, 1961.

Petersen, G. J., et al.: Renal transplantation in Lindau–von Hippel disease. Arch. Surg., *112*:841, 1977.

Fill, W. L., Lamiell, J. M., and Polk, N. O.: The radiographic manifestations of von Hippel–Lindau disease. Radiology, *133*:289, 1979.

KLIPPEL-TRENAUNAY-WEBER SYNDROME

Asymmetric Limb Hypertrophy, Hemangiomata

This entity was originally reported by Klippel and Trenaunay in 1900. Parkes-Weber added the infrequent finding of arteriovenous fistula in 1907. Approximately 140 cases have been published thus far.

ABNORMALITIES

Limbs. Congenital or early childhood hypertrophy of usually one, but occasionally more than one, limb. The hypertrophy may not necessarily coincide with the area of hemangiomatous involvement.

Skin. The hemangiomata vary greatly and include the following types: capillary, cavernous, phlebectasia, and varicosities. These lesions can occur in any area, but are more commonly located on the legs, buttocks, abdomen, and lower trunk. Unilateral distribution predominates, but bilateral involvement is not uncommon.

OCCASIONAL ABNORMALITIES

Limbs. Arteriovenous fistula, lymphangiomatous anomalies, atrophy.

Hands and Feet. Macrodactyly, disproportionate growth of the digits whether large or small, syndactyly, polydactyly, oligodactyly.

Skin. Hyperpigmented nevi and streaks, neonatal and childhood ulcers and vesicles, cutis marmorata, telangiectasia.

Craniofacial. Asymmetric facial hypertrophy, hemangiomata, microcephaly, macrocephaly due to macrencephaly, intracranial calcifications, and eye abnormalities such as glaucoma, cataracts, and heterochromia.

Viscera. Visceromegaly; hemangiomata of the intestinal tract, urinary system, mesentery, and pleura; aberrant major blood vessels, lymphectasia.

Performance. Mental deficiency and/or seizures, usually only in patients having facial hemangiomatosis.

Growth. Small stature, tall stature.

Other. Enlargement of the genitalia, intravascular clotting problems, lipodystrophy.

NATURAL HISTORY. The usual patient with this syndrome does relatively well. There may be disproportionate growth, which requires epiphyseal fusion or removal of the appropriate phalanx. Joint discomfort is not uncommon, and arthritic-type problems may develop. Leg swelling can be bothersome, and ulcers and other chronic skin difficulties may occur. Those few patients with accompanying arteriovenous fistulae require surgical intervention. Rarely, amputation is necessary, particularly if the extremity reaches gigantic proportions or secondary clotting difficulties occur. Hemangiomata of the viscera, brain, eyes, and other areas should always be looked for in this extremely variable disorder.

ETIOLOGY. Unknown. Sporadic occurrence.

References

Klippel, M., and Trenaunay, P.: Du naevus variqueux osteo-hypertrophique. Arch. Gen. Med., *185*:641, 1900.

Parkes-Weber, F.: Angioma formation in connection with hypertrophy of limbs and hemi-hypertrophy. Br. J. Dermatol., *19*:231, 1907.

Kuffer, F. R., et al.: Klippel-Trenaunay syndrome, visceral angiomatosis, and thrombocytopenia. J. Pediatr. Surg., *3*:65, 1968.

Furukawa, T., et al.: Sturge-Weber and Klippel-Trenaunay syndrome with nevus of Ota and Sto. Arch. Dermatol., *102*:640, 1970.

Lindenauer, S. M.: Congenital arteriovenous fistula and the Klippel-Trenaunay syndrome. Ann. Surg., *174*:248, 1971.

Stephan, M. J., et al.: Macrocephaly in association with unusual cutaneous angiomatosis. J. Pediatr., *87*:353, 1975.

Baskerville, P. A., et al.: The Klippel-Trenaunay syndrome: Clinical, radiological and haemodynamic features and management. Br. J. Surg., *72*:232, 1985.

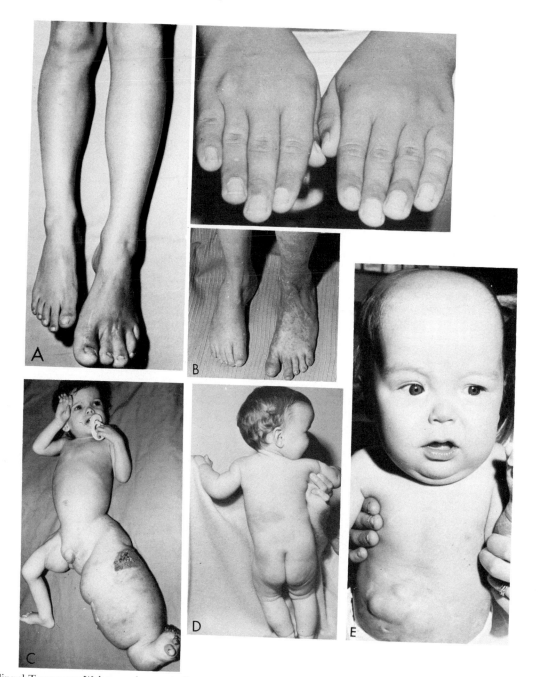

Klippel-Trenaunay-Weber syndrome. *A,* Fourteen year old showing asymmetric hypertrophy in legs, hands (note left fifth finger), and feet, with abnormal vasculature, as is evident in the dorsum of the left foot. *B,* Feet of a mentally deficient microcephalic boy showing left-sided hemangiomatous involvement and macrodactyly. *C,* Mentally normal girl with involvement of clitoris and right thigh and severe involvement of left leg with secondary intravascular clotting. The left leg was amputated, plastic surgery was done in the other involved areas, and the patient is vastly improved. *D,* Mentally normal girl with macrocephaly and hemangiomata in left trunk and lower limb. *E,* Young, normally functioning infant with macrocephaly and cavernous hemangioma in right upper abdomen.

PROTEUS SYNDROME

Hemihypertrophy, Subcutaneous Tumors,
Macrodactyly

This disorder was initially set forth as a clinical entity in 1983 by Wiedemann, who utilized the term proteus (after the Greek God Proteus, the polymorphous) to characterize the variable and changing phenotype of this condition. It has been suggested by Dr. Michael Cohen, Dalhousie University, Halifax, Nova Scotia, that John Merrick, the elephant man, most likely had the proteus syndrome.

ABNORMALITIES
Growth. Asymmetric overgrowth affecting any structure. Increased stature. Weight decreased for height age. Macrocephaly.
Skin and Subcutaneous Tissue. Generalized thickening. Hyperpigmented areas that appear to represent epidermal nevi. Lipomata. Lymphangiomata. Hemangiomata.
Skeletal. Hemihypertrophy. Bony prominences over skull. Angulation defects of knees. Scoliosis.
Hands and Feet. Macrodactyly. Soft tissue hypertrophy, which may appear as gyriform, changes particularly over plantar surfaces of feet.

OCCASIONAL ABNORMALITIES. Elongation of
neck and trunk. Broad, depressed nasal bridge. Ptosis. Strabismus. Epibulbar dermoid. Enlarged eyes. Myopia. Cataracts. Nystagmus. Pectus excavatum. Elbow ankylosis. Mental deficiency. Seizures. Lung abnormality. Muscle atrophy. Pelvic lipomatosis. Café-au-lait spots. Hyperostosis of external auditory canals and on alveolar ridges. Spondylomegaly. Megaspondylodysplasia. Coarse ribs and scapula. Cystic malformation of lungs.

NATURAL HISTORY. Frequently normal at birth, the characteristic features become obvious over the first year of life. Generally progressive throughout childhood, growth of the hamartomata and the generalized hypertrophy usually cease after puberty. Intellectual performance is usually normal. Morbidity is significant. Of 11 patients evaluated by Clark et al., two required amputation of a leg; six had fingers or toes removed; and two women had breast implants and reconstruction.

ETIOLOGY. Unknown. All cases have been sporadic events in otherwise normal families.

References

Cohen, M. M., and Hayden, P. W.: A newly recognized hamartomatous syndrome. Birth Defects, *15*(5B):291, 1979.
Wiedemann, H. R., et al.: The proteus syndrome: Partial gigantism of the hands and/or feet, nevi, hemihypertrophy, subcutaneous tumors, macrocephaly or other skull anomalies and possible accelerated growth and visceral affections. Eur. J. Pediatr., *140*:5, 1983.
Burgio, G. R., and Wiedemann, H. R.: Further and new details on the proteus syndrome. Eur. J. Pediatr., *143*:71, 1984.
Clark, R. D., et al.: Proteus syndrome: An expanded phenotype. Am. J. Med. Genet., (in press).

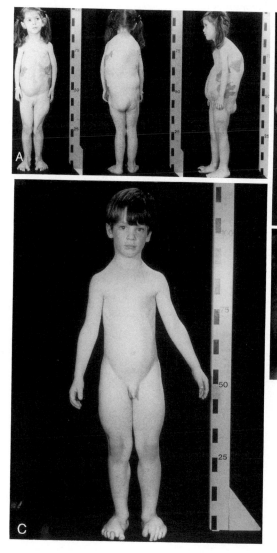

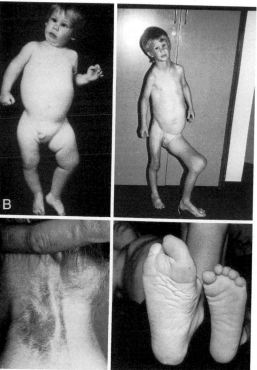

Proteus syndrome. *A*, Four and one-half year old girl with Proteus syndrome. Note the large, simple ears; the soft tissue masses, which have distorted the abdomen, left thigh, and back; and the splayed toes. The hemangiomata over the abdomen are flat, but dark vesicles are erupting. *B*, A boy with Proteus syndrome at eight months and at four years and eight months of age. Note the progression of the soft tissue tumors and leg asymmetry. Note also the linear sebaceous nevus on the back of the neck, the hypertrophied, overlapping toes, and the thickened, rugated plantar surface. *C*, Five year old mildly affected boy with increased subcutaneous tissue over the thighs and broad feet with splayed toes. (From Clark, R. D., et al.: Am. J. Med. Genet., *27*:99, 1987.)

MAFFUCCI SYNDROME

Enchondromatosis, Hemangiomata

Maffucci, in 1881, described a patient with dyschondroplasia and multiple cutaneous hemangiomata. More than 100 similar cases have been recorded subsequently.

ABNORMALITIES. Onset from the neonatal period to adolescence.

Skeletal. Variable early bowing of the long bones, with asymmetric retarded growth. Enchondromata (40 per cent unilateral) primarily in the hands, feet, and tubular long bones.

Vascular. Hemangiomata, most frequently located in the dermis and subcutaneous fat adjacent to the areas of enchondromatosis, but may occur anywhere. Types of hemangiomata are capillary, cavernous, and especially phlebectasia, which often have a grape-like appearance. Thrombosis of the dilated blood vessels with phlebolith formation occurs in 43 per cent of cases.

OCCASIONAL ABNORMALITIES. Lymphangiectasis, lymphangiomata, hemangiomata of the mucous membranes and gastrointestinal tract, other tumors, both malignant and benign and of mesodermal and nonmesodermal origin.

NATURAL HISTORY. The patients usually appear normal at birth, but within the first four years, hemangiomata appear, 25 per cent during the first year. Subsequent enchondromata formation is noted by adolescence. The disorder can be mild, but it is often severe enough to require multiple surgical procedures and occasionally amputation. About 26 per cent have fractures related to enchondromata. The risk of chondrosarcomatous change is about 15 per cent.

ETIOLOGY. Unknown. Sporadic occurrence.

References

Maffucci, A.: Di un caso di encondroma ed angioma multiplo: Contribuzione alla genesi embrionale dei tumor. Movimento Med. Chir., 3:399, 1881.

Bean, W. B.: Dyschondroplasia and hemangiomata (Maffucci's syndrome) II. Arch. Intern. Med., 102:544, 1958.

Lewis, R. J., and Ketcham, A. S.: Maffucci's syndrome. J. Bone Joint Surg. [Am.], 55:1465, 1973.

Sun, Te-Ching, et al.: Chondrosarcoma in Maffucci's syndrome. J. Bone Joint Surg. [Am.], 67-A:1214, 1985.

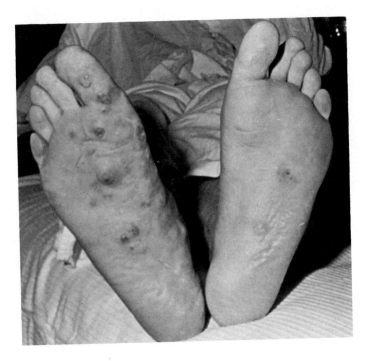

Maffucci syndrome. Note the enlarged right foot and the vascular lesions. These pictures were taken just following the removal of this man's right arm because of chondrosarcomatous change in an area of enchondromata. He had also had gastrointestinal bleeding episodes secondary to lower intestinal hemangiomata.

OSTEOCHONDROMATOSIS SYNDROME

(Ollier Disease, Enchondromatosis)

*Asymmetric Enchondromata
with Local Growth Deficiency*

Ollier described this disorder in 1899, and well over 100 cases have been reported.

ABNORMALITIES

Skeletal. Rounded masses of hyaline cartilage lead to fan-like radiolucencies in metaphyses, later diaphyses, and sometimes epiphyses. Usually bilateral but asymmetric, with limited growth of affected bones, which are most commonly the tubular long bones and sometimes the pelvis.

NATURAL HISTORY. The extremity may be short at birth, with no evidence of enchondromata. Asymmetric growth usually first noted at one to four years of age, with little progression after adolescence. The patients are prone to fractures.

An unknown, probably low risk of developing chondrosarcoma exists. Reactivation of growth in adult life should raise concern regarding malignant degeneration.

ETIOLOGY. Unknown. Usually sporadic, but does occur rarely in more than one member of a family.

References

Ollier, L.: De la Dyschondroplasia. Bull. Soc. Chir. (Lyon), *3*:22, 1899.

Margolis, J.: Ollier's disease. Arch. Intern. Med., *103*:279, 1959.

Mainzer, F., Minagi, H., and Steinbach, H. L.: The variable manifestations of multiple enchondromatosis. Radiology, *99*:377, 1971.

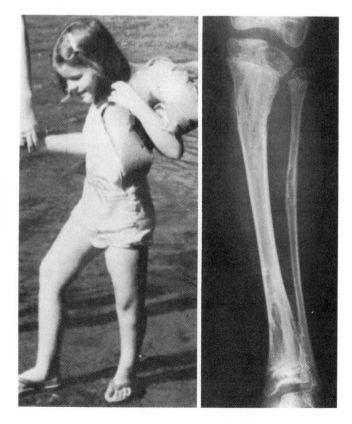

Osteochondromatosis syndrome. Six year old and roentgenogram of her left tibia. She had onset of leg shortness at two years of age. By 16 years of age she had suffered several fractures of the left leg and had developed scoliosis.

PEUTZ-JEGHERS SYNDROME

Mucocutaneous Pigmentation, Intestinal Polyposis

In 1896, Hutchinson described the pigmentary changes in an individual who later died of intussusception. Peutz clearly set forth the disease in 1921, and Jeghers et al. further established this disease entity in 1949. More than 180 cases have been documented.

ABNORMALITIES

Pigmentation. Vertical bands of epidermal pigment presenting as blue-gray or brownish spots on lips, buccal mucous membrane, perioral area, and sometimes digits and elsewhere.

Polyposis. Hamartomatous muscularis mucosae polyps in jejunum, sometimes in other mucus-secreting intestinal mucosa, and occasionally in nasopharynx, bladder, and bronchial mucosa.

Other Tumors. Rare granulosa cell tumor of ovary, sometimes associated with precocious puberty.

NATURAL HISTORY. The pigmentary spots appear from infancy through early childhood and tend to fade in the adult. Seventy per cent of patients have some gastrointestinal problem by age 20 years, most commonly colicky abdominal pain (60 per cent), intestinal bleeding (25 per cent), or both. Intussusception, which may spontaneously recede, is the most serious complication, and iron deficiency anemia may result from chronic blood loss. There is a definite but low risk of malignant transformation in the polyps, with carcinoma of the jejunum, duodenum, and stomach having been reported, as well as ovarian and testicular neoplasms. Almost one half of the patients with malignancy have been younger than 30 years of age. Clubbing of the fingers may occasionally occur in this disease.

ETIOLOGY. Autosomal dominant with a high degree of penetrance.

References

Hutchinson, J.: Pigmentation of the lips and mouth. Arch. Surg., 7:290, 1896.

Peutz, J. L. A.: Very remarkable case of familial polyposis of mucous membrane of intestinal tract and nasopharynx accompanied by peculiar pigmentation of skin and mucous membrane. Ned. Maanschr. Geneesk., *10*:134, 1921.

Jeghers, H., McKusick, V. A., and Katz, K. H.: Generalized intestinal polyposis and melanin spots of the oral mucosa, lips, and digits. A syndrome of diagnostic significance. N. Engl. J. Med., *241*:993, 1949.

Bartholomew, L. G., et al.: Intestinal polyposis associated with mucocutaneous pigmentation. Surg. Gynecol. Obstet., *115*:1, 1962.

Papaioannou, A., and Critselis, A.: Malignant changes in Peutz-Jeghers syndrome. N. Engl. J. Med., *298*:694, 1973.

Tovar, J. A., et al.: Peutz-Jeghers syndrome in children: Report of two cases and review of the literature. J. Ped. Surg. 18:*1*, 1983.

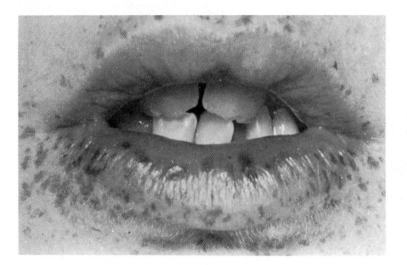

Peutz-Jeghers syndrome. Spotty pigmentation of lips and periorbital area in a child with intestinal polyps. (From Sheward, J. D.: Brit. Med. J., *1*:921, 1962.)

RUVALCABA-MYHRE SYNDROME

Macrocephaly, Polyposis of Colon,
Pigmentary Changes of the Penis

This disorder in two unrelated males was reported by Ruvalcaba et al. in 1980.

ABNORMALITIES

Growth. Macrosomia at birth, with normal adult stature.

Performance. Hypotonia. Severe mental deficiency in the initial two patients described. Normal I.Q. in three others.

Craniofacies. Macrocephaly, with ventricles of normal size.

Eyes. Prominent Schwalbe lines, prominent corneal nerves.

Intestines. Ileal and colonic hamartomatous polyps, similar to those found in Peutz-Jeghers syndrome; partial colectomy in one case at three years.

Penis. Tan, nonelevated spots on glans penis and shaft, first noted at two years of age.

OCCASIONAL ABNORMALITIES. Seizures, diabetes, exotropia, acanthosis nigricans and verruca vulgaris–type facial skin changes, café au lait spots, tongue polyps, lipoma, pectus excavatum, supernumerary nipples.

ETIOLOGY. Unknown. Autosomal dominant inheritance probable, based on mild expression in the mother of an affected male.

COMMENT. Electromyography in three patients showed evidence of a myopathic process, and muscle biopsy in four patients revealed a lipid storage myopathy with increased number of neutral lipid droplets.

References

Ruvalcaba, R. H. A., Myhre, S., and Smith, D. W.: A syndrome with macrencephaly, intestinal polyposis and pigmentary penile lesions. Clin. Genet., *18*:413, 1980.

DiLiberti, J. H., et al.: A new lipid storage myopathy observed in individuals with the Ruvalcaba-Myhre-Smith syndrome. Am. J. Med. Genet., *18*:163, 1984.

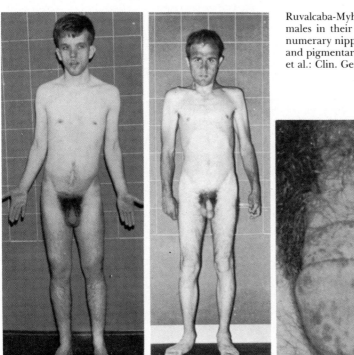

Ruvalcaba-Myhre syndrome. Two unrelated affected males in their twenties, showing macrocephaly, supernumerary nipples (left), scar from early colectomy (left), and pigmentary skin lesions. (From Ruvalcaba, R. H. A., et al.: Clin. Genet. *18:*413, 1980.)

GARDNER SYNDROME

Polyposis of Colon, Epidermal Cysts, Osteomata

Gardner and Richards set forth a complete evaluation of this disease in 1953. The hamartomatous lesions generally do not become evident until later childhood. More than 600 cases have been reported.

ABNORMALITIES

Intestine. Adenomatous polyps of colon, rectum, and occasionally stomach and small intestine.

Skin. Epidermal inclusion and/or sebaceous cysts, especially on back, scalp, and face. Sometimes fibromata, invasive desmoid, or both.

Bone. Osteomata of calvarium, mandible, face, and elsewhere, leading to bone deformation and cortical thickening.

Dentition. Dentigerous cysts, supernumerary teeth, delayed eruption of teeth.

Other. Multiple patches of congenital hypertrophy of retinal pigment epithelium.

OCCASIONAL ABNORMALITIES. Other hamartomata, including odontoma, leiomyoma, lipoma, trichoepithelioma, neurofibroma, carcinoma of thyroid, ampulla of Vater, and duodenal bulb. Desmoids are also likely to develop (41 per cent). Scoliosis.

NATURAL HISTORY. Hamartomata usually become evident between ten and 20 years of age; thereafter, there is grave danger of malignant change in the colonic adenomata, with the majority of affected individuals developing carcinoma of the colon between 19 and 50 years of age. The risk is of sufficient magnitude to warrant prophylactic colectomy in late childhood. Mesenteric fibromatosis and severe adhesions represent potential postoperative problems. The presence of congenital hypertrophy of the retinal pigment epithelium in some but not all families with the usual features of Gardner syndrome suggests genetic heterogeneity for this disorder. In those families in which the ocular defect is present, it can be helpful with recognition of the disorder prior to the development of other features.

ETIOLOGY. Autosomal dominant with high degree of penetrance.

References

Gardner, E. J., and Richards, R. C.: Multiple cutaneous and subcutaneous lesions occurring simultaneously with hereditary polyposis and osteomatosis. Am. J. Hum. Genet., *5*:139, 1953.

Weary, P. E., et al.: Gardner's syndrome. A family group study and review. Arch. Dermatol., *90*:20, 1964.

Leichtling, J. J.: Gardner's syndrome. Mt. Sinai J. Med. (N.Y.), *38*:311, 1971.

Pauli, R. M., Pauli, M. E., and Hall, J. G.: Gardner syndrome and periampullary malignancy. Am. J. Med. Genet., *6*:205, 1980.

Lewis, R. A., et al.: The Gardner syndrome. Significance of ocular features. Ophthalmology, *91*:916, 1984.

OSLER HEMORRHAGIC TELANGIECTASIA SYNDROME

(Hereditary Hemorrhagic Telangiectasia)

Epistaxes, Multiple Telangiectases

This entity was set forth in 1901 by Osler. The telangiectases contain dilated vessels having only an endothelial wall with no elastic tissue and a tendency toward arteriovenous fistulae. Over 264 affected families have been reported, and the incidence is about 1:50,000.

ABNORMALITIES

Vessels. Pinpoint, spider, and/or nodular telangiectases most commonly on tongue, mucosa of lips, face, conjunctiva, ears, fingertips, nail beds, and nasal mucous membrane; occasionally in gastrointestinal tract, bladder, vagina, uterus, lungs, liver, and/or brain.

OCCASIONAL ABNORMALITIES. Arteriovenous
fistulae in lungs, cirrhosis of liver, cavernous angiomata, port wine stain, and aneurysms. Vascular anomalies in brain.

NATURAL HISTORY. Epistaxes often occur in
childhood, and the telangiectases become apparent in later childhood and tend to enlarge, giving rise to increased frequency of hemorrhage. Intermittent brain hemorrhages may give rise to seizures, transient hemipareses, visual disturbances, and/or speech problems. Generally aggravated by pregnancy.

ETIOLOGY. Autosomal dominant with varying
expression.

References

Osler, W.: On a family form of recurring epistaxis, associated with multiple telangiectases of skin and mucous membrane. Bull. Hopkins Hosp., *12*:333, 1901.

Bird, R. M., et al.: Family reunion: study of hereditary hemorrhagic telangiectasia. N. Engl. J. Med., *257*:105, 1957.

Schaumann, B., and Alter, M.: Cerebrovascular malformations in hereditary hemorrhagic telangiectasia. Minn. Med., *56*:951, 1973.

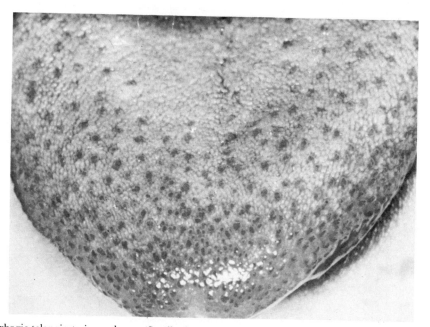

Osler hemorrhagic telangiectasia syndrome. Small telangiectases in the tongue of a girl who presented with cyanotic plethora secondary to multiple arteriovenous fistulae in the lung.

MULTIPLE NEUROMA SYNDROME

(Multiple Endocrine Neoplasia, Type 2b)

*Multiple Neuromata of Tongue,
Lips +/− Medullary Thyroid Carcinoma,
+/− Pheochromocytoma*

Initially felt to represent part of the spectrum of multiple endocrine neoplasia type II, this disorder is now recognized as a distinct entity referred to as type 2b.

ABNORMALITIES

Mucosa. Neuromata extending from lips to rectum and manifest by prominent lips, nodular tongue, involvement of nasal, laryngeal, and intestinal mucous membranes; thickened, anteverted eyelids.

Other Tumors. Medullary thyroid carcinoma, pheochromocytoma.

Skeletal. Marfanoid habitus, pes cavus, slipped femoral capital epiphyses, pectus excavatum, scoliosis.

Other. Tendency toward coarse-appearing facies.

OCCASIONAL ABNORMALITIES.

Slit lamp examination may reveal medullated nerve fibers in the cornea. Cutaneous neuromata and/or neurofibromata. Parathyroid hyperplasia; hypotonia. Developmental delay.

NATURAL HISTORY.

Oral neuromata are usually evident in childhood, with medullary thyroid carcinoma and/or pheochromocytoma becoming serious risks after adolescence. When medullary thyroid carcinoma is implicated, a total thyroidectomy should usually be done because the lesion is often multicentric. When pheochromocytoma is implicated, a thorough exploration should be accomplished, since it is often bilateral and may also be extra-adrenal. Constipation with megacolon often severe enough to suggest Hirschsprung's disease and/or diarrhea frequently develop before the endocrine neoplasms are detected.

ETIOLOGY.

Autosomal dominant inheritance with variable expression is implied, with the majority of cases presumed to be fresh mutations.

COMMENT.

An abnormal response to histamine skin test possibly related to diffuse enlargement of cutaneous nerves has been reported in patients with this disorder.

References

Gorlin, R. J., et al.: Multiple mucosal neuromas, pheochromocytoma and medullary carcinoma of the thyroid—a syndrome. Cancer, *22*:293, 1968.

Schimke, R. N., et al.: Syndrome of bilateral pheochromocytoma, medullary thyroid carcinoma and multiple neuromas. N. Engl. J. Med., *279*:1, 1968.

Carney, J. A., et al.: Alimentary tract ganglioneuromatosis. A major component of the syndrome of multiple endocrine neoplasia, type 2b. N. Engl. J. Med., *295*:1287, 1976.

Carney, J. A., et al.: Abnormal cutaneous innervation in multiple endocrine neoplasia, type 2b. Ann. Int. Med., *94*:362, 1981.

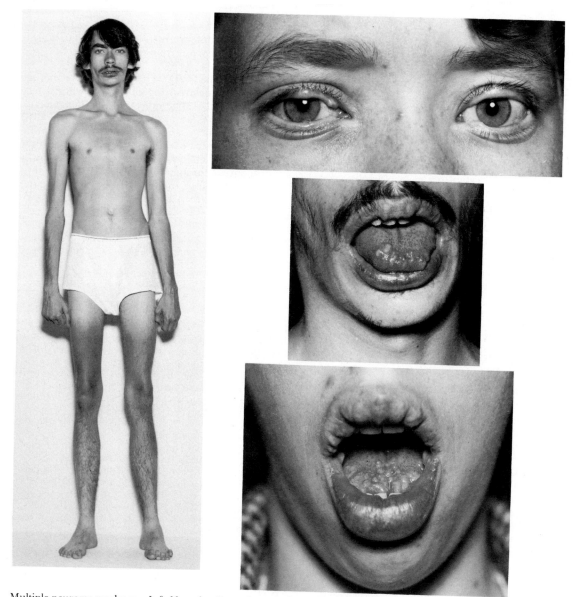

Multiple neuroma syndrome. *Left,* Note the slim asthenic habitus. *Right,* Multiple neuromata involving the conjunctiva and tongue and contributing to the prominent lips. (Courtesy of A. B. Hayles, Mayo Clinic, Rochester, Minnesota.)

GORLIN SYNDROME

Basal Cell Nevus (Carcinoma) Syndrome

Basal Cell Nevi, Broad Facies, Rib Anomalies

Though this condition had been previously described, it was Gorlin and Goltz who recognized the full extent of this pattern of malformation in 1960. Subsequently, more than 300 cases have been reported.

ABNORMALITIES

Performance. Variable mild to moderate mental deficiency, aberrant neurologic function and behavior.

Craniofacial. Frontoparietal bossing. Broad nasal bridge, mild prognathism.

Dentition. Dyskeratotic cysts of mandible, occasionally maxilla. Misshapen and/or carious teeth.

Hands. Short metacarpals, especially the fourth.

Thorax. Bifid, synostotic, and/or partially missing ribs. Scoliosis.

Skin. Basal cell nevi over neck, upper arms, trunk, and face, prone to become carcinomata. Punctate dyskeratotic pits on palms and soles. Milia, especially facial.

Ectopic Calcification. Falx cerebri, falx cerebelli.

Ovaries. Development of calcified ovarian fibromata.

OCCASIONAL ABNORMALITIES. Macrocephaly.

Internal strabismus, cataract, coloboma of iris, prominent medullated retinal nerve fibers, retinal atrophy, glaucoma, chalazion, inner canthal folds, telecanthus, hypertelorism, cleft lip with or without cleft palate, bony bridging of sella turcica, cervical and/or thoracic vertebral fusion, "marfanoid" build, arachnodactyly, hydrocephalus, small genitalia, bicornuate uterus, hypogonadism, cryptorchidism, postaxial polydactyly. Medulloblastoma, fibromata, lipomata, neurofibromata of skin, cardiac tumors, eyelid carcinomas. Anosmia.

Lymphomesenteric cysts that tend to calcify. Agenesis of corpus callosum.

NATURAL HISTORY. The basal cell nevi nodules gradually appear during childhood, with increase at adolescence. The nevi on the face may be papillomatous and are likely to occur around the lids. Malignant change is particularly likely after the second decade. The jaw cysts enlarge, especially in later childhood, and may recur following curettage. A constant vigil must be maintained for malignant transformation of the nevi or other tumors that are a common feature of this syndrome.

ETIOLOGY. Autosomal dominant, full penetrance. Older paternal age is a factor in fresh mutational cases.

References

Binkley, G. W., and Johnson, H. H., Jr.: Epithelioma adenoides cysticum: Basal cell nevi, agenesis of the corpus callosum and dental cysts. A clinical and autopsy study. Arch. Dermatol., *63*:73, 1951.

Gorlin, R. J., and Goltz, R. W.: Multiple nevoid basal-cell epithelioma, jaw cysts, and bifid ribs. A syndrome. N. Engl. J. Med., *262*:908, 1960.

Gorlin, R. J., et al.: The multiple basal-cell nevi syndrome. Cancer, *18*:89, 1965.

Ferrier, P. E., and Hinrichs, W. L.: Basal-cell carcinoma syndrome. Am. J. Dis. Child., *113*:538, 1967.

Codish, S. D., Kraszeski, J., and Pratt, K.: CNS developmental anomaly in basal cell nevus syndrome. Neuropaediatrie, *4*:338, 1973.

DeJong, P. T. V. M., et al.: Medullated nerve fibers: a sign of multiple basal cell nevi (Gorlin's) syndrome. Arch. Ophthalmol., *103*:1833, 1985.

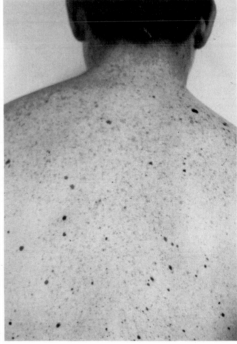

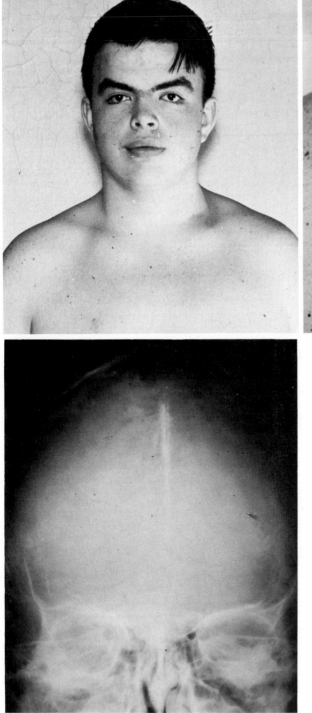

Gorlin syndrome. Fifteen year old. Note mineralization in falx cerebri. (From Ferrier, P. E., and Hinrichs, W. L.: Am. J. Dis. Child., *113*:538, 1967.)

MULTIPLE LENTIGINES SYNDROME

(LEOPARD Syndrome)

Multiple Lentigines, Pulmonic Stenosis,
Mild Hypertelorism, Deafness

Gorlin et al. recognized the multiple defect nature of this disorder and utilized the acronym LEOPARD to denote the **L**entigines, **E**KG abnormalities, **O**cular hypertelorism, **P**ulmonic stenosis, **A**bnormalities of genitalia, **R**etardation of growth, and **D**eafness. More than 70 cases have been described.

ABNORMALITIES

Cutaneous. Multiple 1- to 5-mm dark lentigines, especially on neck and trunk.

Cardiac. Mild pulmonic stenosis. Hypertrophic obstructive cardiomyopathy. Electrocardiographic changes of prolonged P-R and QRS, abnormal P waves.

Other. Mild growth deficiency, mild ocular hypertelorism, prominent ears, mild to moderate sensorineural deafness, winged scapulae, pectus excavatum or carinatum, late adolescence. Cryptorchidism.

OCCASIONAL ABNORMALITIES.

Mental deficiency, mandibular prognathism, café au lait spots, unilateral renal and/or gonadal agenesis or hypoplasia, hypogonadism, hypospadias, hyposmia, subaortic stenosis.

NATURAL HISTORY.

Lentigines differ from freckles in being darker of color, usually present at birth, and not related to sunlight exposure. They often increase in number with age and may occur in any cutaneous area. Many of the other features of the disorder are not readily apparent and must be searched for; examples are the deafness and cardiac findings. Hypogonadism may be secondary to hypogonadotropism; hence, these individuals should be followed closely at the age of adolescence in order to determine whether sex hormone replacement therapy is indicated.

ETIOLOGY.

Autosomal dominant with wide variability in expression, including lack of lentigines in an occasional patient.

References

Gorlin, R. J., Anderson, R. C., and Blaw, M.: Multiple lentigines syndrome. Am. J. Dis. Child., *117*:652, 1969.

Sommer, A., et al.: A family study of the LEOPARD syndrome. Am. J. Dis. Child., *121*:520, 1971.

Swanson, S. L., Santen, R. J., and Smith, D. W.: Multiple lentigines syndrome. J. Pediatr., *78*:1037, 1971.

Voron, D. A., Hatfield, H. A., and Kalkhoff, R. K.: Multiple lentigines syndrome. Case report and review of the literature. Am. J. Med., *60*:447, 1976.

St. John Sutton, M. G., et al.: Hypertrophic obstructive cardiomyopathy and lentiginosis: A little known neural ectodermal syndrome. Am. J. Cardiol., *47*:214, 1981.

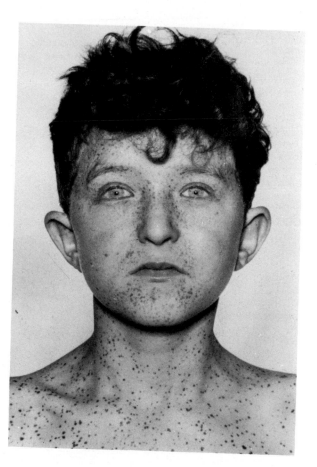

Multiple lentigines syndrome. Adolescent boy showing lentigines, prominent ears, and mild ocular hypertelorism. (From Gorlin, R. J., et al.: Am. J. Dis. Child., *117*:652, 1969.)

GOLTZ SYNDROME

*Poikiloderma with Focal Dermal Hypoplasia,
Syndactyly, Dental Anomalies*

This mesoectodermal disorder was recognized as a distinct entity by Goltz et al. in 1962, although well-described cases had been reported prior to that time. More than 50 cases have been documented.

ABNORMALITIES

Skin. Linear areas of hypoplasia with altered pigmentation, telangiectasis, lipomatous nodules projecting through localized areas of skin atrophy. Angiofibromatous nodules around lips and anus.

Nails. Dystrophic nails, narrow and/or hypoplastic.

Dentition. Hypoplasia of teeth, enamel hypoplasia, late eruption, and/or irregular placement.

Extremities. Syndactyly of fingers and/or toes, especially third and fourth fingers.

Eyes. Strabismus, coloboma, microphthalmos, and/or aniridia.

OCCASIONAL ABNORMALITIES. Moderate short stature, joint hypermotility, mental retardation, microcephaly, bulbar angiofibroma of eye, partial alopecia, congenital heart defects, hernia, skeletal asymmetry, scoliosis, hypoplasia or aplasia of clavicle, failure of pubic bone fusion, polydactyly, adactyly, hypoplasia of digit, cleft hand. Expansile, tumor-like bone lesions.

NATURAL HISTORY. The skin lesions are usually present at birth, although the skin lipomata and the lip and anal papillomata may develop later. No effective therapy is known except plastic surgery for the syndactyly and removal of the papillomata when indicated.

ETIOLOGY. Wodniansky reported partial expression in the mother and sibling of a patient. All other cases have been sporadic. The majority of cases have been females. The present hypothesis is that this is a single gene effect, usually lethal in the male; most cases represent fresh mutations, a situation similar to incontinentia pigmenti. There are many similarities between incontinentia pigmenti and Goltz syndrome, and it is tempting to consider the possibility that both diseases represent genetic alterations of a similar system.

References

Jenner, M.: Naeviforme, Poikilodermie—artige Hautveränderungen mit Missbildungen-(Schwimmhautbildungen an den Fingern, Papillome am Anus). 2 bl. Hautkr., 27:468, 1928.

Wodniansky, P.: Über die Formen der congenitalen Poikilodermie. Arch. Klin. Exp. Dermatol., 205:331, 1957.

Goltz, R. W., et al.: Focal dermal hypoplasia. Arch. Dermatol., 86:708, 1962.

Gorlin, R. J., et al.: Focal dermal hypoplasia syndrome. Acta Dermatovener. (Stockholm), 43:421, 1963.

Holden, J. D., and Akers, W. A.: Goltz's syndrome: focal dermal hypoplasia. A combined mesoectodermal dysplasia. Am. J. Dis. Child., 114:292, 1967.

Joannides, T., et al.: Giant cell tumor of bone in focal dermal hypoplasia. Br. J. Radiol., 56:684, 1983.

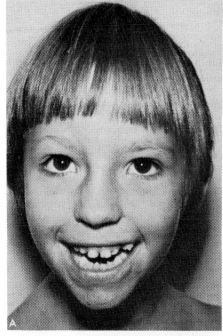

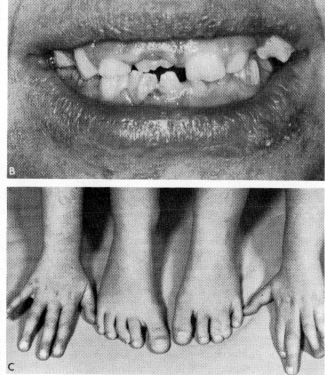

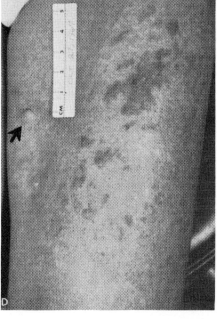

Goltz syndrome. *A*, Eleven year old girl. *B*, Late eruption of teeth with dental hypoplasia and malformation. *C*, Note the syndactyly of the left hand and foot. *D*, Thigh, showing irregular areas of altered pigmentation and of fatty herniation through loci of focal dermal hypoplasia (arrow).

DYSKERATOSIS CONGENITA SYNDROME

*Hyperpigmentation of Skin,
Leukoplakia, Nail Dystrophy, Pancytopenia*

Cole originally described this condition in 1930 and later summarized the findings. Over 50 cases have been reported.

ABNORMALITIES. Although hyperpigmentation of the skin may be present from birth, most of the abnormalities become apparent between five and 15 years of age. Growth deficit is mentioned, but poorly documented.

Skin. Irregular reticular brownish-gray pigmentation, with patchy atrophic areas of hypopigmentation. Hyperkeratosis and hyperhidrosis of palms and soles. May have bullae, telangiectasis.

Mucous Membranes. Premalignant leukoplakia may be found on lips, mouth, anus, urethra, and conjunctiva.

Eyes. Blepharitis, ectropion, and nasolacrimal obstruction with excessive tearing.

Nails. Dystrophy, which may progress to absence of nail.

Dentition. Carious, malaligned.

Hair. Tends to be sparse and fine; occasionally premature graying.

Hematologic. Pancytopenia.

Bone. Osteoporosis, possibly with relative fragility.

Genitalia. Testicular hypoplasia.

Other. Esophageal, anal, urethral, ureteral, and vaginal strictures and stenosis.

OCCASIONAL ABNORMALITIES. Mental deficiency. Hepatic cirrhosis. Immunologic abnormalities, including reduced antibody, tighter response to Vi antigen, failure to respond to skin sensitization, primary thymic dysplasia, hypogammaglobulinemia, impaired rosette formation by lymphocytes, and/or decreased lymphocytic response to mitogenic substances. Hodgkin's disease, adenocarcinoma of pancreas, deafness.

NATURAL HISTORY. The problem in affected tissues tends to become more severe with age, and most patients die before the fourth decade as a consequence of either pancytopenia or malignant transformation in the mucous membranes. When present, leukoplakic lesions should be excised as representing premalignant change.

ETIOLOGY. X-linked recessive inheritance in majority of familial cases. However, both autosomal recessive and autosomal dominant inheritance have been documented.

COMMENT. The dermatologic term dyskeratosis congenita obviously depicts only one feature of this abiotrophic type of disease with hamartomatous features, in which the affected individual develops hypoplasia and dysplasia in the skin, mucous membranes, marrow, and other tissues. The sibling of one patient and the niece of another patient died of leukemia, the latter case raising the question of whether there may be an increased likelihood of leukemia in the heterozygote carrying this mutant gene.

Considering the total pattern of abnormality, dyskeratosis congenita is clearly a different entity from the Fanconi syndrome of pancytopenia with congenital malformations.

References

Cole, H. N., Cole, H. N., Jr., and Lascheid, W. P.: Dyskeratosis congenita. Relationship to poikiloderma atrophicans vasculare and to aplastic anemia of Fanconi. Arch. Dermatol., 76:712, 1957.

Georgouras, K.: Dyskeratosis congenita. Aust. J. Derm., 8:36, 1965.

Addison, J., and Rice, M. S.: The association of dyskeratosis congenita and Fanconi's anemia. Med. J. Aust., 1:797, 1965.

Connor, J. M., and Teague, R. H.: Dyskeratosis congenita. Report of a large kindred. Br. J. Derm., 105:321, 1981.

DeBoeck, K., et al.: Thrombocytopenia: First symptom in a patient with dyskeratosis congenita. Pediatrics, 67:898, 1981.

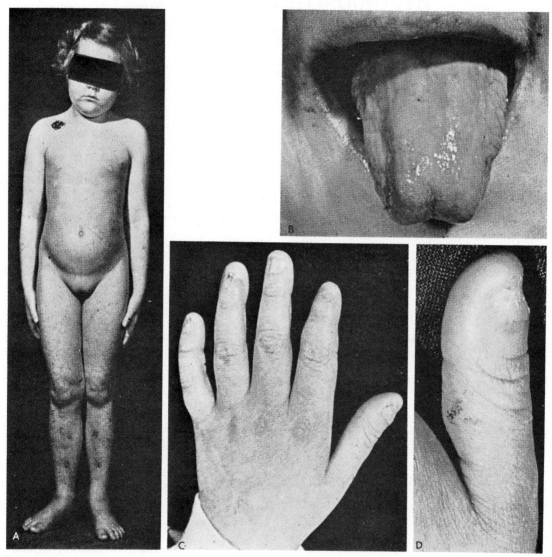

Dyskeratosis congenita syndrome. Eight year old patient showing reticulated skin pigmentation *(A)*, smooth tongue without leukoplakia as yet *(B)*, and nail hypoplasia to aplasia *(C and D)*. (Courtesy of K. Georgouras, Sydney, Australia.)

Q. ECTODERMAL DYSPLASIAS

HYPOHIDROTIC ECTODERMAL DYSPLASIA SYNDROME

Defect in Sweating, Alopecia, Hypodontia

There are a number of ectodermal dysplasia syndromes, of which only a few are represented in this text. The division into hypohidrotic and hidrotic categories on the basis of the extent of the deficit of sweat glands is in no way absolute. Just as there is variable hypoplasia of hair follicles, there is variable hypoplasia of sweat glands.

Thurman described this entity in 1848. In 1875, Charles Darwin set forth the following concise commentary about this disease: "I may give an analogous case, communicated to me by Mr. W. Wedderhorn of a Hindoo family in Scinde, in which ten men, in the course of four generations, were furnished, in both jaws taken together, with only four small and weak incisor teeth and with eight posterior molars. The men thus affected have very little hair on the body, and became bald early in life. They also suffer much during hot weather from excessive dryness of the skin. It is remarkable that no instance has occurred of a daughter being thus affected." In 1929, Weech clearly separated this condition from other clinical problems having ectodermal dysplasia as a feature. Over 130 cases had been reported by 1956.

ABNORMALITIES

Skin. Thin and hypoplastic, with decreased pigment and tendency toward papular changes on face; thin, wrinkled eyelids.

Skin Appendages. Hair: fine, dry, and hypochromic; sparse to absent. Sweat glands: hypoplasia to absence of eccrine glands; apocrine glands more normally represented. Sebaceous glands: hypoplasia to absence.

Mucous Membranes. Hypoplasia, with absence of mucous glands in oral and nasal membranes. Mucous glands may also be absent from bronchial mucosa.

Dentition. Hypodontia to anodontia. Anterior teeth tend to be conical in shape.

Craniofacial. Low nasal bridge, small nose with hypoplastic alae nasi, full forehead, prominent supraorbital ridges. Prominent lips.

OCCASIONAL ABNORMALITIES. Hoarse voice, hypoplasia to absence of mammary glands and/or nipples, absence of tears, failure to develop nasal turbinates, mild to moderate nail dystrophy, eczematous change in skin, asthmatic symptoms.

NATURAL HISTORY. Hyperthermia as a consequence of inadequate sweating not only is a serious threat to life but may be the cause of mental deficiency, which is an occasional feature of this disease. Living in a cool climate and cooling by water when overheated are important measures. The hypoplasia of mucous membranes plus thin nares may require frequent irrigation of the nares to limit the severity of purulent rhinitis. Otitis media and lung infection may also be consequences of the mucous membrane defect. Mucous glands have been hypoplastic to absent not only in the respiratory tract but in esophageal and colonic mucosa as well. Early roentgenologic evaluation may reveal the extent of dental deficit, and dentures are usually necessary. Though the patient is often hairless at birth, some hair may develop. For cosmetic purposes, a wig may merit consideration.

ETIOLOGY. X-linked recessive. Previous reports indicated that about 10 per cent of presumed heterozygous females show some overt expression. Utilizing direct visualization of dermal ridge sweat pores, Frias and Smith noted a diminished frequency of sweat pores in five of six heterozygous mothers of affected males, the latter having an absence of sweat pores. More recently, streaks devoid of sweat glands have been demonstrated along the lines of Blaschko, forming a v-shape over the back of carrier females. The majority of heterozygous females show some expression for the disease.

References

Thurman, J.: Two cases in which the skin, hair and teeth were very imperfectly developed. Medico-Chir. Trans., *31*:71, 1848.

Darwin, C.: The Variations of Animals and Plants under Domestication, 2nd ed. London, John Murray, 1875.

Weech, A. A.: Hereditary ectodermal dysplasia (congenital ectodermal defect). A report of two cases. Am. J. Dis. Child., *37*:766, 1929.

Lowry, R. B., Robinson, G. C., and Miller, J. R.: Hereditary ectodermal dysplasia. Symptoms, inheritance patterns, differential diagnosis, management. Clin. Pediatr., *5*:395, 1966.

Frias, J. L., and Smith, D. W.: Diminished sweat pores in hypohidrotic ectodermal dysplasia: A new method for assessment. J. Pediatr., *72*:606, 1968.

Happle, R., and Frosch, P. J.: Manifestations of the lines of Blaschko in women heterozygous for X-linked hypohydrotic ectodermal dysplasia. Clin. Genet., *27*:468, 1985.

Illustrations on pages 478 and 479

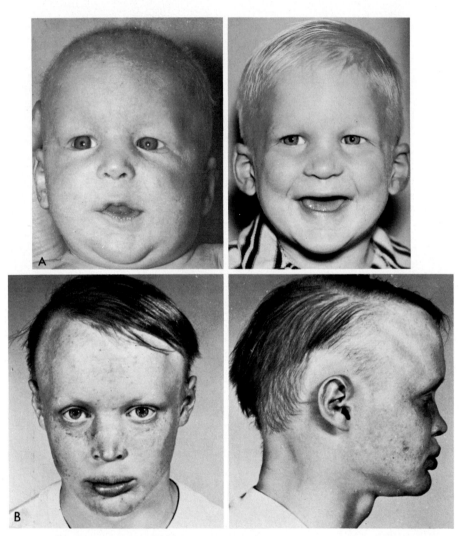

Hypohidrotic ectodermal dysplasia syndrome. *A*, Young infant; diagnosis made after hyperthermic episode. Same boy at two years of age. *B*, Older boy. The hypoplasia of the skin contributes to the prominent appearance of the lips. Note the midfacial hypoplasia.

Illustration continued on opposite page

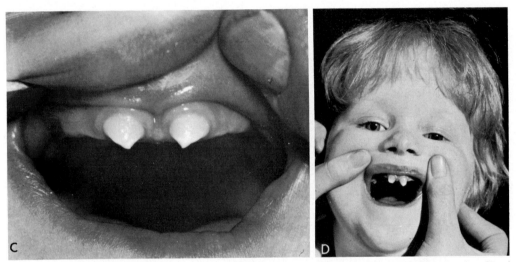

C, Hypoplasia of alveolar ridge in two year old. Hypoplastic conical incisors. *D*, Partial expression in a female.

AUTOSOMAL RECESSIVE HYPOHIDROTIC ECTODERMAL DYSPLASIA SYNDROME

Passarge et al. emphasized an autosomal recessive type of hypohidrotic ectodermal dysplasia, and Gorlin et al. summarized the findings in 18 such pedigrees. The clinical features have not been distinguishable from the X-linked hypohidrotic ectodermal dysplasia, except for the fact that females are as severely affected as males. The natural history is similar to that of X-linked hypohidrotic ectodermal dysplasia, although the patients may have a greater problem with ozena (foul, purulent nasal discharge). The parents have been normal.

References

Passarge, E., Nuzum, C.T., and Schubert, W.K.: Anhidrotic ectodermal dysplasia as autosomal recessive trait in an inbred kindred. Humangenetik, *3*:181, 1966.

Gorlin, R.J., Old, T., and Anderson, V.E.: Hypohidrotic ectodermal dysplasia in females. A critical analysis and argument for genetic heterogeneity. Z. Kinderheilkd, *108*:1, 1970.

Bartlett, R.C., Eversole, L.R., and Adkins, R.S.: Autosomal recessive hypohidrotic ectodermal dysplasia: Dental manifestations. Oral Surg., *33*:736, 1972.

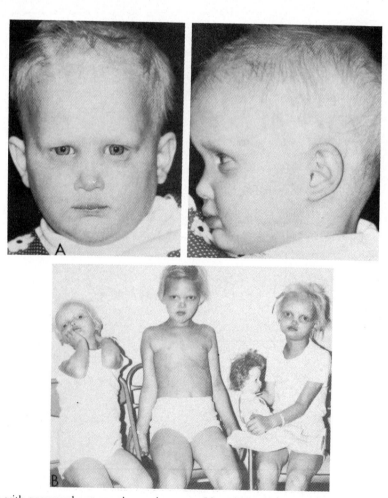

A, Female infant with presumed autosomal recessive type of hypohidrotic ectodermal dysplasia. *B*, Three affected sisters. (*B* From Passarge E., et al.: Humangenetik, *3*:181, 1966.)

RAPP-HODGKIN ECTODERMAL DYSPLASIA SYNDROME

(Hypohidrotic Ectodermal Dysplasia, Autosomal Dominant Type)

Hypohidrosis, Oral Clefts, Dysplastic Nails

Rapp and Hodgkin reported three affected individuals in 1968, and Summitt and Hiatt added one additional case.

ABNORMALITIES

Growth. Variable growth deficiency.
Skin. Thin, with hypohidrosis and sparse, fine hair. Pili torti.
Nails. Small, narrow, dysplastic.
Dentition. Hypodontia with small, conical teeth.
Face. Low nasal bridge, narrow nose, maxillary hypoplasia. High forehead.
Mouth. Small. Variable cleft of lip, palate, uvula.
Genitalia. Hypospadias.

NATURAL HISTORY. Liable to have hyperthermia in early childhood. Frequent occurrence of purulent conjunctivitis and otitis media, the latter presumably related to palatal incompetence.

ETIOLOGY. Autosomal dominant, although X-linked dominant inheritance is not excluded. Sweat pores present, but markedly reduced in number on the palms.

References

Rapp, R. S., and Hodgkin, W. E.: Anhidrotic ectodermal dysplasia: Autosomal dominant inheritance with palate and lip anomalies. J. Med. Genet., 5:269, 1968.

Summitt, R. L., and Hiatt, R. L.: Hypohidrotic ectodermal dysplasia with multiple associated anomalies. Birth Defects, 7(8):121, 1971.

Wannarachue, N., Hall, B. D., and Smith, D. W.: Ectodermal dysplasia and multiple defects (Rapp-Hodgkin type). J. Pediatr., 81:1217, 1972.

Silengo, M. C., et al.: Distinctive hair changes (pili torti) in Rapp-Hodgkin ectodermal dysplasia syndrome. Clin. Genet., 21:297, 1982.

Schroeder, H. W., and Sybert, V. P.: Rapp-Hodgkin ectodermal dysplasia. J. Pediatr., 110:72, 1987.

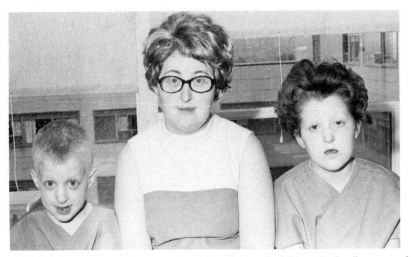

Rapp-Hodgkin ectodermal dysplasia syndrome. Affected mother and children in family reported by Rapp and Hodgkin. The mother is wearing a wig. Note the narrow nose, small mouth, and features of ectodermal dysplasia. (From Rapp, R. S., and Hodgkin, W. E.: J. Med. Genet., 5:269, 1968.)

TRICHO-DENTO-OSSEOUS SYNDROME

(TDO Syndrome)

Kinky Hair, Enamel Hypoplasia, Sclerotic Bone

Lichtenstein et al. defined this disorder in 107 individuals from one large kindred. Robinson et al. had previously described an autosomal dominant disorder with curly hair and enamel hypoplasia, +/− nail hypoplasia. Although it is not possible to be certain from the reported cases, the overall similarities suggest that they are the same disorder.

ABNORMALITIES

Hair. Kinky at birth.

Dentition. Small, widely spaced, pitted teeth with poor enamel, increased pulp chamber size (taurodontism).

Facies. Frontal bossing, dolichocephaly, squarish jaw.

Bone. Mild to moderate increased bone density, most evident in lateral roentgenograms of skull.

Nails. Brittle, with superficial peeling (about 50 per cent).

OCCASIONAL ABNORMALITY. Partial craniosynostosis.

NATURAL HISTORY. The hair sometimes straightens with age. The teeth become eroded and discolored, are prone to periapical abscesses, and are lost by the second to third decade. The sclerotic bone appears to be secondary to closely compacted lamellae and is rarely associated with any clinical symptomatology.

ETIOLOGY. Autosomal dominant. Elevated serum acid phosphatase level has been documented, although the significance of the finding is unknown.

References

Robinson, G. C., Miller, J. R., and Worth, H. M.: Hereditary enamel hypoplasia. Its association with characteristic hair structure. Pediatrics, *37*:489, 1966.

Lichtenstein, J., et al.: The Tricho-Dento-Osseous (TDO) syndrome. Am. J. Hum. Genet., *24*:569, 1972.

Shapiro, S. D., et al.: Tricho-Dento-Osseous syndrome. Am. J. Med. Genet., *16*:225, 1983.

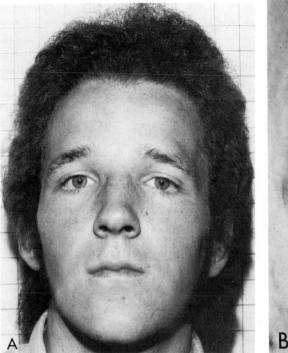

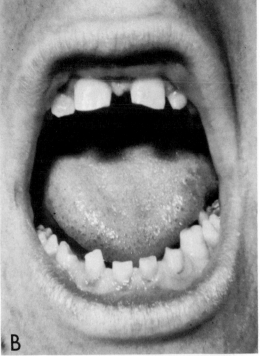

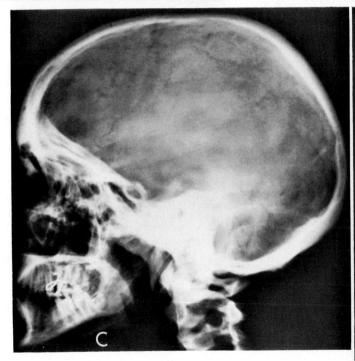

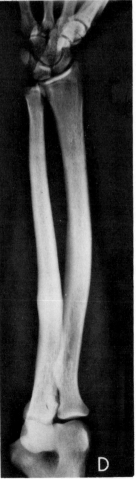

Tricho-dento-osseous syndrome. *A* to *D*, Young adult. Note the kinky hair, hypodontia, and increased bone density, especially at the base of the skull. (From Lichtenstein, J. R., et al.: Am. J. Hum. Genet., *24:*569, 1972.)

CLOUSTON SYNDROME

Nail Dystrophy, Dyskeratotic Palms and Soles,
Hair Hypoplasia

Clouston in 1939 reported 119 individuals in a French-Canadian family. Rajagopalan and Tay described an affected Chinese pedigree in 1977. Over 200 instances have been described.

ABNORMALITIES

Skin. Thick dyskeratotic palms and soles. Hyperpigmentation over knuckles, elbows, axillae, areolae, and pubic area.

Hair. Hypoplasia to alopecia (61 per cent).

Nails. Hypoplasia to aplasia, dysplasia.

Eyes. Strabismus.

OCCASIONAL ABNORMALITIES. Cataract, dull
mentality, short stature, thickened skull, tufting of terminal phalanges.

ETIOLOGY. Autosomal dominant.

References

Joachim, H.: Hereditary dystrophy of the hair and nails in six generations. Ann. Intern. Med., *10*:400, 1936.

Clouston, H. R.: The major forms of hereditary ectodermal dysplasia (with an autopsy and biopsies on the anhidrotic type). Can. Med. Assoc. J., *40*:1, 1939.

Wilkey, W. D., and Stevenson, G. H.: A family with inherited ectodermal dystrophy. Can. Med. Assoc. J., *53*:226, 1945.

Gold, R. J. M., and Scriver, C. R.: Properties of hair keratin in an autosomal dominant form of ectodermal dysplasia. Am. J. Hum. Genet., *24*:549, 1972.

Rajagopalan, K. V., and Tay, C. H.: Hydrotic ectodermal dysplasia: study of a large Chinese pedigree. Arch. Dermatol., *113*:481, 1977.

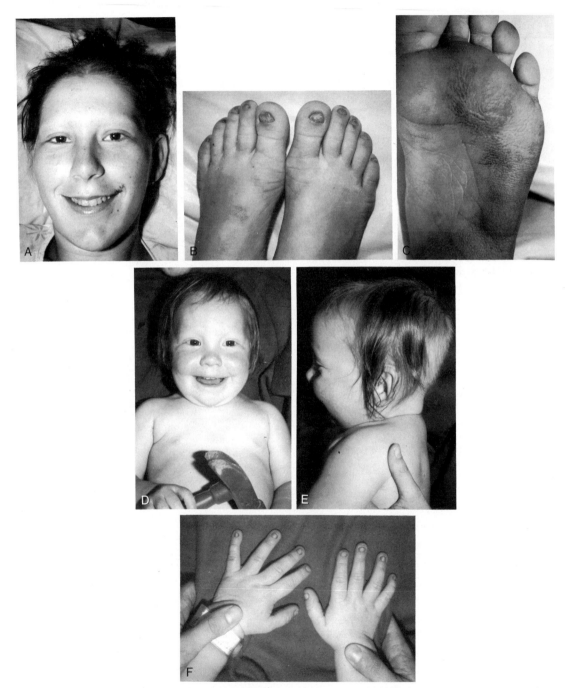

Clouston syndrome. *A* to *F,* Nineteen year old mother and her 22 month old daughter. Note the sparse hair, dysplastic nails, and dyskeratotic soles.

PACHYONYCHIA CONGENITA SYNDROME

Thick Nails, Hyperkeratosis, Foot Blisters

Pachyonychia congenita is an ectodermal dysplasia described by Jadassohn and Lewandowsky, in which there is excessive keratin and occasionally extra teeth.

ABNORMALITIES

Nails. Progressive thickening of anterior half. The nails may eventually be hypoplastic or even absent.

Skin. Patchy to complete hyperkeratosis of palms and soles, callosities of feet, palmar and plantar bullae formation in areas of pressure. Keratosis pilaris with tiny cutaneous horny excrescences. Epidermal cysts filled with loose keratin on face, neck, and upper chest.

Mucous Membranes. Leukokeratosis of mouth and tongue, especially in positions of increased trauma. Scalloped tongue edge.

Dentition. Erupted teeth at birth, lost by four to six months. Early eruption of primary teeth and early loss of secondary teeth due to severe caries.

OCCASIONAL ABNORMALITIES. Corneal thickening, cataracts, thickening of tympanic membrane, hyperhidrosis. Dry and sparse hair. Osteomata. Intestinal diverticula. Large joint arthritis. Bushy eyebrows. Hoarseness secondary to marked laryngeal obstruction.

NATURAL HISTORY. Manifestations are not present at birth. Usually the nails are grossly thickened by one year of age. Complete surgical removal of the nails is sometimes merited, although any matrix left behind will reform abnormal nails. Severe recurrent upper respiratory symptoms frequently lead to hospitalization.

ETIOLOGY. Autosomal dominant, with wide variability in expression. predominantly found in Slavs and Jews of Slavonic origin. The basic mechanism of the disease is unknown; however, vacuolization of the cytoplasm of nail matrix cells may be of significance.

References

Jadassohn, J., and Lewandowsky, F.: Pachyonychia congenita, keratosis disseminata circumscripta (folliculosis): tylomata; leukokeratosis linguae. Ikonographia Dermatologica, Tab., *629*, 1906.

Soderquist, N. A., and Reed, W. B.: Pachyonychia congenita with epidermal cysts and other congenital dyskeratoses. Arch. Dermatol., *97*:31, 1968.

Young, L. L., and Lenox, J. A.: Pachyonychia congenita. A long-term evaluation. Oral Surg., *36*:663, 1973.

Stieglitz, J. B., and Centerwall, W. R.: Pachyonychia congenita. (Jadassohn-Lewandowsky syndrome): A seventeen-member, four-generation pedigree with unusual respiratory and dental involvement. Am. J. Med. Genet., *14*:21, 1983.

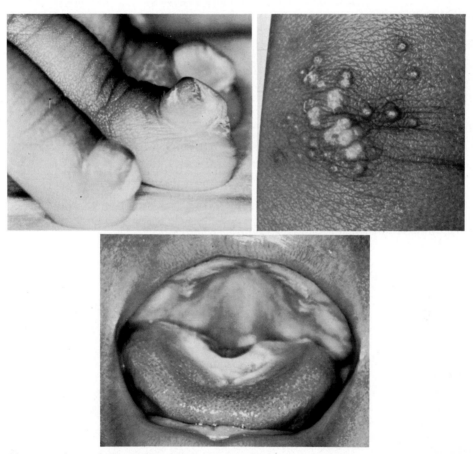

Pachyonychia congenita syndrome. Negro infant showing altered nails, cutaneous hyperkeratoses at knee, and leukokeratotic lesions on tongue and lateral palate.

PACHYDERMOPERIOSTOSIS SYNDROME

Thick Coarse Skin, Clubbing

This disorder was originally described by Friedreich in 1868 and further clarified by Touraine et al. in 1935.

ABNORMALITIES

Skin. Development of coarse, thick, oily skin, especially over upper face and scalp, with secondary cutis verticis gyrata and sometimes ptosis of the eyelids. Hyperhidrosis of hands and feet, peripheral vascular stasis. Seborrheic hyperplasia with thick stratum corneum.
Limbs. Clubbing with periostosis, most pronounced at tendinous insertions. Joint and muscle discomfort.

OCCASIONAL ABNORMALITIES. Papular mucinosis, large keloids. Resorption of distal phalanges of hands and feet.

NATURAL HISTORY. Earliest age of onset is about three years, with accentuation at adolescence and for a decade or so thereafter; more severe in males.

ETIOLOGY. Autosomal dominant, with wide variance in expression.

References

Friedreich, N.: Hyperostose des gesammten Skelettes. Virchow Arch. Path. Anat., *43*:83, 1868.
Touraine, A., Solente, G., and Golé, L.: Un syndrome ostéodermopathique: La pachydermie plicaturée avec pachypériostose des extrémités. Presse Med., *43*:1820, 1935.
Rimoin, D. L.: Pachydermoperiostosis (idiopathic clubbing and periostosis). Genetic and physiologic considerations. N. Engl. J. Med., *272*:923, 1965.
Hedayati, H., Barmada, R., and Skosey, J. L.: Acrolysis in pachydermoperiostosis. Arch. Intern. Med., *140*:1087, 1980.

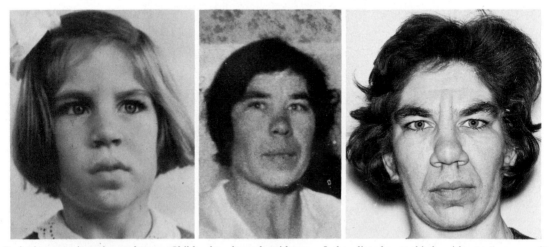

Pachydermoperiostosis syndrome. Child who showed evidence of the disorder at birth with an "acromegal" appearance. Although she was large as a child, her adult height was 5 feet, 6 inches. She had amenorrhea with a rudimentary uterus and small ovaries. The middle photo shows her at 30 years of age, with progression in the thickening of skin and hirsutism. Her mother, shown to the right, was similarly but less severely affected. (From Ursing, B.: Acta. Med. Scand., *188:*157, 1970.)

XERODERMA PIGMENTOSA SYNDROME

Undue Sunlight Sensitivity, Atrophic and Pigmentary Skin Changes, Actinic Skin Tumors

Xeroderma pigmentosa occurs in about one in 60,000 to 100,000 individuals.

ABNORMALITIES

Skin. Sunlight sensitivity with first exposure. Progressive skin atrophy with irregular pigmentation, telangiectases, angiomata, keratoses, and development of basal cell and squamous cell carcinomata, and less often keratocanthoma, adenocarcinoma, melanoma, neuroma, sarcoma, and angiosarcoma.

Eye. Photophobia. Recurrent conjunctivitis leading to keratitis and keratoconus and scarring leading to entropion, ectropion, or symblepharon.

Neurologic. Slowly progressive neurologic abnormalities sometimes associated with mental deterioration. Cerebral atrophy. Choreoathetosis, ataxia, and spasticity.

NATURAL HISTORY. Progressive disfigurement and tumors often by three to four years of age. Most patients die of malignancy before 20 years.

ETIOLOGY. Autosomal recessive. The majority of affected patients have a defect in the excision repair of ultraviolet radiation–induced DNA lesions. The defect is due to homozygosity for one of at least eight different mutations. Thus, XP patients fall into one of eight complementation groups (A through G plus a variant). Groups A, C, and D are most common. CNS problems are found in group A patients, who show the lowest level of DNA repair, whereas group C patients, who show the highest level of repair, are usually without overt neurologic disorders and have a longer life span. The severity of the skin and eye lesions relates more to the degree of sun exposure. The defect can be identified in cultured fibroblasts from amniocentesis.

The DeSanctis-Cacchione syndrome is a disorder that includes xeroderma pigmentosa, mental retardation, and hypogonadism. The XP complementation group is uncertain.

References

Rook, A., Wilkinson, D. S., and Ebling, F. J. G. (eds.): Textbook of Dermatology. Oxford and Edinburgh, Blackwell Scientific Publications, 1968.

Regan, J. D., et al.: Xeroderma pigmentosa: A rapid sensitive method for prenatal diagnosis. Science, *174*:147, 1971.

Pawsey, S. A., et al.: Clinical, genetic and DNA repair studies on a consecutive series of patients with xeroderma pigmentosa. Q. J. Med., *48*:179, 1979.

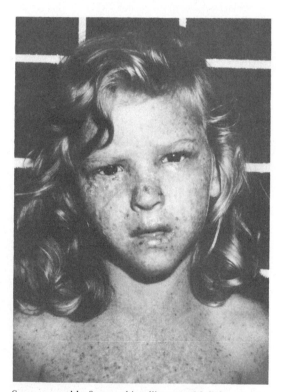

Seven year old of normal intelligence with light-sensitive xeroderma pigmentosa. (Courtesy of Dr. Robert Summitt, University of Tennessee College of Medicine, Memphis.)

SENTER SYNDROME

Ichthyosiform Erythroderma, Sensorineural Deafness

Senter et al. reported this disorder in a child in 1978 and recognized 12 similar patients from the literature.

ABNORMALITIES

Performance. Sensorineural deafness.

Growth. Postnatal growth deficiency.

Skin. Ichthyosiform erythroderma with mild lamellar ichthyosis and hyperkeratosis with thickened palms and soles. Variable alopecia. Decreased sweating.

Nails. Variable nail dystrophy.

Dentition. Variable malformations of teeth.

Eyes. Six of 12 patients developed inflamed vascularized corneas, which were replaced by transplants that also became vascularized.

Other. Cryptorchidism, variable flexion contractures. Tight heel cords.

ETIOLOGY. Unknown. One instance of affected siblings of normal parentage raises the possibility of autosomal recessive inheritance.

References

Senter, T. P., et al.: Atypical ichthyosiform erythroderma and congenital sensorineural deafness—a distinct syndrome. J. Pediatr., *92*:68, 1978.

Cram, D. L., Resneck, J. S., and Jackson, W. B.: A congenital ichthyosiform syndrome with deafness and keratitis. Arch. Dermatol., *115*:467, 1979.

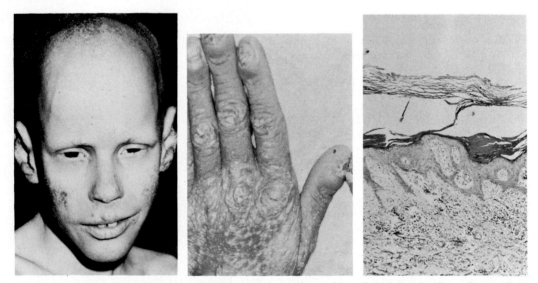

Senter syndrome. Eight year old showing alopecia, nail dystrophy, and lamellar ichthyosis. (From Senter, T. P., et al.: J. Pediatr., *92*:68, 1978.)

R. ENVIRONMENTAL AGENTS

FETAL ALCOHOL EFFECTS
(Fetal Alcohol Syndrome)

*Prenatal Onset Growth Deficiency,
Microcephaly, Short Palpebral Fissures*

In 1968, Lemoine of Nantes, France, recognized the multiple effects that alcohol can have on the developing fetus, including the more severe end of the spectrum, the fetal alcohol syndrome. Lemoine's report was not well accepted, and the disorder was independently rediscovered in 1973 by Jones et al. in the offspring of chronically alcoholic women. It is now appreciated as the most common major teratogen to which the fetus is liable to be exposed. In Gothenburg, Sweden, the studies of Olegaard et al. have shown that one in 300 babies is born with fetal alcohol effects, with one half of these having the fetal alcohol syndrome. They estimate that 10 to 20 per cent of mental deficiency with an I.Q. in the 50 to 80 range is a result of alcohol, and one in six cases of cerebral palsy is the result of heavy alcohol exposure in utero. Studies in Seattle and in Northern France have shown the incidence to be greater than one in 1000 babies born. Hence, ethanol is of major public health concern as a teratogen.

In 1973, Jones et al. delineated this disorder in eight unrelated children, all born to women who were severe chronic alcoholics prior to and during their pregnancy. Additional studies have confirmed the initial observations.

ABNORMALITIES. Variable features from among the following:

Growth. Pre- and postnatal onset growth deficiency.

Performance. Average I.Q. of 63. Fine motor dysfunction manifested by weak grasp, poor eye-hand coordination, and/or tremulousness. Irritability in infancy, hyperactivity in childhood.

Craniofacial. Mild to moderate microcephaly, short palpebral fissures, maxillary hypoplasia. Short nose, smooth philtrum with thin and smooth upper lip.

Skeletal. Joint anomalies including abnormal position and/or function, altered palmar crease patterns. Small distal phalanges. Small fifth fingernails.

Cardiac. Heart murmur, frequently disappearing by one year of age. Ventricular septal defect most common, followed by auricular septal defect.

OCCASIONAL ABNORMALITIES. Ptosis of eyelid, frank microphthalmia, cleft lip +/− cleft palate, micrognathia, protruding auricles, mildly webbed neck, short neck, cervical vertebral malformations (10 to 20 per cent), rib anomalies, tetralogy of Fallot, coarctation of the aorta, renal anomaly (10 to 20 per cent), strawberry hemangiomata, hypoplastic labia majora. Short fourth and fifth metacarpal bones. Meningomyelocele, hydrocephalus.

NATURAL HISTORY. There may be tremulousness in the early neonatal period. Postnatal linear growth tends to remain retarded, and the adipose tissue is thin. This often creates a "failure to thrive" interpretation. These individuals tend to be irritable as young infants, hyperactive as children, and more social as young adults. A ten year follow-up of eight of the 11 children initially diagnosed with this disorder indicates that four are mildly mentally retarded and are attending school in a combination of regular and remedial classes and four are severely handicapped. Problems with dental malalignment and malocclusion, eustachian tube dysfunction, and myopia have developed with time. The severity of the maternal alcoholism and the extent and severity of the pattern of malformation seem to be most predictive of ultimate prognosis.

ETIOLOGY. Ethanol or its byproducts. The least significant effect recognized at two drinks per day has been slightly smaller birth size (approximately 160 g smaller than average). It is not until four to six drinks per day are consumed that additional subtle clinical features begin to become evident. Most of the children believed to have fetal alcohol syndrome have been born of frankly alcoholic women whose intake is eight to ten drinks or more per day.

Text continued on page 494

Illustrations on pages 492 and 493

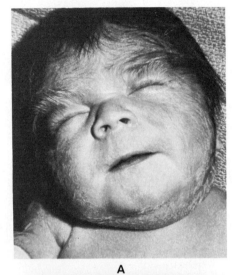

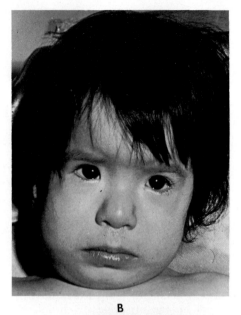

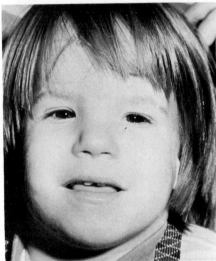

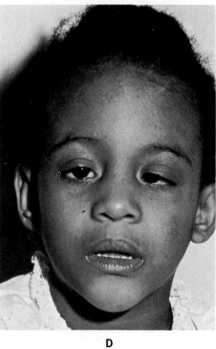

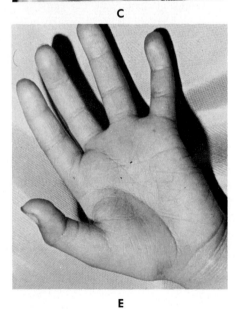

Fetal alcohol effects. Affected children of chronic alcoholic women; at birth (A), one year (B), two and one half years (C), and three years and nine months (D). Note the short palpebral fissures for all children, strabismus (B and D), ptosis of the eyelid (D), and facial hirsutism in the newborn (A). The hand shows mildly altered upper palmar crease patterning (E). (A from Jones, K. L., and Smith, D. W.: Lancet, 2:999, 1973; B–E from Jones, K. L., et al.: Lancet, 1:1267, 1973.)

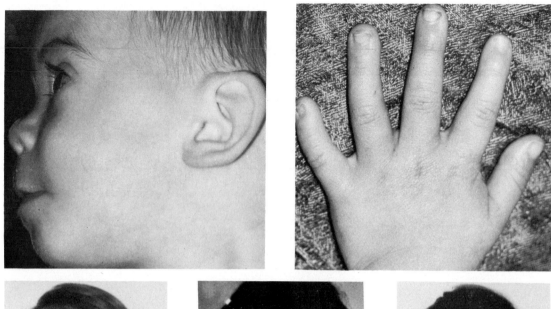

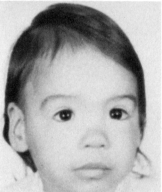

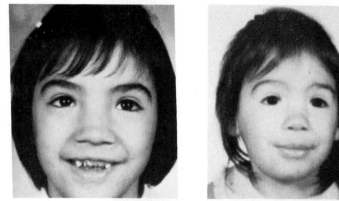

Fetal alcohol effects. *Upper,* Profile of an infant, showing short, upturned nose, thin upper lip, relatively small mandible, and prominent crus across concha of ear. There may be small nails, mild syndactyly, and relatively short fourth and fifth metacarpals. *Middle,* Change in facies in the same child from 18 months to two and one-half years to seven years of age. *Lower,* Twenty-two year old with fetal alcohol syndrome, still showing short palpebral fissures, smooth philtrum, and smooth upper lip. He is a pleasant individual, with an I.Q. of 65.

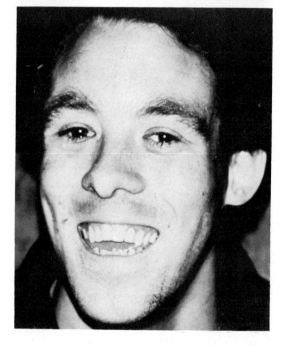

The risk of a serious problem in the offspring of a chronically alcoholic woman has been estimated to be 30 to 50 per cent, the greatest risk being for varying degrees of mental deficiency.

COMMENT. The most serious consequence of heavy prenatal alcohol exposure is the problem of brain development and function. Beyond diminished brain cell number and intelligence, there can be problems of malformation, which include heterotopias (faulty migration) of neurons and frank malformation of early brain.

References

Lemoine, P., et al.: Les enfants de parents alcoholiques. Ovest. Med., *21*:476, 1968.

Jones, K. L., et al.: Pattern of malformation in offspring of chronic alcoholic mothers. Lancet, *1*:1267, 1973.

Jones, K. L., and Smith, D. W.: Recognition of the fetal alcohol syndrome in early infancy. Lancet, *2*:999, 1973.

Jones, K. L., et al.: Outcome in offspring of chronic alcoholic women. Lancet, *1*:1076, 1974.

Majewski, F., et al.: Zur Klinik und Pathogenese der Alkohol-Embryo. Bericht über 68 Fälle. Munch. Med. Wochenschr., *118*:1635, 1976.

Clarren, S. K., and Smith, D. W.: The fetal alcohol syndrome; a review of the world literature. N. Engl. J. Med., *198*:1063, 1978.

Olegaard, R., et al.: Effects on the child of alcohol abuse during pregnancy. Acta Paediatr. Scand., *275* (Suppl.):112, 1979.

Smith, D. W.: The fetal alcohol syndrome. Hosp. Practice, *10*:121, 1979.

Jones, K. L.: Fetal alcohol syndrome. Pediatr. Review, *8*:122, 1986.

FETAL HYDANTOIN EFFECTS

(Fetal Dilantin Syndrome, Fetal Hydantoin Syndrome)

Although data suggesting the possible teratogenic effects of anticonvulsants were first presented by Meadow in 1968, convincing epidemiologic evidence of the association between hydantoins and congenital abnormalities awaited the studies of Fedrick and of Monson et al. Further studies by Speidel and Meadow and by Hill et al. have revealed a pattern of malformation that may include digit and nail hypoplasia, unusual facies, and growth and mental deficiencies.

ABNORMALITIES. Varying combinations of the following, with the fetal hydantoin syndrome representing the broader, more severe end of the spectrum.

Growth. Mild to moderate growth deficiency, usually of prenatal onset, but may be accentuated in the early postnatal months.

Performance. Occasional borderline to mild mental deficiency. Performance in childhood may be better than that anticipated from progress in early infancy.

Craniofacial. Wide anterior fontanel, metopic ridging, ocular hypertelorism, broad, depressed nasal bridge, short nose with bowed upper lip, broad alveolar ridge, cleft lip and palate.

Limbs. Hypoplasia of distal phalanges with small nails, especially postaxial digits; low arch dermal ridge patterning of hypoplastic fingertips; digitalized thumb; dislocation of hip.

Other. Short neck, rib anomalies, widely spaced small nipples, umbilical and inguinal hernias, pilonidal sinus, coarse profuse scalp hair, hirsutism, low-set hair line, abnormal palmar crease. Strabismus.

OCCASIONAL ABNORMALITIES. Microcephaly, brachycephaly, positional foot deformities, strabismus, coloboma, ptosis, slanted palpebral fissures, webbed neck, pulmonary or aortic valvular stenosis, coarctation of aorta, patent ductus arteriosus, cardiac septal defects, single umbilical artery, pyloric stenosis, duodenal atresia, anal atresia, renal malformation, hypospadias, micropenis, ambiguous genitalia, cryptorchidism, symphalangism, syndactyly, holoprosencephaly malformation sequence.

NATURAL HISTORY. The infants not uncommonly have relative failure to thrive during the early months for reasons unknown. Some improvement may be seen in the growth of nails and distal phalanges. The mild degrees of mental deficiency are the greatest concern. Those with the fetal hydantoin syndrome who show multiple hydantoin effects have an average I.Q. of 71.

ETIOLOGY. Although only the effects of phenytoin (Dilantin) have been sufficiently studied to warrant definite conclusions, closely related compounds should be regarded as potentially harmful to the fetus. Furthermore, there is evidence that combinations of hydantoins plus barbiturates may increase the risk to the fetus. The risk of the hydantoin-exposed fetus having the fetal hydantoin syndrome is about 10 per cent, and the risk for having some effects of the disorder is an additional 33 per cent. No dose response curve has been demonstrated, nor has a "safe" dose been found below which there is no increased teratogenic risk. Numerous studies now suggest that susceptibility of the fetus to the teratogenic effects of hydantoins depends on the fetal genotype. Inherited defects in phenytoin arene oxide detoxification may contribute.

References

Meadow, S. R.: Anticonvulsant drugs and congenital abnormalities. Lancet, 2:1296, 1968.

Aase, J. M.: Anticonvulsant drugs and congenital abnormalities. Am. J. Dis. Child., 127:758, 1970.

Speidel, B. D., and Meadow, S. R.: Maternal epilepsy and abnormalities of the fetus and newborn. Lancet, 2:839, 1972.

Fedrick, J.: Epilepsy and pregnancy: A report from the Oxford Record Linkage Study. Br. Med. J., 2:442, 1973.

Monson, R. R., et al.: Diphenylhydantoin and selected congenital malformations. N. Engl. J. Med., 289:1049, 1973.

Hill, R. M., et al.: Infants exposed in utero to antiepileptic drugs. Am. J. Dis. Child., 127:645, 1974.

Hanson, J. W., and Smith, D. W.: The fetal hydantoin syndrome. J. Pediatr., 87:285, 1975.

Hanson, J. W., et al.: Risks to the offspring of women treated with hydantoin anticonvulsant, with emphasis on the fetal hydantoin syndrome. J. Pediatr., 89:662, 1976.

Phelen, M. C., Pellock, J. M., and Nance, W. E.: Discordant expression of fetal hydantoin syndrome in heteropaternal dizygotic twins. N. Engl. J. Med., 307:99, 1982.

Buehler, B.: Epoxide hydralase activity and fetal hydantoin syndrome. Proc. Greenwood Genet. Center, 2:277, 1983.

Finnell, R. H., and Chernoff, G. F.: Editorial comment: Genetic background: The elusive component in the fetal hydantoin syndrome. Am. J. Med. Genet., 19:459, 1984.

Strickler, S. M., et al.: Genetic predisposition to phenytoin-induced birth defects. Lancet, 2:746, 1985.

Illustrations on pages 496 to 499

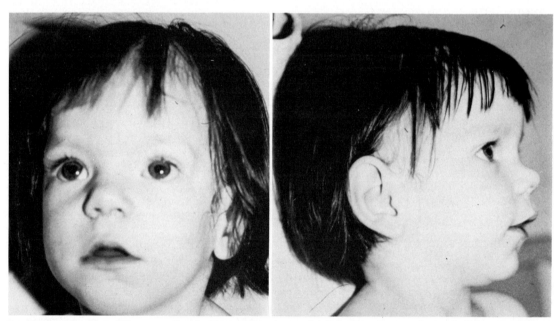

Fetal hydantoin effects. Fifteen month old with growth and mental deficiencies whose mother took diphenylhydantoin and phenobarbital throughout pregnancy. Note the hypoplastic nails and phalanges, mild ptosis, relatively low and broad nasal bridge, and coarse hair. (Courtesy of J. Hanson, University of Iowa, Iowa City.)

Illustration continued on opposite page

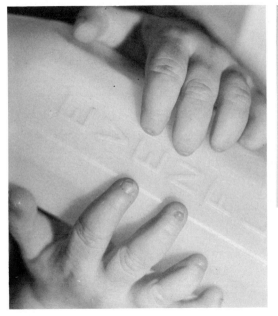

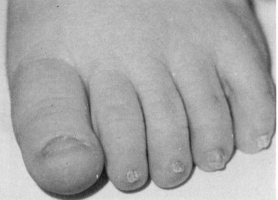

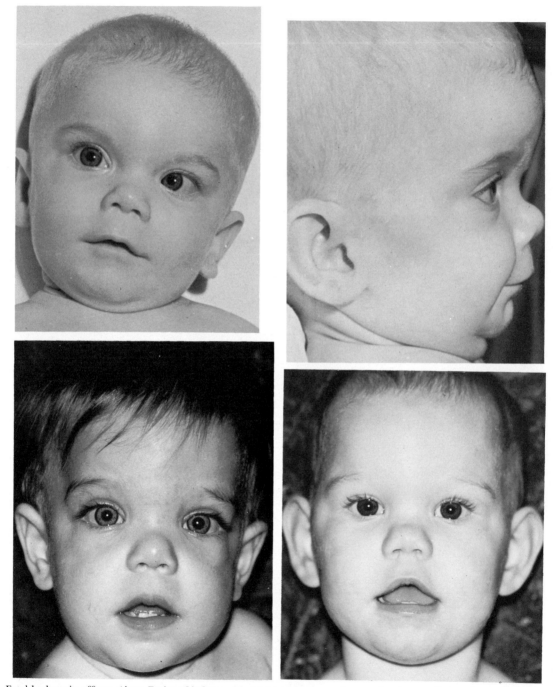

Fetal hydantoin effects. *Above,* Facies of infants with fetal hydantoin syndrome, showing small nose, low nasal bridge with hypertelorism, strabismus, and bowed upper lip. The child in the lower right was exposed to high levels of both alcohol and hydantoin.

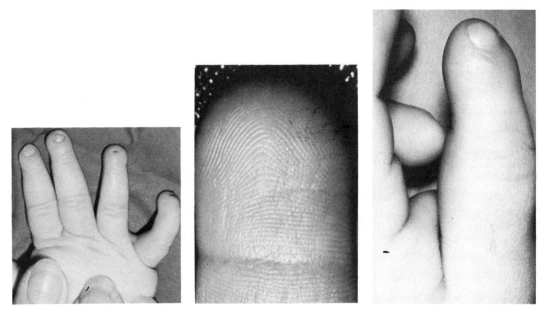

Fetal hydantoin effects. Nail hypoplasia, most severe on ulnar side, low arch dermal ridge patterning, and occasional finger-like thumb.

FETAL TRIMETHADIONE EFFECTS

(Fetal Trimethadione Syndrome, Tridione Syndrome)

In 1970, German et al. reported significant abnormalities among the offspring of four women treated with trimethadione or paramethadione. Feldman et al. summarized the results of 53 pregnancies in which the mother was treated during the first trimester with either trimethadione or paramethadione.

ABNORMALITIES. Varying features from among the following:
Performance. Mental deficiency, speech disorders.
Growth. Prenatal onset growth deficiency.
Craniofacial. Mild brachycephaly. Mild midfacial hypoplasia, short upturned nose with broad and low nasal bridge, prominent forehead, mild synophrys with unusual upslant to eyebrows. Strabismus, ptosis, epicanthal folds. Cleft lip and palate, high arched palate, micrognathia. Poorly developed rectangular or cupped and overlapping helix.
Cardiovascular. Septal defects, tetralogy of Fallot.
Genitourinary. Ambiguous genitalia, hypospadias, clitoral hypertrophy.
Limbs. Simian crease.

OCCASIONAL ABNORMALITIES. Facial hemangiomata, webbed neck, scoliosis, transposition of the great vessels, hypoplastic heart, pyloric stenosis, renal anomalies, umbilical and inguinal hernias, hearing and visual deficits, dislocated hip.

NATURAL HISTORY. Mental deficiency and serious cardiac defects give many cases a poor prognosis.

ETIOLOGY. Both trimethadione and its congener paramethadione have been associated with a similar constellation of defects. Of the 53 pregnancies reviewed by Feldman et al., 13 resulted in spontaneous abortion, and 83 per cent of the live-born infants had at least one major malformation, 14 of which led to death.

COMMENT. The frequency and severity of defects associated with maternal use of these drugs during pregnancy are high enough to warrant consideration of early elective termination of pregnancy.

References

German, J., Lowal, A., and Ehlers, K. H.: Trimethadione and human teratogenesis. Teratology, 3:349, 1970.
Zackai, E., et al.: The fetal trimethadione syndrome. J. Pediatr., 87:280, 1975.
Feldman, G. L., Weaver, D. D., and Lovrien, E. W.: The fetal trimethadione syndrome. Am. J. Dis. Child, 131:1389, 1977.

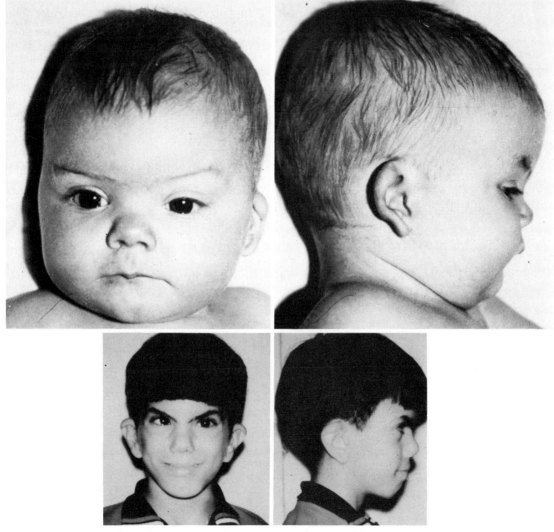

Fetal trimethadione effects. *Above,* Five month old with tetralogy of Fallot whose mother took trimethadione throughout pregnancy. Note ear malformation, hypoplastic midface, and unusual eyebrow configuration. (Courtesy of J. Hanson, University of Iowa, Iowa City.) *Below,* Ten year old with speech delay whose mother took trimethadione during pregnancy. Note ear malformation, unusual slant to eyebrows, and strabismus. (Courtesy of E. Zackai, Philadelphia Children's Hospital.)

FETAL VALPROATE EFFECTS

Concern was raised regarding prenatal valproic acid exposure in 1982 by Robert and Guiband, who documented an association between maternal ingestion of valproic acid and meningomyelocele in the offspring. DiLiberti et al. and Hanson et al. set forth a broader pattern of malformation in 1984.

ABNORMALITIES

Craniofacies. Narrow bifrontal diameter. High forehead. Epicanthal folds connecting with an infraorbital crease or groove; telecanthus; broad, low nasal bridge with short nose and anteverted nostrils. Midface hypoplasia. Long philtrum with a thin vermilion border. Relatively small mouth.

Cardiovascular. Aortic coarctation. Hypoplastic left heart. Aortic valve stenosis. Interrupted aortic arch. Secundum type atrial septal defect. Pulmonary atresia without ventricular septal defect. Perimembranous ventricular septal defect.

Limbs. Long, thin fingers and toes. Hyperconvex fingernails.

Other. Meningomyelocele. Cleft lip.

OCCASIONAL ABNORMALITIES.
Growth and mental deficiencies. Supernumerary nipples. Hypospadius. Inguinal and umbilical hernias. Broad chest. Bifid rib. Triphalangeal thumbs.

NATURAL HISTORY. Insufficient data are available to make any definitive conclusions regarding the long-term effects of prenatal valproic acid exposure.

ETIOLOGY. Prenatal valproic acid exposure. In a recent study of 14 prospectively ascertained infants exposed prenatally to valproic acid alone, almost half were distressed during labor, and 28 per cent had low Apgar scores. Four of the 14 had a pattern of malformation consistent with the fetal valproate syndrome.

References

Robert, E., and Guiband, P.: Maternal valproic acid and congenital neural tube defects. Lancet, 2:934, 1982.

DiLiberti, J. H., et al.: The fetal valproate syndrome. Am. J. Med. Genet., 19:473, 1984.

Hanson, J. W., et al.: Effects of valproic acid on the fetus. Pediatr. Res., 18:306A, 1984.

Ardinger, H. H., Clark, E. B., and Hanson, J. W.: Cardiac malformations associated with fetal valproic acid exposure. David W. Smith Meeting; Malformations and Morphogenesis; Santa Fe, New Mexico, 1985.

Jager-Roman, E., et al.: Fetal growth, major malformations, and minor anomalies in infants born to women receiving valproic acid. J. Pediatr., 108:997, 1986.

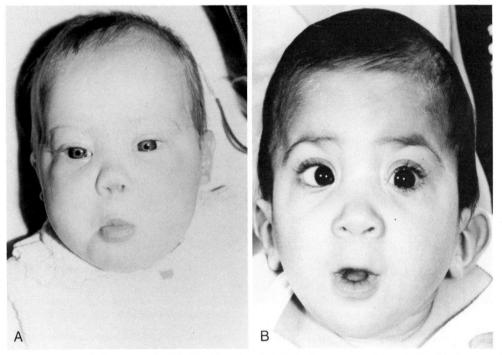

Fetal valproate effects. *A*, Seven month old girl with epicanthal folds that connect with an infraorbital crease, short nose, long philtrum, and small mouth. *B*, Ten month old boy with a short nose, long philtrum with a thin vermillion border, and a relatively small mouth. (From Diliberti, J. H., et al.: Am. J. Med. Genet., *19:*473, 1984.)

FETAL WARFARIN EFFECTS

(Warfarin Embryopathy, Fetal Warfarin Syndrome)

Nasal Hypoplasia, Stippled Epiphyses,
Coumarin Derivative Exposure in First Trimester

Isolated reports of infants who, in retrospect, were affected by warfarin were followed in 1975 by simultaneous recognition of this association in five infants. At least 29 infants are known to have been affected.

ABNORMALITIES

Facies. Nasal hypoplasia and depressed nasal bridge (29/29), often with a deep groove between the alae nasi and nasal tip.

Skeletal. Stippling of uncalcified epiphyses (24/24), particularly of axial skeleton, at the proximal femora and in the calcanei; stippling disappears after the first year.

Limbs. Mild hypoplasia of the nails and shortened fingers (12/24).

Growth. Low birth weight (10/23); most demonstrate catch-up growth.

Performance. Significant retardation in 5/16.

OCCASIONAL ABNORMALITIES. CNS and eye abnormalities, including microcephaly, hydrocephalus, Dandy-Walker malformation, agenesis of corpus callosum; optic atrophy, microphthalmia, Peter anomaly of eye. Severe rhizomelia, scoliosis, congenital heart defect.

NATURAL HISTORY. Infants often present with upper airway obstruction, which is relieved by the placement of an oral airway. Seven infants have died and five are significantly retarded; the others have done well except for persistent cosmetic malformation of the nose. The stippling is incorporated into the calcifying epiphyses and has resulted in few problems.

ETIOLOGY. Although the critical period of coumarin exposure is between six and nine weeks' gestation, controversy exists regarding second and third trimester exposure. Previous studies have suggested that the central nervous system abnormalities are associated with exposure limited to the second or third trimester and are related to secondary disruption of CNS architecture most likely due to hemorrhage. However, a recent case report suggests that prenatal coumarin exposure between the eighth and twelfth weeks of gestation can lead to CNS abnormalities, indicating a direct teratogenic effect on CNS morphogenesis. Furthermore, three recent prospective studies of children exposed during the second and third trimesters revealed no evidence of central nervous system or eye abnormalities, suggesting that the incidence of CNS problems in babies born to women receiving coumarin limited to the later two trimesters must be exceedingly low.

COMMENT. An estimate of the overall risk in pregnancies in which coumarin derivatives are used is that about two thirds will have a normal outcome, with the others ending in the birth of infants with fetal warfarin syndrome and CNS effects or in spontaneous abortion.

The fetal warfarin syndrome shares many features with various forms of chondrodysplasia punctata. It is critical that this differentiation be made for counseling purposes.

References

DiSaia, P. J.: Pregnancy and delivery of a patient with a Starr-Edwards mitral valve prosthesis. Report of a case. Obstet. Gynecol., *28*:469, 1966.

Kerber, I. J., Warr, O. S., and Richardson, C.: Pregnancy in a patient with a prosthetic mitral valve. J.A.M.A., *203*:223, 1968.

Becker, M. H., et al.: Chondrodysplasia punctata. Is maternal warfarin a factor? Am. J. Dis. Child., *129*:356, 1975.

Pettifor, J. M., and Benson, R.: Congenital malformations associated with the administration of oral anticoagulants during pregnancy. J. Pediatr., *86*:459, 1975.

Shaul, W. L., Emery, H., and Hall, J. G.: Chondrodysplasia punctata and maternal warfarin use during pregnancy. Am. J. Dis. Child., *129*:360, 1975.

Hall, J. G., Pauli, R. M., and Wilson, K. M.: Maternal and fetal sequelae of anticoagulation during pregnancy. Am. J. Med., *68*:122, 1980.

Kaplan, L. C.: Congenital Dandy Walker malformation associated with first trimester warfarin: A case report and literature review. Teratology, *32*:333, 1985.

Iturbe-Alessio, I., et al.: Risks of anticoagulant therapy in pregnant women with artificial heart valves. N. Engl. J. Med., *315*:1390, 1986.

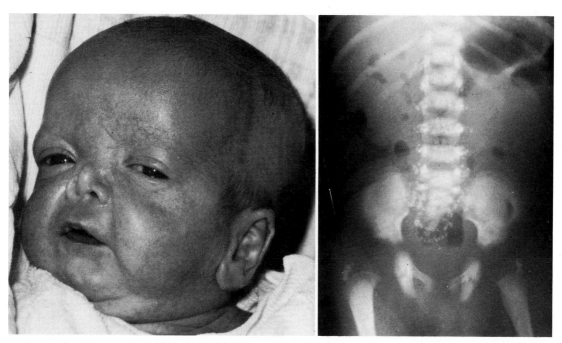

Fetal warfarin effects. Patient at five days of age. Note hypoplastic nose with low nasal bridge and broad, flat face. Roentgenogram at one day of age showing stippling along the vertebral column, in the sacral area, and in proximal femurs. Stippling was also noted in the cervical vertebrae, acromion process, and tarsal bones. (From Shaul, W. L., Emery, H., and Hall, J. G.: Am. J. Dis. Child., *129*:360, 1975.)

FETAL AMINOPTERIN EFFECTS

Cranial Dysplasia, Broad Nasal Bridge,
Low-Set Ears

The folic acid antagonist aminopterin has occasionally been utilized as an abortifacient during the first trimester of pregnancy. Thiersch first noted abnormal morphogenesis in three abortuses and one full-term offspring of mothers who received aminopterin from four to nine weeks following the presumed time of conception. Subsequently, other cases have been published, including an account of toxicity secondary to methotrexate, the methyl derivative of aminopterin. The apparent dosage of the folic acid antagonist has ranged from 12 to 30 mg, and it was taken between four and ten weeks of gestation. The similar pattern of malformation has consisted of cranial dysplasia, foot anomalies, and other less consistent defects.

ABNORMALITIES. Variable features, based on five cases.
Growth. Prenatal onset growth deficiency. Microcephaly.
Craniofacial. Severe hypoplasia of frontal bone, parietal bones, temporal or occipital bones, wide fontanels, and synostosis of lambdoid or coronal sutures. Upsweep of frontal scalp hair. Broad nasal bridge, shallow supraorbital ridges, prominent eyes, micrognathia, cleft palate, low-set ears, maxillary hypoplasia, epicanthal folds.
Limbs. Relative shortness, especially of forearm (mesomelia). Talipes equinovarus, hypodactyly, synostosis.

OCCASIONAL ABNORMALITIES. Cleft palate, dislocation of hip, retarded ossification of pubis and ischium, rib anomalies, short thumbs, partial syndactyly of third and fourth fingers, single crease on fifth finger, dextroposition of the heart, hypotonia.

NATURAL HISTORY. Although fetal or early postnatal death has been the more usual outcome, at least several patients have survived beyond the first year of age. One was described as slow in growth but within normal limits in mental and motor performance at 15 months of age. E. B. Shaw of San Francisco has observed a 17 year old affected girl with normal intelligence.

References

Thiersch, J. B.: Therapeutic abortions with a folic acid antagonist, 4-aminopteroylglutamic acid (4-amino P.G.A.) administered by the oral route. Am. J. Obstet. Gynec., *63*:1298, 1952.

Milunsky, A., Graef, J. W., and Gaynor, M. F., Jr.: Methotrexate induced congenital malformations with a review of the literature. J. Pediatr., *72*:790, 1968.

Shaw, E. B., and Steinbach, H. L.: Aminopterin-induced fetal malformation. Am. J. Dis. Child., *115*:477, 1968.

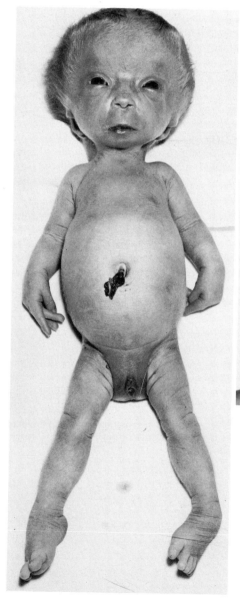

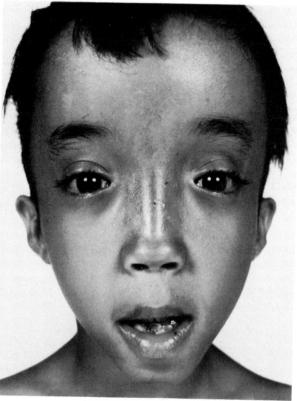

Fetal aminopterin effects. *Left*, Affected newborn weighing 1.3 kg at 42 weeks' gestation (From Warkany, J., et al.: Am. J. Dis. Child., *97*:274, 1959.) *Right*, Affected boy. (Courtesy of Dr. Noreen L. Rudd, Toronto.)

RETINOIC ACID EMBRYOPATHY

(Accutane Embryopathy)

CNS Defects, Microtia, Cardiac Defects

First licensed in the United States in September, 1982, with the brand name Accutane, isotretinoin (13-*cis*-retinoic acid) was initially recognized to be a human teratogen one year later. Lammer et al. have recently estimated the risk for major malformations in prenatally exposed children and have set forth the spectrum of structural defects. Of 21 affected infants, 17 had defects of the craniofacies, 12 had cardiac defects, 18 had altered morphogenesis of the CNS, and seven had anomalies of thymic development.

ABNORMALITIES

Craniofacial. Bilateral microtia and/or anotia with stenosis of the external ear canal. Accessory parietal sutures. A narrow sloping forehead. Micrognathia, U-shaped (Robin) palatal cleft. Flat depressed nasal bridge and ocular hypertelorism.

Cardiovascular. Conotruncal malformations, including transposition of the great vessels, tetralogy of Fallot, double-outlet right ventricle, truncus arteriosus communis, and supracristal ventricular septal defect. Aortic arch interruption (type B). Retroesophageal right subclavian artery. Aortic arch hypoplasia.

Central Nervous System. Hydrocephalus. Microcephaly. Structural errors of cortical and cerebellar neuronal migration and gross malformations of posterior fossa structures, including cerebellar hypoplasia, agenesis of the vermis, cerebellar microdysgenesis, and megacisterna.

Other. Thymic abnormalities.

NATURAL HISTORY. Among the 21 affected infants evaluated by Lammer et al., three were stillborn and 9 were live-born infants who died secondary to cardiac defects, brain malformations, or combinations of the two. Information regarding the nine affected infants who survived the neonatal period is unknown. In particular, no data are available regarding developmental performance in prenatally exposed infants.

ETIOLOGY. Isotretinoin (Accutane). Twenty-two per cent of 36 prospectively ascertained pregnancies resulted in a first trimester spontaneous abortion, 3 per cent in a malformed stillborn infant, and 11 per cent in a live-born infant with at least one major malformation. None of the abortuses were evaluated regarding malformations. All affected infants were prenatally exposed to Accutane between postconceptual days seven and 124. Daily dosage of Accutane has averaged from 0.5 to 1.5 mg per kg of maternal body weight. There is no evidence to suggest that maternal use of isotretinoin prior to conception is teratogenic.

References

Rosa, F. W.: Teratogenicity of isotretinoin. Lancet, *2*:513, 1983.

Fernoff, P. M., and Lammer, E. J.: Craniofacial features of isotretinoin embryopathy. J. Pediatr., *105*:595, 1984.

Lott, I. T., et al.: Fetal hydrocephalus and ear anomalies associated with maternal use of isotretinoin. J. Pediatr., *105*:597, 1984.

Lammer, E. J., et al.: Retinoic acid embryopathy. N. Engl. J. Med., *313*:837, 1985.

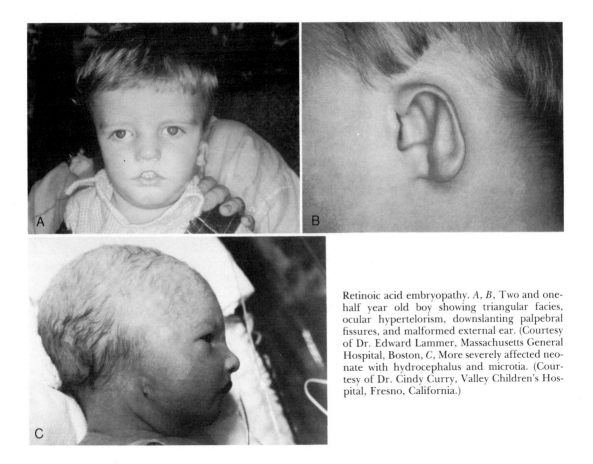

Retinoic acid embryopathy. *A, B,* Two and one-half year old boy showing triangular facies, ocular hypertelorism, downslanting palpebral fissures, and malformed external ear. (Courtesy of Dr. Edward Lammer, Massachusetts General Hospital, Boston, *C,* More severely affected neonate with hydrocephalus and microtia. (Courtesy of Dr. Cindy Curry, Valley Children's Hospital, Fresno, California.)

FETAL RUBELLA EFFECTS

(Fetal Rubella Syndrome)

Deafness, Cataracts, Patent Ductus Arteriosus

Gregg, in 1941, first called attention to the permanent residua of fetal rubella acquired from the mother during the first trimester of gestation. Culture of the viral agent during the severe 1964 epidemic resulted in an appreciation of the "expanded rubella syndrome" as the consequence of widespread chronic disease. The effects range from deafness, one of the most common residua, to the more complete fetal rubella syndrome.

ABNORMALITIES. Fetal death may occur. The following are the tissues that are affected and the consequent abnormalities noted in the 1964 epidemic. The asterisks (*) indicate permanent residua.

Tissue	Abnormalities
General hypoplasia	Growth deficiency
Central nervous system	*Mental deficiency, microcephaly
Cochlea	*Deafness
Lens	*Cataract
Other parts of eye	*Glaucoma, corneal opacity, chorioretinitis, microphthalmia, strabismus
Blood vessels	*Patent ductus arteriosus, peripheral pulmonic stenosis, fibromuscular proliferation with thickened intima of medium and large arteries
Myocardium	*Septal defects, myocardial disease

Early infancy

Tissue	Abnormalities
Marrow elements	Thrombocytopenia, anemia
Reticuloendothelial	Hepatosplenomegaly
Liver	Obstructive jaundice
Bone	Osteolytic metaphyseal lesions
Lung	Interstitial pneumonia

OCCASIONAL ABNORMALITIES. Renal disease, hemolytic anemia, large anterior fontanel, late eruption of teeth, hypospadias, cryptorchidism, meningocele, dermatoglyphic alterations. Diabetes mellitus. Hypopituitarism.

NATURAL HISTORY. The frequency of fetal infection from mothers having rubella during the first trimester is about 50 per cent. The risks associated with rubella still exist in the second trimester, especially growth deficiency, deafness, mental deficiency, and peripheral pulmonic stenosis. Cultures for rubella virus in the excretions of patients were positive in 63 per cent of neonates with evidence of the rubella syndrome; 31 per cent of the cultures were still positive at five to seven months, 7 per cent at ten to 13 months, and none past the age of three years. However, rubella virus was recovered from a cataract removed from a three year old child. Thus, the disease is chronic, and although the neonate has prenatal antibodies to the rubella agent, the intracellular rubella virus may persist for a long period of time.

The occurrence of residual defects, especially of mental deficiency (60 per cent have I.Q.s below 90 and 20 per cent below 70), was much higher in the 1964 epidemic than in those of the past, in which deafness was the most common residuum of fetal rubella (31 per cent).

Prevention of maternal rubella by widespread administration of attenuated rubella vaccine is completely merited. Beyond this, the occurrence of validated maternal rubella during the first half of pregnancy should induce serious consideration of early termination of that pregnancy.

ETIOLOGY. Rubella virus. The agent may remain in the tissues and cause pathology years after birth. One example is the later development of diabetes mellitus due to long-term, chronic viropathy in the islets of Langerhans of the pancreas.

References

Gregg, N. M.: Congenital cataract following German measles in the mother. Trans. Ophthalmol. Soc. Aust., *3*:35, 1941.

Cooper, L. Z., and Krugman, S.: Diagnosis and management: congenital rubella. Pediatrics, *37*:335, 1966.

Menser, M. A., Dods, L., and Harley, J. D.: A twenty-five-year follow-up of congenital rubella. Lancet, *2*:1347, 1967.

Hardy, J. B.: Clinical and developmental aspects of congenital rubella. Arch. Otolaryngol., *98*:230, 1973.

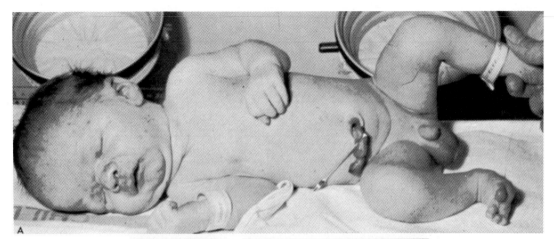

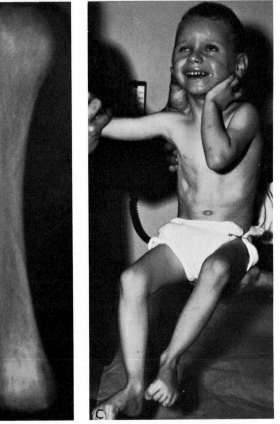

Fetal rubella effects. *A*, Neonate, clinically sick with lethargy, petechiae, and hepatosplenomegaly. (From Smith D. W.: J Pediatr., *70*:517, 1967.) *B*, Osseous lesions in the femur of five day old baby. Note coarse trabecular pattern and subperiosteal rarefaction. *C*, Child, three years and nine months old, with height age of two years and nine months and mental deficiency. The patient has cataracts, chorioretinitis, hearing impairment, and cryptorchidism—all the apparent residua of congenital rubella.

FETAL METHYL MERCURY EFFECTS

Methyl mercury has been shown to be teratogenic, especially to the developing brain.

ABNORMALITIES
Growth. Variable growth deficiency.
CNS and Performance. Variable microcephaly. Aberrant muscle tone, deafness, blindness.

NATURAL HISTORY. Prenatal exposure usually leaves permanent sequelae of all gradations.

ETIOLOGY. Methyl mercury exposure in utero. The levels in the fetus and in the young infant, who may receive additional mercury through breast milk, tend to be higher than the maternal levels. Sources of maternal exposure have included fish from contaminated water (the Minimata Bay disaster in Japan), flour made from methyl mercury–treated seed grain (at least 6,530 people affected in Iraq), or meat eaten from animals reared on such seed grain (New Mexico). The adult symptomatology is dose-related, ranging from paresthesias to ataxia to dysarthria to visual problems and deafness and finally to death at ingestion levels of 25 to 200 mg of methyl mercury. There may be a latent period of several weeks to two to three months between ingestion and symptomatology; hence, a fetus might be exposed before it is appreciated that the mother is affected. The methyl mercury readily crosses the placenta, and the impact on the developing brain can cause severe mental deficiency.

References

Harada, Y.: Congenital Minimata disease. *In* Minimata Disease—Study Group of Minimata Disease. Kumamoto, Japan, Kumamoto University, 1968, pp. 93–117.

Bakir, F., et al.: Methylmercury poisoning in Iraq. Science, *181*:230, 1973.

Koos, B. J., and Longo, L. D.: Mercury toxicity in the pregnant woman, fetus and newborn infant. Am. J. Obstet. Gynecol., *126*:390, 1976.

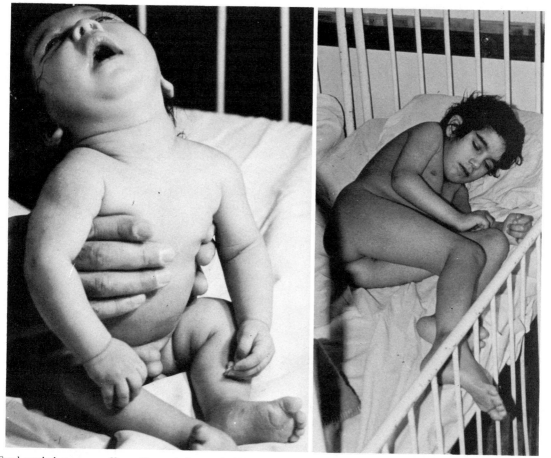

Fetal methyl mercury effects. Young infant and child with severe developmental deficiency due to in-utero methyl mercury exposure, their Iraqi mothers having eaten bread made from methyl mercury–treated seed grain. (Courtes of Dr. S. Elhassani.)

FETAL VARICELLA EFFECTS

*Cicatricial Skin, Limb Hypoplasia,
Mental Deficiency with Seizures*

LaForet and Lynch first described multiple defects in the child of a woman who had varicella during early gestation. Strabstein et al. summarized five cases, and Dudgeon has personally evaluated at least eight additional cases.

ABNORMALITIES

Performance. Mental deficiency, +/− seizures in the majority, with cortical atrophy.
Growth. Variable prenatal growth deficiency.
Eyes. Chorioretinitis.
Limbs. Hypoplasia of limb, +/− rudimentary digits, +/− paralysis with atrophy of limb.
Skin. Cutaneous scars.

OCCASIONAL ABNORMALITIES. Cataracts, microphthalmia, optic atrophy.

NATURAL HISTORY. The frequency of fetal infection from mothers having varicella during pregnancy is low. In a study by Enders, all live-born children born to 45 prospectively ascertained women who had seriologically proven primary varicella between the first and seventh months of pregnancy were normal. Paryani and Arvin identified the fetal varicella syndrome in one of 11 infants born to women with first trimester varicella and in none of 27 infants whose mothers had varicella in the second or third trimester. Of those affected, at least 50 per cent have died in early infancy, and the majority of the survivors have had mental deficiency with seizures. The cicatricial skin presumably represents the residuum of early infected bullous skin lesions.

ETIOLOGY. Most cases have occurred in the wake of maternal varicella during the period of eight to 19 weeks' gestation.

References

LaForet, E. G., and Lynch, C. L., Jr.: Multiple congenital defects following maternal varicella. N. Engl. J. Med., *236*:534, 1947.

Strabstein, J. C., et al.: Is there a congenital varicella syndrome? J. Pediatr., *64*:239, 1974.

Dudgeon, P., Institute of Child Health, The Hospital for Sick Children, London. Personal communication, June, 1977.

Enders, G.: Varicella-zoster virus infection in pregnancy. Prog. Med. Virol., *29*:166, 1984.

Paryani, S. G., and Arvin, A. M.: Intrauterine infection with varicella-zoster virus after maternal varicella. N. Engl. J. Med., *314*:1542, 1986.

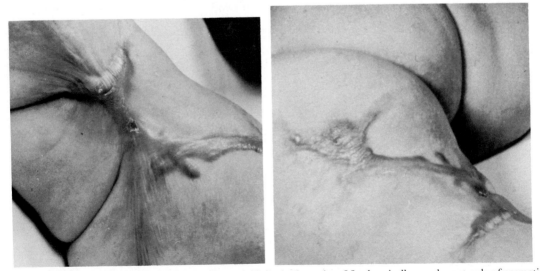

Fetal varicella effects. Severe cicatricial skin changes in limbs in the wake of fetal varicella may be not only of cosmetic concern but also associated with tissue deficits in the surrounding region. (Courtesy of Dr. Phillip Dudgeon, The Hospital for Sick Children, London.)

FETAL IODINE DEFICIENCY EFFECTS

(Endemic Cretinism)

Mental Deficiency, Spastic Diplegia, Deafness

Endemic cretinism has been clearly shown to be the consequence of severe iodine deficiency during the first half of gestation, affecting brain development and function.

ABNORMALITIES. These occur in all gradations of severity.

CNS. Mental deficiency, spastic diplegia, neurogenic deafness, strabismus, nystagmus.

OCCASIONAL ABNORMALITIES. Goiter, signs of hypothyroidism.

NATURAL HISTORY. The deafness, mental deficiency, and spastic diplegia do not respond to the administration of either thyroid hormone or iodine.*

ETIOLOGY. Severe maternal iodine deficiency (less than 20 µg per day) during the first half of gestation. Administration of iodized oil or other sources of iodine prior to pregnancy totally prevents the disorder. It occurs in areas of severe iodine intake deficiency, such as once existed in the Alpine regions of Switzerland, France, and Northern Italy and that still exist in some mountainous areas of New Guinea, the Himalayas of Southeast Asia, the Andes, and Zaire, including Idjwi Island. These are areas of endemic iodine-deficiency goiter, which is the most common effect that the deficiency has on the adult. However, iodine appears to be necessary, in an as yet unknown fashion, for normal brain morphogenesis during the first third to half of gestation. During this time, severe iodine deficiency may result in fetal iodine deficiency effects, a condition that is not a result of fetal hypothyroidism.

---

*Recent studies indicate that there is a motor performance defect affecting the entire population of children with this deficiency.

References

Connolly, K. J., Pharoah, P. O. D., and Hetzel, B. S.: Fetal iodine deficiency and motor performance during childhood. Lancet, 2:1149, 1979.

Hetzel, B. S., and Hay, I. D.: Thyroid function, iodine nutrition, and fetal brain development. Clin. Endocrinol., 11:445, 1979.

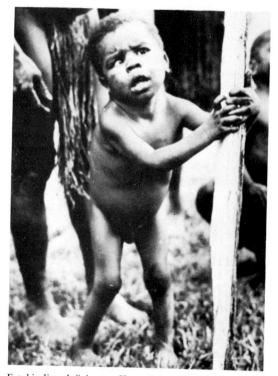

Fetal iodine deficiency effects. Young boy with cretinism, showing strabismus, vacant facies, and leg deformities secondary to neurologic deficits. (From Hetzel, B. S.: Med. J. Aust., 2:615, 1970.)

HYPERTHERMIA-INDUCED SPECTRUM OF DEFECTS

A number of animal studies have shown severe maternal hyperthermia during the first one third to one half of gestation to be teratogenic. The most extensive studies have been those of Edwards on the guinea pig. He showed that maternal hyperthermia of 1.5°C above normal tends to stop the growth of neuronal mitotic cells in the ependymal layer of the developing brain, and elevation of 3.0°C or more tends to kill such cells. The residual impact varies with the timing, severity, and duration of the maternal hyperthermia. Since the neuronal cell populations may not recover from such an antimitotic insult, the most consistent features have been problems of growth, development, and dysfunction of the brain. These have included neural tube defects when the hyperthermia was induced at the time of neural tube closure. Shortly thereafter, in the period corresponding to four to six weeks of human development, severe hyperthermia (2 to 3°C elevation for one hour daily) caused microcephaly, with "dumb" offspring who were often hypotonic with microphthalmia and other less consistent defects. (The degree of microcephaly is shown in the accompanying figure.) Hyperthermia at the equivalent of seven to 14 human weeks caused problems in spinal cord morphogenesis with consequent neurogenic contractures less consistently.

The studies in the human are limited at this point in time. However, the preliminary findings bear similarity to the nature of defects produced by hyperthermia in the animal studies. The nature of the defects relates to the timing of the hyperthermia rather than to its cause. Most of the relevant cases have been tentatively related to febrile illness, with the patient having a temperature of 38.9°C or higher, most commonly 40°C or above. The duration of the high fever has been one day or more, usually several days, which is unusual in the first third of gestation. The illness has varied, with influenza, pyelonephritis, and streptococcal pharyngitis being the most common. Two cases were considered secondary to severe hyperthermia induced by prolonged sauna bathing (30 to 45 minutes), and one case was thought to be related to very hot, prolonged tub bathing. The latter three cases are extraordinary in the duration of heat exposure.

Retrospective human studies of more than 170 cases of neural tube defect, including anencephaly, meningomyelocele, and occipital encephalocele, have disclosed an overall history of maternal hyperthermia during the week of neural tube closure (21 to 28 days) in approximately 10 per cent of the cases, whereas no such history was determined in the controls. These findings are compatible with the hypothesis that hyperthermia is one cause for neural tube defects in the human.

Table 1–1 summarizes the retrospective findings of 24 dysmorphic patients of previously unknown etiology in whom there was a maternal history of unusual hyperthermia during the first trimester. The similarities among these patients with a history of hyperthermia of comparable timing are striking, as is the similarity of the findings in these human cases to the experimentally hyperthermia-induced defects in the guinea pig. All of the cases manifested some form of CNS deficit. Structural abnormalities included microcephaly (occasional), and there was necropsy evidence of neuronal heterotopias and/or polymicrogyria. Function deficits included mental deficiency, seizures, micropenis interpreted as secondary to luteinizing hormone (LH) insufficiency and therefore a sign of hypothalamic dysfunction, and variable neuromuscular alterations of tone. The most consistent neuromuscular alteration was hypotonia, with about one half of the patients having hyperactive reflexes (hypotonic diplegia). Defects of facial morphogenesis were noted in the majority of cases in which the hyperthermia was said to have occurred between four and seven weeks' gestation (8 of 11). Some of these facial defects may be secondary to the CNS involvement, causing microphthalmia, problems in frontal brain growth resulting in a small midface, and deficit of movement leading to micrognathia. However, the instances of cleft lip and palate and the defects in ear morphogenesis more clearly suggest that hyperthermia may affect facial morphogenesis as well as brain development. Other dysmorphic features were minor limb abnormalities, including syndactyly, in four of 23 cases.

The more recent findings of other investigators tend to support the concept of unusual hyperthermia being a teratogenic influence in the human. Of greatest significance is the study of Shiota, who documented a 14 per cent incidence of "febrile" illness during early pregnancy in the mothers of 113 embryos with neural tube defects who were aborted therapeutically. The embryos were obtained through the Congenital Anomaly Research Center of Kyoto University. The history of maternal fever was documented before or immediately after the fetal loss, before the neural tube defect was documented. However, much more investigation is required. To date there has not been an adequate prospective study from which

Table 1–1. **PREDOMINANT DEFECTS IN 24 DYSMORPHIC OFFSPRING FOR WHOM A RETROSPECTIVE HISTORY OF MATERNAL HYPERTHERMIA BETWEEN 4 AND 14 WEEKS POST CONCEPTION WAS ELICITED**

Problems	Gestational Timing of Hyperthermia*		Proportion of Total
	4–7 Weeks	8–14 Weeks	
CNS			
Structural			
Neuronal heterotopias	2/2	2/2	100%
Microphthalmia	6/11	1/13	29%
Microcephaly	1/10	1/13	9%
Functional			
Mental deficiency	8/8	11/11	100%
Hypotonicity†	5/10	7/13	52%
(Hypotonic diplegia)	(2/10)	(4/13)	26%
Hypertonicity	3/10	3/10	30%
Neurogenic contractures	2/11	3/13	21%
Seizures	5/8	2/11	33%
Micropenis (LH deficiency)	2/7	0/6	15%
FACIAL			
Microphthalmia	6/11	1/13	29%
Micrognathia	5/11	1/13	25%
Midfacial hypoplasia	3/11	1/13	17%
External ear anomalies	3/11	1/13	17%
Cleft lip and/or palate	3/11	0/13	13%

*Denominator includes only those patients for whom the timing of exposure could be pinpointed to within a two week period and for whom the abnormality could be evaluated.
†Reflexes not mentioned in six instances.

one could derive risk data concerning the developing offspring subjected to a given level of hyperthermia at a given time of gestation.

In addition to potential dysmorphogenesis in early gestation, maternal hyperthermia has been associated with an increase in spontaneous abortion, stillbirth, and prematurity.

References

Edwards, M. J.: Congenital defects in guinea pigs following induced hyperthermia during gestation. Arch. Pathol., *84*:42, 1967.

Edwards, M. J.: Congenital defects in guinea pigs: Prenatal retardation of brain growth of guinea pigs following hyperthermia during gestation. Teratology, *2*:239, 1969.

Edwards, M. J.: The experimental production of arthrogryposis multiplex congenita in guinea pigs by maternal hyperthermia during gestation. J. Pathol., *104*:221, 1971.

Kilham, L., and Ferm, V. H.: Exencephaly in fetal hamsters following exposure to hyperthermia. Teratology, *14*:323, 1976.

Lyle, J. G., Edwards, M. J., and Jonson, K. M.: Critical periods and the effects of prenatal heat stress on the learning and brain growth of mature guinea pigs. Biobehavior Review, *1*:1, 1977.

Chance, P. I., and Smith, D. W.: Hyperthermia and meningomyelocele and anencephaly. Lancet, *1*:769, 1978.

Miller, P., Smith, D. W., and Shepard, T.: Maternal hyperthermia as a possible cause of anencephaly. Lancet, *1*:519, 1978.

Halperin, L. R., and Wilroy, R. S.: Maternal hyperthermia and neural tube defects. Lancet, *2*:212, 1978.

Smith, D. W., Clarren, S. K., and Harvey, M. A.: Hyperthermia as a possible teratogenic agent. J. Pediatr., *92*:878, 1978.

Clarren, S. K., et al.: Hyperthermia—a prospective evaluation of a possible teratogenic agent in man. J. Pediatr., *95*:81, 1979.

Fisher, N. L., and Smith, D. W.: Hyperthermia as a possible cause for occipital encephalocele. Clin. Res., *28*:116A, 1980.

Shiota, K.: Neural tube defects and maternal hyperthermia in early pregnancy: Epidemiology in a human embryo population. Am. J. Med. Genet., *12*:281, 1982.

Edwards, M. J., Department of Veterinary Medicine, University of Sydney, Australia. Personal communication.

Illustrations on pages 518 and 519

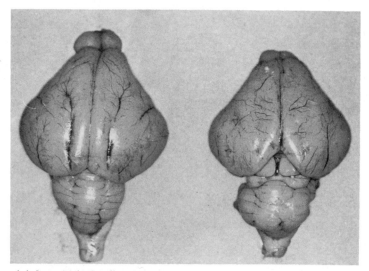

Hyperthermia-induced defects. *Right,* Smaller (14 per cent less) size brain of guinea pig whose mother's temperature was raised for one hour daily 2 to 3°C above euthermia from days 18 to 25 of gestation contrasted with a normal guinea pig brain to the left. Note the especially small frontal area. This was considered to be the reason for the shorter snout (maxilla). (Courtesy of Dr. Marshall Edwards, University of Sydney School of Veterinary Medicine.)

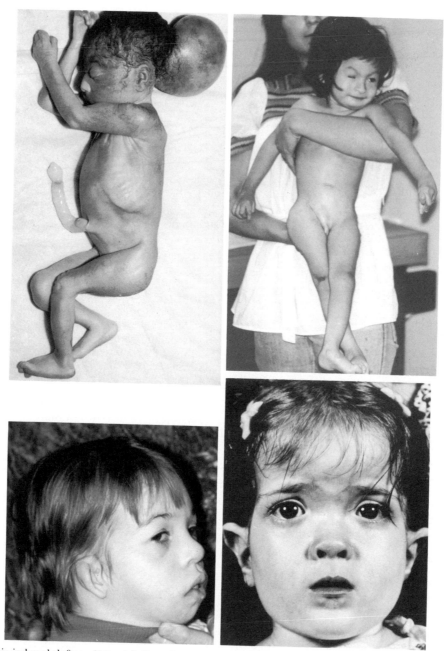

Hyperthermia-induced defects. *Upper left*, Encephalocele; maternal history of high fever between days 23 and 25 of gestation. *Upper right*, Eighteen month old severely retarded boy with hypotonic diplegia, micropenis, unilateral microphthalmia, cleft palate, and micrognathia. Maternal fever of 40° to 41°C between the fourth and fifth weeks of gestation. *Lower left*, Twelve year old severely retarded girl with hypotonic diplegia, midface hypoplasia, micrognathia, incomplete ear morphogenesis, and a cardiac defect. Maternal "flu" with high fever between the sixth and eighth weeks of gestation. *Lower right*, Fourteen month old with moderate hypotonic diplegia and developmental deficiency, who has a hypoplastic midface with mild ocular hypertelorism, low nasal bridge, and prominent auricles. Maternal fever of 40°C between the seventh and eighth weeks of gestation. (Lower right from Pleet, H., Graham, J. M., Jr., and Smith, D. W.: J. Pediatr 67:785, 1981.)

MATERNAL PKU FETAL EFFECTS

*Mental Deficiency, Microcephaly, Retarded Growth,
Increased Incidence of Structural Defects*

In 1963, Mabry et al. reported maternal phenylketonuria (PKU) as a cause of mental retardation. Affected children have normal phenylalanine hydroxylase activity but are presumably damaged during pregnancy by the elevated phenylalanine level in their mothers. The actual mechanism by which the imbalanced prenatal amino acid environment produces these defects is still a matter of speculation.

The majority of the structural defects, including growth deficiency, probably occur during organogenesis and appear to result from the toxic effect of an abnormally high phenylalanine level, which is concentrated on the fetal side of the placenta to a gradient of 3:2. During the later stage of gestation, there is interference with CNS myelination and maturation. Controlled phenylalanine intake during pregnancy is being attempted with varied results.

ABNORMALITIES
Performance. Mental deficiency in the vast majority, with I.Q.s often below 50.
CNS. Frequent mild manifestations of dysfunction. Increased muscle tone with pigeon-toed gait in seven of 11 patients; seizures.
Growth. Pre- and postnatal growth deficiency.
Craniofacial. Mild to moderate microcephaly is seen in most cases, and at times, there is characteristic round facies with prominent glabella and epicanthal folds. Strabismus. Long, underdeveloped philtrum with thin upper lip, small upturned nose, and maxillary and mandibular hypoplasia.
Cardiac. Variable defects. Of 14 affected patients, two died in the neonatal period secondary to cardiac defects, one had multiple structural anomalies, including a cardiac defect, one had coarctation of the aorta, and three had heart murmurs.

The recent findings of Lenke and Levy confirm earlier impressions and are delineated in Table 1–2.

OCCASIONAL ABNORMALITIES.
Cervical and sacral spine anomalies, cleft lip and palate, esophageal atresia, microphthalmia, irritability, overactivity.

Table 1–2. **ABNORMALITIES CAUSED BY MATERNAL PKU EFFECTS**

Abnormality	20 mg/dl or more	16–19 mg/dl
Spontaneous abortions	24% (297)*	30% (66)
Mental retardation in the offspring	92% (172)	73% (37)
Microcephaly	73% (138)	68% (44)
Congenital heart disease	12% (225)	15% (46)
Birthweight, 2500 g or less	40% (89)	52% (33)

*Size of sample is indicated in parentheses.
1 mmol/l = 16.6 mg/dl

ETIOLOGY. Phenylketonuria is an autosomal recessive disorder. Children of a homozygous female are obligatory heterozygotes; they do not have a phenylalanine hydroxylase deficiency, but if the father is a PKU carrier, the offspring carries a 50 per cent risk of having PKU in addition to maternal effects. The diagnosis is confirmed by finding an elevated phenylalanine level in maternal blood.

COMMENT. An increasing number of women of normal intelligence with treated PKU are entering childbearing age, and there is growing concern about the effects of maternal metabolic dysfunction upon the fetus. There is some evidence that the fetus may be affected when the maternal phenylalanine level is as low as 4 to 10 mg/dl. The severity of the effects parallels the increasing levels of phenylalanine in maternal blood.

References

Mabry, C. C., et al.: Maternal phenylketonuria: Cause of mental retardation in children without the metabolic defect. N. Engl. J. Med., *269*:1404, 1963.
Zaleski, L. A., Casey, R., and Zaleski, W. A.: Maternal phenylketonuria: dietary treatment during pregnancy. Can. Med. Assoc. J., *121*:1591, 1979.
Lenke, R. R., and Levy, H. L.: Maternal phenylketonuria and hyperphenylalaninemia; International survey of treated and untreated pregnancies. N. Engl. J. Med., *303*:1202, 1980.
Lipson, A., et al.: Maternal hyperphenylalaninemia fetal effects. J. Pediatr., *104*:216, 1984.

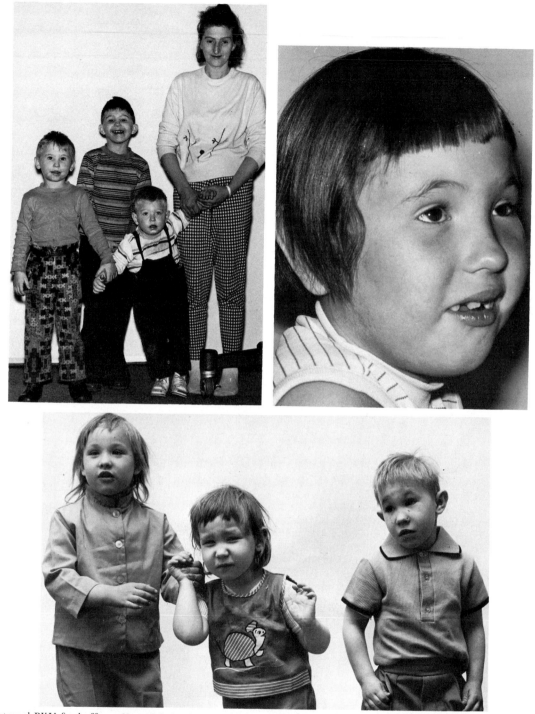

Maternal PKU fetal effects. *Upper left,* Mother with PKU and three affected offspring, none with PKU. *Upper right,* Affected girl. *Lower,* Three affected siblings of PKU mother. In addition to the relative microcephaly, note the subtle similarity in the facies, including the poorly defined philtrum. (Courtesy of Dr. Witheld Zaleski, University of Saskatoon, Department of Pediatrics.)

S. MISCELLANEOUS SYNDROMES

COFFIN-SIRIS SYNDROME

*Hypoplastic to Absent Fifth Finger and Toenails,
Coarse Facies*

Coffin and Siris reported three patients with this disorder in 1970, and Weiswasser et al. reported an additional case in 1973. Also, several of the patients described by Senior might represent examples of this syndrome. More than ten cases have been reported.

ABNORMALITIES
Growth. Prenatal onset of mild to moderate growth deficiency.
Performance. Mental deficiency, moderate to severe hypotonia.
Craniofacial. Mild microcephaly. Coarse facies with full lips.
Limbs. Hypoplastic to absent fifth finger and toenails, with lesser hypoplasia in other digits. Lax joints with radial dislocation at elbow. Coxa valga. Small patellae.
Hair. General hirsutism with tendency to have sparse scalp hair.

OCCASIONAL ABNORMALITIES. Ptosis of eyelids, hypotelorism, preauricular skin tag, hemangioma, cryptorchidism, hernias, short sternum, cardiac defect (patent ductus arteriosus, ventricular septal defect, atrial septal defect, tetralogy of Fallot, patent foramen ovale with aberrant pulmonary vein). Gastrointestinal anomalies (gastric and duodonal ulcer, neonatal intussusception, intestinal malrotation, gastric outlet obstruction secondary to redundant gastric mucosa). Short forearm, vertebral anomalies, cleft palate, Dandy-Walker anomaly of brain, hypoplasia or partial agenesis of corpus collosum, and in one patient abnormal olivae and arcuate nuclei and cerebellar heterotopias.

NATURAL HISTORY. Feeding problems and recurrent upper and lower respiratory tract infections are frequent during early life.

ETIOLOGY. Occurrence in siblings of unaffected parents has raised the question of autosomal recessive inheritance. Similar nail hypoplasia has been noted in some babies born of women who received phenytoin (Dilantin) therapy during pregnancy.

References

Coffin, G. S., and Siris, E.: Mental retardation with absent fifth fingernail and terminal phalanx. Am. J. Dis. Child., *119*:433, 1970.

Senior, B.: Impaired growth and onychodysplasia. Short children with tiny toenails. Am. J. Dis. Child., *122*:7, 1971.

Weiswasser, W. H., et al.: Coffin-Siris syndrome: Two new cases. Am. J. Dis. Child., *125*:838, 1973.

Carey, J. C., and Hall, B. D.: The Coffin-Siris syndrome. Am. J. Dis. Child., *132*:667, 1978.

DeBassio, W. A., Kemper, T. L., and Knoelel, J. E.: Coffin-Siris syndrome: Neuropathologic findings. Arch. Neurol., *42*:350, 1985.

Bodurtha, J., et al.: Distinctive gastrointestinal anomaly associated with Coffin-Siris syndrome. J. Pediatr., *109*:1015, 1986.

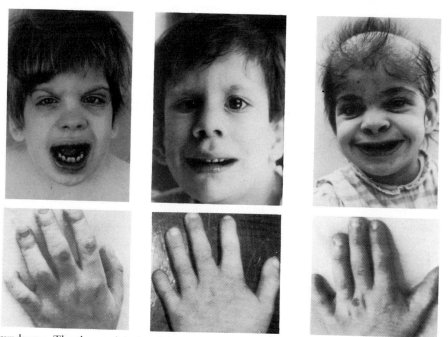

Coffin-Siris syndrome. The three original patients. (From Coffin, G. S., and Siris, E.: Am. J. Dis. Child., *119*:433, 1970.)

BÖRJESON-FORSSMAN-LEHMANN SYNDROME

Large Ears, Hypogonadism,
Severe Mental Deficiency

In 1961, Börjeson et al. described an entity of X-linked mental deficiency, epilepsy, hypogonadism, obesity, and dysmorphic facies seen in three related males and three of their less severely affected female relatives. In 1978, an unrelated case was reported by Weber et al. Recently, five additional males from two unrelated families and several of their variably affected female relatives have been identified and studied to document the full spectrum of this disorder.

ABNORMALITIES

Growth. Height usually less than fiftieth percentile. Moderate obesity may decrease in later life.

Performance. Severe mental deficiency, with an I.Q. of 10 to 40. Supraspinal hypotonia. Markedly abnormal EEG, with very poor alpha rhythms. Seizures may be present.

Craniofacial. Microcephaly. Coarse facies with prominent supraorbital ridges and deep-set eyes. Large (7.5 to 9 cm) but normally formed ears.

Eyes. Nystagmus, ptosis, and poor vision, with a variety of retinal and/or optic nerve abnormalities.

Genitalia. Small penis with small and soft or undescended testes and delayed secondary sexual characteristics. Hypogonadism appears to be hypogonadotropic.

Skeletal. Variable radiographic abnormalities: thick calvarium, small cervical spinal canal, mild scoliosis, kyphosis, Scheuermann-like vertebral changes, metaphyseal widening of the long bones and hands, hypoplastic distal and middle phalanges, thin cortices.

Other. Autopsy findings suggest that CNS anomalies are due to a primary abnormality of neuronal migration. Chromosomes have been normal in all studied cases. Hands are noted to be soft and fleshy with tapering fingers.

NATURAL HISTORY. From birth, these patients are hypotonic, with severe developmental delay. Walking may begin as late as four to six years and remains awkward. Speech is limited to a few phrases at most. There is no known unusual susceptibility to health problems, although bronchopneumonia was responsible for the demise of two of the original patients at the ages of 20 and 44 years. Life span is presumed to be normal. A sheltered environment is necessary because of severe limitations of nervous system performance.

ETIOLOGY. X-linked recessive inheritance inferred from impressive kindreds, in which all affected males are related through common female relatives. Female heterozygotes fall into a spectrum of those without any observable features to those with the abnormalities of growth and craniofacial, ocular, and skeletal features characteristic of this syndrome. Performance ranges from moderate mental retardation (I.Q. of 56 to 70) to above average intelligence. No test has been determined to identify apparently normal carrier females.

Features of this syndrome are suggestive of a storage disorder, but no abnormalities in enzyme activities have been detected in skin fibroblast cultures.

References

Börjeson, M., Forssman, H., and Lehmann, O.: Combination of idiocy, epilepsy, hypogonadism, dwarfism, hypometabolism, and morphologic peculiarities inherited as an X-linked recessive syndrome. Proc. 2nd Int. Congr. Ment. Retard., Vienna (1961), Part I, 1963, p. 188.

Börjeson, M., Forssman, H., and Lehmann, O.: An X-linked, recessively inherited syndrome characterized by grave mental deficiency, epilepsy, and endocrine disorder. Acta Med. Scand., *171*:13, 1962.

Brun, A., Börjeson, M., and Forssman, H.: An inherited syndrome with mental deficiency and endocrine disorder. A patho-anatomical study. J. Ment. Defic. Res., *18*:317, 1974.

Weber, F. T., et al.: Primary hypogonadism in the Börjeson-Forssman-Lehmann syndrome. J. Med. Genet., *15*(1):63, 1978.

Robinson, L. K., et al.: The Börjeson-Forssman-Lehmann syndrome. Am. J. Med. Genet., *15*:457, 1983.

Ardinger, H. H., Hanson, J. W., Zellweger, H. U.: Börjeson-Forssman-Lehmann syndrome. Further delineation in five cases. Am. J. Med. Genet., *19*:653, 1984.

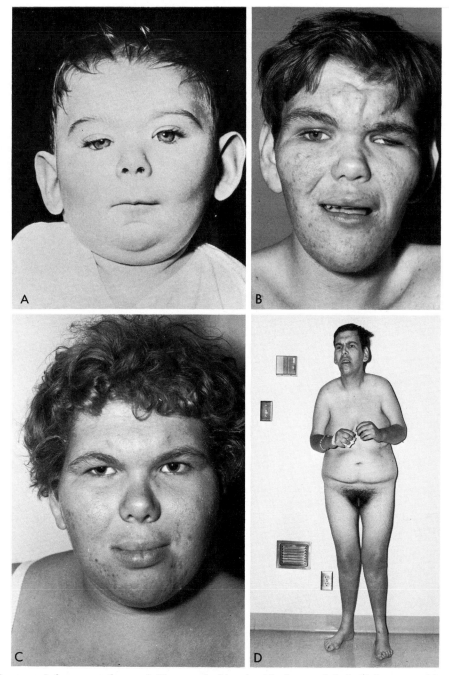

Börjeson-Forssman-Lehmann syndrome. *A*, Ten month old male with characteristic facial features and large ears. *B*, Unrelated 24 year old male. *C*, Twenty-three year old sister of patient shown in *B*, with mild mental deficiency and characteristic facies. *D*, Twenty-seven year old maternal cousin of patients shown in *B* and *C*, demonstrating obesity and hypogenitalism.

ARTERIOHEPATIC DYSPLASIA

(Alagille Syndrome)

Cholestasis, Peripheral Pulmonic Stenosis, Peculiar Facies

In 1973, Watson and Miller reported five families with 21 affected individuals. Since that time, at least 30 more cases have been described. Males and females are affected equally.

ABNORMALITIES

General. Growth retardation.

Craniofacial. Deep-set eyes, broad forehead, bulbous nose, prominent chin.

Eyes. Posterior embryotoxon (prominence of Schwalbe's line).

Cardiac. Peripheral pulmonic stenosis.

Skeletal. Vertebral defects, including hemivertebrae, "butterfly" vertebrae, and spina bifida occulta. Rib anomalies.

Hepatic. Paucity of intrahepatic bile ducts. Cholestasis without cirrhosis. Hypercholesterolemia.

OCCASIONAL ABNORMALITIES

General. Mild mental retardation.

CNS. Areflexia.

Eyes. Retinal degeneration. Strabismus.

Cardia. Atrial septal defect. Ventricular septal defect. Patent ductus arteriosus. Coarctation of the aorta.

Hands. Short distal phalanges.

Renal. Decreased creatinine clearance, increased blood urea nitrogen, increased serum uric acid. Horseshoe kidney.

Genitalia. Hypogonadism.

Endocrine. Decreased growth hormone. Increased testosterone. Hypothyroidism.

NATURAL HISTORY. Most patients present with neonatal jaundice, which clears by age four. Cholestasis (elevated serum bile acids), manifested by pruritus, is lifelong. Cirrhosis never develops, and liver damage is mild.

The peripheral pulmonic stenosis is generally asymptomatic. Although the majority of patients have a normal life span, death prior to five years of age due to cardiac failure or renal failure or both has recently been reported in a few cases.

ETIOLOGY. Autosomal dominant.

References

Watson, G. H., and Miller, V.: Arteriohepatic dysplasia: Familial pulmonary arterial stenosis with neonatal liver disease. Arch. Dis. Child., *48*:459, 1973.

Alagille, D., et al.: Hepatic ductular hypoplasia associated with characteristic facies, vertebral malformations, retarded physical, mental and sexual development, and cardiac murmur. J. Pediatr. *86*:63, 1975.

Henriksen, N. T., et al.: Hereditary cholestasis combined with peripheral pulmonary stenosis and other anomalies. Acta Paediatr. Scand., *66*:7, 1977.

Riely, C. A., et al.: A father and son with cholestasis and peripheral pulmonic stenosis. J. Pediatr., *92*:406, 1978.

Shulman, S. A., et al.: Arteriohepatic dysplasia (Alagille syndrome): Extreme variability among affected family members. Am. J. Med. Genet., *19*:325, 1984.

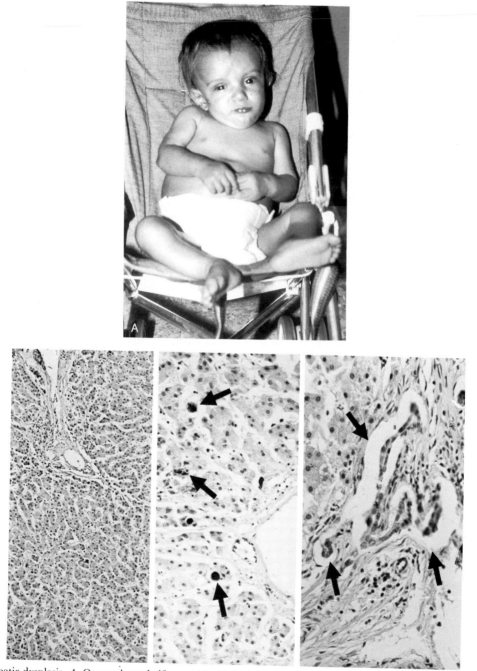

Arteriohepatic dysplasia. *A,* One and one-half year old with broad forehead and prominent chin. *B,* Three histologic sections of the liver from a patient with arteriohepatic dysplasia. On the left is a low-power view showing fine fibrosis and nodularity; higher power views in the middle and on the right reveal a paucity of intrahepatic bile ducts. The arrows denote bile stasis *(middle section)* and bile ducts *(right section).*

MELNICK-NEEDLES SYNDROME

Prominent Eyes, Bowing of Long Bones,
Ribbon-like Ribs

This disorder was reported by Melnick and Needles in 1966, and subsequently, a number of affected families have been reported with this osteodysplasia.

ABNORMALITIES

Craniofacial. Small facial bones with prominent eyes, full cheeks, and small mandible. Late closure of fontanels, dense base of skull, lag in paranasal sinus development.

Limbs. Short upper arms and distal phalanges. Bowing of radius and tibia. Flaring of distal humerus, tibia, and fibula. Coxa valga.

Other Skeletal. Relatively small thoracic cage with irregular ribbon-like ribs and short clavicle with narrow shoulders, pectus excavatum. Tall vertebrae with anterior concavity in thoracic region. Iliac flaring.

OCCASIONAL ABNORMALITY. Dislocation of hip. Ureteral stenosis leading to hydronephrosis.

NATURAL HISTORY. Small face with prominent and hyperteloric-appearing eyes. Abnormal gait and bowing may be the first evident signs of the disorder. Dental malocclusion is frequent, and with time, osteoarthritis of the back and/or hip may become a problem. A contracted pelvis in the female may make vaginal delivery difficult. Stature is usually normal. Frequent respiratory infections may be due to the small thoracic cage. Pulmonary hypertension has occurred.

ETIOLOGY. With the exception of two severely affected stillborn males born to typically affected women, all individuals have been female. Three instances of female to female transmission have been documented. Whether this disorder is due to an X-linked or autosomal dominant gene lethal in the male is unknown at present.

References

Melnick, J. C., and Needles, C. F.: An undiagnosed bone dysplasia. Am. J. Roentgenol. Radium Ther. Nucl. Med., *97:*39, 1966.

Coste, F., Maroteaux, P., and Chouraki, L.: Osteoplasty (Melnick-Needles syndrome). Ann. Rheum. Dis., *27:*360, 1968.

Maroteaux, P., Chouraki, L., and Coste, F.: L'ostéodyplasie (Melnick-Needles syndrome). Presse Méd., *76:*715, 1968.

Gorlin, R. J., and Knier, J.: Letter to the editor: X-linked or autosomal dominant, lethal in the male, inheritance of the Melnick-Needles (osteodysplasty) syndrome? A reappraisal. Am. J. Med. Genet., *13:*465, 1982.

von Oeyen, P., et al.: Omphalocele and multiple severe congenital anomalies associated with osteodysplasty (Melnick-Needles syndrome). Am. J. Med. Genet., *13:*453, 1982.

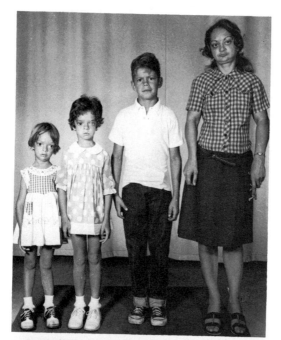

Melnick-Needles syndrome. *Left*, Affected mother and two daughters; note the facies and lower limbs. The boy is not affected. (Courtesy of Dr. William Nyhan, University of California, San Diego.) *Below*, Facies of an affected young woman. (Courtesy of Dr. Manuel Hernandez, Madrid, Spain.)

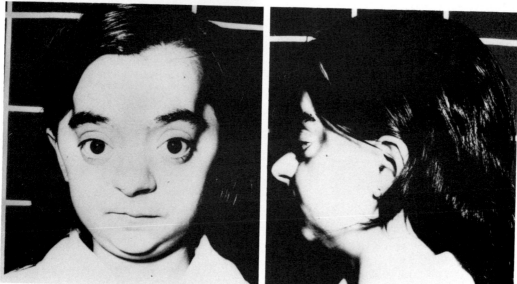

BARDET-BIEDL SYNDROME

Retinal Pigmentation, Obesity, Polydactyly

The variable manifestations of this syndrome were initially described by Bardet and Biedl in the 1920s. Subsequently, more than 300 cases have been reported. This disorder is clearly different from the condition described in 1865 by Laurence and Moon, although it was referred to as the Laurence-Moon-Biedl syndrome in the third edition of this book.

PRINCIPAL ABNORMALITIES

Obesity	83%
Mental deficiency	80%
Polydactyly, syndactyly, or both	75%
Retinitis pigmentosa	68%
Genital hypoplasia, hypogonadism, or both	60%

OTHER ABNORMALITIES. Renal defects (including a chronic glomerulonephritis type of lesion) and hypertension. Cardiac defects. Urologic anomalies. Occasional defects include nystagmus, strabismus, diabetes insipidus, clinodactyly of the fifth finger. Cystic dilatation of intrahepatic and common bile ducts. Hirsuitism. Ovarian stromal hyperplasia. Moderate shortness of stature.

NATURAL HISTORY. The natural history of this condition is poorly outlined in the literature. The mental deficiency is usually mild to moderate, and the retinal degeneration generally results in problems with night vision during childhood, even by three years of age. Only about 15 per cent of patients show an atypical retinal pigmentation by five to ten years of age. Central vision is lost, followed by loss of peripheral vision. By age 20, 73 per cent of patients are blind. There may be neurologic evidence of spinocerebellar degeneration or cranial nerve palsy. Obesity is usually present from early infancy. The hypogonadism has been described as primary germinal hypoplasia and also as hypogonadotropic in type. It is important to appreciate that some of the patients undergo spontaneous changes in adolescence.

ETIOLOGY. Autosomal recessive.

COMMENT. The extent of abnormality may vary considerably between affected siblings, and it may be impossible to make the diagnosis of Bardet-Biedl syndrome in an isolated case demonstrating only a part of the syndrome, especially only mental retardation, obesity, and genital hypoplasia.

References

Bardet, G.: Sur un syndrome d'obesité infantile avec polydactylie et rétinite pigmentaire. (Contribution à l'étude des formes cliniques de l'obesité hypophysaire.) Faculté de Medicine de Paris, Thesis, 470, 1920.

Biedl, A.: Ein Geschwisterpaar mit adiposo-genitaler Dystrophie. Dtsch. Med. Wochenschr., *48*:1630, 1922.

Klein, D., Ammann, F.: The syndrome of Laurence-Moon-Bardet-Biedl and allied diseases in Switzerland: Clinical, genetic and epidemiological studies. J. Neurol. Sci., *9*:479, 1969.

Hurley, R. M., et al.: The renal lesion of the Laurence-Moon-Biedl syndrome. J. Pediatr., *87*:206, 1975.

Haning, R. V., et al.: Virilism as a late manifestation in the Bardet-Biedl syndrome. Am. J. Med. Genet., *7*:279, 1980.

Schachat, A. P., and Maumenee, I. H.: Bardet-Biedl syndrome and related disorders. Arch. Ophthalmol., *100*:285, 1982.

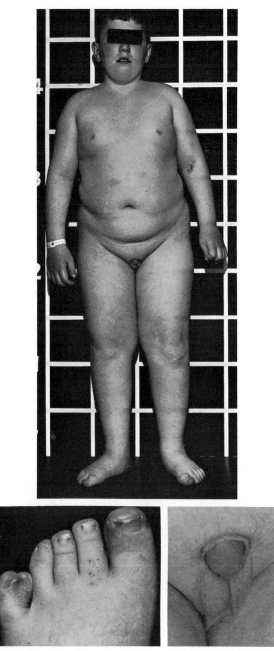

Bardet-Biedl syndrome. Ten year old male with retinal pigmentation and renal insufficiency. Obesity from birth.
I.Q. of 52.

RIEGER EYE MALFORMATION SEQUENCE

(Mesodermal Dysgenesis of the Iris, Goniodysgenesis)

Iris Dysplasia, Abnormal Pupils, Glaucoma; Primary Defect in the Differentiation of Mesodermal Tissue Layers in the Anterior Chamber

The Rieger eye malformation is a structural defect of the anterior chamber consisting of iris hypoplasia, a prominent Schwalbe line, and iris adhesions that attach to the Schwalbe line. Since Rieger's description of this anomaly in 1935, approximately 190 individuals with the malformation have been reported in the European and American literature. About 15 per cent of the patients presented with associated congenital glaucoma, whereas an additional 40 per cent developed increased ocular pressure later in life.

A vast array of nonocular abnormalities have been reported in association with this defect. The most frequently cited association is the constellation of dental abnormalities, midfacial hypoplasia, and the Rieger eye malformation; this pattern is labeled the Rieger syndrome. The Rieger eye malformation sequence may also occur as one feature in at least several other distinctive syndromes. These disorders include chromosomal syndromes (partial 3p trisomy, 4p deletion) and four mendelian conditions distinct from the classic Rieger syndrome.

The defect may occur by itself or as a part of a broader pattern of malformation. The anterior chamber of the eye is felt to develop by the separation of two dissimilar mesodermal tissue layers. This defect may be an alteration in the differentiation of these tissues with abnormal laying down of cells.

References

Allen, L., Burian, H. M., and Braley, A. E.: A new concept of the development of the anterior chamber angle. Arch. Ophthalmol., *53*:783, 1955.

Alkemade, P. P.: Dysgenesis Mesodermalisis of the Iris and Cornea. Assen, The Netherlands, Royal van Gorcum Publisher, 1969.

Fitch, N., and Kaback, M.: The Axenfeld syndrome and the Rieger syndrome. J. Med. Genet., *15*:30, 1978.

Carey, J. C., et al.: Heterogeneity of the Rieger eye malformation. Clin. Res., *28*:116A, 1980.

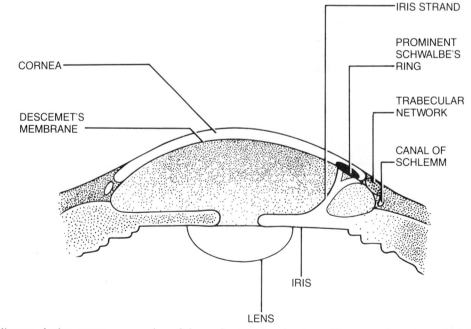

This diagram depicts a transverse section of the ocular anterior chamber with a normal angle on the left and the Rieger eye malformation on the right.

RIEGER SYNDROME

Iris Dysplasia, Hypodontia

Rieger described this association of anomalies in 1935. The Rieger eye malformation sequence may occur as an isolated anomaly or as one feature in a number of different syndromes. Its occurrence with hypodontia and occasionally other features has been described as the Rieger syndrome.

ABNORMALITIES
Facial. Dysplasia of iris including hypoplasia, mesenchymal tissue filling in the angle of the anterior chamber, aberrant synechiae of iris. Broad nasal bridge, maxillary hypoplasia, thin upper lip, everted lower lip.
Dentition. Hypodontia, partial anodontia, or both.
Other. Hypospadias, protrusion of umbilical skin.

OCCASIONAL ABNORMALITIES. Eye: glaucoma, microcornea, corneal opacity, ectopia lentis, aniridia, optic atrophy. Mental deficiency. Conductive deafness.

ETIOLOGY. Autosomal dominant with rather wide variance in expression.

References

Rieger, H.: Beiträge zur Kenntnis seltener Missbildungen der Iris. Arch. Ophthalmol., *133*:602, 1935.

Busch, G., Weiskopf, J., and Busch, K. T.: Dysgenesis mesodermalis et ectodermalis Rieger oder Riegerische Krankheit. Klin. Monatsbl. Augenheilkhd., *136*:513, 1960.

Pearce, W. G., and Kerr, C. B.: Inherited variation in Rieger's malformation. Br. J. Ophthalmol., *49*:530, 1965.

Jorgenson, R. J., et al.: The Rieger syndrome. Am. J. Med. Genet., *2*:307, 1978.

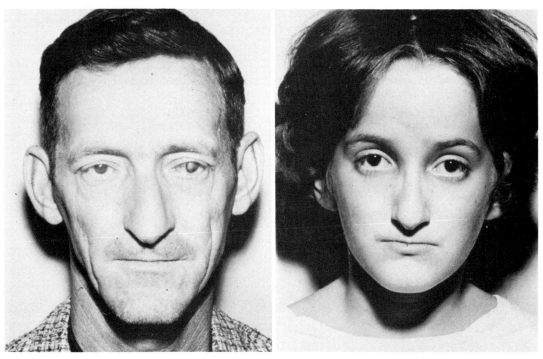

Rieger syndrome. Father and daughter with iris dysplasia. The daughter has two irregular pupils on the right and three on the left. The father has severe loss of vision, with corneal opacification secondary to glaucoma. Both have hypodontia, maxillary hypoplasia with malocclusion, and a short philtrum. In addition, the daughter had sagittal craniosynostosis.

CEREBRO-COSTO-MANDIBULAR SYNDROME

*Rib-Gap Defect with Small Thorax,
Severe Micrognathia*

This disorder was initially described by Smith et al. in 1966, and over 30 cases have been reported.

ABNORMALITIES

Performance. Mental deficiency is frequent among the survivors.

Growth. Prenatal onset of growth deficiency. Birth weight 2.5 to 2.9 kg.

Facies. Severe micrognathia with glossoptosis and short to cleft soft palate.

Thorax. Bell-shaped small thorax with gaps between posterior ossified rib and anterior cartilaginous rib, especially fourth to tenth ribs. Anomalous rib insertion to vertebrae.

Other. Inconsistent observations of redundant skin, abnormal tracheal cartilaginous rings, vertebral anomalies, elbow hypoplasia, hearing loss.

OCCASIONAL ABNORMALITIES. Microcephaly. Fifth finger clinodactyly.

NATURAL HISTORY. Forty per cent die in the first year, one half of these in the first month due to respiratory insufficiency. Of those who survive, feeding and speech difficulties are common, as well as mental deficiency in 50 per cent of cases. The rib gap defects resolve into pseudoarthroses with time.

ETIOLOGY. Autosomal recessive inheritance is implied by the occurrence of three offspring from normal parentage. However, Leroy et al. reported an affected mother and her two affected children, suggesting autosomal dominant inheritance for some cases of this disorder.

References

Smith, D. W., Theiler, K., and Schachenmann, G.: Rib-gap defect with micrognathia, malformed tracheal cartilages, and redundant skin: A new pattern of defective development. J. Pediatr., *69*:799, 1966.

Doyle, J. F.: The skeletal defects of the cerebro-costo-mandibular syndrome. Ir. J. Med. Sci., Ser. 7, *2*:595, 1969.

McNicholl, B., et al.: Cerebro-costo-mandibular syndrome. A new familial developmental disorder. Arch. Dis. Child., *45*:421, 1970.

Silverman, F. N., et al.: Cerebro-costo-mandibular syndrome. J. Pediatr., *97*:406, 1980.

Tachibina, K., et al.: Cerebro-costo-mandibular syndrome. Hum. Genet., *54*:283, 1980.

Leroy, J. G., et al.: Cerebro-costo-mandibular syndrome with autosomal dominant inheritance. J. Pediatr., *99*:441, 1981.

Smith, K. G., and Sekar, K. C.: Cerebro-costo-mandibular syndrome. Clin. Pediatr., *24*:223, 1985.

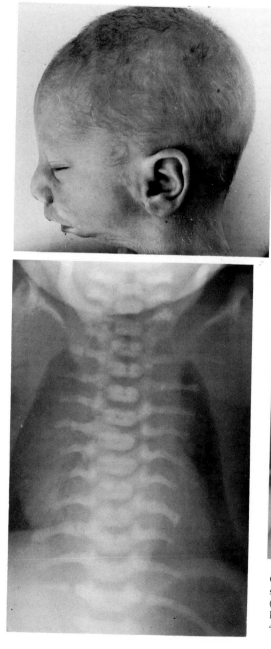

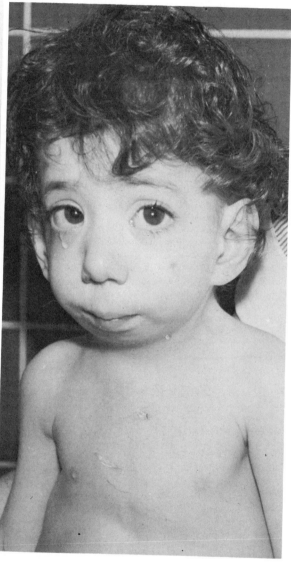

Cerebro-costo-mandibular syndrome. *Left,* Newborn showing severe micrognathia and incompletely ossified aberrant ribs. (From Smith, D. W., et al.: J. Pediatr., *69*:799, 1966.) *Right,* Four year old. (From McNicholl, B., et al.: Arch. Dis. Child., *45*:421, 1970.)

JARCHO-LEVIN SYNDROME

(Spondylothoracic Dysplasia)

Jarcho and Levin described this disorder in 1938, and subsequently, at least 17 cases have been recognized.

ABNORMALITIES
Craniofacial. Prominent occiput; tendency to have broad forehead, wide nasal bridge, anteverted nares, and upslant to palpebral fissures.
Thorax and Spine. Short thorax with diminished ribs and multiple vertebral defects, short neck.
Limbs. Impression of long digits with camptodactyly and syndactyly.

OCCASIONAL ABNORMALITIES. Cryptorchidism. Hydronephrosis with ureteral obstruction. Bilobed bladder. Absent external genitalia. Anal and urethral atresia. Uterus didelphys. Cerebral polygyria. Single umbilical artery.

NATURAL HISTORY. Although the majority of affected individuals die in early infancy as a result of respiratory insufficiency secondary to the small thoracic volume, a small number have lived beyond one year of age.

ETIOLOGY. Autosomal recessive. Most reported cases have occurred in Puerto Rican individuals.

References

Jarcho, S., and Levin, P. M.: Hereditary malformations of the vertebral bodies. Johns Hopkins Med. J., 62:216, 1938.

Pérez-Comas, A., and Garcia-Castro, J. M.: Occipito-facial-cervico-thoracic-abdomino-digital dysplasia: Jarcho-Levin syndrome of vertebral anomalies. J. Pediatr., 85:388, 1974.

Poor, M. A., et al.: Nonskeletal malformations in one of three siblings with Jarcho-Levin syndrome of vertebral anomalies. J. Pediatr., 103:270, 1983.

Cassidy, S. B., Herson, V., and Tibbets, J.: Natural history of Jarcho-Levin syndrome (spondylo-thoracic dysplasia). Proc. Greenwood Genet. Center., 3:92, 1984.

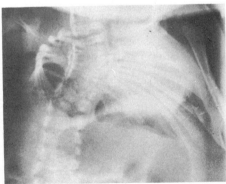

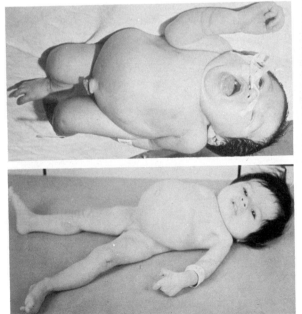

Jarcho-Levin syndrome. Affected neonate and young infant, with roentgenogram of the former. (From Pérez-Comas, A., and Garcia-Castro, J. M.: J. Pediatr., 85:388 1974.)

LEPRECHAUNISM SYNDROME
(Donohue Syndrome)

Prenatal Adipose Deficiency,
Full Lips, Islet Cell Hyperplasia

This somewhat puzzling disorder was initially described as dysendocrinism by Donohue in 1948. Later, Donohue and Uchida reported two siblings under the term leprechaunism, and since then more than 30 cases have been recorded.

ABNORMALITIES
Growth. Prenatal and postnatal growth deficiency with retarded osseous maturation and marked lack of adipose tissue; mean birth weight, about 2.6 kg.
Facies. Small, with prominent eyes, wide nostrils, thick lips, large ears. Gingival hyperplasia.
Endocrine. Large phallus, breast hyperplasia (female), Leydig cell hyperplasia (male), follicular development with cystic ovary, hyperplasia of islets of Langerhans, hyperglycemia, hyperinsulinemia.
Other. Body and facial hirsutism. Acanthosis nigricans. Nail dysplasia. Wrinkled, loose skin. Pachyderma. Rugation of orifices. Hyperkeratosis. Prominent nipples. Apparent motor and mental retardation. Abdominal distention.

NATURAL HISTORY. Usually severe failure to thrive and frequent infections, with death in early infancy. One patient survived to two and one fourth years of age. Hypoglycemia occurs following prolonged fast. The basic defect in metabolism is undetermined.

ETIOLOGY. Autosomal recessive inheritance is implied by consanguinity and sibship occurrence. D'Ercole et al. consider the prime defect to be lack of cellular response to insulin, causing growth deficiency, hyperglycemia, hyperinsulinemia, and hyperplasia of the islets of Langerhans.

References

Donohue, W. L.: Dysendocrinism. J. Pediatr., *32*:739, 1948.
Donohue, W. L., and Uchida, I.: Leprechaunism. A euphemism for a rare familial disorder. J. Pediatr., *45*:505, 1954.
Salmon, M. A., and Webb, J. N.: Dystrophic changes associated with leprechaunism in a male infant. Arch. Dis. Child., *38*:530, 1963.
D'Ercole, J. A., et al.: Leprechaunism: studies on the relationship between hyperinsulinism, insulin resistance, and growth retardation. J. Clin. Endocrinol. Metab., *48*:495, 1979.
Roth, S. L., et al.: Cutaneous manifestations of leprechaunism. Arch. Dermatol., *117*:531, 1981.

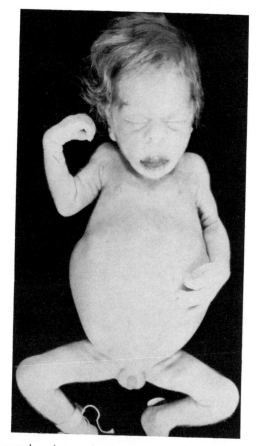

Leprechaunism syndrome. Necropsy photo of neonate with hyperglycemia and hyperinsulinemia who showed cellular unresponsiveness to insulin and who had islet cell hyperplasia at necropsy. (Courtesy of Dr. J. A. D'Ercole and Dr. Louis Underwood, University of North Carolina School of Medicine, Chapel Hill.)

BERARDINELLI LIPODYSTROPHY SYNDROME

(Generalized Lipodystrophy)

Lipoatrophy, Phallic Hypertrophy, Hepatomegaly, Hyperlipemia

Berardinelli reported this unusual lipodystrophic syndrome in 1954. Although more than 25 cases have been recorded subsequently, the metabolic defect responsible for this inborn error of metabolism has not been determined.

ABNORMALITIES
Performance. Mental deficiency as a variable feature.
Growth. Accelerated growth and maturation, enlargement of hands and feet, phallic enlargement, hypertrophy of muscle with excess glycogen, lack of adipose from early life.
Skin. Coarse with hyperpigmentation, especially in axillae. Variable acanthosis nigricans.
Hair. Hirsutism with curly scalp hair.
Vascular. Large superficial veins.
Liver. Hepatomegaly with excess neutral fat and glycogen and eventual cirrhosis.
Plasma. Hyperlipemia (neutral fats). Hyperinsulinism. Insulin-resistant nonketotic hyperglycemia may develop. Hyperglucagonemia.

OCCASIONAL ABNORMALITIES.
Cardiomegaly, corneal opacities, hyperproteinemia, hyperinsulinemia. Polycystic ovarian disease.

NATURAL HISTORY.
The accelerated growth and hyperlipemia are most prominent in early childhood, and hyperglycemia may develop in later childhood. The oldest reported patient, 16 years of age, was diabetic. Cirrhosis of the liver with esophageal varices may become a fatal complication.

COMMENT.
Although the accelerated growth and maturation plus the muscle hypertrophy and enlargement of the phallus are suggestive of androgen effect, neither androgens nor gonadotropins are elevated, and the hirsutism does not include pubic and axillary hair. Oserd et al. found that mononuclear leukocytes from affected patients bound less insulin than cells from controls, suggesting that altered insulin receptors are responsible for the insulin resistance and decreased synthesis of triglycerides.

ETIOLOGY.
Autosomal recessive, as indicated by sibship occurrence and parental consanguinity.

References

Berardinelli, W.: An undiagnosed endocrinometabolic syndrome: report of two cases. J. Clin. Endocrinol. Metab., *14*:193, 1954.

Seip, M., and Trygstad, O.: Generalized lipodystrophy. Arch. Dis. Child., *38*:447, 1963.

Senior, B., and Gellis, S. S.: The syndromes of total lipodystrophy and of partial lipodystrophy. Pediatrics, *33*:593, 1964.

Oserd, S., et al.: Decreased binding of insulin to its receptor in patients with congenital generalized lipodystrophy. N. Engl. J. Med., *296*:245, 1977.

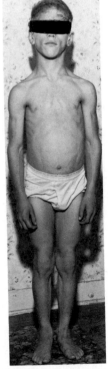

Berardinelli lipodystrophy syndrome. Preadolescent age boy showing hypertrophied muscle and relative lack of subcutaneous fat. (Courtesy of Central Wisconsin Colony and Training School.)

DISTICHIASIS-LYMPHEDEMA SYNDROME

Double Row of Eyelashes, Lymphedema

ABNORMALITIES

Eyes. Extra row of eyelashes, replacing meibomian glands.

Limbs. Lymphedema, predominantly from knee downward.

OCCASIONAL ABNORMALITIES.
Epidural spinal cysts $+/-$ secondary vertebral anomalies. Partial ectropion of lower lid, epicanthal folds, pterygium colli. Submucous cleft palate. Bifid uvula.

NATURAL HISTORY.
The extra eyelashes may cause irritative ocular problems. The lymphedema usually becomes evident between the ages of five and 20 years, especially at the time of adolescence. The possibility of epidural cysts with secondary neurologic or other complications must always be considered in this disorder. Eyelash removal or surgery for the lymphedema is difficult to accomplish with good results, and hence, treatment is generally withheld unless grossly indicated.

ETIOLOGY.
Autosomal dominant inheritance.

References

Falls, H. F., and Dertesz, E. D.: A new syndrome combining pterygium colli with developmental anomalies of the eyelids and lymphatics of the lower extremities. Trans. Am. Ophthalmol. Soc., 62:248, 1964.

Ribinow, M., Johnson, G. F., and Verhagen, A. D.: Distichiasis-lymphedema. A hereditary syndrome of multiple congenital defects. Am. J. Dis. Child., 119:343, 1970.

Hoover, R. E., and Kelley, J. S.: Distichiasis and lymphedema: A hereditary syndrome with possible multiple defects—A report of a family. Trans. Ophthalmol. Soc., 69:293, 1971.

Holmes, L. B., Fields, J. P., and Zabriskiek, J. B.: Hereditary late onset lymphedema. Pediatrics, 61:575, 1978.

Schwartz, J. F., O'Brien, M. S., and Hoffman, J. C.: Hereditary spinal arachnoid cysts, distichiasis, and lymphedema. Ann. Neurol., 7:340, 1980.

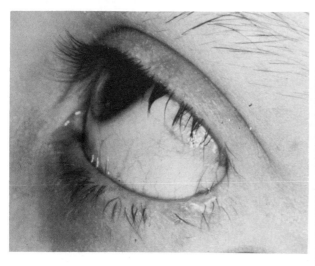

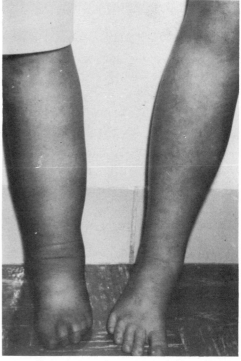

Distichiasis in the eye of this teen-age girl and lymphedema in her leg *(on right)* and more severely so in that of her affected mother *(on left)*.

FABRY SYNDROME

(Anderson-Fabry Disease, Angiokeratoma Corporis Diffusum)

Dark Nodular Angiectases,
Attacks of Burning Pain, Renal Insufficiency

This disease was originally described by Fabry. Its basis has since been recognized as the cellular accumulation of ceramide trihexoside as a consequence of the deficiency of ceramide trihexosidase, the enzyme that normally degrades this neutral glycolipid.

ABNORMALITIES IN AFFECTED MALES

General. Attacks of burning pain in hands and feet.

Cutaneous. Minute dark nodular angiectases in clusters around umbilicus, on genitalia, knees, hips, mucous membranes, and so forth.

Eyes. Superficial corneal opacities.

Renal. Proteinuria; variable red cells, white cells, and casts in urine; progressive renal insufficiency.

CNS. May have seizures, headache, dizziness, hemiplegia, and other presumed reactions to cerebrovascular disease.

Cardiac. Glycolipid infiltration of myocardium, conduction tissues, valves, and endothelium.

OCCASIONAL ABNORMALITIES. Diarrhea, epistaxes, hemoptysis, anemia secondary to blood loss, saccular retinal vessels, hypertrophic obstructive cardiomyopathy, varicosities, edema of ankles, hands, and face, hypohydrosis. Central nervous system problems may include mental deficiency, optic atrophy, myoclonus, spastic paraplegia, and/ or dementia. Thick lips, coarse facies. Chronic airflow obstruction secondary to the accumulation of ceramide trihexoside in airway epithelium.

NATURAL HISTORY. The skin angiectases, though often present in earlier childhood, are usually not noted until after ten years of age. The burning pain, sometimes associated with fever, may start in childhood; it occurs in attacks precipitated by heat, cold, exercise, or fever. Chronic airflow obstruction occurs secondary to the accumulation of ceramide trihexoside in airway epithelium. Renal insufficiency progresses to a fixed specific gravity of the urine, and the mean age of survival is 42 years.

ETIOLOGY. X-linked with full penetrance in the hemizygous male. There is variable mild expressivity in the heterozygous female, who may show mild corneal opacities and who has a value of ceramide trihexosidase that is intermediate between that of the affected male and the normal person.

References

Fabry, J.: Ein Beitrag zur Purpura haemorrhagica nodularis. Arch. Derm. Syph., *43*:187, 1898.

Optiz, J. M., et al.: The genetics of angiokeratoma corporis diffusum (Fabry's disease) and its linkage relations with the Xg locus. Am. J. Hum. Genet., *17*:325, 1965.

Brady, R. O., et al.: Enzymatic defect in Fabry's disease. Ceramide trihexosidase deficiency. N. Engl. J. Med., *276*:1163, 1967.

Wallace, H. G.: Anderson-Fabry disease. Br. J. Dermatol., *88*:1, 1973.

Rosenberg, D. M., et al.: Chronic airflow obstruction in Fabry's disease. Am. J. Med., *68*:898, 1980.

Colucci, W. S., et al.: Hypertrophic obstructive cardiomyopathy due to Fabry's disease. N. Engl. J. Med., *307*:926, 1982.

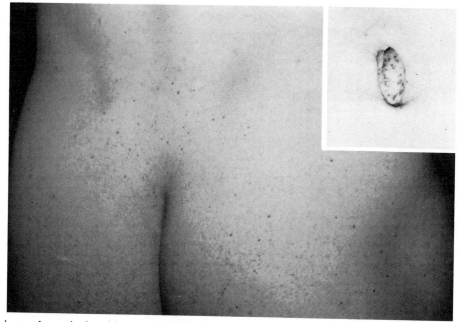

Fabry syndrome. Lower back and buttock area of older child, showing small dark nodular lesions, which are especially prominent in the umbilicus (inset). (From R. Summitt, University of Tennessee College of Medicine, Memphis.)

CHÉDIAK-HIGASHI SYNDROME

*Partial Albinism, Large Granules
in Leukocytes*

César originally described this disorder in 1943, and later Chédiak and Higashi each independently recognized the disease. More than 40 cases have been reported.

ABNORMALITIES

Partial Albinism. Gray sheen to light-colored hair, diminished uveal and retinal pigmentation with photophobia and nystagmus.

Hematologic and Reticuloendothelial. Neutropenia with tendency toward lymphocytosis, anemia, and thrombocytopenia. Large cytoplasmic inclusions in leukocytes, promyeloblasts, myeloblasts, and other granule-containing cells. Lymphoid-histiocytic cell infiltration with variable hepatosplenomegaly and lymphadenopathy.

OCCASIONAL ABNORMALITIES. Mental deficiency; seizures; peripheral neuropathy; corneal opacity; hyperhidrosis; buccal ulcerations; neonatal icterus; hyperlipemia.

NATURAL HISTORY. The majority of affected individuals die in early childhood as the result of recurring infection or a peculiar malignant lymphoma. Survival to adulthood can occur but is unusual.

ETIOLOGY. Autosomal recessive with high frequency of consanguinity. The heterozygote may show enlarged cytoplasmic inclusions in leukocytes.

COMMENT. Electron microscopy has provided evidence of the leukocyte cytoplasmic granules being swollen lysosomes; the melanocytes contain giant melanosomes, which may explain the partial albinism. Windhorst et al. have interpreted this evidence as being indicative of a disease of the limiting membranes. A decrease in natural killer activity of peripheral leukocytes has been demonstrated. These natural killer cells are thought to have a role in surveillance against tumors.

References

César, A. B.: Neutropenia crónica maligna familiar con granulaciones atípicas de los leucocitos. Bol. Soc. Cub. Ped., *15*:900, 1943.

Chédiak, M.: Nouvelle anomalie leucocytaire de caractère constitutionnel et familial. Rev. Hématol., 7:362, 1952.

Windhorst, D. B., Zelickson, A. S., and Good, R. A.: Chédiak-Higashi syndrome: hereditary gigantism of cytoplasmic organelles. Science, *151*:81, 1966.

Blume, R. S., and Wolff, S. M.: The Chédiak-Higashi syndrome; Studies in four patients and review of the literature. Medicine, *51*:247, 1972.

Roder, J. C., et al.: A new immunodeficiency disorder in humans involving NK cells. Nature, *284*:553, 1980.

T. MISCELLANEOUS SEQUENCES

LATERALITY SEQUENCES

In addition to reversal of the sides, with partial to complete situs inversus, there can be bilateral left- or right-sidedness.

The primary defect in both is a failure of normal asymmetry in morphogenesis. The basic problem would presumably be present prior to 30 days of development. The accompanying chart sets forth the differences as well as the similarities between the patterns due to predominantly left-sided bilaterality and due to right-sided bilaterality. Among other differences, the spleen dramatically reflects the variant laterality in the two. With left-sided bilaterality there is polysplenia (usually bilateral spleens plus rudimentary extra splenic tissue), and with right-sided bilaterality there is asplenia or a hypoplastic spleen. The defect in lateralization leading to the failure of normal asymmetry in morphogenesis is most likely etiologically heterogeneous. As such, although usually sporadic, autosomal dominant, autosomal recessive, and X-linked recessive inheritance have all been documented.

BILATERAL LEFT-SIDEDNESS SEQUENCE (polysplenia syndrome). The sex incidence is about equal. The cardiac anomalies are usually not as severe as with bilateral right-sidedness.

BILATERAL RIGHT-SIDEDNESS SEQUENCE (asplenia syndrome, Ivemark syndrome, triad of spleen agenesis, defects of heart and vessels, and situs inversus). This is two to three times more common in males than in females. The complex cardiac anomalies, usually giving rise to cyanosis and early cardiac failure, are the major cause of early death. The possibility of gastrointestinal problems must also be considered, especially as related to the aberrant mesenteric attachments. Renal anomalies are also more frequent (25 per cent). Survivors have had an increased frequency of cutaneous, respiratory, and other infections, possibly related to the asplenia. Tests to detect asplenia include valuation of red blood cells for Howell-Jolly bodies and Heinz bodies.

COMMENT. Both bilateral left-sidedness and bilateral right-sidedness are pathogenetically similar, most likely the result of a primary defect in lateralization leading to failure of normal asymmetric development.

References

Freedom, R. M.: The asplenia syndrome. J. Pediatr., *81*:1130, 1972.

Van Mierop, L. H. S., Gessner, I. H., and Schiebler, G. L.: Asplenia and polysplenia syndromes. Birth Defects, *8*:74, 1972.

Arnold, G. L., Bixler, D., and Gerod, D.: Probable autosomal recessive inheritance of polysplenia, situs inversus and cardiac defects in an Amish family. Am. J. Med. Genet., *16*:35, 1983.

Illustration on following page

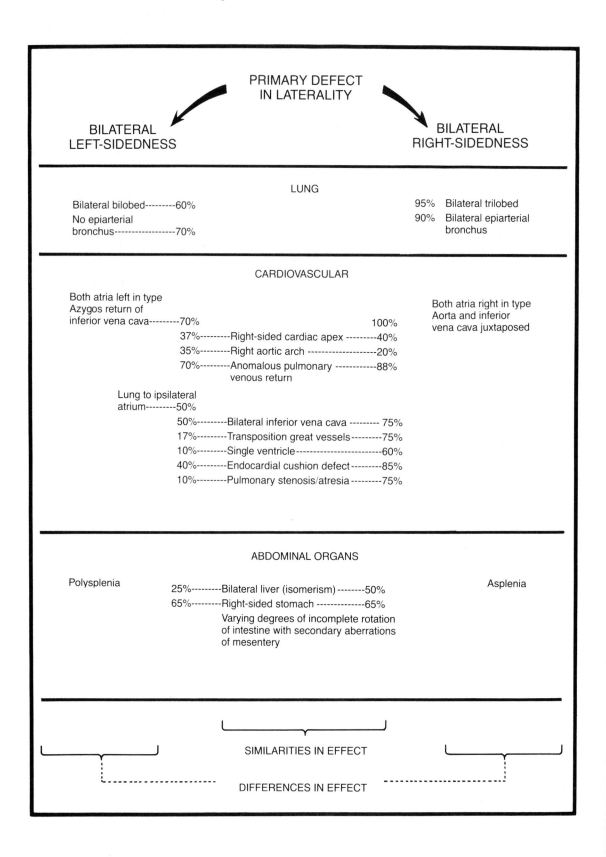

KARTAGENER SYNDROME

Situs Inversus, Sinusitis, Bronchiectasis

Described by Kartagener in 1933, this syndrome accounts for about one tenth of the cases of bronchiectasis and about one sixth of the cases of situs inversus.

ABNORMALITIES

Organ Orientation. Situs inversus, partial to complete, with gross defects in cardiac septation in some patients; occasional asplenia. (See Laterality Sequences.)

Respiratory Tract. Absence of frontal sinus development. Lack of aeration of mastoids. Thick, tenacious mucus with problems of infection and stasis. Conductive deafness.

NATURAL HISTORY. Provided the patient does not have a lethal cardiac anomaly, there is variable age of onset and severity of chronic middle ear infection, rhinitis (sometimes with nasal polyps), sinusitis, pneumonia, chronic cough, and follicular bronchiectasis. *Haemophilus influenzae* and *Diplococcus pneumoniae* are the more common bacterial pathogens. Over 90 per cent of patients are symptomatic during childhood. The initial presentation of chronic rhinitis with wheezing and rales may falsely suggest an allergic problem. Middle ear problems frequently result in deafness. Partial lung resections may eventually be indicated for bronchiectasis. Occasional patients have had low IgA levels, but this does *not* appear to be the cause of this congenital defect in the function and integrity of the respiratory epithelium.

ETIOLOGY. Autosomal recessive inheritance implied. Abnormal respiratory cilia as well as immotile sperm indicate a problem in the morphogenesis of these specialized motile structures. Affected males are usually sterile, whereas affected females have decreased fertility.

References

Kartagener, M.: Zur Pathogenese der Bronkiektasien. Bronkiektasien bei situs viscerum inversus. Beitr. Klin. Tuberk., *83*:489, 1933.

Mayo, P.: Kartagener's syndrome. J. Thorac. Cardiovasc. Surg., *42*:39, 1961.

Holmes, L. B., Blennerhassett, J. B., and Austen, K. F.: A reappraisal of Kartagener's syndrome. Am. J. Med. Sci., *255*:13, 1968.

Hartline, J. V., and Zelkowitz, P. S.: Kartagener's syndrome in childhood. Am. J. Dis. Child., *121*:349, 1971.

Afzelius, A. B.: Kartegener's syndrome and abnormal cilia. N. Engl. J. Med., *297*:1011, 1977.

HOLOPROSENCEPHALY SEQUENCE

Arhinencephaly-Cebocephaly-Cyclopia:
Primary Defect—In Prechordal Mesoderm

During the third week of fetal development, the prechordal mesoderm migrates forward into the area anterior to the notochord and is necessary for the development of the midface as well as having an inductive role in the morphogenesis of the forebrain. The consequences of prechordal mesoderm defect are varying degrees of deficit of midline facial development, especially the median nasal process (premaxilla), and incomplete morphogenesis of the forebrain. Cyclopia represents a severe deficit in early midline facial development, and the eyes become fused, the olfactory placodes consolidate into a single tube-like proboscis above the eye, and the ethmoid and other midline bony structures are missing. With cyclopia, there is failure in the cleavage of the prosencephalon, with grossly incomplete morphogenesis of the forebrain. Less severe deficits result in hypotelorism and varying degrees of inadequate midfacial and incomplete forebrain development that are more common than cyclopia and frequently include cleft lip and palate. The important clinical point is that incomplete midline facial development, such as hypotelorism or absence of the philtrum or nasal septum, suggests the possibility of a serious anomaly in brain development and function.

Although the cause is unknown and the defects are isolated in the vast majority of cases, certain chromosomal aberrations, including trisomy 13, 18p−, and 13q− syndromes, as well as the Meckel-Gruber syndrome, should be considered. In addition, there exists an autosomal dominant form of holoprosencephaly. Therefore parents of an affected child should be checked for mild manifestations such as a single central incisor. Finally, holoprosencephaly has been seen in the offspring of diabetic mothers.

The prognosis for central nervous system function in individuals with this type of defect is very poor, and the author recommends limitation of medical assistance toward survival in patients in whom the forebrain is obviously severely affected.

References

Adelmann, H. B.: The problem of cyclopia. Part II. Q. Rev. Biol., *11*:284, 1936.

DeMeyer, W., Zeman, W., and Palmer, C. G.: The face predicts the brain: diagnostic significance of median facial anomalies for holoprosencephaly (arhinencephaly). Pediatrics, *34*:256, 1964.

Cohen, M. M.: An update on the holoprosencephalic disorders. J. Pediatr., *101*:865, 1982.

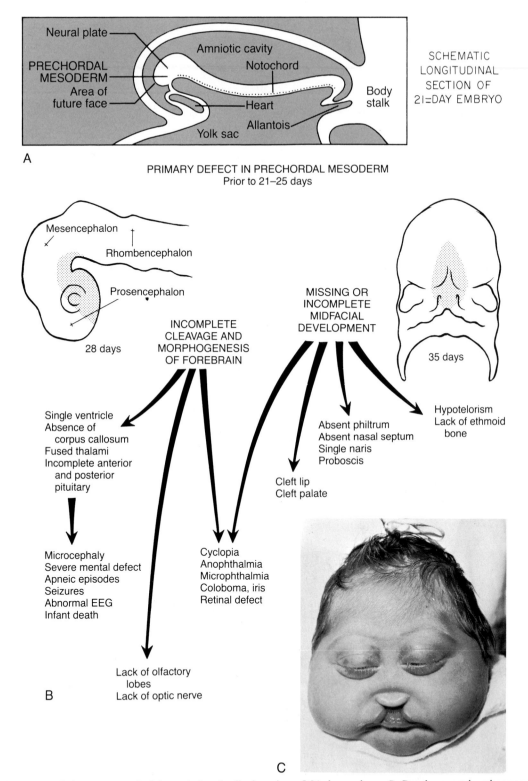

Holoprosencephaly sequence. *A*, Schematic longitudinal section of 21 day embryo. *B*, Developmental pathogenesis of the sequence. *C*, Affected individual.

MENINGOMYELOCELE, ANENCEPHALY, INIENCEPHALY SEQUENCES

Primary Defect—In Neural Tube Closure

The initiating malformation appears to be a defect in closure of the neural groove to form an intact neural tube, which is normally completely fused by 28 days. Anencephaly represents a defect in closure at the anterior portion of the neural groove. The secondary consequences are as follows: (1) the unfused forebrain develops partially and then tends to degenerate; (2) the calvarium is incompletely developed; and (3) the facial features and auricular development are secondarily altered to a variable degree, including cleft palate, frequent abnormality of the cervical vertebrae, and occasional incomplete development of the anterior pituitary.

Defects of closure at the mid- or caudal neural groove can give rise to meningomyelocele and other secondary defects, as depicted. The early form of one such lesion is illustrated below.

Defects of closure in the cervical and upper thoracic region can culminate in the iniencephaly sequence, in which secondary features may include retroflexion of the upper spine with short neck and trunk, cervical and upper thoracic vertebral anomalies, defects of thoracic cage, anterior spina bifida, diaphragmatic defects with or without hernia, and hypoplasia of lung and/or heart.

There appear to be multiple etiologies for defects of neural tube closure, including early amnion rupture and possibly hyperthermia. Most commonly no mode of etiology is appreciated, and the recurrence risk is about 4 per cent for parents who have had one affected child. Liberation of alpha fetoprotein into the amniotic fluid from the anencephaly or meningomyelocele that is not skin-covered allows for early amniocentesis detection, which may be augmented by sonography and/or radiography.

References

Giroud, A.: Causes and morphogenesis of anencephaly. Ciba Foundation Symposium on Congenital Malformations, 1960, pp. 199–218.

Lemire, R. J., Shepard, T. H., and Alvord, E. C., Jr.: Caudal myeloschisis (lumbo-sacral spina bifida cystica) in a five millimeter (horizon XIV) human embryo. Anat. Rec., *152*:9, 1965.

Lemire, R. J., Beckwith, J. B., and Shepard, T. H.: Iniencephaly and anencephaly with spinal retroflexion. Teratology, *6*:27, 1972.

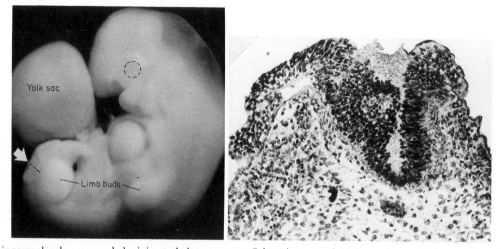

Meningomyelocele, anencephaly, iniencephaly sequences. Otherwise normal 28 day embryo with incomplete closure of the posterior neural groove (arrow), which shows aberrant growth of cells to the side in a transverse section (right). Had this embryo survived, it would presumably have developed a meningomyelocele. (From Lemire, R.: Anat. Rec., *152*:9, 1965.)

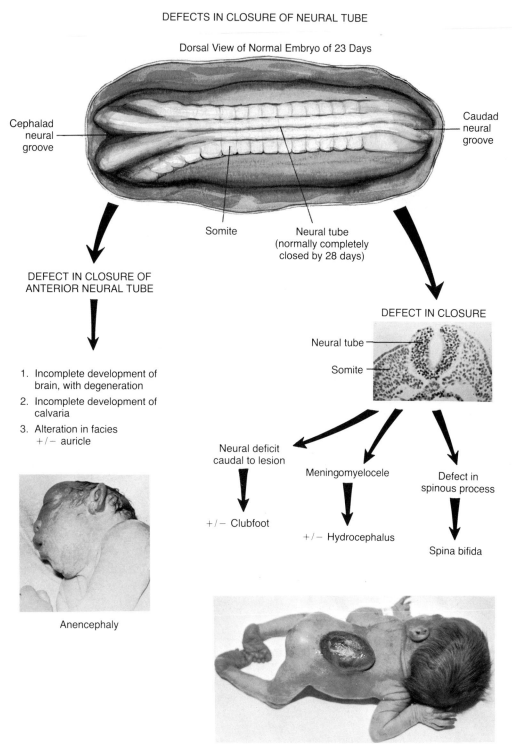

DEFECTS IN CLOSURE OF NEURAL TUBE

Dorsal View of Normal Embryo of 23 Days

Cephalad neural groove

Caudad neural groove

Somite

Neural tube (normally completely closed by 28 days)

DEFECT IN CLOSURE OF ANTERIOR NEURAL TUBE

DEFECT IN CLOSURE

Neural tube

Somite

1. Incomplete development of brain, with degeneration
2. Incomplete development of calvaria
3. Alteration in facies
   + / − auricle

Neural deficit caudal to lesion

Meningomyelocele

Defect in spinous process

+ / − Clubfoot

+ / − Hydrocephalus

Spina bifida

Anencephaly

Meningomyelocele with partially epithelialized sac

Developmental pathogenesis of anencephaly and meningomyelocele.

OCCULT SPINAL DYSRAPHISM SEQUENCE

(Tethered Cord Malformation Sequence)

Following closure of the neural groove at about 28 days, the cell mass caudal to the posterior neuropore tunnels downward and forms a canal in a process that gives rise to the most distal portions of the spinal cord—the filum terminale and conus medullaris. Failure of normal morphogenesis in this region leads to a spectrum of structural defects that cause orthopedic or urologic symptoms through tethering or compression of the sacral nerve roots, with restriction of the normal cephalic migration of the conus medullaris. Defects involve structures derived from both mesodermal and ectodermal tissue and include mesodermal hamartomata, sacral vertebral anomalies, hyperplasia of the filum terminale, and structural alterations of the distal cord itself. In most situations, there is a cutaneous marker at the presumed junction between the caudal cell mass and the posterior neuropore. Markers consist of tufts of hair, skin tags, dimples, lipomata, and aplasia cutis congenita.

The recognition of the surface manifestations of such a malformation sequence at birth should ideally lead to further evaluation and/or management. Roentgenograms of the spine may or may not show any abnormality. Since air or contrast myelography may be technically difficult to accomplish in early infancy, a direct surgical approach may often be warranted. Early management will prevent neuromuscular lower limb and/or urologic problems such as retention, incontinence, and/or infection secondary to continued tractional tethering of the cord and nerve roots. If the physician waits for signs of such serious complications, the neurologic damage may not be reversible. A 4 per cent incidence of open neural tube defects has been documented in first degree relatives of probands.

References

Anderson, F. M.: Occult spinal dysraphism: Diagnosis and management. J. Pediatr., *73*:163, 1968.

Carter, C. O., Evans, K. A., and Till, K.: Spinal dysraphism: Genetic relation to neural tube malformations. J. Med. Genet., *13*:343, 1976.

Tavafoghi, V., et al.: Cutaneous signs of spinal dysraphism. Arch. Dermatol., *114*:573, 1978.

Higginbottom, M. C., et al.: Aplasia cutis congenita: cutaneous marker of occult spinal dysraphism. J. Pediatr., *96*:687, 1980.

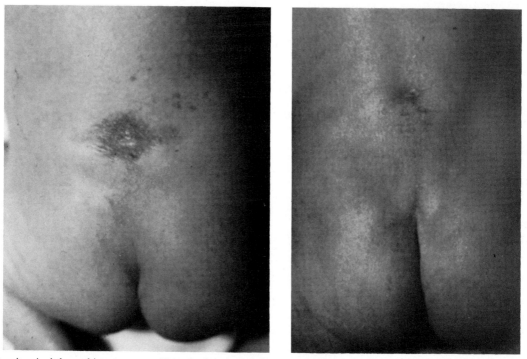

Occult spinal dysraphism sequence. Note the location of these lesions, which were the clues that resulted in surgical correction of tethered cord in early infancy. In addition to the flat hemangioma *(left)*, the mound of connective tissue *(right)*, and the localized absence of skin (both), surface anomalies may consist of lipomas, deep dimples, hair tufts, and skin tags. (From Higginbottom, M. C., et al.: J. Pediatr, *96*:687, 1980.)

SEPTO-OPTIC DYSPLASIA SEQUENCE

De Morsier recognized the association between the absence of the septum pellucidum and hypoplasia of the optic nerves and called it septo-optic dysplasia. The clinical spectrum of altered development and function arising from this defect has been reported by Hoyt and others to include hypopituitary dwarfism. The presumed developmental pathogenesis is depicted to the right.

ABNORMALITIES. Based on 17 cases.

Eyes. Hypoplastic optic nerves, chiasm, and infundibulum with pendular nystagmus and visual impairment, occasionally including field defects.

Hypothalamic. Secondary hypopituitarism, varying from isolated growth hormone deficiency to panhypopituitarism.

Other. Agenesis of septum pellucidum in about half of cases.

OCCASIONAL ABNORMALITIES. Trophic hormone hypersecretion, including growth hormone, corticotropin, and prolactin. Sexual precocity.

NATURAL HISTORY. Visual impairment, including partial to complete amblyopia, is frequent, and funduscopic evaluation discloses hypoplastic optic discs. Hypopituitarism of hypothalamic origin is a frequent feature and merits hormone replacement therapy. Kaplan found this sequence to be the most frequently recognized single defect in children with pituitary growth hormone deficiency. Most affected individuals are of normal intelligence, though mental deficiency does occur.

Features of the septo-optic dysplasia sequence may occur as a part of a broader pattern of early brain defect, such as the holoprosencephaly type of defect, in which case the prognosis for brain function and survival is poor.

ETIOLOGY. Unknown. Though this defect is usually a sporadic occurrence, the author has evaluated one case in which the otherwise normal mother had unilateral amblyopia with a hypoplastic optic disc. In addition, two first cousins with hypopituitarism have been reported, one of whom had septo-optic dysplasia.

References

de Morsier, G.: Études sur les dysraphies crânioencéphaliques. III. Agénésie du septum lucidum avec malformation du tractus optique. La dysplasie septo-optique. Schweiz. Arch. Neurol. Neurochir. Psychiatr., 77:267, 1956.

Hoyt, W. F., et al.: Septo-optic dysplasia and pituitary dwarfism. Lancet, 1:893, 1970.

Kaplan, S., University of California School of Medicine, San Francisco; personal communication.

Brook, C. G. D., Sanders, M. D., and Hoare, R. D.: Septo-optic dysplasia. Br. Med. J., 3:811, 1972.

Haseman, C. A., et al.: Sexual precocity in association with septo-optic dysplasia and hypothalamic hypopituitarism. J. Pediatr., 92:748, 1978.

Blethen, S. L., and Weldon, V. V.: Hypopituitarism and septo-optic "dysplasia" in first cousins. Am. J. Med. Genet., 21:123, 1985.

Margalith, D., Tze, W. J., and Jan, J. E.: Congenital optic nerve hypoplasia with hypothalamic-pituitary dysplasia. Am. J. Dis. Child., 139:361, 1985.

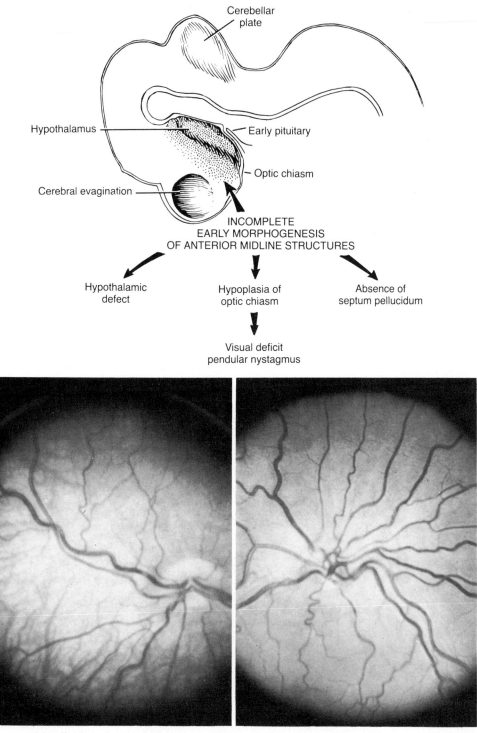

Above, Presumed localization of early single defect (stippled area) as shown in sagittal view of 38 day brain. *Below,* Photos of retinae of four year old patient with the septo-optic dysplasia sequence who had reduced vision, pendular nystagmus, and growth deficiency secondary to pituitary growth hormone deficiency. Note the hypoplastic optic nerve heads and aberrant vascular arrangement.

ATHYROTIC HYPOTHYROIDISM SEQUENCE

(Hypothyroidism Sequence)

Primary Defect—In Development of Thyroid Gland

Athyrotic hypothyroidism is usually a sporadic occurrence in an otherwise normal child. Severe hypothyroidism does not give rise to growth deficiency until after birth. Postnatally, morphogenesis and function are grossly impaired as a metabolic consequence of the lack of thyroid hormone. Adequate thyroid hormone replacement therapy, at least ¾ grain of U.S.P. desiccated thyroid per day for the affected infant, will allow for a complete return to physical normality for age. However, the detrimental effect of the hypothyroid state on morphogenesis and function of the brain is irreparable. Therefore, the earlier a diagnosis is made and adequate thyroid hormone therapy instituted, the better is the prognosis for mental function. The routine newborn screening for thyroxine (T_4) or thyroid-stimulating hormone (TSH) levels has allowed for early detection and treatment of the hypothyroid young infant, and as a result intelligence is usually in the normal range.

ABNORMALITIES. The following are some of the early signs that may allow for detection of the hypothyroid baby early in life. There is usually prenatal onset of osseous immaturity, as evidenced by large fontanels and immature facial bone structure (see illustration). Myxedema causes full subcutaneous tissues—most evident in the lower eyelids—with enlarged muscle mass and hoarse cry. Klein summarized the relative frequency of signs and symptoms that had been noted prior to three months of age in 31 patients with congenital hypothyroidism.

General

Feeding problems	39%
Decreased activity	39%
Constipation	52%
Neonatal jaundice	16%

Cutaneous-Vascular

Cold to touch	19%
Dry skin	45%
Mottling	58%

Myxedema

Enlarged tongue	45%
Hoarse cry	39%

Other

Umbilical hernia	58%

References

Wilkins, L.: The Diagnosis and Treatment of Endocrine Disorders in Childhood and Adolescence. Springfield, Ill., Charles C Thomas, 1965.

Smith, D. W., and Popich, G.: Large fontanels in congenital hypothyroidism. J. Pediatr., *80*:753, 1972.

Klein, A. H., Pittsburgh. Personal communication.

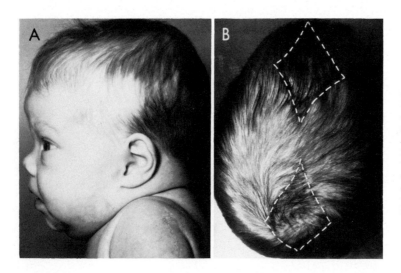

Evidence of osseous immaturity in a 3 month old infant with athyrotic hypothyroidism. *A*, Immature facies with low nasal bridge. Note also the full subcutaneous tissues. *B*, Immaturity of osseous calvarium, with outer limits of large fontanels indicated. The bone age as determined from roentgenograms of the knee and foot was interpreted as being at about an 8 month fetal level.

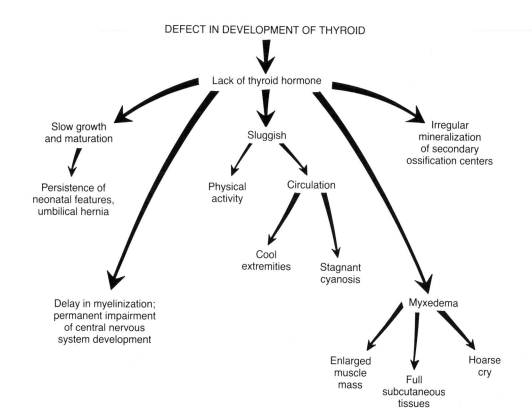

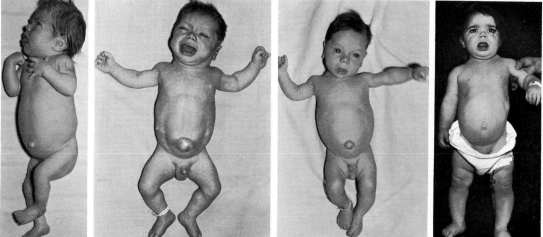

Age: 2 months
Height age: 1 month
Bone age: birth

Age: 9 months
Height age: 2 months
Bone age: birth

After 3 weeks of
thyroid replacement

Age: 3 years, untreated
Height age: 12 months
Bone age: 3 months

Above, Developmental pathogenesis of athyrotic hypothyroidism. *Below*, Athyrotic patients.

DiGEORGE SEQUENCE

*Primary Defect—Fourth Branchial Arch and
Derivatives of Third and Fourth Pharyngeal Pouches*

This pattern of malformation was emphasized by DiGeorge and variably includes defects of development of the thymus, parathyroids, and great vessels. Conley et al. have observed 19 cases at necropsy. The illustration shows the presumed developmental pathogenesis. The DiGeorge sequence may occur by itself, but in about 60 per cent of cases it is one feature of a broader pattern of malformation.

ABNORMALITIES. Varying features from among the following:

Thymus. Hypoplasia to aplasia, with deficit of cellular immunity allowing for severe infectious disease.

Parathyroids. Hypoplasia to absence, allowing for severe hypocalcemia and seizures in early infancy.

Cardiovascular. Aortic arch anomalies, including right aortic arch, interrupted aorta, conotruncal anomalies such as truncus arteriosus and ventricular septal defect, patent ductus arteriosus, and tetralogy of Fallot.

Facial. Tendency to have hypertelorism, short philtrum, downslanting palpebral fissues, ear anomalies.

OCCASIONAL ABNORMALITIES. Mental deficiency of mild to moderate degree. Esophageal atresia, choanal atresia, imperforate anus, diaphragmatic hernia.

NATURAL HISTORY. The majority of patients die within the first month. The most common cause of death is the cardiovascular defect, the second most common is infectious disease, and the third is seizures relative to hypocalcemia. Detection of any feature of this sequence should lead to concern as to the other features.

ETIOLOGY. Unknown. Although usually a sporadic occurrence in otherwise normal families, this pattern is etiologically heterogeneous. It has been associated with prenatal alcohol exposure and more recently in two familial cases with partial monosomy of the proximal long arm of chromosome 22. It is unclear at present what percentage of patients with DiGeorge sequence have a deletion of the number 22 chromosome.

References

Lobdell, D. H.: Congenital absence of the parathyroid glands. Arch. Pathol., 67:412, 1959.

Kretschmer, R., Say, B., Brown, D., and Rosen, F. S.: Congenital aplasia of the thymus gland (DiGeorge's syndrome). N. Engl. J. Med., 279:1295, 1968.

Freedom, R. M., Rosen, F. S., and Nadas, A. S.: Congenital cardiovascular disease and anomalies of the third and fourth pharyngeal pouch. Circulation, 46:165, 1972.

Conley, M. E., et al.: The spectrum of the DiGeorge syndrome. J. Pediatr., 94:883, 1979.

Greenberg, F., et al.: Familial DiGeorge syndrome and associated partial monosomy of chromosome 22. Hum. Genet., 65:317, 1984.

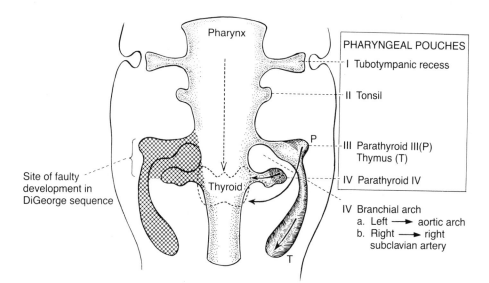

Schematic appearance of anterior foregut and its derivatives at around the fifth week of development, showing the presumed site of defect in the DiGeorge sequence.

KLIPPEL-FEIL SEQUENCE

*Short Neck with Low Hairline and Limited
Movement of Head; Primary Defect—Early
Development of Cervical Vertebrae*

In this malformation sequence, originally described by Klippel and Feil in 1912, the cervical vertebrae are usually fused, though hemivertebrae and other defects may also be found. There may also be secondary webbed neck, torticollis, and/or facial asymmetry. The frequency is about 1:42,000 births, and 65 per cent of patients are female. The sequence may be a part of a serious problem in early neural tube development, as is found in iniencephaly, cervical meningomyelocele, syringomyelia, or syringobulbia. Primary or secondary neurologic deficits may occur, such as paraplegia, hemiplegia, cranial or cervical nerve palsies, and synkinesia.

The following defects have occurred in a nonrandom association in patients with the Klippel-Feil sequence: deafness, either conductive or neural, noted in as many as 30 per cent, congenital heart defects, the most common being a ventricular septal defect; and mental deficiency, cleft palate, rib defects, the Sprengel sequence, scoliosis, and renal abnormalities.

Because of the neck immobility, affected individuals are more liable to have fracture of the neck and should therefore avoid violent trauma.

Usually a sporadic occurrence of unknown etiology, this sequence has rarely been found in siblings. A close evaluation of the immediate family is indicated, since autosomal dominant inheritance with variable expression in affected individuals has been noted, although this is presumably rare.

References

Klippel, M., and Feil, A.: Un cas d'absence des vertébres cervicales, avec cage thoracique remontant jusqu'à la base du crâne (cage thoracique cervicale) Mouv. Inconogr. Salpêt., *25*:223, 1912.

Gorlin, R. J., and Pindborg, J. J.: Syndromes of the Head and Neck. New York, McGraw-Hill Book Co., 1963, pp. 335–338, 401.

Morrison, S. G., Perry, L. W., and Scott, L. P., III: Congenital brevicollis (Klippel-Feil syndrome) and cardiovascular anomalies. Am. J. Dis. Child., *115*:614, 1968.

Palant, D. J., and Carter, B. L.: Klippel-Feil syndrome and deafness. Am. J. Dis. Child., *123*:218, 1972.

Hensinger, R. W., Lang, J. E., and MacEwen, G. D.: Klippel-Feil syndrome. J. Bone Joint Surg., *56-A*:1246, 1974.

Infant with the Klippel-Feil sequence.

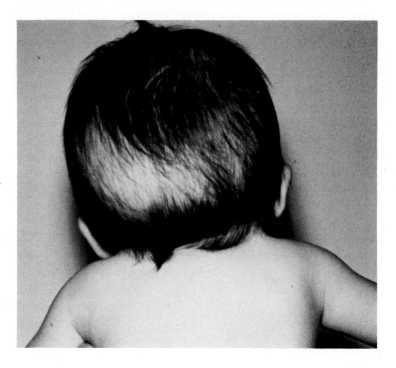

JUGULAR LYMPHATIC OBSTRUCTION SEQUENCE

The lymphatic channels in each upper quadrant drain into the jugular lymphatic sac, which, at about 40 days of development, opens into the jugular vein on that side. Failure of development of this communication results in stasis of the lymph fluid, which causes a host of consequences referred to as the jugular lymphatic obstruction sequence. The distended jugular lymph sac results in an excess of skin in the neck region with alteration in the zone of hair growth and the hair directional patterning plus elevation and sometimes protrusion of the lower auricle. The accumulating peripheral lymphedema causes full subcutaneous tissues with relative overgrowth of the overlying skin, prominent fingertip pads, and narrow hyperconvex nails, which are often deeply set at the base. The lack of lymphatic drainage results in an increased volume of fluid in the venous system, resulting in large veins.

This is apparently a lethal anomaly unless the communication between the jugular lymph sac and the jugular vein develops by mid- to late fetal life. Once the link does occur, the distended jugular lymph sac collapses, leaving redundant overlying skin folds that are referred to as a pterygium colli. The drainage from the subcutaneous areas leaves relatively redundant skin, which is especially notable in the facies. The peripheral lymphedema may not have completely receded by birth, causing puffy hands and feet.

The jugular lymphatic obstruction sequence accounts for many of the features of the surviving individuals with the XO Turner syndrome and may be the predominant cause of the high early fetal lethality in this disorder. However, the sequence is a nonspecific defect and may occur in a number of disorders.

The lymphatic channels in the lower quadrants drain into the iliac lymph sacs, which are analogous to the jugular lymph sacs. A lag in the communication with the venous system results in peripheral lymphedema in the lower limbs and sometimes the genital region. If the iliac lymph sacs are grossly distended, there may be distention of the abdomen. Decompression by communication with the venous system may yield a residuum of redundant abdominal skin, which is one cause of the so-called "prune belly."

References

Töndury, G., and Kubik, S.: Zur Ontogenese des lymphatischen systems. Handbuch der Allgemeinen Pathologie. Berlin, Springer-Verlag, 1975, pp. 2–38.

Van der Putte, S. C.: The development of the lymphatic system in man. Adv. Anat. Embryol., *51*:1, 1975.

Van der Putte, S. C.: Lymphatic malformation in human fetuses. A study of fetuses with Turner's syndrome or status Bonnevie-Ullrich. Virchows Arch. (Path. Anat.), *376*:233, 1977.

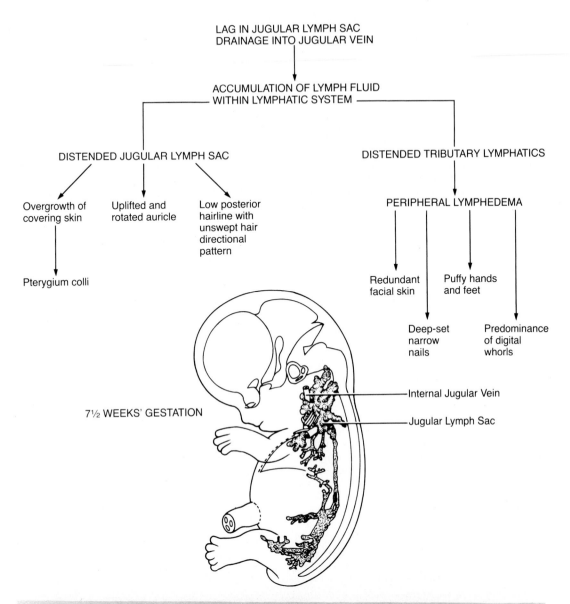

LAG IN JUGULAR LYMPH SAC
DRAINAGE INTO JUGULAR VEIN

ACCUMULATION OF LYMPH FLUID
WITHIN LYMPHATIC SYSTEM

DISTENDED JUGULAR LYMPH SAC

Overgrowth of
covering skin

Uplifted and
rotated auricle

Low posterior
hairline with
unswept hair
directional
pattern

Pterygium colli

DISTENDED TRIBUTARY LYMPHATICS

PERIPHERAL LYMPHEDEMA

Redundant
facial skin

Puffy hands
and feet

Deep-set
narrow
nails

Predominance
of digital
whorls

7½ WEEKS' GESTATION

Internal Jugular Vein

Jugular Lymph Sac

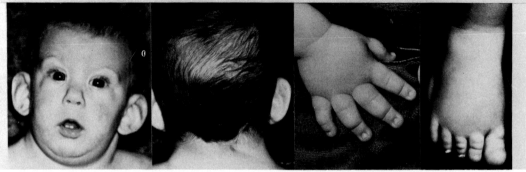

Presumed genesis of the jugular lymphatic obstruction sequence. The jugular lymph sac, shown here in a seven and one-half week embryo, normally opens into the jugular vein by about 40 days. Late communication may yield a number of residua engendered during the period of lymphatic obstruction.

EARLY URETHRAL
OBSTRUCTION SEQUENCE

Early urethral obstruction is most commonly the consequence of urethral valve formation during the development of the prostatic urethra. Less commonly, it is due to urethral atresia, bladder neck obstruction, or distal urethral obstruction. With urine formation occurring, by seven to eight weeks of fetal life, there is a progressive back-up of urine flow, leading to the consequences shown in the flow diagram. The male to female ratio of 20:1 in this disorder is a result of the predominant malformations being in the development of the penile urethra. Cryptorchidism occurs secondary to the bulk of the distended bladder, preventing full descent of the testes. The back pressure usually limits full renal morphogenesis and may result in dilatation of the renal tubules, which by histologic section examination may be interpreted as renal "cysts." The compressive mass of the bladder may limit full rotation of the colon and may even compress the iliac vessels to the point of causing partial defects or vascular disruption of the lower limb(s). The oligohydramnios will give rise to all the secondary phenomena of the oligohydramnios deformation sequence.

Severe early urethral obstruction is often lethal by mid- to late fetal life unless the bladder ruptures and is thereby decompressed. The bladder rupture may occur through a patent urachus, an obstructing urethral "valve," or the wall of the bladder or ureter. Following decompression, the fetus will be left with a "prune belly."

Unfortunately, most of those who survive to term have incurred severe renal damage and are unable to live long after birth. Those who do survive may be assisted by urologic procedures to aid urinary drainage and control urinary tract infection. Respiration and bowel movements may be eased by wrapping the abdomen with a "belly binder." With advancing age, the hypoplastic abdominal musculature will usually improve in volume and strength to the point of being no serious problem.

The recurrence risk for the disorder is dependent on the specific cause of the urethral obstruction, and these data have not yet been determined. This defect most commonly occurs in an otherwise normal individual, but may be but one feature of a broader pattern of malformation, such as the VATER association (see page 602).

Early fetal diagnosis is possible, since sonography will show the distended bladder by ten weeks from conception. This defect should lend itself to early fetal surgery, with the placement of a catheter from the bladder to the amniotic space being helpful until after birth, when the primary malformation may be repaired.

References

Stumme, E. G.: Ueber die symmetrischen kongenitalen Bauchmuskel defeckte und über die Kombination derselben mit anderen Bildunganomalien des Rumfes. Mitt. Grenzigebeite Med. Chir., 6:548, 1903.

Silverman, F. N., and Huang, N.: Congenital absence of the abdominal muscles. Am. J. Dis. Child., 80:91, 1950.

Lattimer, J. K.: Congenital deficiency of abdominal musculature and associated genitourinary anomalies. J. Urol., 79:343, 1958.

Pagon, R. A., Smith, D. W., and Shepard, T. H.: Urethral obstruction malformation complex: A cause of abdominal muscle deficiency and the "prune belly." J. Pediatr., 94:900, 1979.

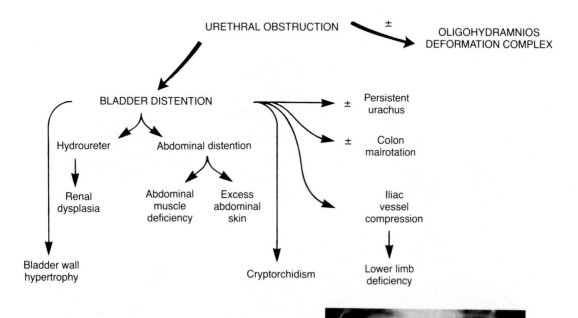

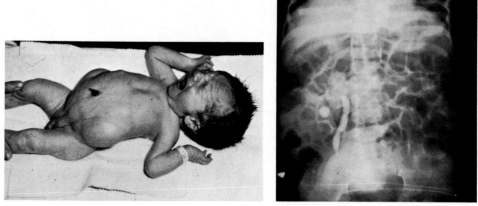

Developmental pathogenesis of early urethral obstruction sequence.

Illustration continued on following page

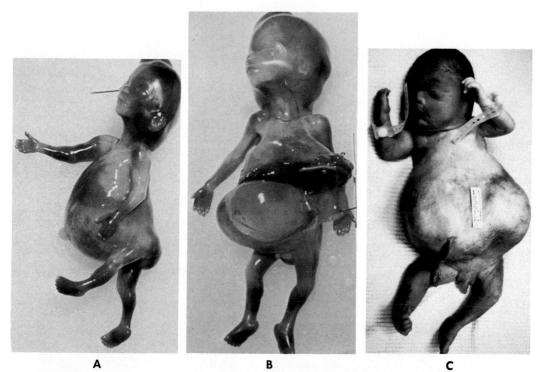

A   **B**   **C**

Early urethral obstruction sequence. *A, B,* Ten week fetus before and after abdomen was opened, showing distended bladder due to urethral obstruction. (Courtesy of Dr. Thomas Shepard, University of Washington, Seattle.) *C, D,* Older stillborn fetus with bilobed, thickened, massively distended bladder due to urethral obstruction. Vascular occlusion to legs resulted in ischemia and altered morphogenesis of the feet. (Courtesy of Cindy Dolan, Spokane, Washington.) *E, F,* Prenatal rupture of prostatic urethral obstruction decompressed the abdomen, leaving a "prune belly" as one residuum. (*F* courtesy of Dr. Jaime L. Frias, University of Nebraska, Omaha.)

Illustration continued on opposite page

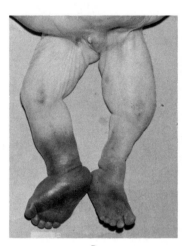

D

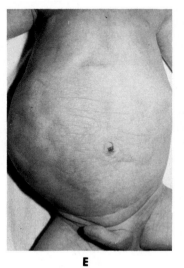

E

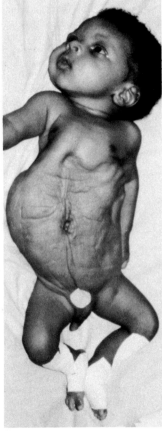

F

EXSTROPHY OF BLADDER SEQUENCE

Primary Defect—In Infraumbilical Mesoderm

Normally the bladder portion of the cloaca and the overlying ectoderm are in direct contact (the cloacal membrane) until the infraumbilical mesenchyme migrates into the area at about the sixth to seventh week of fetal development, giving rise to the lower abdominal wall, genital tubercles, and pubic rami. A failure of the infraumbilical mesenchyme to invade the area allows for a breakdown in the cloacal membrane, in similar fashion to that which normally occurs at the oral, anal, and urogenital areas, where mesoderm does not intercede between ectoderm and endoderm. Thus the posterior bladder wall is exposed, in conjunction with defects in structures derived from the infraumbilical mesenchyme.

This malformation sequence, six times as likely to occur in the male as in the female, continues to be a difficult one to correct, though encouraging results have followed immediate postnatal primary closure of both the bladder and the pubic rami.

References

Wyburn, G. M.: The development of the infraumbilical portion of the abdominal wall, with remarks on the aetiology of ectopia vesicae. J. Anat., *71*:201, 1937.

Muecke, E. C.: The role of the cloacal membrane in exstrophy: the first successful experimental study. J. Urol., *92*:659, 1964.

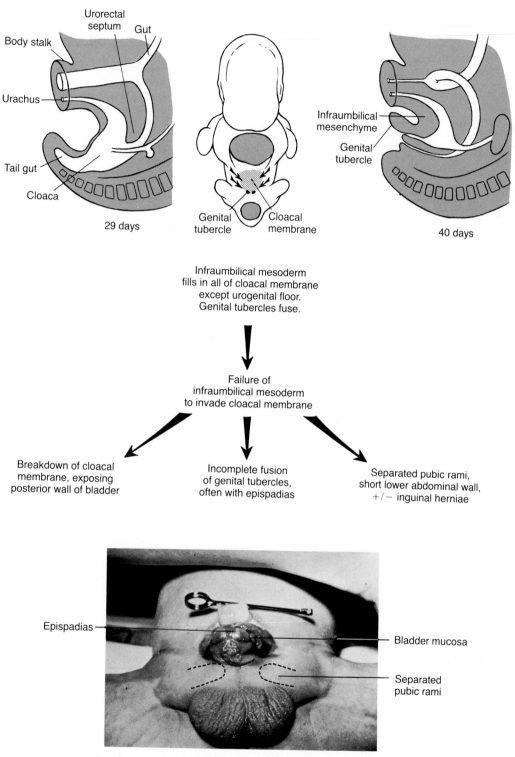

Developmental pathogenesis of exstrophy of bladder sequence.

EXSTROPHY OF CLOACA SEQUENCE

Primary Defect—Early Mesoderm
That Will Contribute to Infraumbilical Mesenchmye,
Cloacal Septum, and Lumbosacral Vertebrae

The remarkable similarity among otherwise normal individuals with this bizarre type of defect suggests a similar mode of developmental pathology having its inception as a single localized defect—theoretically in the early development of the mesoderm, which will later contribute to the infraumbilical mesenchyme, cloacal septum, and caudal vertebrae. The consequences are (1) failure to cloacal septation, with the persistence of a common cloaca into which the ureters, ileum, and a rudimentary hindgut open; (2) complete breakdown of the cloacal membrane with exstrophy of the cloaca, failure of fusion of the genital tubercles and pubic rami, and often omphalocele; and (3) incomplete development of the lumbosacral vertebrae with herniation of a grossly dilated central canal of the spinal cord (hydromyelia), yielding a soft, cystic, skin-covered mass over the sacral area, sometimes asymmetric in its positioning. The rudimentary hindgut may contain two appendices, and there is no anal opening. The small intestine may be relatively short. Cryptorchidism is a usual finding in the male. Affected females have unfused müllerian elements with completely bifid uterine horns and short, duplicated, or atretic vaginas. Most patients have a single umbilical artery, and anomalies of the lower limbs are occasionally present.

Surgical intervention has been carried out. However, considering the overall problem of urinary and fecal incontinence plus the incomplete genital development, the author believes that a decision toward surgical partial correction should be undertaken only after careful consideration with the family.

References

Spencer, R.: Exstrophia splanchnica (exstrophy of the cloaca). Surgery, 57:751, 1965.

Zwiren, G. T., and Patterson, J. H.: Exstrophy of the cloaca: report of a case treated surgically. Pediatrics, 35:687, 1965.

Beckwith, J. B.: The congenitally malformed. VII. Exstrophy of the bladder and cloacal exstrophy. Northwest Med., 65:407, 1966.

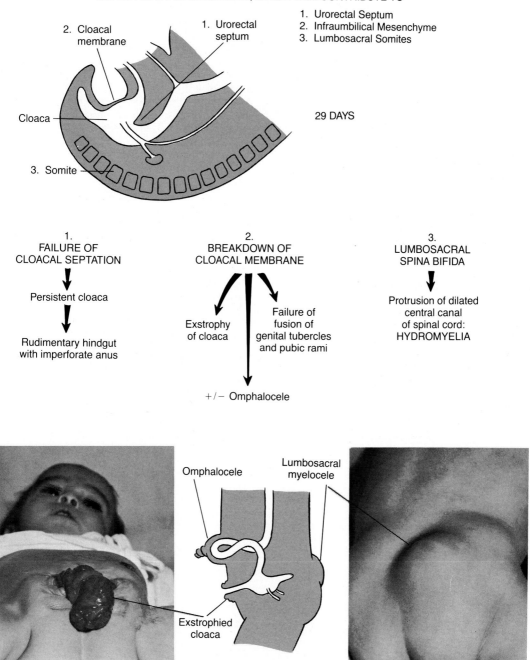

DEFECT IN EARLY MESODERM, WHICH WILL CONTRIBUTE TO

1. Urorectal Septum
2. Infraumbilical Mesenchyme
3. Lumbosacral Somites

2. Cloacal membrane

1. Urorectal septum

Cloaca

29 DAYS

3. Somite

| 1. FAILURE OF CLOACAL SEPTATION | 2. BREAKDOWN OF CLOACAL MEMBRANE | 3. LUMBOSACRAL SPINA BIFIDA |

Persistent cloaca

Exstrophy of cloaca

Failure of fusion of genital tubercles and pubic rami

Protrusion of dilated central canal of spinal cord: HYDROMYELIA

Rudimentary hindgut with imperforate anus

+ / − Omphalocele

Omphalocele

Lumbosacral myelocele

Exstrophied cloaca

Above, Developmental pathogenesis of exstrophy of cloaca sequence. *Below, left,* Infant with exstrophy of the cloaca (prolapsed intestine). Note separation of scrotal folds and genital tubercle.

ROKITANSKY SEQUENCE

Vaginal Atresia and Rudimentary Uterus;
Primary Defect—In Lower
Paramesonephric Ducts (Müllerian Ducts)

The paramesonephric ducts normally fuse caudally at about eight weeks of fetal development and thereafter form the uterus, cervix, and the upper part of the vagina. A single defect in development of the caudal paramesonephric ducts is the presumed explanation for the pattern of anomaly initially reported by Rokitansky, which is characterized by an incomplete to atretic vagina and a rudimentary to bicornuate uterus. The fallopian tubes and ovaries are usually nearly normal with normal secondary sexual characteristics, except for a lack of menstruation. The lower vagina, which is derived from an outpouching from the urogenital sinus, is usually present as a blindly ending pouch. The cause is unknown, with most cases being sporadic. About 4 per cent of cases have been familial, with affected female siblings.

Associated anomalies include defects in other derivatives of the mesonephric ridge. About one third to one half of the patients have a renal anomaly such as renal agenesis, hypoplasia, or double ureters. Also, about 10 per cent of patients have a vertebral and/or rib anomaly.

The Rokitansky malformation sequence may be a part of a broader pattern of malformation. For example, Winter et al. reported four sisters; three had vaginal atresia, all had unilateral or bilateral renal agenesis, and the two survivors had conductive deafness.

References

Rokitansky, K.: Über sog. Verdoppelung des Uterus. Med. Jahrb. des Osterreich. Staates, *26*:39, 1838.

Bryan, A. L., Nigro, J. A., and Counseller, V. S.: One hundred cases of congenital absence of the vagina. Surg. Gynecol. Obstet., *88*:79, 1949.

Anger, D., Hemet, J., and Ensel, J.: Forme familiale du syndrome de Rokitansky-Kuster-Hauser. Bull. Féd. Soc. Gynécol. Obstet. Lang. Fr., *18*:229, 1966.

Leduc, B., Van Campenjout, J., and Simard, R.: Congenital absence of the vagina. Observations on 25 cases. Am. J. Obstet. Gynecol., *100*:512, 1968.

Winter, J. S. D., et al.: A familial syndrome of renal, genital, and middle ear anomalies. J. Pediatr., *72*:88, 1968.

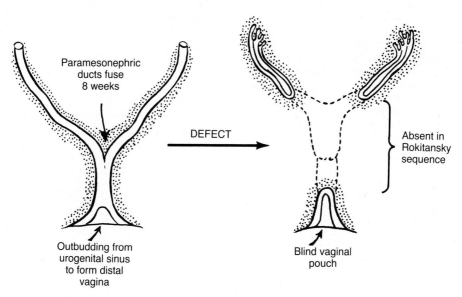

Paramesonephric
ducts fuse
8 weeks

DEFECT

Absent in
Rokitansky
sequence

Outbudding from
urogenital sinus
to form distal
vagina

Blind vaginal
pouch

Presumed derivation of the Rokitansky sequence.

OLIGOHYDRAMNIOS SEQUENCE

(Potter Syndrome)

Primary Defect—Development of Oligohydramnios

Renal agenesis, which must occur prior to 31 days of fetal development, will secondarily limit the amount of amniotic fluid and thereby result in further anomalies during prenatal life. The renal agenesis may be the only primary defect, or it may be one feature of a more extensive caudal axis anomaly. Other types of urinary tract defects such as polycystic kidneys or obstruction may also be responsible for oligohydramnios and its consequences. Another cause is chronic leakage of amniotic fluid from the time of midgestation. Regardless of the cause, the secondary effects of oligohydramnios are the same and would appear to be the result of compression of the fetus, as depicted below. The cause of death is respiratory insufficiency, with a lack of the late development of alveolar sacs. A similar lag in late development of the lung is observed with diaphragmatic hernia or asphyxiating thoracic dystropy. In both of these latter situations, there is external compression of the developing lung; this is considered the most likely cause in oligohydramnios, as shown in the figure.

When the oligohydramnios is secondary to agenesis or dysgenesis of both kidneys or agenesis of one kidney and dysgenesis of the other, renal ultrasonagraphic evaluation of both parents and siblings of affected infants should be performed, since 9 per cent of first degree relatives had asymptomatic renal malformations in a study by Roodhooft et al.

References

Potter, E. L.: Bilateral renal agenesis. J. Pediatr., *29*:68, 1946.

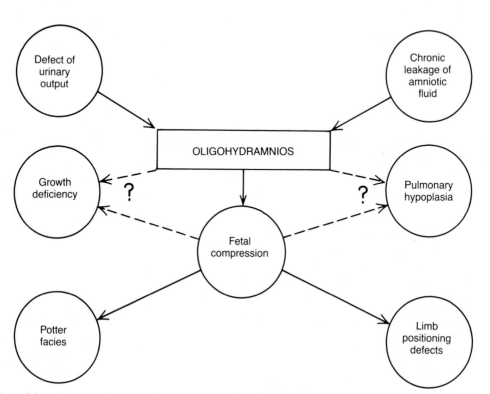

Depiction of the origin and effects of oligohydramnios. The oligohydramnios sequence is implied to be secondary to fetal compression.

Bain, A. D., and Scott, J. S.: Renal agenesis and severe urinary tract dysplasia. A review of 50 cases with particular reference to the associated anomalies. Br. Med. J., *1*:841, 1960.

Thomas, I. T., and Smith, D. W.: Oligohydramnios, cause of the non-renal features of Potter's syndrome, including pulmonary hypoplasia. J. Pediatr., *84*:811, 1974.

Roodhooft, A. M., Birnholz, J. C., and Holmes, L. B.: Familial nature of congenital absence and severe dysgenesis of both kidneys. N. Engl. J. Med., *310*:1341, 1984.

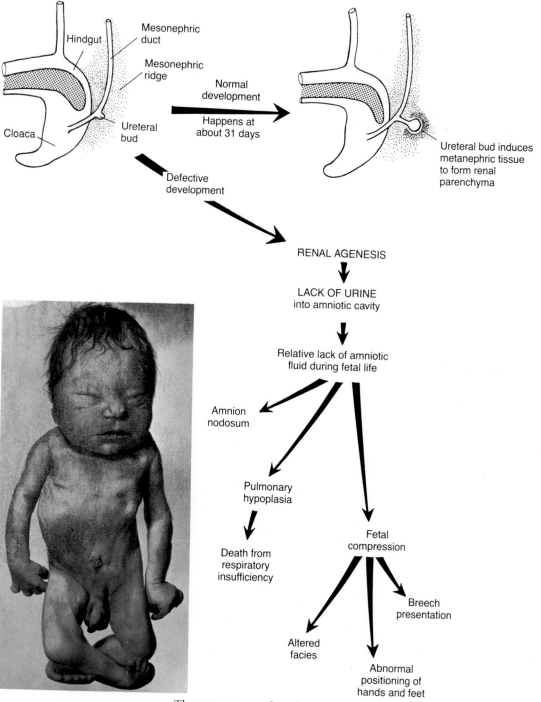

The consequences of renal agenesis.

SIRENOMELIA SEQUENCE

This defect has previously been thought to be the consequence of a wedge-shaped early deficit of the posterior axis caudal blastema, allowing for fusion of the early limb buds at their fibular margins with absence or incomplete development of the intervening caudal structures. However, Stevenson et al. have shown recently that sirenomelia and its commonly associated defects are produced by an alteration in early vascular development. Rather than blood returning to the placenta through the usual paired umbilical arteries arising from the iliac arteries, blood returns to the placenta through a single large vessel, a derivative of the vitelline artery complex, which arises from the aorta just below the diaphragm. The abdominal aorta distal to the origin of this major vessel is always subordinate and usually gives off no tributaries, especially renal or inferior mesenteric arteries, before it bifurcates into iliac arteries. This vascular alteration leads to a "vitelline artery steal" in which blood flow and thus nutrients are diverted from the caudal structures of the embryo to the placenta. Resultant defects include a single lower extremity with posterior alignment of knees

and feet, arising from failure of the lower limb bud field to be cleaved into two lateral masses by an intervening allantois; absence of sacrum and other defects of vertebrae; imperforate anus and absence of rectum; absence of external and internal genitalia; renal agenesis; and absence of the bladder. Based on the variable alterations that could exist in blood flow, a variable spectrum of abnormalities occurs in structures dependent on the distal aorta for nutrients. Thus, as with other disruptive vascular defects, no two cases of sirenomelia are ever exactly the same.

References

Wolff, E.: Les bases de la tératogénèse expérimentale des vertèbres amniotes, d'après les résultats de méthodes directes. Arch. Anat. Histol. Embryol. (Strasb.), *22*:1, 1936.

Stevenson, R. E., et al.: Vascular steal: The pathogenetic mechanism producing sirenomelia and associated defects of the viscera and soft tissues. Pediatrics, *78*:451, 1986.

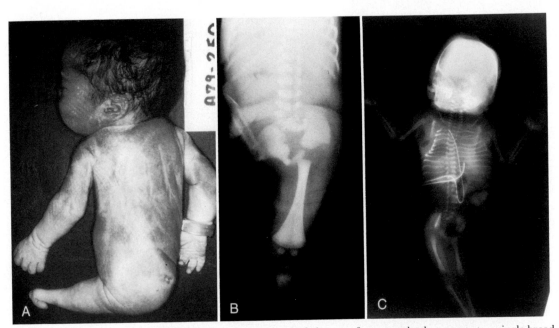

A, Stillborn infant with sirenomelia. *B*, *C*, The bones in the single leg vary from completely separate to a single broad femur with two distal ossification centers and a broad tibia with two ossification centers.

CAUDAL DYSPLASIA SEQUENCE

(Caudal Regression Syndrome)

This disorder has previously been grouped with sirenomelia, which was thought to represent its most severe form. Recent evidence suggests that the two are pathogenetically unrelated. Whereas sirenomelia and its associated defects are produced by an early vascular alteration leading to a "vitelline artery steal," the caudal dysplasia sequence is most likely heterogeneous with respect to its etiology and developmental pathogenesis.

Structural defects of the caudal region observed in this pattern of malformation include the following to variable degrees: incomplete development of the sacrum and, to a lesser extent, the lumbar vertebrae; absence of the body of the sacrum leading to flattening of the buttocks, shortening of the intergluteal cleft, and dimpling of the buttocks; disruption of the distal spinal cord leading secondarily to neurologic impairment, varying from incontinence of urine and feces to complete neurologic loss; and extreme lack of growth in the caudal region resulting from decreased movement of the legs secondary to neurologic impairment. The most severely affected infants have flexion and abduction at the hips and popliteal webs secondary to lack of movement. Talipes equinovarus and calcaneovalgus deformities are common.

Occasional abnormalities include renal agenesis, imperforate anus, cleft lip, cleft palate, microcephaly, and meningomyelocele.

NATURAL HISTORY. In the most severely affected individuals, prognosis is poor. Urologic and orthopedic management is required in the vast majority of those who survive.

ETIOLOGY. Unknown. Sixteen per cent have occurred in offspring of diabetic mothers. Although usually sporadic, a few instances of affected siblings born to unaffected parents have been described.

References

Rusnak, S. L., and Driscoll, S. G.: Congenital spinal anomalies in infants of diabetic mothers. Pediatrics, 35:989, 1965.

Passarge, E., and Lenz, W.: Syndrome of caudal regression in infants of diabetic mothers: observations of further cases. Pediatrics, 37:672, 1966.

Gellis, S. S., and Feingold, M.: Picture of the month: caudal dysplasia syndrome. Am. J. Dis. Child., 116:407, 1968.

Price, D. L., Dooling, E. C., and Richardson, E. P.: Caudal dysplasia (caudal regression syndrome). Arch. Neurol., 23:212, 1970.

Finer, N. N., Bowen, P., and Dunbar, L. G.: Caudal regression anomalad (sacral agenesis in siblings. Clin. Genet., 13:353, 1978.

Stewart, J. M., and Stoll, S.: Familial caudal regression anomalad and maternal diabetes. J. Med. Genet., 16:17, 1979.

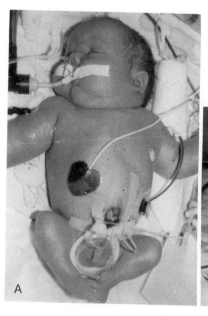

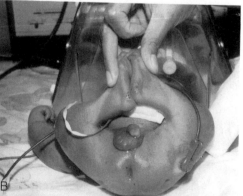

Caudal dysplasia sequence. *A*, Newborn male infant with a normal upper body and a short lower segment. *B*, Note the pterygia in the popliteal region, which are secondary to neurologically related flexion contractures at the knees.

EARLY AMNION RUPTURE
SEQUENCE

Though the structural defects consequent to early amnion rupture were reported by Portal in 1685, it was not until more recent times that analogous defects have been produced experimentally by early rupture of the amnion in the rat by Poswillo, Kino, and Kennedy and Persaud and that the full spectrum of defects that occur in the human have been appreciated by Torpin, Jones et al., Higginbottom et al., Graham et al., and Miller et al. As shown in the figures, early rupture of the amnion may cause problems in morphogenesis because of early compression of the embryo. Such early compression may result in molded deformation, e.g., scoliosis and foot deformities. It may also cause edema, hemorrhage, and resorptive necrosis with disruption of previously normal tissues, as has been experimentally produced by amnion rupture at the time of early limb morphogenesis. The compression may also distort early limb morphogenesis, causing polydactyly, and may result in incomplete morphogenesis of normally developing structures, producing, for example, syndactyly due to incomplete separation of the digits. The early compression and/or aberrant amniotic attachments may limit the space and movement of the fetus and result in a short umbilical cord. Aberrant amnion bands, strands, and sheets can cause disruption of morphogenesis in the craniofacial region, abdominal wall, and/or limbs. They can also result in incompletion of normal stages of morphogenesis, can

limit mobility, and can lead to mechanical postural deformations. The nature and severity of the consequences of early amnion rupture relate to the timing of the event, as indicated in Table 1–3. From the earliest types of defects, such as anencephaly, to the later problems, such as the oligohydramnios deformation sequence due to chronic long-term leakage of amniotic fluid, the clinician encounters all gradations in the spectrum of defects that may occur as a result of early amnion rupture. No two affected fetuses will have exactly the same features, and there is no single feature, including amniotic bands, that consistently occurs. Examination of the placenta and membranes may be most helpful. Aberrant bands or strands of amnion may be noted, and/or there may be the rolled-up remnants of the amnion at the placental base of the umbilical cord.

Most of the early amnion rupture cases are spontaneous abortuses, are stillborn, or die soon after birth. More than half of those affected have not initially had a correct diagnosis. All too commonly, the "diagnosis" is of one or more of the secondary major defects, upon which the counseling and recurrence risk are fallaciously based. Among "anencephaly" cases, for example, a minimum of three of 79 studied by Holmes et al. were early amnion rupture sequence cases, as were a minimum of three of 56 cases in the study by Lemire et al. Added together, these findings indicate that at least 4 per cent of "anencephaly"

Table 1–3. **ABNORMALITIES FOUND IN EARLY AMNION RUPTURE SEQUENCE**

Fetal Timing	Craniofacial	Limbs	Other
3 weeks	Anencephaly Facial distortion, proboscis Unusual facial clefting Eye defects, encephalocele, meningocele	—	Placenta attached to head and/or abdomen
5 weeks	Usual cleft lip Choanal atresia	Limb reduction Polydactyly Syndactyly	Abdominal wall defects Thoracic wall defects Scoliosis
7 weeks and onward	Cleft palate (Robin deformation sequence) Ear deformation Craniostenosis	Amniotic bands Amputation Hypoplasia Pseudosyndactyly Distal lymphedema Foot deformation Dislocation of hip	Short umbilical cord Omphalocele
Later	Oligohydramnios deformation sequence	—	—

cases are, in reality, early amnion rupture sequence, with anencephaly as one feature of the disorder. The combination of several consequences of early amnion rupture may be mistakenly considered as a syndrome diagnosis. This has happened in the combinations of abdominal or thoracic wall defects and associated limb defects, which have been termed cyllosoma and pleurosomus. Most of these cases simply represent one part of the broad spectrum of defects due to early amnion rupture and should not be considered as specific separate diagnoses.

Early amnion rupture and its consequences are not rare. Certainly among spontaneous abortuses it is one of the more common recognizable patterns of structural defect. Among neonates, it is estimated that about 1 in 2000 have some problem secondary to early amnion rupture.

ABNORMALITIES. Abnormalities are listed in Table 1–3.

NATURAL HISTORY AND MANAGEMENT. The natural history varies with the severity of the problem. As mentioned, most of the early amnion rupture cases are early lethals, such as abortuses, stillborns, or early postnatal deaths. There is an occasional instance in which the face may show disruptive clefting and distortion without serious involvement of the brain. For such an infant, full plastic surgical repair measures are merited, since the brain can be normal. The most common survivors with amnion rupture problems are those who have amnion constrictive bands and/or amputations of the limb. These infants are usually quite normal except for the obvious limb problems. Occasionally, plastic surgery may be indicated, especially for the partially constrictive, deep residual groove that encircles a limb and is associated with partial limitation of vascular and/or lymphatic return from the distal limb. In such instances, a Z-plasty of the skin may be done to relieve the partial constriction, as well as for cosmetic improvement.

If there has been chronic amnion leakage, the neonate may show features of the oligohydramnios deformation sequence, including incomplete development of the lung, with respiratory insufficiency and development of hyaline membrane disease. Every attempt should be made to oxygenate and support such an infant, since, with continued lung morphogenesis, the prognosis can be excellent.

Because the result of early amnion rupture is external compression and/or disruption, there are rarely any internal anomalies. Hence, the features evident by surface examination are usually the only abnormalities. For example, if the calvarium appears to be normal in shape and form, the brain can be assumed to be normal.

ETIOLOGY. The etiology has been, with rare exceptions, idiopathic. Those rare exceptions are known or presumed to be caused by trauma and include two examples of attempted early termination of pregnancy by using a coat hanger and one incident of a woman falling from a horse while pregnant. It has generally been a sporadic event in an otherwise normal family, and hence the recurrence risk is usually stated as being negligible.

References

Portal, P.: La Pratique des Accouchements. Paris, 1685.

Torpin, R.: Amniochorionic mesoblastic fibrous strings and amniotic bands: Associated constricting fetal malformations or fetal death. Am. J. Obstet. Gynecol., 91:65, 1965.

Poswillo, D.: Observations of fetal posture and causal mechanisms of congenital deformity of the palate, mandible and limbs. J. Dent. Res., 45(Suppl. 3):2, 1966.

Torpin, R.: Fetal Malformations Caused by Amnion Rupture During Gestation. Springfield, Ill., Charles C Thomas, 1968.

Jones, K. L., et al.: A pattern of craniofacial and limb defects secondary to aberrant tissue bands. J. Pediatr., 84:90, 1974.

Kino, Y.: Clinical and experimental studies of the congenital constriction band syndrome, with emphasis on its etiology. J. Bone Joint Surg., 57(5):636, 1975.

Holmes, L. B., Driscoll, S. G., and Atkins, L.: Etiology heterogeneity for neural tube defects. N. Engl. J. Med., 294:365, 1976.

Kennedy, L. A., and Persaud, T. V. N.: Pathogenesis of developmental defects induced in the rat by amniotic sac puncture. Acta Anat., 97:23, 1977.

Lemire, R. J., Beckwith, J. B., and Warkany, J.: Anencephaly. New York, Raven Press, 1978.

Higginbottom, M. C., et al.: The amniotic band disruption complex: Timing of amniotic rupture and variable spectra of consequent defects. J. Pediatr., 95:544, 1979.

Pagon, B., et al.: Body wall defects with reduction limb anomalies. A report of 15 cases. Birth Defects Original Article Series, 15(5A):171, 1979.

Graham, J. M., et al.: Limb reduction anomalies and early in-utero limb compression. J. Pediatr., 96:1052, 1980.

Miller, M. E., et al.: Compression-related defects from early amnion rupture: Evidence for mechanical teratogenesis. J. Pediatr., 98:292, 1981.

Illustrations on pages 578 to 583

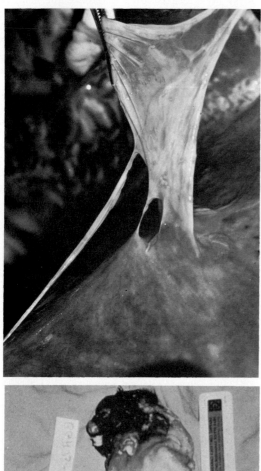

Aberrant attachments of amnion to chorion, with amnionic strand evident in the placenta of an infant with severe early amnion rupture sequence.

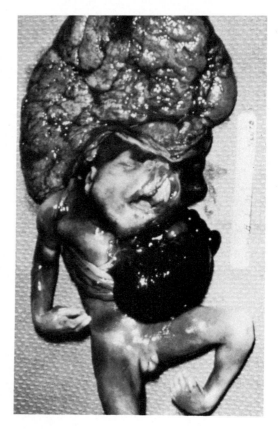

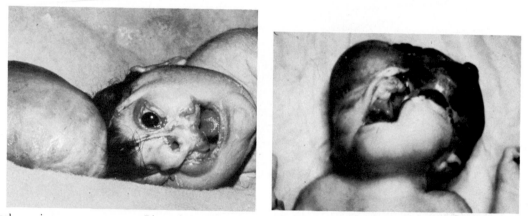

Early amnion rupture sequence. Disruptions of early craniofacial morphogenesis include instances with severe defects of the brain, asymmetric encephalocele, and band disruption of facial development. These bands can extend upward from the mouth, nose, and/or occasionally from other parts of the face. The head may be attached to the placenta. The affected individual may show multiple other effects such as band amputation (opposite page left) and body wall disruption (opposite page right).

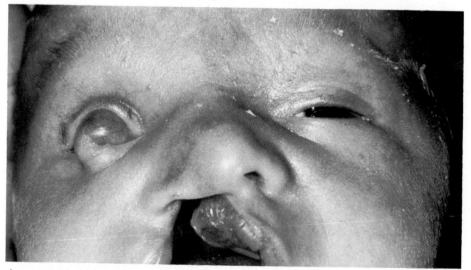

Early amnion rupture sequence. The amnionic bands are often gone by the time of birth, leaving only the residual effects. In this example, there was presumably a band from the mouth that extended upward and prevented closure of the lip, resulting in an aberrant disruption of the lower eyelid region, with cutaneous-type epithelialization over the eye and the aberrant hair directional patterning in the right lateral eyebrow. This is the same patient shown in the lower right on the next page.

Illustration continued on following page

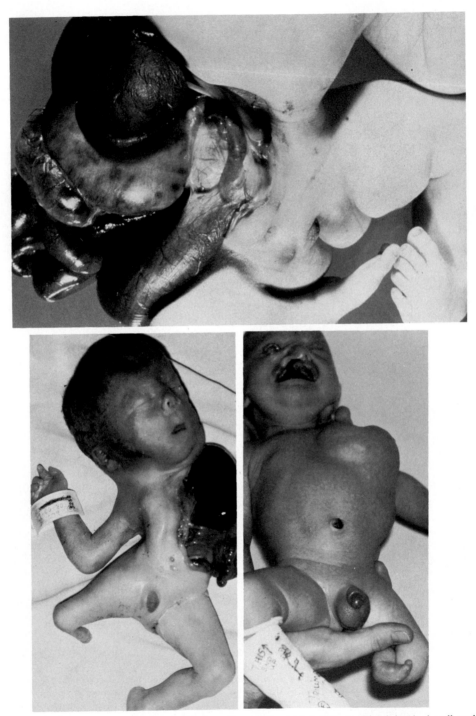

Early amnion rupture sequence. Early compressive effects may yield deficits in the abdominal wall and/or limb reduction deficiencies of all gradations. The body wall defect may occasionally be skin covered, as is the case in the lower right photo. There was an amnionic band attachment to the center of the thoracic defect in the latter instance.

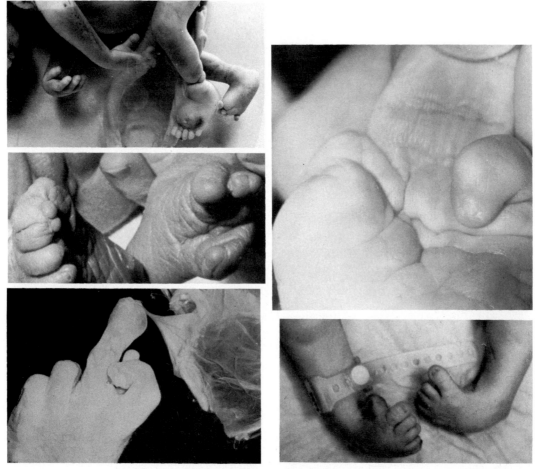

Early amnion rupture sequence. Secondary limb problems include band-related constriction, band-related pseudo-syndactyly (mid-left photo), compression or band-related deficiencies, and compression or band-related distortion. The lower left photo shows distortion with altered growth of a finger to which the amnion is still attached. Early compression may result in incomplete separation of the digits (syndactyly) or aberration in early finger rays with polydactyly, as shown in the photo to the right. (Courtesy of Cindy Dolan, Spokane, Washington.)

Illustration continued on following page

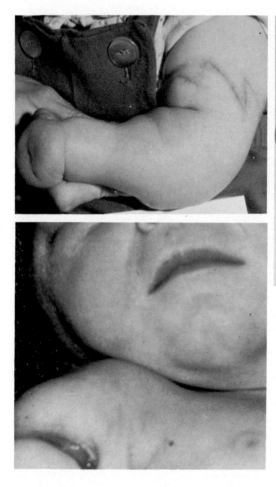

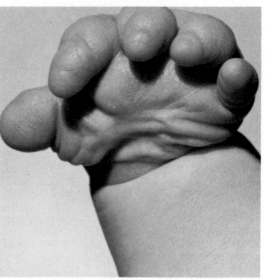

Early amnion rupture sequence. A severe amnionic band constriction may result in hypoplasia and/or edema in the distal limb, as shown in the upper left and right photos. (Courtesy of Dr. Allan MacFarlane, Fairbanks, Alaska.) This infant had a multiple Z-plasty plastic surgical repair in order to improve partially the postnatal status of this amnionic band–induced limb deficiency. The neonate shown below had a severe band-induced constriction in the upper right arm, presumably engendered at 15 weeks when her mother began to have persistent amnionic fluid leakage, with consequent oligohydramnios yielding the excess of loose, redundant facial skin.

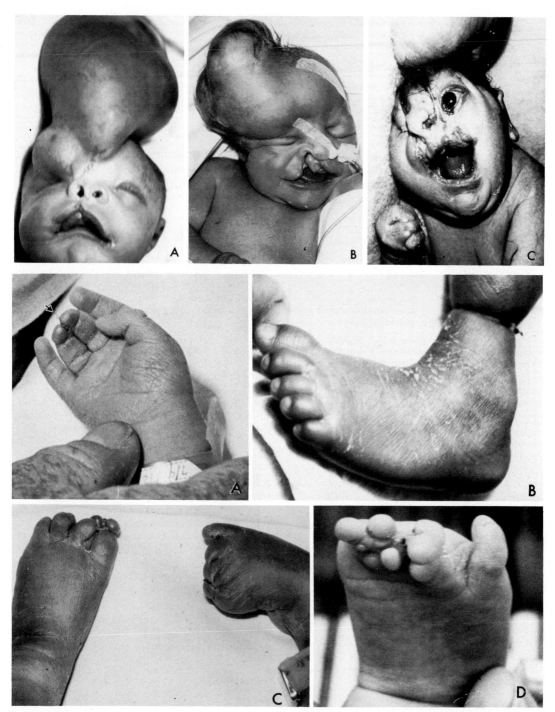

Early amnion rupture sequence. *Above*, Asymmetric encephaloceles and disruption of facial morphogenesis presumed to be secondary to aberrant tissue bands. The same patients had limb anomalies secondary to bands. *A*, Note the notch in the upper lip. *B*, Note the striking asymmetry of the encephalocele. *C*, Note the disruptive tissue bands extending upward from the apices of the facial clefts. *Below*, Variable limb anomalies secondary to aberrant bands. *A*, The arrow denotes the broken band that caused the pseudosyndactyly. *B*, Band constricting the ankle. *C*, *D*, Pseudosyndactyly, amputation, and disruption of toe morphogenesis. (From Jones, K. L., et al.: J. Pediatr., *84*:90, 1974.)

U

U. SPECTRA OF DEFECTS

FACIO-AURICULO-VERTEBRAL SPECTRUM

(First and Second Branchial Arch Syndrome, Oculoauricular Vertebral Dysplasia, Hemifacial Microsomia, Goldenhar Syndrome)

The predominant defects in this nonrandom association of anomalies represent problems in morphogenesis of the first and second branchial arches, sometimes accompanied by vertebral anomalies and/or ocular anomalies. The occurrence of epibulbar dermoid with this pattern of anomaly, especially when accompanied by vertebral anomaly, was designated as the Goldenhar syndrome, and the predominantly unilateral occurrence was designated as hemifacial microsomia. However, the occurrence of various combinations and gradations of this pattern of anomalies, both unilateral and bilateral, with or without epibulbar dermoid, and with or without vertebral anomaly, has suggested that hemifacial microsomia and the Goldenhar syndrome may simply represent gradations in severity of a similar error in morphogenesis. The frequency of occurrence is estimated to be 1:3000 to 1:5000, and there is a slight (3:2) male predominance.

ABNORMALITIES. Variable combinations of the following, tending to be *asymmetric* and 70 per cent unilateral.
Facial. Hypoplasia of malar, maxillary, and/or mandibular region, especially ramus and condyle of mandible and temporomandibular joint. Lateral cleft-like extension of corner of mouth (macrostomia). Hypoplasia of facial musculature.
Ear. Microtia, accessory preauricular tags and/or pits, most commonly in a line from the tragus to the corner of the mouth. Middle ear anomaly with variable deafness.
Oral. Diminished to absent parotid secretion. Anomalies in function or structure of tongue. Malfunction of soft palate.
Vertebral. Hemivertebrae or hypoplasia of vertebrae, most commonly cervical but may also be thoracic or lumbar.

OCCASIONAL ABNORMALITIES
Eye. Epibulbar dermoid, lipodermoid, notch in upper lid, strabismus, microphthalmia.

Ear. Inner ear defect with deafness.
Oral. Cleft lip, cleft palate.
Cardiac. Ventricular septal defect, patent ductus arteriosus, tetralogy of Fallot, and coarctation of aorta, in decreasing order.
Other. Mental deficiency (I.Q. below 85 in 13 per cent). Branchial cleft remnants in anterior-lateral neck, laryngeal anomaly, hypoplasia to aplasia of lung. Occipital encephalocele. Renal, limb, and/or rib anomalies. Prenatal growth deficiency. Low scalp hairline.

NATURAL HISTORY. Cosmetic surgery is strongly indicated. Most of these patients are of normal intelligence. Mental deficiency is more common in association with microphthalmia. Deafness should be tested for at an early age.

ETIOLOGY. Unknown. Usually sporadic. Estimated recurrence in first degree relatives is about 2 per cent, although minor features of this disorder may be more commonly noted in relatives. When unilateral it tends to be right-sided. Summitt has reported one family with dominant inheritance of varying degrees of this pattern of anomalies, indicating heterogeneity of cause.

References

Goldenhar, M.: Associations malformatives de l'oeil et de l'oreille. J. Genet. Hum., 1:243, 1952.
Gorlin, R. J., and Pindborg, J. J.: Oculo-auriculo-vertebral dysplasia. In Gorlin, R. J., and Pindborg, J. J. (eds.): Syndromes of the Head and Neck. New York, McGraw-Hill Book Co., 1964, p. 419.
Summitt, R. L.: Familial Goldenhar syndrome. Birth Defects, 5:106, 1969.
Pashayan, H., Pinsky, L., and Fraser, F. C.: Hemifacial microsomia-oculo-auriculo-vertebral dysplasia. A patient with overlapping features. J. Med. Genet., 7:185, 1970.
Baum, J. L., and Feingold, M.: Ocular aspects of Goldenhar's syndrome. Am. J. Ophthalmol., 75:250, 1973.

Budden, S. S., and Robinson, G. C.: Oculoauricular vertebral dysplasia. Its association with sensorineural deafness and other abnormalities. Am. J. Dis. Child., *125*:431, 1973.

Converse, J. M., et al.: On hemifacial microsomia. The first and second branchial arch syndrome. Plast. Reconstr. Surg., *51*:268, 1973.

Mellow, D. H., Richardson, J. E., and Douglas, D. M.: Goldenhar's syndrome—oculoauriculo-vertebral dysplasia. Arch. Dis. Child., *48*:537, 1973.

Rollnick, B. R., et al.: Oculoauriculovertebral dysplasia and variants. Phenotypic characteristics of 294 patients. Am. J. Med. Genet., *26*:361, 1987.

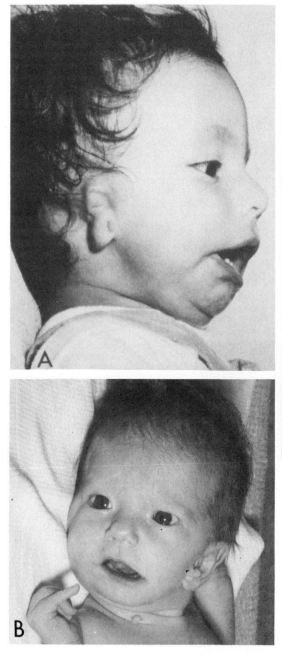

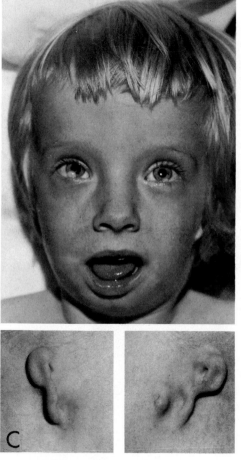

Facio-auriculo-vertebral spectrum *A*, Right-sided "hemifacial microsomia." Note the macrostomia and micrognathia. *B*, Asymmetric bilateral involvement, with left-sided facial weakness. Note the skin tag, which contained cartilage, in the anterior left neck. There were slight epibulbar dermoids, and there was transposition of the great vessels of the heart. *C*, Two and one-half year old. A laryngeal cyst was excised when the patient was four months of age. She has a 40- to 50-decibel hearing deficit by air conduction but normal reception by bone conduction. Note the epibulbar lipodermoids.

Illustration continued on following page

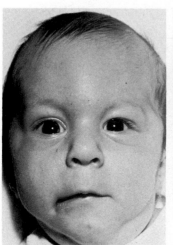
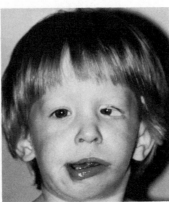
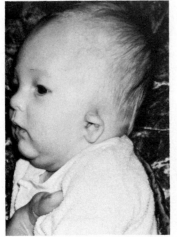
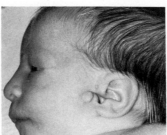

Facio-auriculo-vertebral spectrum. Variation in severity of effects on the eye region, corners of the mouth, nasal region, mandible, and auricular region.

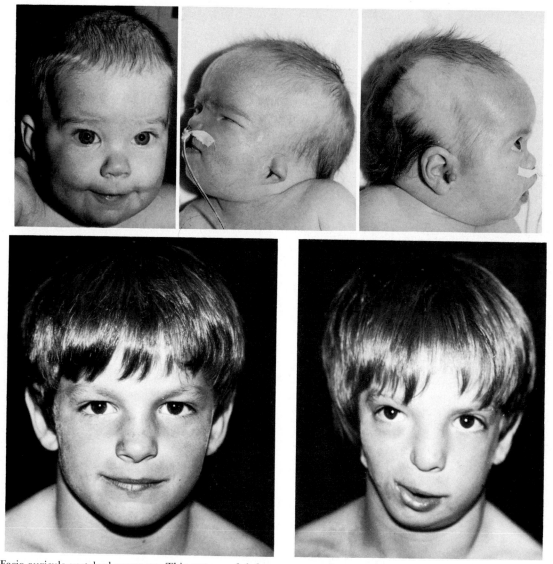

Facio-auriculo-vertebral spectrum. This pattern of defect appears to be more common in monozygotic (MZ) twins and usually affects only one of them. These two sets of MZ twins not only illustrate this but provide an excellent illustration (left) of how the individual on the right would have appeared if this problem in facial morphogenesis had not occurred. (*Above*, courtesy of Dr. Uta Burck, Institut für Humangenetik, Universität Hamburg; *below*, courtesy of Dr. Jaime Frias, University of Nebraska Medical School, Omaha.)

OROMANDIBULAR-LIMB HYPOGENESIS SPECTRUM

(Hypoglossia-Hypodactyly Syndrome, Aglossia-Adactyly Syndrome, Glossopalatine Ankylosis Syndrome, Moebius Syndrome, Charlie M. Syndrome, Facial-Limb Disruptive Spectrum)

Limb Deficiency, Hypoglossia, Micrognathia

In 1932, Rosenthal described aglossia and associated malformations. More recently, Kaplan et al. have emphasized a "community" or spectrum of disorders and have suggested some common elements in modes of developmental pathology.

ABNORMALITIES. Various combinations from among the following features:

Craniofacial. Small mouth, micrognathia, hypoglossia, variable clefting or aberrant attachments of tongue; mandibular hypodontia; cleft palate; cranial nerve palsies including Moebius sequence; broad nose; telecanthus; lower eyelid defect; facial asymmetry.

Limbs. Hypoplasia of varying degrees, to point of adactyly. Syndactyly.

Other. Brain defect, especially of cranial nerve nuclei, causing Moebius sequence. Splenogonadal fusion.

NATURAL HISTORY. Early feeding and speech difficulties may occur. Orthopedic and/or plastic surgery may be indicated for the limb problems. Intelligence and stature are generally normal. Serious problems with hyperthermia can occur in children with four-limb amputation.

ETIOLOGY. Unknown, usually sporadic. The hypothesis that the abnormalities are the disruptive consequence of hemorrhagic lesions has experimental backing from the studies of Poswillo. The presumed vascular problem is more likely to occur in distal regions, such as the distal limbs, tongue, and occasionally parts of the brain.

References

Rosenthal, R.: Aglossia congenita. A report of the condition combined with other congenital malformations. Am. J. Dis. Child., *44*:383, 1932.

Poswillo, D.: The pathogenesis of the first and second branchial arch syndrome. Oral Surgery, *35*:302, 1973.

Kaplan, P., Cummings, C., and Fraser, F. C.: A "community" of face-limb malformation syndromes. J. Pediatr., *89*:241, 1976.

Pauli, R. M., and Greenlaw, A.: Limb deficiency and splenogonadal fusion. Am. J. Med. Genet., *13*:81, 1982.

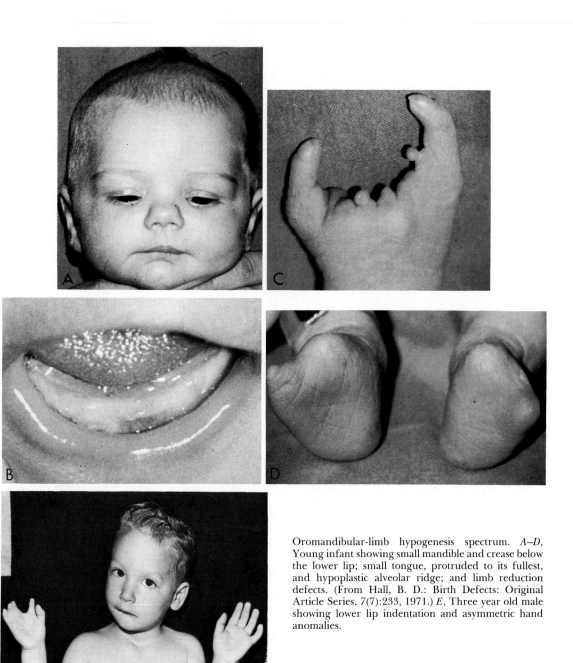

Oromandibular-limb hypogenesis spectrum. *A–D,* Young infant showing small mandible and crease below the lower lip; small tongue, protruded to its fullest, and hypoplastic alveolar ridge; and limb reduction defects. (From Hall, B. D.: Birth Defects: Original Article Series, 7(7):233, 1971.) *E,* Three year old male showing lower lip indentation and asymmetric hand anomalies.

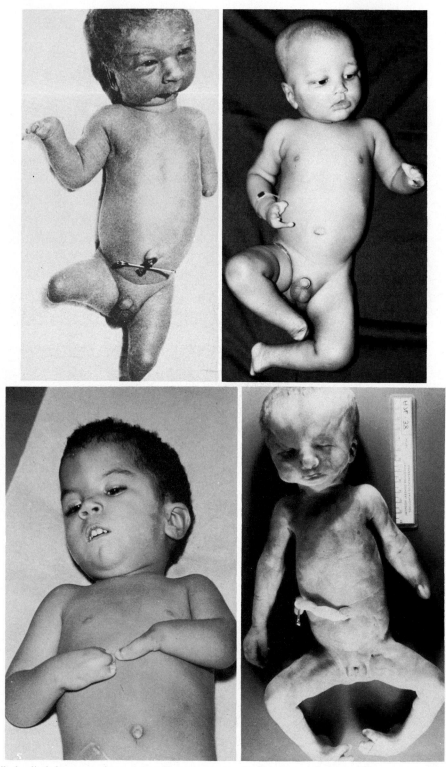

Oromandibular-limb hypogenesis spectrum. No one instance is the same as the next. There are varying degrees of limb deficiency, hypoglossia, and/or micrognathia.

MONOZYGOTIC (MZ) TWINNING AND STRUCTURAL DEFECTS— GENERAL

Monozygotic (MZ) twinning occurs in about one per 200 births and, as such, represents the most common aberration of morphogenesis noted in the human. The frequency of MZ twin conceptuses is probably appreciably higher than 1:200. Livingston and Poland found a threefold excess of MZ twins among spontaneous abortuses versus live-born twins, with the ratio of MZ to DZ (dizygotic) being 17:1 in the abortuses versus 0.8:1 in the live-born twins. Most of these MZ aborted twins had structural defects and may represent the early lethal effect of the types of structural defects that have been noted to occur with excess frequency in MZ twins.

Structural defects occur two to three times more commonly in live-born MZ twins than in DZ twins or singletons. The origin and nature of these defects are summarized in Table 1–4, and the first three categories are individually set forth in the following subsections. The fourth category of deformation due to in-utero crowding, which is not increased in MZ versus DZ twins, is set forth in *Smith's Recognizable Patterns of Human Deformation* and will not be detailed here.

MZ twinning may occur soon after conception, and this type may even have separate placentas. The development of two embryonic centers in the blastocyst by four to five days of gestation yields twins with monochorionic-diamnionic membranes, the most common type of MZ twinning. The final potential timing for the induction of MZ twinning is by 15 to 16 days of development, with the formation of more than one Hensen node and primitive streak in the embryonic plate. This will result in monochorionic-monoamnionic twins, who account for about 4 per cent of MZ twins.

In addition to the problems that were alluded to concerning MZ twins, there appears to be an increased likelihood of fetal death in one or more of MZ twins who develop in a monoamnionic sac, at least partially because of cord entanglements leading to vascular problems. There is also an overall excess of perinatal mortality in MZ twins. The primary cause is prematurity, but the excess of structural defects also contributes to this high mortality.

The value and importance of examining the placenta for the condition of the membranes, vascular interconnections between the twins, and evidence of a decreased twin should be obvious.

The etiologies for MZ twinning are largely unknown. A single gene, dominant type of inheritance has been implicated in an occasional family. Experimental studies have implied environmental factors, such as late fertilization of the ovum in the rabbit and vincristine administration in the rat.

Table 1–4. ORIGIN AND TYPES OF STRUCTURAL DEFECTS IN MZ TWINS

Origin	Types of Defects
A. ? The same causative factor that gave rise to MZ twinning	Early malformations or malformation sequences
B. Incomplete twinning	Conjoined twins
C. Consequence of vascular placental shunts	
1. Artery-artery	Disruptions, including acardiac and amorphous twins
2. Artery-vein	Twin-twin transfusion, causing unequal size, unequal hematocrit, and/or other problems
3. Death of one twin with thromboplastin or embolic release to co-twin	Vascular disruptive defects
D. Constraint in fetal life	Deformations due to uterine constraint

A. MZ TWINS AND EARLY MALFORMATIONS

The excess of early types of malformation among MZ twins may be the consequence of the same etiology that gave rise to the MZ twinning aberration of morphogenesis. For example, Stockard was able to produce both MZ twinning *and* early malformation such as cyclopia by early environmental insults (alterations of oxygen level and temperature) to the developing Atlantic minnow (*Fundulus*). The findings of Schinzel et al. are in keeping with this hypothesis. They found that the malformations in MZ twins were predominantly early defects, presumably engendered at the same time as the MZ twinning. The incidence of associated early malformations was greatest in the monochorionic-monoamnionic cases, which would usually have been induced at the time of embryonic plate development and hence would theoretically be more likely to have associated early malformations. The early types of defects that have been considered to be of excess frequency in MZ twins are as follows:

1. Sacrococcygeal teratoma.
2. Sirenomelia.
3. The VATER association (see page 602).
4. Exstrophy of the cloaca malformation sequence.
5. Holoprosencephaly malformation sequence.
6. Anencephaly.

About 5 to 20 per cent of such cases are concordant; thus, the majority are nonconcordant. When one twin has the more severe degree of a malformation sequence, the other twin may show lesser degrees of the same type of initiating defect.

These early defects are individually presented in this text. Most are early lethals and cause spontaneous abortion. This is probably a partial explanation of the excess of MZ twins among spontaneous abortuses.

Recurrence risk counseling should involve the total problem, namely, the MZ twinning plus the associated malformation sequence. To our knowledge, this risk is of low to negligible magnitude, although the specific etiologies for this type of problem are unknown.

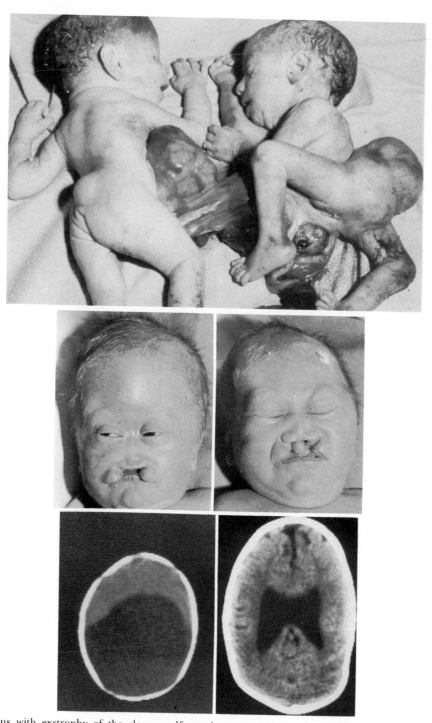

Above, MZ twins with exstrophy of the cloaca malformation sequence. Note that the severity of the individual components of this malformation sequence, such as the skin-covered myelocele, varies from one twin to the other. *Middle and below,* Holoprosencephaly malformation sequence of varying severity in MZ twins (8 days), with CAT scans showing single ventricle on the left (died at 18 days) and more normal ventricular development on the right. (Middle and bottom photos courtesy of Dr. Uta Burck, Institut für Humangenetik, Universität Hamburg.)

B. CONJOINED TWINS

Conjoined twins may be viewed as examples of incomplete twinning and occur in about 1 per cent of MZ twins. Although it is feasible that two closely placed embryonic centers in the four to five day old blastocyst could result in conjoined twins, it seems more likely that they originate at the primitive streak stage of the embryonic plate (15 to 17 days). Current experimental techniques in animals have not been successful in producing conjoined twins.

The most common type of conjoined twins is termed thoracopagus, in which the twins are joined at the thorax. Juncture at the head, buttocks, and less commonly, other anatomic sites also occurs. Partial to complete duplication of only the upper or lower body parts may also take place.

As with MZ twins in general, there is a higher incidence of early malformations in conjoined twins. Disregarding the incidence of anomalies related to the sites of juncture, there is a 10 to 20 per cent occurrence of major early defects. As with separate MZ twins, the malformations in conjoined twins are often not concordant. The high frequency of associated malformations in conjoined twins may relate to the timing of the defect, which is presumed to be at the embryonic plate–primitive streak stage of development.

The likelihood of particular types of early malformation occurring in certain kinds of conjoined twins is increased very nonrandomly. For example, the dicephalic conjoined twin frequently has anencephaly, most commonly affecting only one of the heads. Whether this relates to differences in early blood flow to the respective heads remains to be determined. The recurrence risk for conjoined twins appears to be negligible.

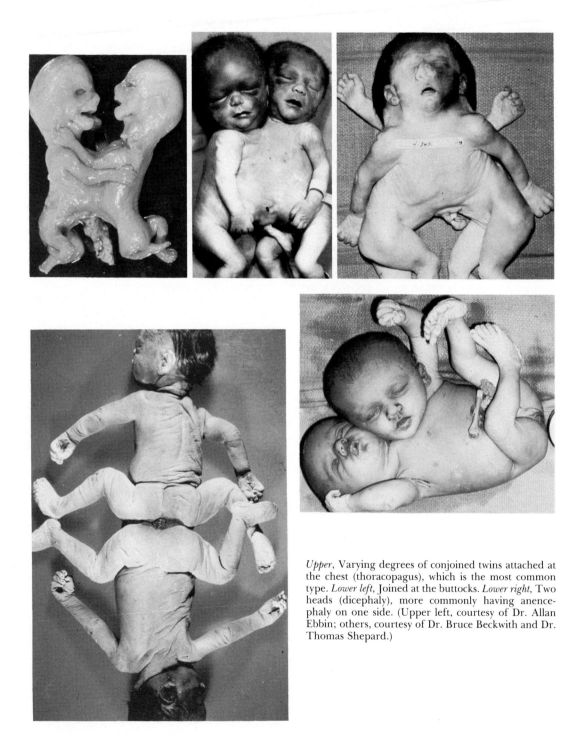

Upper, Varying degrees of conjoined twins attached at the chest (thoracopagus), which is the most common type. *Lower left,* Joined at the buttocks. *Lower right,* Two heads (dicephaly), more commonly having anencephaly on one side. (Upper left, courtesy of Dr. Allan Ebbin; others, courtesy of Dr. Bruce Beckwith and Dr. Thomas Shepard.)

C. Placental Vascular Shunts in MZ Twins—General

Benirschke has indicated that the great majority of monochorionic (single placenta) twins have a conjoined placenta with vascular interconnections. These develop on a chance basis and are usually evident on the fetal surface of the placenta where the major vessels course between the fetuses and the major cotyledons. The magnitude of inter-twin vascular shunts may be judged by the caliber of the connecting vessels, which relates to the amount of flow they have carried. Much of the early in-utero mortality and excess of structural defects in MZ twins may well relate to the secondary consequences of these vascular connections between the twins. Some of the types of shunts and their adverse effects on one or both of the MZ twins are set forth subsequently.

C–1. ARTERY-ARTERY TWIN DISRUPTION SEQUENCE

Benirschke emphasized the dire consequences that could result from a sizable artery-artery placental shunt, usually accompanied by a vein-vein shunt. The tendency will be for the arterial pressure of one twin to overpower that of the other, usually early in morphogenesis. The "defeated" recipient then has reverse flow from the co-twin. This sends "used" arterial blood from the donor into the iliac vessels of the recipient, perfusing the lower part of the body more than the upper part. The results are a host of disruptions, with deterioration of previously existing tissues as well as incomplete morphogenesis (malformation) of tissues that are in the process of formation. The variably missing tissues include the head, heart, upper limbs, lungs, pancreas, and upper intestine. Rudiments of early disrupted tissues may be found in the residuum. The extent of disruption may be even broader, leaving as the residuum an "amorphous" twin. There is every gradation, from amorphia to acardia to less severe degrees of disruption, with no one case being identical to another. Examples of some of the gradations of severity are shown in the accompanying figure.

The donor twin may have an excessive cardiac load resulting in cardiomegaly and even cardiac decompensation, with secondary liver dysfunction, hypoalbuminemia, and edema. Sometimes this may progress to the level of hydrops.

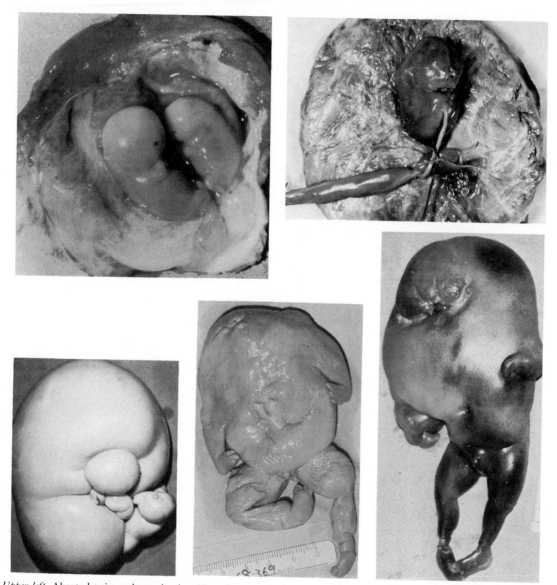

Upper left, Aborted twin embryos in situ. Note the growth deficiency, especially in the head and upper limbs of the twin to the right. This may well represent the early stage of artery-to-artery disruptive transfusion from the twin on the left to the one on the right, the early genesis of the acardiac situation. (Courtesy of Dr. Lewis Holmes, Massachusetts General Hospital, Boston.) *Upper right,* Amorphous acardiac, partially embedded in the placenta and not detected by the delivering physician. Note the twisted cord (held up by the probe) that partially occluded vascular flow for both the acardiac fetus and the surviving fetus. (Courtesy of Dr. Mason Barr, Jr., University of Michigan Medical School, Ann Arbor.) *Lower,* Gradations of severity, from amorphous twin to acephalic, with upper limb deficiency due to artery-artery shunt and reverse circulation from co-twin. (Courtesy of Dr. Thomas Shepard, University of Washington School of Medicine, Seattle.)

C–2. ARTERY-VEIN TWIN TRANSFUSION SEQUENCE

Artery-vein transfusion may result in problems such as those summarized in Table 1–5. The excessive volume in the recipient twin not only tends to lead to increased growth and an enlarged heart but also causes increased kidney size and excess urine output, with resultant polyhydramnios. The high hematocrit may constitute a serious risk of vascular problems and merits early postnatal management. The transfuser twin, being hypovolemic, tends to have diminished renal blood flow, smaller kidneys, and oligohydramnios (when the twins are diamnionic). There may even be evidence of transient renal insufficiency in the smaller twin during the first days after birth, as the kidneys have been hypofunctional since before birth.

Tan et al. have found that 18 per cent of MZ twins are discrepant in size and hematocrit at birth; hence, this is not a rare occurrence.

Treatment may be warranted soon after birth to provide each affected twin with a more normal hematocrit. There are several means of accomplishing this. The author has had experience with continuous exchange transfusion from one MZ twin to the other, reversing the order of the transfuser and the recipient with each 10 ml syringe exchange of blood, after having first adjusted somewhat for the hypervolemia in one twin and the hypovolemia in the other. The exchange is continued until they are of comparable color. In one such exchange (using a three-way stopcock), the initial hematocrits were 13.0 g/dl and 23.5 g/dl, and after the exchange transfusion, they were 17.0 g/dl and 17.5 g/dl, respectively.

Table 1–5. **PROBLEMS SECONDARY TO ARTERIOVENOUS TWIN-TWIN TRANSFUSION**

Feature	Donor Twin	Recipient Twin
Growth	Smaller size	Larger size
Hematocrit	Low	High
Blood volume	Hypovolemia	Hypervolemia
Renal blood flow and renal size	Diminished	Increased
Amnionic fluid	Oligohydramnios	Polyhydramnios
Heart size	Diminished	Increased

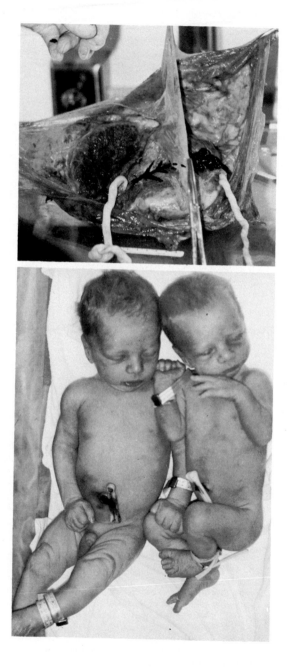

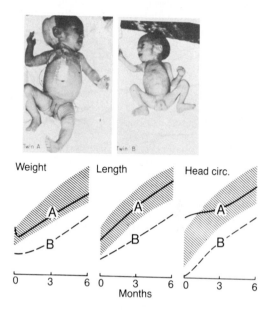

Weight   Length   Head circ.

Months

Left, Discrepant size of MZ twins as the result of an arteriovenous shunt in the monochorionic-diamnionic placenta. The direction of the flow is shown by the arrows, from the anemic transfuser at the right to the plethoric, overgrown recipient at the left. The hypovolemic smaller twin had transient evidence of renal insufficiency in the first days after birth. *Above,* Marked discrepancy in size at birth. Note the rapid initial drop in the hypervolemic recipient's (twin A) weight after birth. She was given a shunt for "hydrocephalus"; however, in the opinion of the author, this represented large head size secondary to hypervolemia. The smaller donor twin (twin B) had evidence of transient renal insufficiency soon after birth, which resolved. She continued to grow at a slow rate. Postnatal growth in the smaller twin has varied from full catch-up to no catch-up and may be dependent on the in-utero age of onset of the growth deficiency; the earlier the growth deficiency, the less likely it will be for catching-up growth to occur. The larger twin B developed a porencephalic cyst presumably secondary to the plethora, and a vascular problem as a consequence. No aggressive therapy had been pursued relative to the plethora.

C–3. COMPLICATIONS IN AN MZ TWIN FROM THE
IN-UTERO DEATH OF THE CO-TWIN

Benirschke first implicated death of an MZ co-twin (stillborn or fetus papyraceus) as a potential cause for problems in the surviving twin as a consequence of thromboplastin gaining access to the survivor's circulation and causing disseminated intravascular coagulation. The other possibility is that emboli from the deceased co-twin enter the circulation of the survivor. Either mechanism can give rise to areas of ischemia and disruption, with subsequent loss of tissue. Some of the defects occurring in the co-twin of the deceased MZ twin are the following:

1. Disseminated intravascular coagulation.
2. Aplasia cutis.
3. Porencephalic cyst to hydranencephaly.
4. Limb amputation.
5. Intestinal atresia.
6. Gastroschisis.

Melnick has concluded from the Collaborative Perinatal Project (50,000 deliveries) that about 3 per cent of near-term MZ twins have a deceased co-twin, and about one third of the survivors, or 1 per cent of MZ twin births, have severe brain defects as a consequence of the foregoing mechanisms. The surviving infants with porencephalic cysts and/or hydranencephaly are usually severely mentally deficient with microcephaly, spastic diplegia, and seizures.

References

General

Stockard, C. R.: Developmental rate and structural expression: an experimental study of twins, "double monsters," and single deformities and the interaction among embryonic organs during their origin and development. Am. J. Anat., 28:115, 1921.
Benirschke, K.: Twin placenta in perinatal mortality. N.Y. State J. Med., 61:1499, 1961.
Benirschke, K., and Driscoll, S. G.: The placenta in multiple pregnancy. Handbuch Pathol. Histol., 7:187, 1967.
Bomsel-Helmreich, O.: Delayed ovulation and monozygotic twinning in the rabbit. Acta Genet. Med. Gemellol., 23:19, 1974.
Myrianthopoulos, N. C.: Congenital malformations in twins. Acta Genet. Med. Gemellol., 24:331, 1976.
Harvey, M. A. S., Huntley, R. M., and Smith, D. W.: Familial monozygotic twinning. J. Pediatr., 90:246, 1977.
Kaufman, M. H., and O'Shea, K. S.: Induction of monozygotic twinning in the mouse. Nature, 276:707, 1978.
Schinzel, A. A. G. L., Smith, D. W., and Miller, J. R.: Monozygotic twinning and structural defects. J. Pediatr., 95:921, 1979.

Livingston, J. E., and Poland, B. J.: A study of spontaneously aborted twins. Teratology, 21:139, 1980.

Early Malformations in MZ Twins

Stockard, C. R.: Developmental rate and structural expression: an experimental study of twins, "double monsters," and single deformities and the interaction among embryonic organs during their origin and development. Am. J. Anat., 28:115, 1921.
Gross, R. E., Clatworthy, H. W., and Mecker, J. A.: Sacrococcygeal teratomas in infants and children. Surg. Gynecol. Obstet., 92:341, 1951.
Davies, J., Chazen, E., and Nance, W. E.: Symmelia in one of monozygotic twins. Teratology, 4:367, 1971.
Mohr, H. P.: Misibiludungen bei Zwilligen. Ergeb. Inn. Med. Kinderheilkd., 33:1, 1972.
Smith, D. W., Bartlett, C., and Harrah, L. M.: Monozygotic twinning and the Duhamel anomalad (imperforate anus to sirenomelia): A nonrandom association between two aberrations in morphogenesis. Birth Defects, 12:53, 1976.
Schinzel, A. A. G. L., Smith, D. W., and Miller, J. R.: Monozygotic twinning and structural defects. J. Pediatr., 95:921, 1979.
Livingston, J. E., and Poland, B. J.: A study of spontaneously aborted twins. Teratology, 21:139, 1980.

Conjoined Twins

Riccardi, V. M., and Bergmann, C. A.: Anencephaly with incomplete twinning (diprosopus). Teratology, 16:137, 1977.
Schinzel, A. A. G. L., Smith, D. W., and Miller, J. R.: Monozygotic twinning and structural defects. J. Pediatr., 95:921, 1979.

Vascular Shunts Between MZ Twins

Confalonieri, C.: Gravidanza gemellare monocoriale biamniotica con feto papiraceo ed atresia intestinale congenita nell'altro feto. Riv. Ost. Ginec. Prat., 33:199, 1951.
Naeye, R. L.: Human intrauterine parabiotic syndrome and its complications. N. Engl. J. Med., 268:804, 1963.
Hague, I. U., and Glassauer, F. E.: Hydranencephaly in twins. N.Y. State J. Med., 69:1210, 1969.
Moore, C. M., McAdams, A. J., and Sutherland, J.: Intrauterine disseminated intravascular coagulation: a syndrome of multiple pregnancy with a dead twin fetus. J. Pediatr., 74:523, 1969.
Saier, F., Burden, L., and Cavanagh, D.: Fetus papyraceus. An unusual case with congenital anomaly of the surviving fetus. Obstet. Gynecol., 45:271, 1975.
Balvour, R. P.: Fetus papyraceus. Obstet. Gynecol., 47:507, 1976.
Weiss, D. B., Aboulafia, Y., and Isackson, M.: Gastroschisis and fetus papyraceus in double ovum twins. Harefuah, 91:392, 1976.
Benirschke, K., and Harper, V.: The acardiac anomaly. Teratology, 15:311, 1977.

Mannino, F. L., Jones, K. L., and Benirschke, K.: Congenital skin defects and fetus papyraceus. J. Pediatr., *91*:559, 1977.

Melnick, M.: Brain damage in survivor after death of monozygotic co-twin. Lancet, *2*:1287, 1977.

Schinzel, A. A. G. L., Smith, D. W., and Miller, J. R.: Monozygotic twinning and structural defects. J. Pediatr., *95*:921, 1979.

Tan, K. L., et al.: The twin transfusion syndrome. Clin. Pediatr., *18*:111, 1979.

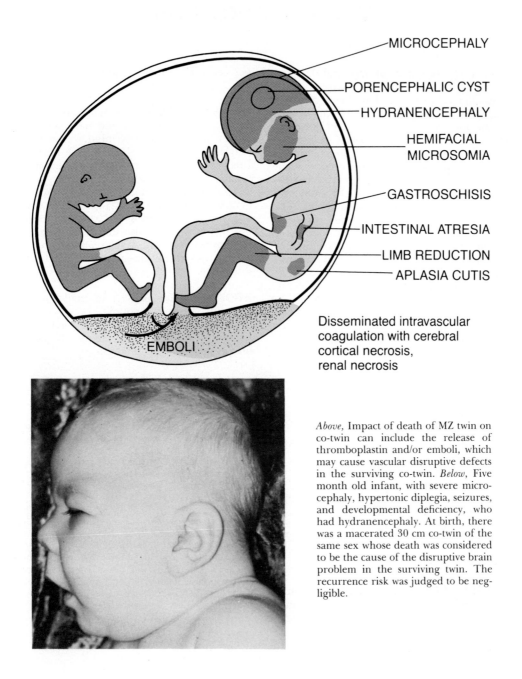

MICROCEPHALY

PORENCEPHALIC CYST

HYDRANENCEPHALY

HEMIFACIAL MICROSOMIA

GASTROSCHISIS

INTESTINAL ATRESIA

LIMB REDUCTION

APLASIA CUTIS

EMBOLI

Disseminated intravascular coagulation with cerebral cortical necrosis, renal necrosis

Above, Impact of death of MZ twin on co-twin can include the release of thromboplastin and/or emboli, which may cause vascular disruptive defects in the surviving co-twin. *Below,* Five month old infant, with severe microcephaly, hypertonic diplegia, seizures, and developmental deficiency, who had hydranencephaly. At birth, there was a macerated 30 cm co-twin of the same sex whose death was considered to be the cause of the disruptive brain problem in the surviving twin. The recurrence risk was judged to be negligible.

V. MISCELLANEOUS ASSOCIATIONS

VATER ASSOCIATION

A nonrandom association of vertebral defects, imperforate anus, and esophageal atresia with tracheo-esophageal fistula has long been appreciated. Say and Gerald noted the association of imperforate anus, vertebral defects, and polydactyly, and Say et al. extended the latter to include polyoligodactyly. The spectrum was broadened by Quan and Smith to include *V*ertebral defects, *A*nal atresia, *T-E* fistula with esophageal atresia, and *R*adial and *R*enal dysplasia, and the acronym VATER association was utilized to designate this complex. Cardiac defects and a single umbilical artery as well as prenatal growth deficiency were also nonrandom features of this pattern of anomalies, and these were emphasized by Temtamy and Miller, who utilized the acronym VATERS association, with the *V* standing for both vertebral defects and ventricular septal defect and the *S* designating single umbilical artery. The general spectrum of the pattern in a total of 34 cases is presented below, as summarized by Temtamy and Miller.

ABNORMALITIES. Thirty-four cases with three or more VATER association defects.

Vertebral anomalies	70%
Ventricular septal defects and other cardiac defects	53%
Anal atresia with or without fistula	80%
T-E fistula with esophageal atresia	70%
Radial dysplasia, including thumb or radial hypoplasia, preaxial polydactyly, syndactyly	65%
Renal anomaly	53%
Single umbilical artery	35%

OTHER LESS FREQUENT DEFECTS. Prenatal growth deficiency, postnatal growth deficiency, ear anomaly, large fontanels, defect of lower limb (23 per cent), rib anomaly, defects of external genitalia.

NATURAL HISTORY. Though many of these patients may fail to thrive and have slow developmental progress in early infancy related to their defects, the majority of them have normal brain function and thus merit vigorous attempts toward rehabilitation, surgical and otherwise.

This spectrum of anomalies may occur as a part of a broader pattern, such as the trisomy 18 or 13q− syndromes, in which case the prognosis is not favorable. It is also important to appreciate that cases with radial dysplasia and cardiac defect may be mistakenly designated as the Holt-Oram syndrome.

ETIOLOGY. This pattern of malformation has generally been a sporadic occurrence in an otherwise normal family. The etiology is unknown. It has been more frequently seen in the offspring of diabetic mothers.

References

Say, B., and Gerald, P. S.: A new polydactyly, imperforate anus, vertebral anomalies syndrome. Lancet, 2:688, 1968.

Say, D., et al.: A new syndrome of dysmorphogenesis-imperforate anus associated with poly-oligodactyly and skeletal (mainly vertebral) anomalies. Acta Paediatr. Scand., 60:197, 1971.

Silver, W., et al.: The Holt-Oram syndrome with previously undescribed associated anomalies. Am. J. Dis. Child., 124:911, 1972.

Quan, L., and Smith, D. W.: The VATER association, *V*ertebral defects, *A*nal atresia, *T-E* fistula with esophageal atresia, *R*adial and *R*enal dysplasia: A spectrum of associated defects. J. Pediatr., 82:104, 1973.

Temtamy, S. A., and Miller, J. D.: Extending the scope of the VATER association: Definition of a VATER syndrome. J. Pediatr., 85:345, 1974.

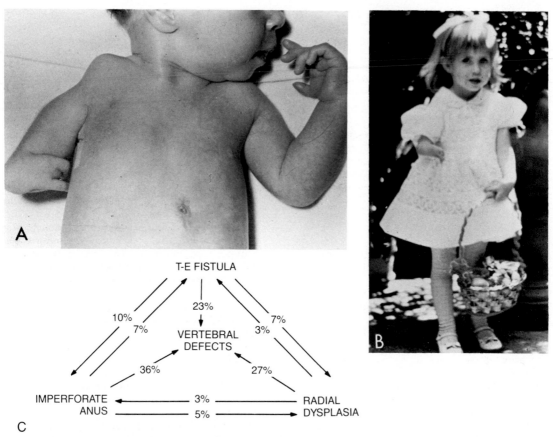

T-E FISTULA

10%   23%   7%
7%   →   3%

VERTEBRAL
DEFECTS

36%   27%

IMPERFORATE ← 3% ———— RADIAL
ANUS ———— 5% ————→ DYSPLASIA

C

A, Young infant with vertebral anomalies, anal atresia, esophageal atresia with T-E fistula, radial aplasia on the right, and thumb hypoplasia on the left. *B,* Same patient at two years of age, with normal intelligence. *C,* Relative frequencies of some of the other VATER association defects when the patient is ascertained by virtue of having one of the defects. (From Quan, L., and Smith, D. W.: J. Pediatr., *82:*104, 1973.)

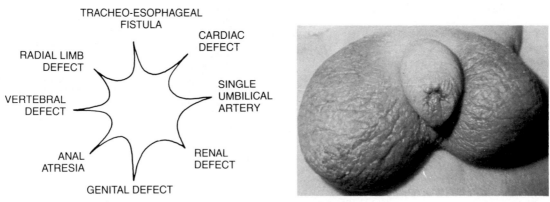

TRACHEO-ESOPHAGEAL
FISTULA

CARDIAC
DEFECT

RADIAL LIMB
DEFECT

SINGLE
UMBILICAL
ARTERY

VERTEBRAL
DEFECT

ANAL
ATRESIA

RENAL
DEFECT

GENITAL DEFECT

Left, Expanded VATER association of defects, including genital anomaly *(right).*

MURCS ASSOCIATION

Müllerian Duct,
Renal and Cervical Vertebral Defects

The MURCS association, as described in 30 patients by Duncan et al. in 1979, consists of a nonrandom association of *MÜ*llerian duct aplasia, *R*enal aplasia, and *C*ervicothoracic *S*omite dysplasia.

ABNORMALITIES

Growth. Small stature.

Skeletal. Cervicothoracic vertebral defects, especially from C5 to T1 (80 per cent), sometimes to the extent of being termed the Klippel-Feil malformation sequence.

Genitourinary. Absence of vagina; absence to hypoplasia of uterus (96 per cent, but there is an ascertainment bias for this defect; sometimes referred to as the Rokitansky malformation sequence). Renal agenesis and/or ectopy (88 per cent).

OCCASIONAL ABNORMALITIES. Moderate frequency of rib anomalies, upper limb defects, and Sprengel scapular anomaly. Infrequent features include deafness, external ear defects, facial asymmetry, cleft lip and palate, micrognathia, and gastrointestinal defects.

NATURAL HISTORY. Most patients are ascertained because of primary amenorrhea or infertility associated with normal secondary sexual characteristics. Rarely, the MURCS association may be diagnosed in the course of an investigation for a renal malformation or because of multiple malformations. Small stature is frequent, with adult stature usually being less than 152 cm.

DIFFERENTIAL DIAGNOSIS WITH VATER ASSOCIATION. Although the MURCS and VATER associations both may have vertebral, genital, and upper limb abnormalities, they are usually distinct clinical entities.

In the MURCS association, the vertebral malformations occur consistently in the cervicothoracic region as compared with the anomalous vertebrae of VATER patients, which are more frequently found in the lower thoracic, lumbar, and sacrococcygeal spine.

Although the renal agenesis/ectopy and the uterovaginal dysplasia of the MURCS association can be found in VATER association patients, they occur less frequently, and most of the other types of upper and lower urinary tract and external genital anomalies that may occur in VATER association patients are not usually found in the MURCS association.

Upper limb abnormalities are found in 24 per cent of VATER association patients but are unusual in the MURCS association.

ETIOLOGY. The etiology is not known, and it is usually a sporadic disorder in an otherwise normal family. One hypothesis for the pathogenesis of the MURCS association has been proposed that attributes the associated defects to an early alteration of the blastema of the lower cervical and upper thoracic somites, upper limb buds, and pronephric ducts, all of which have an intimate spatial relationship in early development.

References

Griffin, J. E., et al.: Congenital absence of the vagina. Ann. Intern. Med., *85*:224, 1976.

Duncan, P. A.: Embryologic pathogenesis of renal agenesis associated with cervical vertebral anomalies (Klippel-Feil phenotype). Birth Defects, *13*(3D):91, 1977.

Duncan, P. A., and Shapiro, L. R.: MURCS and VATER associations: Vertebral and genitourinary malformations with distinct embryologic pathogenetic mechanisms. Teratology, *19*:24A, 1979.

Duncan, P. A., et al.: The MURCS association: Müllerian duct aplasia, renal aplasia, and cervicothoracic somite dysplasia. J. Pediatr., *95*:399, 1979.

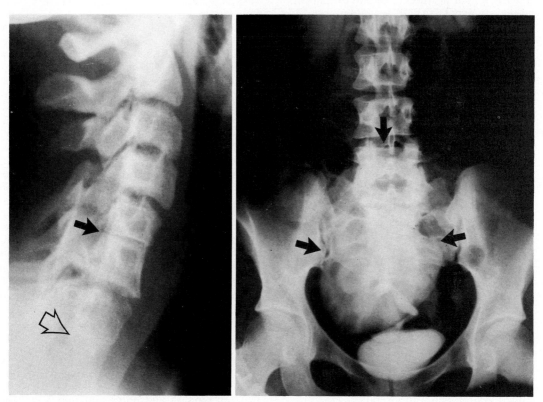

Examples of the types of defects found in individuals with the MURCS association include partial to complete cervical vertebral fusion *(left,* arrows) and ectopic pelvic single large kidney on IVP *(right,* arrows).

CHARGE ASSOCIATION

Choanal atresia appears to be nonrandomly associated with multiple congenital anomalies in patients with normal chromosomes. This association was first summarized by Hall, and many similar anomalies have been observed in patients ascertained for ocular coloboma. The spectrum was broadened by Pagon et al. to include *C*oloboma, *H*eart disease, *A*tresia choanae, *R*etarded growth and development and/or CNS anomalies, *G*enital anomalies and/or hypogonadism, and *E*ar anomalies and/or deafness. This latter report utilized the acronym CHARGE association, reported 21 new cases, and summarized the findings in 41 previously reported cases. Other medically significant associated anomalies have included renal anomalies, tracheoesophageal fistula, facial palsy, micrognathia, cleft lip, cleft palate, and omphalocele.

ABNORMALITIES. Sixty-two cases with four or more of the seven major CHARGE association defects.

Colobomatous malformation sequence (ranging from isolated iris coloboma without visual impairment to clinical anophthalmos; retinal coloboma most common)	80%
Heart defect (tetralogy of Fallot, patent ductus arteriosus, double outlet right ventricle with an atrioventricular canal, ventricular septal defect, atrial septal defect, right-sided aortic arch)	–
Atresia choanae (membranous and/or bony)	58%
Growth deficiency (usually postnatal)	87%
Mental deficiency (ranging from mild to profound with several patients at autopsy demonstrating arhinencephaly variants and several adults demonstrating hypogonadotrophic hypogonadism reminiscent of Kallmann syndrome)	94%
Genital hypoplasia (in males)	75%
Ear anomalies and/or deafness (ranging from small ears without malformation of the pinna to cup-shaped, lop ears; either sensorineural or mixed sensorineural and conductive deafness, ranging from mild to profound)	88%

OTHER FINDINGS. Micrognathia, including Robin malformation sequence; cleft lip; cleft palate; facial palsy; feeding difficulties resulting from poor suck and velopharyngeal incompetence; DiGeorge sequence; renal anomalies; omphalocele; tracheoesophageal fistula; rib anomalies; ptosis; ocular hypertelorism; microcephaly; anal atresia and/or stenosis.

NATURAL HISTORY. In some instances, the severity of these defects has been such that death has occurred during the perinatal period, the result of either respiratory insufficiency, intractable hypocalcemia, or congenital heart disease. Though prenatal growth deficiency has been present in some cases, most patients have been the appropriate size for gestational age, with linear growth shifting down to or below the third percentile during the first six months of life. Most patients have shown some degree of mental deficiency and/or CNS defects, and visual or auditory handicaps may further compromise cognitive function.

The CHARGE association shows some phenotypic overlap with VATER association and also shares some phenotypic features with recognized chromosomal syndromes such as trisomy 13, trisomy 18, 4p− syndrome, and cat eye syndrome. In addition, choanal atresia can be one feature of a variety of monogenic disorders, such as Apert syndrome, Crouzon syndrome, Saethre-Chotzen syndrome, or Treacher Collins syndrome. The nature of the associated defects is sufficient to distinguish CHARGE association from these latter conditions.

ETIOLOGY. Unknown. Many of the anomalies present in the CHARGE association may derive from altered morphogenesis during the second month of gestation. The choanae are formed between days 35 and 38 of gestation, when the bucconasal membrane ruptures as the epithelia lining the oral and nasal cavities come into contact with each other. Colobomata result from failure of the fetal fissure to close during the fifth week of gestation. Cardiac septation begins with the appearance of the septum primum from the midline of a common atrium at about day 32, proceeds through fusion of the mid-atrioventricular canal at approximately day 38, and is reasonably complete by day 45, when the outflow tracts, valves, and membranous ventricular septum have been formed. Holoprosencephaly variants may reflect altered morphogenesis during the fourth to fifth weeks of gestation and may result in hypogonadotrophic hypogonadism, growth deficiency, and

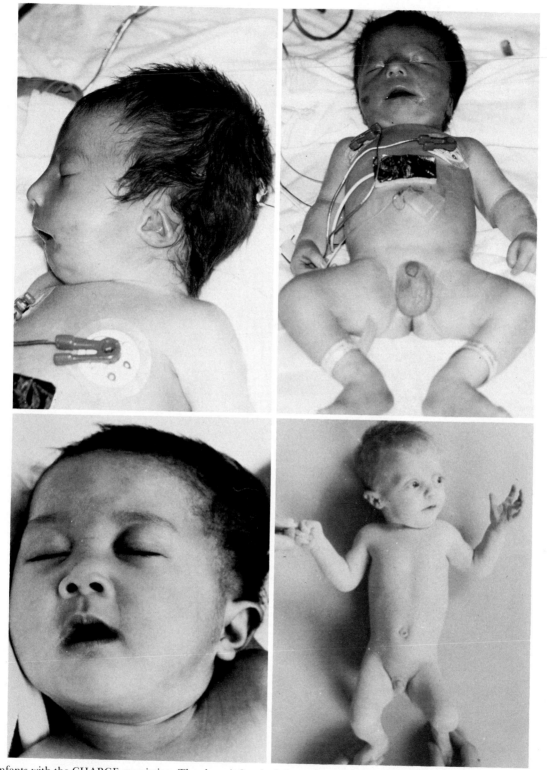

Infants with the CHARGE association. The above infant had choanal atresia, aberrant auricles, micrognathia, a short neck with low hairline, a cardiac defect, hypertonicity, seizures, and a micropenis. (The lower two infants, courtesy of Dr. Bryan Hall, University of Kentucky, Lexington.)

mental retardation. External ear morphogenesis occurs during the sixth week of gestation, shortly after the cochlea begins to form on day 36 (its full length being established by 75 days of gestation). Thus, the defects seen in the CHARGE association might be attributed to arrested development between days 35 and 45 post conception.

The causes for such arrested development are probably heterogeneous. There have been instances in which familial recurrence of some of the associated anomalies has suggested a possible genetic etiology, but reduced reproductive fitness has made this possibility difficult to evaluate. The normal parents of an affected child appear to have a low but not negligible recurrence risk.

References

Hall, B. D.: Choanal atresia and associated multiple anomalies. J. Pediatr., *95*:395, 1979.

Hittner, H. M., et al.: Colobomatous microphthalmia, heart disease, hearing loss, and mental retardation—a syndrome. J. Pediatr. Ophthalmol. Strabismus, *16*:122, 1979.

Pagon, R. A., et al.: Coloboma, congenital heart disease, and choanal atresia with multiple anomalies. CHARGE association. J. Pediatr., *99*:1981.

August, J. P., et al.: Hypopituitarism and the CHARGE association. J. Pediatr., *103*:424, 1983.

Koletzko, B., and Majewski, F.: Congenital anomalies in patients with choanal atresia: CHARGE association. Eur. J. Pediatr., *142*:271, 1984.

ALPHABETICAL LISTING OF SYNDROMES

2

Approaches to Categorical Problems of
growth deficiency, mental deficiency, arthrogryposis, ambiguous external genitalia

Many patients with specific patterns of malformation may initially be evaluated by the clinician because of a categorical problem such as growth deficiency or mental deficiency. The physician is challenged to arrive at a specific overall diagnosis that will be of value in the management of and prognosis and counsel for that particular patient and family. This chapter sets forth approaches toward a specific diagnosis for several of the more common or more difficult categorical types of problems. It is designed to provide an overall diagnostic point of view, placing the patterns of malformation in relevant perspective to other types of disorders in which such a problem may occur.

Each categorical problem is considered from the standpoint of normal morphogenesis, mechanisms by which abnormal morphogenesis may occur, and the clinical man-

614

ner of proceeding toward a specific overall diagnosis. These approaches are designed to be rational for the particular problem and germane for the specific patient.

APPROACH TO GROWTH DEFICIENCY

Normal Growth

Assuming proper skeletal organization and ossification, adult stature and the age at which it is achieved are the respective consequences of the following phenomena:

1. *Mitotic* rate and thereby rate of increasing cell number, especially in the epiphyses.

2. *Maturational* rate of the skeletal system toward final epiphyseal ossification, which can be assessed as "bone age."

Both of these processes are influenced by many genes (polygenic). Some of these genes are apparently located on the sex chromosomes. For example, the XY male tends to be taller than the XX female, even in childhood, and the XYY individual is generally taller than the XY male. The XX female matures more rapidly and at a more consistent rate than the XY male and thus reaches the advent of adolescence and final height attainment at an earlier chronologic age than the male.

The genetically determined potential for stature and pace of maturation are dependent upon an adequate supply of certain nutrients, vitamins, hormones, and oxygen to the skeletal cells. The dramatic trend toward increasing size and pace of maturation during the past 100 years is most likely related to better nutrition and relatively less chronic disease during childhood.

Causes of Growth Deficiency

Growth deficiency, although a valuable clinical sign, is a highly nonspecific one. Five general categories of growth deficiency are presented subsequently, each having somewhat different overall characteristics in terms of growth pattern, mode of evaluation to-

ward a specific diagnosis, prognosis for eventual stature, and/or management. The first two categories are variants of normal growth, and the other three represent abnormalities in the growth process. This classification, with the exception of prenatal infectious disease, is summarized in Table 2–1.

Variants of Normal

Familial Short Stature. Familial short stature is characterized by an otherwise normal small child who is maturing at a normal rate, as indicated by "bone age," with a family history of small stature in otherwise normal close relatives. Such individuals are usually within normal limits for size at birth, have a consistently slow pace of linear growth during childhood, reach adolescence at a usual age, and are relatively short in final stature.

Familial Slow Maturation. Familial slow maturation is characterized by a slowly maturing child who is short for chronologic age but not for maturational age (bone age), with a family history of slow maturation. The latter is indicated by late advent of adolescence and final height attainment in one or more close relatives. Such individuals are usually within normal limits for size at birth, with slowing in the pace of growth and maturation becoming evident during late infancy

Table 2–1. CLASSIFICATION OF GROWTH DEFICIENCY

Features	Normal Variants	
	Familial Short Stature	Familial Slow Maturation
Onset of growth deficiency	Postnatal	Postnatal (early childhood)
Rate of maturation	Normal	Slow
Family history	Short stature	Slow maturation
Final stature	Short	Normal limits
Therapy to increase eventual stature	None	None

Features	Abnormals*	
	Primary Skeletal Growth Deficiency	Secondary Growth Deficiency
Onset of growth deficiency	Usually prenatal	Usually postnatal
Rate of maturation	Variable, usually normal	Usually retarded
Associated anomalies	Frequent	Unusual, except when causative anomaly
Malproportionment	Frequent	Unusual, except for rickets
General modes of etiology	Chromosomal abnormalities	Environmental
	Mutant gene syndromes, including the osteochondrodysplasias	Defect in nonskeletal organ, including endocrine
	Syndromes of unknown etiology	Metabolic disorders
		Chronic infectious disease
Therapy to increase eventual stature	None at present	Specific treatment can result in "catch-up" growth

*Prenatal infectious disease and fetal alcohol syndrome are not included.

or early childhood. They have a late onset of a normal adolescence and usually achieve a final height within the normal range, but at a late chronologic age.

Abnormal Growth

Aside from the rare and rather obvious situation of sexual precocity leading to rapid growth and accelerated maturation with an early and relatively short final height attainment, the other growth deficiency disorders can be grouped into three general categories.

Primary Skeletal Growth Deficiency. The implication for this category is that of a primary intracellular problem that affects the growth of the skeletal system. The growth deficiency is usually of prenatal onset and is often accompanied by malproportionment or defects in skeletal molding. The same problem that affects cellular growth and morphogenesis in the skeleton may have affected other tissues as well. Thus the patient often presents with a *pattern* of multiple malformations, the recognition of which may allow for a concise overall diagnosis.

Postnatal growth generally proceeds at a consistently slow pace. Although the anomalous skeletal development may lead to difficulty in the interpretation of "bone age," maturation usually advances at a near-normal rate, and adolescence is achieved at a usual age. As yet, there is no known therapy for increasing the eventual stature of persons with any one of the disorders within this category. The prognosis for stature can best be inferred from knowledge of the final height attainment of other patients with the same disorder.

Many of the patterns of malformation presented in this text have primary growth deficiency as one feature. These include chromosomal abnormality syndromes, osteochondrodysplasias and many other mutant gene syndromes, plus a number of syndromes of unknown etiology. For a few of them, such as the Hurler syndrome, the Hunter syndrome, and X-linked spondyloepiphyseal dysplasia, the growth deficiency does not become manifest until months or years after birth.

Secondary Skeletal Growth Deficiency. The implication for this category is that the skeletal cells are normal. The growth deficiency is *secondary* to a problem outside the skeletal system that limits its capacity for growth. The problem may exist in the delivery of nutrients, hormones, or oxygen to the skeletal cells or in the maintenance of extracellular homeostasis. Specific types of secondary growth deficiency disorders are listed in Table 2–2. It is unusual for these types of problems to give rise to growth deficiency during fetal life,* and hence the onset of growth deficiency is usually *postnatal*. As illustrated in Figure 2–1, defects in the development and function of the brain, pituitary, thyroid, heart, lungs, liver, intestines, or kidneys seldom have a serious effect on prenatal growth but can cause postnatal growth deficiency. Since the growth problem is of postnatal onset, there usually are no associated malformations, except for an anomaly that may be responsible for the growth deficiency. Furthermore, the skeletal system is normally proportioned and modeled, except in the case of rickets.

Skeletal maturation is usually retarded to about the same extent as linear growth, with the exception of primary hypothyroidism, in which case osseous maturation is usually relatively more retarded than is linear growth.

When the cause of the secondary growth deficiency is recognized and rectified, one may witness the amazing phenomenon of catch-up growth, an acceleration of growth and maturation toward expectancy for chronologic age. This phenomenon dramatically emphasizes the fact that there is no primary growth problem within the skeletal system. The extent of catch-up growth varies in accordance with the age of onset, duration, and nature of the growth problem—plus the adequacy of therapy.

Prenatal Infectious Disease. Certain prenatally acquired infectious diseases such as toxoplasmosis, cytomegalic inclusion disease, and rubella may give rise to a chronic disease that can adversely affect growth, presumably by direct involvement of the skeletal system. The onset of growth deficiency is prenatal. Such babies often demonstrate other signs of prenatal infectious disease such as hepatosplenomegaly, brain dysfunction, and in the case of rubella, the patient may have cataracts and cardiac and/or auditory defects. There

---

*Mild degrees of prenatal secondary growth deficiency may occur with maternal toxemia, malnutrition, or heavy cigarette smoking, and prenatal onset of serious persisting growth deficiency may occur in the offspring of women with chronic alcoholism.

Table 2–2. **SECONDARY GROWTH DEFICIENCY**

Problem	Reason for Growth Deficiency	Diagnostic Studies
Nutritional a. Inadequate intake b. Partial intestinal obstruction c. Malabsorption	Nutritional deficiency	Response to adequate intake GI radiographic studies Absorption, GI enzyme studies
Deprivation syndrome	Neglect, abuse, nutritional	Response to environmental change Home and family investigation
Mental deficiency, usually severe	Unknown	Exclude other causes of mental deficiency
Cardiac defect a. Large left to right shunt b. Cyanotic type	?Rapid circulation time ?Hypoxia, sluggish circulation	Cardiac evaluation
Respiratory insufficiency	?Hypoxia	Usually obvious
Renal dysfunction	Acidosis Polyuria with dehydration Rickets	Urine pH, serum electrolytes, CO_2, urine concentrating ability Serum calcium, phosphorus
Pituitary growth hormone deficiency	?Diminished lipolysis and amino acid transport to cell	Stimulated serum growth hormone values
Hypothyroidism	Deficit in energy metabolism	Serum thyroxine or protein-bound iodine
Chronic serious infectious disease (not upper-respiratory)	Unknown	
Metabolic disorders such as hypercalcemia, hypophosphatemic rickets, hypokalemia, galactosemia, glycogen storage disease, salt-losing congenital adrenal hyperplasia		

Figure 2–1. Serious problems in development and function of the listed tissues usually do not have an adverse effect on prenatal growth, whereas each problem can be the cause of serious postnatal secondary growth deficiency.

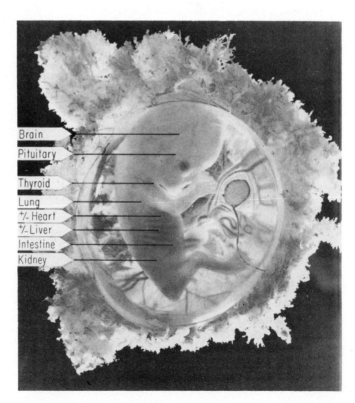

is inadequate knowledge about the eventual growth pattern in such babies, although the growth rate may improve after one to two years of age.

Clinical Approach to Growth Deficiency

Emphasis should be placed on the following:

1. Family history relative to stature and maturational rate.

2. History of patient's growth, plotted on normal grids. Of particular importance is the *age of onset* of growth deficiency and the *rate* of growth. Compare with normals for the mean parental stature when possible.

3. A complete physical evaluation should include height, weight, head circumference, and facial anomalies. Check closely for evidence of malproportionment, including asymmetry. Measure span and upper-to-lower segment ratio when indicated.

4. Based on the findings, most patients can be separated into one of the following three categories:

a. Normal for genetic background. No further studies indicated.

b. Prenatal onset of growth deficiency. Strive to recognize a specific overall syndrome among the primary growth deficiency disorders represented in this text. Also consider prenatal infectious disease, the fetal alcohol syndrome, and the fetal hydantoin syndrome.

c. Postnatal onset of growth deficiency. Generally, obtain a bone age determination (roentgenographs of knee and foot prior to three months, usually just hand and wrist thereafter). Consider such secondary growth deficiency disorders as those set forth in Table 2–2 plus the few primary skeletal growth deficiency syndromes that have a postnatal onset of growth deficiency.

APPROACH TO MENTAL DEFICIENCY

Since knowledge about the development of the central nervous system (CNS) and the causes of mental deficiency is rather incomplete, the following section should be interpreted as being preliminary and tentative.

Normal Development of CNS[5]

At 18 days of fetal development, the thickened neural plate becomes a neural groove, the margins of which join to form the neural tube, which is completely closed by 28 days. Rapid growth takes place anteriorly with formation of the primitive brain vesicles: the prosencephalon (forebrain), mesencephalon (midbrain), and rhombencephalon (hindbrain). By 23 days, the optic outpouchings are occurring from the prosencephalon, and by 33 days, its lateral outpouchings, i.e., the early cerebral hemispheres, are evident. Major brain morphogenesis continues for many months; the cerebellum does not begin its major period of morphogenesis until four to five fetal months. Within the cerebral hemispheres, the inner layer of neuroepithelial cells differentiates to become neuroblasts, which migrate outward in successive waves to form the cortical mantle layers. By ten weeks, the cerebral cortex is quite thin, with only one outer cortical layer in contrast with the

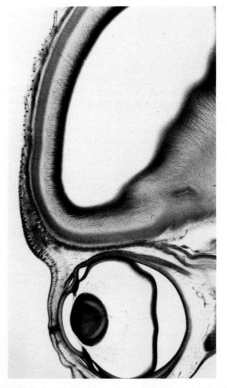

Figure 2–2. Sagittal section of fetal brain at the level of the eye at ten weeks of development. Note the single cortical zone of the cerebral cortex and the relatively large ventricular space. (From Smith, D. W., and Gong, B. T.: Teratology, *9*:17, 1974.)

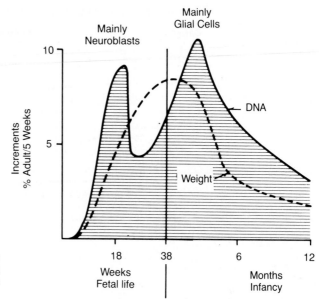

Figure 2–3. Rate of brain growth in terms of new cells (DNA) and weight during the most critical period of brain morphogenesis. (Adapted from Dobbin, J.: Am. J. Dis. Child., *120*:411, 1970.)

relatively large size of the lateral ventricles, as shown in Figure 2–2. Cell numbers are increasing rapidly, with a major addition of neurons at approximately four to five fetal months. New cells are being added well into postnatal life, as indicated in Figure 2–3. Although most of the neurones are present at birth, a major addition of glial cells occurs during the first six postnatal months. Most of the myelinization process, the responsibility of glial cells, occurs during the first year. The "wiring" of the axone networks, so integral to advancing and integrated function, is also occurring; however, less is known about critical periods for these interconnections between neurones. The functional consequences of this rapid brain growth and integration of neurones are reflected in the orderly progression of advancing performance during this time. Brain growth is almost complete by two years, with the organ reaching about 80 per cent of its adult size by this age.

Approach to Problems in Which Mental Deficiency is a Feature

Clinical Subcategorization of Mental Deficiency Relative to Diagnostic Studies

The majority of children with milder degrees of mental deficiency, having intelligence quotients (I.Q.s) in the range of 50 to 70, come from mentally dull and/or socio-economically deprived parents, related to polygenic and/or environmental factors.[6] This group also includes some XXY boys, an occasional XXX girl, some children with malformation syndromes, and some patients with inborn errors of metabolism, milder defects of central nervous system (CNS) development, or residual CNS insults. Among the more severely mentally deficient patients, with I.Q.s below 50, the clinician is more likely to arrive at a precise overall diagnosis. Though the following categorical breakdown of mental deficiency is especially relevant for severely affected patients, it is applicable for all degrees of mental deficiency.

This general subcategorization was designed to be of clinical value to aid in the rational diagnostic evaluation of a given patient with mental deficiency. It is based on findings derived from an appropriate family history, prenatal and birth history, postnatal history, and physical examination, with the latter including a careful search for associated major and minor malformations. It is the author's contention that, having obtained such information, there is no single laboratory study that is indicated for all patients with evidence of mental deficiency. Rather, the next phase of the diagnostic evaluation should be individualized in accordance with the findings from the history and physical

Table 2–3. **CATEGORIZATION OF MENTAL DEFICIENCY**

		Category	Subgroups		Studies to Consider
I	44%	Prenatal Onset of Problem in Morphogenesis	Single defect of brain	14%	Consider CAT scan
			Multiple defect, including brain		
			Chromosomal	12%	Chromosome studies
			Unknown	6%	
			Known syndrome, not chromosomal	6%	
II	?3%	Perinatal Insult to Brain	Trauma		
			Metabolic		
			Infectious		
III	?12%	Postnatal Onset of Problem	Environmental		
			Metabolic disorders, including known inborn errors	4%	Indicated metabolic study
			Infectious		
			Other		
IV	41%	Undecided Age of Onset of Problem			Consider metabolic studies, chromosome study
	?Very Small %	Disorders Which Might Present *Clinically* in Several of the Above Categories	Prenatal infectious disease		Appropriate culture and/or antibody studies
			Hypothyroidism, congenital		P.B.I. or T$_4$

The percentage figures were obtained from Kaveggia et al.[7] and represent the approximate per cent of each category and subgroup from the *total* of 1224 seriously mentally deficient patients in their study.

examination. This subcategorization is predominantly based on the apparent *age of onset of the problem*. Table 2–3 summarizes the subgroups and the types of diagnostic laboratory studies that might merit consideration of each subgroup. These are elaborated upon in the following text.

Category I: Prenatal Problem in Morphogenesis of the Brain. This group is the largest one, making up 44 per cent of 1224 seriously mentally deficient patients evaluated by Kaveggia et al.[7] and 53 per cent of a less severely mentally deficient group reported by Smith and Simons.[8] About one third of this subcategory of patients were considered to have a single primary defect in brain morphogenesis, such as primary microcephaly, hydrocephalus, hydranencephaly, a defect of neural tube closure, or other types of cerebral dysmorphogenesis. The other two thirds had multiple major and/or minor malformations of non-CNS structures, and by inference, the mental deficiency was also considered to be the consequence of a defect in early morphogenesis of the brain. This latter discrimination is often dependent upon a cautious total physical examination with the purpose of detecting minor as well as major anomalies. For example, Smith and Bostian[9] evaluated 50 consecutive patients with idiopathic mental deficiency and found that 42 per cent of them had three or more extra-CNS major and/or minor anomalies of prenatal onset versus none with three or more associated anomalies in 100 concomitantly examined control children without mental deficiency. Within Kaveggia et al.'s[7] multiple defect subcategory, 41 per cent of patients had a chromosomal abnormality, mostly the Down syndrome, 18 per cent had known syndromes of nonchromosomal etiology, and 41 per cent had patterns of malformation of unknown etiology.

Category II: Perinatal Insult to Brain. This group includes kernicterus, severe neonatal hypoglycemia, intracerebral hemorrhage, perinatal hypoxia, and meningitis and sepsis—all more common in the prematurely born infant. Caution should be exerted before assuming that problems of birth and perinatal adaptation are the *primary* cause of mental deficiency in patients who have evidence of *prenatal* onset of a problem in morphogenesis. Such patients, especially those who have a severe defect of early brain development and those with prenatal onset of growth deficiency, are more likely to have problems in neonatal adaptation.

Category III: Postnatal Onset of Problem in Brain Function. These patients generally appear normal as newborns. After a variable period of time, during which they have normal appearance and function, there is a slowing and/or deterioration in developmental progress and performance. This group includes environmental insults such as trauma, meningitis, encephalitis, hypernatremia, water intoxication, severe hypoglycemia, severe hypoxemia, and lead encephalopathy plus certain enzymatic defects of amino acid, carbohydrate, uric acid, mucopolysaccharide, and brain lipid metabolism. Though some of these latter inborn errors of metabolism may have a prenatal onset, only a few of them, such as the Leroy I-cell syndrome or generalized gangliosidosis, have gross clinical manifestations by the time of birth. Thus the *clinical* implication is usually that of a postnatal onset of the problem. Kaveggia et al.[7] found that 4.3 per cent of 1224 seriously mentally deficient patients had established inborn errors of metabolism, of which one third had phenylketonuria.

Category IV: Undecided Age of Onset of the Problem in Brain Function. These are the patients who show no obvious evidence of a prenatal problem in morphogenesis, have no established history of a gross insult to the brain in the perinatal period, and who have been rather consistently slow in postnatal developmental progress without evident cause. They may or may not have other evidence of CNS dysfunction, such as spasticity, hypotonia, seizures, and/or aberrant behavior. This is the second largest group, making up 41 per cent of the series studied by Kaveggia et al.[7]

Disorders That May Present Clinically in Several of the Four Categories

1. *Prenatal infectious disease.* The patient with mental deficiency as a consequence of prenatally acquired infectious disease such as rubella, cytomegalic inclusion disease, or toxoplasmosis may have obvious historical and physical indications of prenatal onset of the disorder, may have had serious problems in perinatal adaptation, or may have had no obvious problems until a later age. Thus, their clinical presentation may be in any one of the above categories.

2. *Congenital hypothyroidism.* Early detection of congenital hypothyroidism, with thyroid hormone replacement, is critical in preventing or at least limiting the adverse effect of hypothyroidism on early brain development.[10] Signs of prenatal onset of osseous immaturity, such as unusually large fontanels[11] and facial immaturity with a short nose, are usually present at birth, and perinatal problems not uncommonly include persisting indirect bilirubinemia, lethargy, and/or poor feeding. Unfortunately, congenital hypothyroidism is seldom detected on the basis of these early signs and symptoms. Most commonly, it is not suspected until postnatal onset of slow growth, sluggish activity, myxedema, and lag of developmental progression become evident. Patients with partial degrees of congenital hypothyroidism may not show signs of myxedema and may have a very subtle postnatal onset of slowness in growth, maturation, and developmental progress, with borderline sluggishness in activity. Thus the clinician could interpret the patients as belonging in any of the above categories, though they obviously belong in Category I (prenatal onset).

Diagnostic Studies in Patients with Mental Deficiency—Their Rational Usage

1. Studies that may resolve the diagnosis.
a. *Chromosome studies.* Indications for chromosome studies are largely limited to appropriate patients in Category I who have multiple malformations and to those in Category IV (undecided) when the clinical findings do not *exclude* the possibility of XXY or XXX.
b. *Studies for inborn errors of metabolism.* Patients with mental deficiency due to an inborn error of metabolic function, most commonly the consequence of a recessively inherited enzyme defect, often have one or more additional clues besides mental deficiency alone. Some of these are set forth in Table 2–4. These patients usually fit into Category III. They appear normal at birth and then at variable postnatal ages develop diffuse nonlateralizing evidence of central nervous system deficit or deterioration of function. A history of intermittent lapses of consciousness, inanition, unexplained hypoglycemia, or recurrent acidosis should each be potential clues toward an inborn error of metabolism. For example, acidosis may be a feature of lactic acidemia, and intermittent loss of consciousness may occur in the severe form of maple syrup urine disease or in hyperammonemia.

Phenylketonuria may be difficult to determine from the clinical findings. When

Table 2–4. **EXAMPLES OF FEATURES IN ADDITION TO MENTAL DEFICIENCY THAT OFTEN OCCUR POSTNATALLY IN CERTAIN INBORN ERRORS OF METABOLISM**[12]

Disorder	Features
Phenylketonuria, classic; autosomal recessive	Light pigmentation; eczema (33%); poor coordination, seizures (25%), autistic behavior
Sanfilippo syndrome (MPS III); autosomal recessive	Developmental lag after 1 year with deterioration toward restless behavior, clumsiness by age 6–7 yrs; development of coarse facies and hair by 2–3 yrs; gum hypertrophy, mild limitation in finger extension
Hurler syndrome (MPS I); autosomal recessive	Developmental lag after 6–10 mos, with deterioration and growth deficiency, coarse facies, stiff joints, gibbus, hepatosplenomegaly, cloudy corneas, rhinitis
Hunter syndrome (MPS II), severe type; X-linked recessive	Developmental lag after 6–12 mos, with growth deficiency, coarse facies, stiff joints, hepatosplenomegaly; no gibbus or cloudy corneas
Galactosemia, severe type; autosomal recessive	Development in early infancy (on cow's milk feeding) of lethargy, hypotonia, hepatomegaly, icterus, hypoglycemia, cataract, with failure to thrive
Lesch-Nyhan syndrome; X-linked recessive	Development after 6–8 mos of spasticity, choreoathetosis, self-mutilation, autistic behavior, growth deficiency; tophi in late childhood
Homocystinuria; autosomal recessive	Mild arachnodactyly, pectus, genu valgus, pes cavus, mild limitation of finger extension; downward lens dislocation, usually by age 10 yrs; wide facial pores, malar flush; thrombotic phenomena, contributing to CNS problems
Argininosuccinicaciduria; autosomal recessive	Onset in first 1–2 yrs of growth deficiency, mild hepatomegaly, skin lesions, dry brittle hair with trichorrhexis nodosa, seizures

it cannot be excluded as a possibility by the overall features, a urine ferric chloride test or a serum phenylalanine determination should be done.

c. *Studies for prenatal infectious disease.* Patients with mental deficiency as the result of congenital rubella, cytomegalic inclusion disease, or toxoplasmosis usually also have one or more of the following features: microcephaly, chorioretinitis, prenatal onset growth deficiency, hepatosplenomegaly, neonatal petechiae, jaundice, and/or deafness. Patients with congenital rubella may also have cataract, cardiac defect, and other anomalies. Those mentally deficient patients who have one or more of these additional findings and whose total findings do not *exclude* the possibility of the disorder being due to prenatal infectious disease should be considered for one or more of the following studies: direct culture of the infectious agent (in early infancy), specific fluorescent IgM antibody determination, and complement-fixation antibody determination.

d. *Thyroid studies.* A protein-bound iodine (P.B.I.) or serum thyroxine determination is merited for the mentally deficient patient who has evidence of osseous immaturity, slow postnatal growth, sluggish physical activity, and myxedematous full-

ness in the tissues. Thyroid studies are *not* indicated in the patient with mental deficiency and short stature who does not show any other clinical indication of having hypothyroidism.

2. Ancillary studies that may assist in the diagnosis.

a. *Computed axial tomography (CAT) scan* may occasionally be indicated in a Category I patient with a primary defect in brain morphogenesis in an effort to delineate the nature and extent of the brain malformation more fully. This may be of particular relevance for hydrocephalus. For other defects, the study may provide a better perspective toward prognosis as well as genetic counseling.

b. *Skull roentgenograms* merit consideration in a patient with clinical signs of craniosynostosis, evidence of increased intracranial pressure, cutaneous signs of tuberous sclerosis or Sturge-Weber malformation sequence, or evidence of prenatal infectious disease, especially toxoplasmosis. Otherwise, there is seldom any clinically relevant information to be derived from this study.

c. *Long bone roentgenograms* may be indicated by clinical findings such as skeletal abnormalities. Bone age determination may be indicated in patients with decelerating growth, especially those in whom the over-

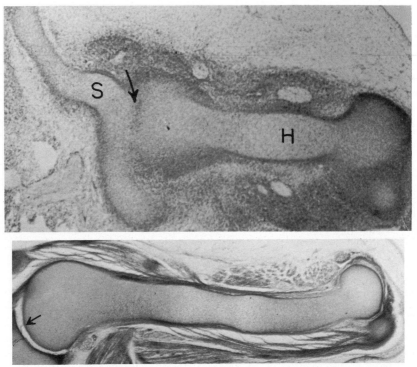

Figure 2–4. Development of scapulo (S)–humoral (H) shoulder joint *(arrow)* at 38 days of development *(above)* and at about 47 days *(below)*. Note that joint morphogenesis occurs secondarily. By the time the joint is formed, functional muscle has differentiated.

all findings are compatible with hypothyroidism, and in patients with excessive rate of growth, but it is of little practical value in patients with prenatal onset of growth deficiency.

d. *Electroencephalograms* may be warranted in patients with a history of seizures or suspected seizure-equivalent.

e. *Fasting blood glucose* level merits consideration in patients with a history suggestive of hypoglycemic signs and symptoms but is not necessarily indicated for all patients with seizures.

f. Other serum chemistries, blood studies, and urinalysis should be performed only as prompted by findings other than mental deficiency in the history or examination.

APPROACH TO ARTHROGRYPOSIS
(Prenatal Onset of Joint Contractures)

Normal Development of Joints

Joint development begins secondarily within the early mesenchymal condensations of the precartilaginous bone at about five and one-half weeks. By seven weeks, many joint spaces exist, and by eight weeks, there is movement of the limbs. Figure 2–4 shows the early development. Motion is essential for the normal development of the joints and their contiguous structures.

Problems That Can Cause Congenital Joint Contractures
(Figure 2–5)

1. *Neurologic abnormality* has been the most common cause of arthrogryposis in the experience of the author. The neurologic disorders that may be responsible for the secondary arthrogryposis include meningomyelocele, anterior motor horn cell deficiency, prenatal spasticity, and certain gross brain defects such as anencephaly, hydranencephaly, and holoprosencephaly.

2. *Muscle problems* such as muscle agenesis, rare fetal myopathies, and occasionally myotonic dystrophy.

3. *Joint and contiguous tissue problems* such as synostosis, lack of joint development, aber-

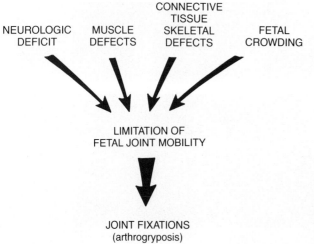

Figure 2–5. The types of problems that can lead to prenatal joint contractures.

rant fixation of joints as in diastrophic dwarfism, aberrant laxity of joints with dislocations as in the Larsen syndrome, and aberrant soft tissue fixations as in the popliteal web syndrome.

4. *Fetal crowding and constraint* as with multiple births or with oligohydramnios in disorders such as renal agenesis or early persisting leakage of amniotic fluid.

Methods of Evaluation

1. *History.* The history relative to arthrogryposis should include information on the onset and character of fetal movements (often diminished), mode of delivery (often breech), and amniotic fluid (oligohydramnios may give rise to fetal crowding).

2. *Total pattern of anomalies.* Non-joint–related anomalies may indicate that the arthrogryposis is part of a multiple defect syndrome such as the trisomy 18 syndrome.

3. *Joint and skeletal evaluation.* Physical and radiologic assessment of joints and skeletal system is indicated. Determine whether the joint fixation is a result of an anatomic anomaly, such as lack of development of a joint or synostosis, or a deficit in functional movement with no primary structural cause. Always check for scoliosis and for hip dislocation.

4. *Evaluation of hand and foot creases.* The palmar and finger creases and the sole creases represent the planes of early flexional function and are evident by 11 to 12 weeks of fetal age. Absent or abnormal creases are secondary to aberrant form or function in the early hand or foot development. They also provide an historical record of the flexional planes of function that have existed and thus facilitate decisions relative to rehabilitation of existing function.

5. *Search for dimples.* When close fetal contact between bone and overlying skin has occurred, there may be failure in the development of subcutaneous and adipose tissue at that locale, thereby causing a dimple. The finding of aberrant dimples implies an early fetal onset of the problem, resulting in aberrant cutaneous-osseous approximation, as shown in Figure 2–6.

6. *Cautious neurologic and muscle assessment.* Attempts to determine whether there is a primary neurologic or muscle problem can be most difficult, since deficit in either one can lead to aberrant function of the other. Electromyographic (EMG) studies occasionally may be of value. In the great majority of patients with arthrogryposis who have abnormal study results, the evidence points toward neuropathy and rarely to a myopathy. Muscle biopsy may only occasionally be of value, since it is difficult to determine whether muscle hypoplasia and/or fibrosis is a primary or secondary phenomenon.

Comment and Management

When a particular diagnosis can be delineated, the management should be specific for that disorder, including a lack of medical intervention for such disorders as the trisomy 18 syndrome. There remain a number of patients with multiple congenital joint contractures for whom no specific diagnosis can presently be clearly determined. Based on a

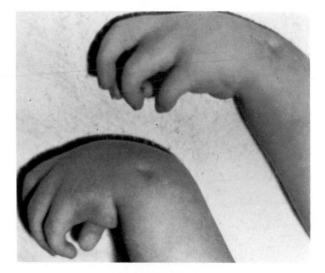

Figure 2–6. Dimples on the dorsum of the wrists, indicating that the aberrant positioning of the hands had been present from early in fetal life. The joint contractures in this infant were considered to be secondary to neurologic deficiency.

study of over 350 patients with congenital contractures of joints, Dr. Judith Hall, University of British Columbia, Vancouver, has made the most significant contribution to our understanding of this problem as well as to an approach to its etiology.

APPROACH TO AMBIGUOUS (PARTIALLY MASCULINIZED) EXTERNAL GENITALIA

Normal Development

Genes on the Y chromosome determine testicular differentiation of the gonad, which at about eight weeks' gestation begins producing testosterone, actively causing masculinization of the external genitalia, with fusion of the labioscrotal folds to form a scrotum, enlargement of the phallus, and fusion of the labia minora folds into a penile urethra, as shown in Figure 2–7. The testes descend into the scrotum by seven to eight fetal months.

Causes of Aberrant Development[16, 17]

Partial masculinization of the external genitalia, including incomplete descent of the testicles, can be secondary to any one of the following problems:

1. Diminished fetal androgen production because of a defect in development and/or function of the testicles.

2. Diminished to absent cellular response to androgen (testosterone) in the male.

3. Primary defect in development of external genitalia in the male, not secondary to hormonal aberration.

4. Partially masculinized external genitalia due to exposure of the XX female to androgen in utero. The androgen may derive either from the fetus (e.g., congenital adrenal hyperplasia) or from the mother during early gestation.

Methods of Evaluation
(Figure 2–8)

1. *Complete examination for associated nongenital anomalies.* If significant nongenital anomalies are present, it is highly unlikely that the patient has congenital adrenal hyperplasia or any other known defect in steroidogenesis. An attempt should then be made to identify the total pattern of malformation from among known syndromes, such as the Smith-Lemli-Opitz syndrome, in which genital anomaly is one feature of a multiple defect disorder.

2. *Determination of genetic sex.*

a. *Buccal smear for X-chromatin.* This procedure will assist in the determination of the number of X chromosomes, the second X tending to be clumped at the nuclear periphery as the "X-chromatin." The usual frequency of X-chromatin–positive cells in the XX individual is 19 to 35 per cent and near zero in the XY individual. However, it is important to appreciate that the frequency of X-chromatin–positive cells in the female may be lower during

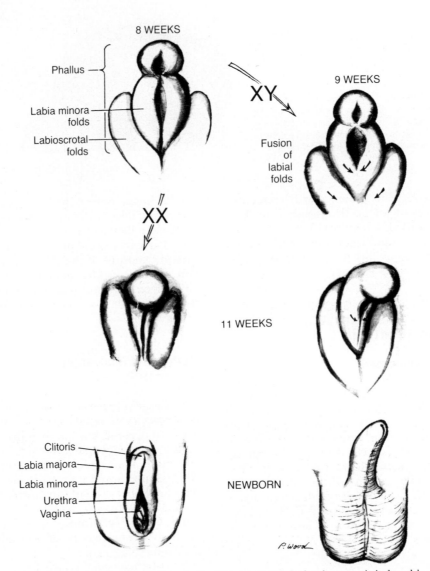

Figure 2–7. Normal morphogenesis of external genitalia. The normal male development is induced by testosterone derived from the fetal testicle. (Illustrations adapted from photos supplied by J. Jirásek, Prague, Czechoslovokia.)

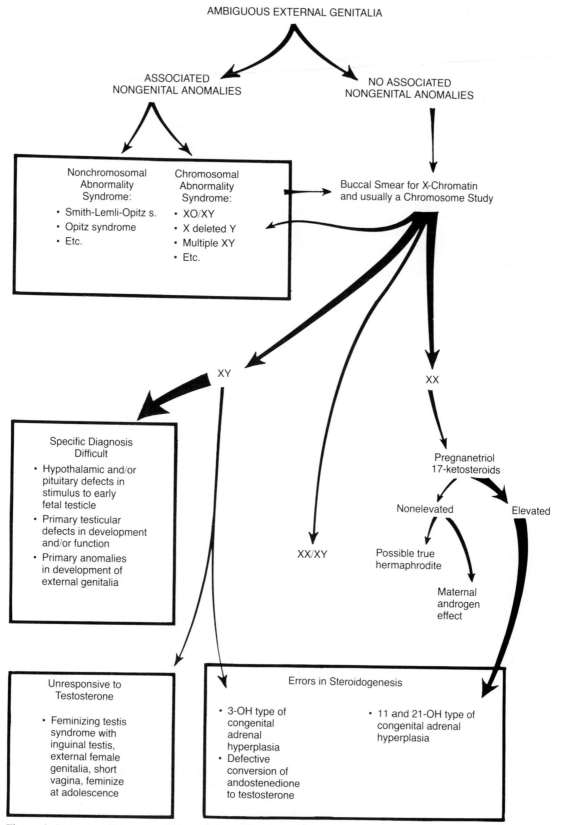

Figure 2–8. Approach toward arriving at a specific overall diagnosis in the patient who has ambiguous external genitalia.

the first two postnatal days or with un-treated congenital adrenal hyperplasia.

b. *Chromosomal study of cultured leukocytes.* Most patients with ambiguous genitalia should have a chromosomal study. Exceptions include those with a known nonchromosomal abnormality syndrome and those X-chromatin–positive females with congenital adrenal hyperplasia or with a history of the mother having been exposed to a known androgen during the first two to three months of gestation. At least 20 cells should be studied because of the possibility of mosaicism, such as XO/XY, XX/XY, and so forth.

3. *Determination of the genital anatomy.*

a. *Gonads.* If no gonads are found in the scrotal area, place a finger over the inguinal canal to prevent the ascent of any inguinal gonad and palpate the inguinal areas carefully, ideally with three fingers. If one or more gonads are found, it is highly unlikely that the patient is a partially masculinized female, since inguinal or lower gonads are usually testes. Only in the situation of inguinal hernia may one find an ovary in the inguinal area.

b. *Phallus.*

1. Assess the length and width of the phallus (see Chapter 7 for standards). If it is a relatively thin phallus, the patient is unlikely to be a female with congenital adrenal hyperplasia, since she would be under "active" androgen stimulation with increased caliber to the phallus.

2. If there is a single opening at the base of the phallus and also a small "pit" on the glans, the former represents the urethral opening and the latter is of no significance.

c. *Urogenital sinus or urethra; vagina; uterus.*

1. When there is only a single opening at the base of the phallus, insert a relatively stiff catheter or sterile probe into it. Direct the catheter tip downward in the direction of the anal opening. If it goes in that direction easily and can be palpated beneath the perineal skin, there is probably a urogenital sinus with both urethral and vaginal orifices, as in the female with congenital adrenal hyperplasia. If it is a "penile" urethra, the catheter will usually go cephalad and cannot be easily palpated in the perineal area.

2. Inject radiopaque material into the sin-gle opening under pressure and obtain a lateral roentgenogram to demonstrate whether there is a vaginal pouch.

3. If a vaginal opening is evident, insert a catheter into it and determine its depth.

4. Uterus. Do a cautious rectal examination with the little finger, feeling for a uterine body. When removing the finger in the neonate, stroke the anterior rectal area outward. If there is a vagina, this maneuver will often result in the extrusion of vaginal mucus from the single urogenital opening.

4. *Hormonal and metabolic studies* are indicated only for patients who do not have associated nongenital anomalies.

a. *XX females.* Ideally, there should be three 24-hour urines for pregnanetriol and 17-ketosteroid determinations in order to exclude congenital adrenal hyperplasia. Daily serum sodium and potassium determinations should be made to detect evidence of salt loss.

b. *XY males.* Although rare, congenital adrenal hyperplasia with defective 3-hydroxylation or other defects that adversely affect the steroidogenesis of testosterone as well as hydrocortisone should be considered, as well as a defect in conversion of androstenedione to testosterone.

Management

The initial evaluation of the newborn baby with ambiguity in the development of the external genitalia, including those with a fully developed penis but no palpable testes, constitutes an emergency situation relative to the sex of rearing. The XX individuals with congenital adrenal hyperplasia (the most common single cause of ambiguous genitalia) and those females partially masculinized in utero by maternal androgen should be raised as females with appropriate cosmetic surgery. Exploratory surgery for gonadal and internal genital anatomy should usually precede a sex of rearing decision in the rare situations of the XX/XY individual or the XX patient who has neither congenital adrenal hyperplasia nor a history compatible with maternally derived, in utero androgen effect. For the great majority of the remaining patients, the sex of rearing is dependent upon whether the phallus can serve as a cosmetically and functionally adequate penis. When this is not possible, the sex of rearing should be female, with appropriate cosmetic surgery. In some of the borderline cases in which the male sex of rearing would seem preferable, the author has utilized a short course of Depo-Testosterone therapy in low dosage, 25 mg every three weeks for three months, in order to enlarge the penis during early infancy.[18] This has resulted in a one and one-half to twofold enlargement of the penis, thus allowing for better parental acceptance (especially paternal) and early cosmetic surgery for hypospadias. The rationale for this therapy is based on the supposition that most of these cases represent inadequate androgen effect from the fetal testicle in bringing about full-size development of the penis; hence, exogenous testosterone is given for a short period of time in order to enlarge the incompletely developed penis. Beyond the phallic enlargement, no other signs of virilization have been noted during this type of short-term, low-dosage course of testosterone. Transient mild to moderate acceleration of growth and skeletal maturation have occurred, tending to return to a normal rate after discontinuing testosterone therapy. Hence, no appreciable effect of this therapy is anticipated in terms of ultimate growth.

The author prefers to have testosterone enlargement of the phallus (when indicated) and/or cosmetic surgery to the external genitalia accomplished before 18 months to two years of age, with the exception of creating a vaginal pouch. The purpose of this approach is to have the external genital anatomy as appropriate as possible for sex rearing before the age when the individual will be fully cognizant of sex and gender orientation.

Because of the risk of tumor and malignancy, removal of intraabdominal testicular tissue is generally indicated unless it appears near-normal and can be brought into the scrotum. This need not necessarily be accomplished during childhood, with the probable exception of the XO/XY mosaic patient. The dysmorphic testicle, such as may be found in XO/XY patients, has a significant risk of tumor development, even prior to adolescence.

References

Growth Deficiency

1. Faulkner, F., ed.: Human Development. Philadelphia, W. B. Saunders Co., 1966.

2. Gardner, L. I., ed.: Endocrine and Genetic Diseases of Childhood and Adolescence. 2nd ed. Philadelphia, W. B. Saunders Co., 1975.
3. Garn, S. M., and Rohmann, C. G.: Interaction of nutrition and genetics in the timing of growth and development. Pediatr. Clin. North Am., *13*:353, 1966.
4. Tanner, J. M., Goldstein, H., and Whitehouse, R. H.: Standards for children's height at ages two to nine years allowing for height of parents. Arch. Dis. Child., *45*:755, 1970.

Mental Deficiency

5. O'Rahilly, R., and Gardner, E.: The timing and sequence of events in the development of human nervous system during the embryonic period proper. Z. Anat. Entwicklungsgesch., *34*:1, 1971.
6. Drillen, C. M., Jameson, S., and Wilkinson, E. M.: Studies in mental handicap, Part I: Prevalence and distribution by clinical type and severity of defect. Arch. Dis. Child., *41*:528, 1966.
7. Kaveggia, E. G., et al.: Diagnostic genetic studies on 1,224 patients with severe mental retardation. Proceedings of the Third Congress of the International Association for Scientific Study of Mental Deficiency. Held at The Hague, Holland, September 4–12, 1973.
8. Smith, D. W., and Simons, F. E. R.: Rational diagnostic evaluation of the child with mental deficiency. Am. J. Dis. Child., *129*:1285, 1975.
9. Smith, D. W., and Bostian, K. D.: Congenital anomalies associated with idiopathic mental retardation. J. Pediatr., *65*:189, 1964.
10. Smith, D. W., Blizzard, R. M., and Wilkins, L.: The mental prognosis in hypothyroidism in infancy and childhood: A review of 128 cases. Pediatrics, *19*:1011, 1957.
11. Smith, D. W., and Popich, G.: Large fontanels in congenital hypothyroidism: A potential clue toward earlier recognition. J. Pediatr., *80*:753, 1972.
12. Holmes, L. B., et al.: Mental Retardation. An Atlas of Diseases with Associated Physical Abnormalities. New York, Macmillan Publishing Co., 1972.

Arthrogryposis

13. Fisher, R. L., et al.: Arthrogryposis multiplex congenita, a clinical investigation. J. Pediatr., *76*:255, 1970.
14. Hall, J. G., Reed, S. D., and Greene, D.: The distal arthrogryposes: Delineation of new entities—Review and nosologic discussion. Am. J. Med. Genet., *11*:185, 1982.
15. Hall, J. G., Reed, S. D., and Driscoll, E. P.: Part I. Amyoplasia: A common sporadic condition with congenital contractures. Am. J. Med. Genet., *15*:571, 1983.

Ambiguous External Genitalia

16. Williams, R. H., ed.: Textbook of Endocrinology, 5th ed. Philadelphia, W. B. Saunders Co., 1974.
17. Summitt, R. L.: Differential diagnosis of genital ambiguity in the newborn. Clin. Obstet. Gynecol., *15*:112, 1972.
18. Guthrie, R. D., Smith, D. W., and Graham, C. B.: Testosterone treatment for the micropenis during early childhood. J. Pediatr., *83*:247, 1973.

3

Morphogenesis and Dysmorphogenesis

Knowledge of normal morphogenesis may assist in the interpretation of structural defects, and the study of structural defects may assist in the understanding of normal morphogenesis. Each anomaly must have a logical mode of development and cause. When interpreting a structural defect, the clinician is looking back to an early stage in development with which he or she has often had little acquaintance. This chapter sets forth some of the phenomena of morphogenesis and the normal stages in early human development, followed by the types of abnormal morphogenesis and the relative timing of particular malformations.

NORMAL MORPHOGENESIS

Phenomena of Morphogenesis

The genetic information that guides the morphogenesis and function of an individual is all contained within the zygote. After the first few cell divisions, differentiation begins to take place, presumably through activation or inactivation of particular genes, allowing cells to assume diverse roles. The entire process is programmed in a timely and sequential order with little allowance for error, especially in early morphogenesis.

Although little is known about the fundamental processes that control morphogenesis, it is worthwhile to mention some of the normal phenomena that occur and to give examples of each.

Cell Migration

The proper migration of cells to a predestined location is critical in the development of many structures. For example, the germ cells move from the yolk sac endoderm to the urogenital ridge, where they interact with other cells to form the gonad.

Control over Mitotic Rate

The size of particular structures, as well as their form, is to a large extent the consequence of control over the rates of cell division.

Interaction Between Adjacent Tissues

The optic cup induces the morphogenesis of the lens from the overlying ectoderm, the ureteric bud gives rise to the development of the kidney from the adjacent metanephric tissue, the notochord is essential for normal development of the overlying neural tissue, and the prechordal mesoderm is important for the normal morphogenesis of the overlying forebrain. These are but a few examples of the many interactions that are essential features in morphogenesis.

Adhesive Association of Like Cells

In the development of a structure such as a long bone, the early cells tend to aggregate closely in condensations, a membrane comes to surround them, and only later do they resemble cartilage cells. The association of like cells is dramatically demonstrated by admixing trypsinized liver and kidney cells in vitro and observing them reaggregate with their own kind.

Controlled Cell Death

Controlled cell death plays a role in normal morphogenesis. Examples include death of tissue between the digits resulting in separation of the fingers and recanalization of the duodenum. The dead cellular debris is engulfed by large macrophages, leaving no trace of the tissue.

Hormonal Influence over Morphogenesis

Androgen effect is one example of a hormonal influence over morphogenesis—in this case, that of the external genitalia. Normally, the individual with a Y chromosome has testosterone from the fetal testicle that induces enlargement of the phallus, closure of the labia minoral folds to form a penile urethra, and fusion of the labioscrotal folds to form a scrotum. Prior to eight weeks, the genitalia appear female in type and will remain so unless androgenic hormone is present.

Mechanical Forces

Mechanical forces play a major role in morphogenesis. The size, growth, and form of the brain and its early derivatives, for example, have a major function in the formation of the calvarium and upper face. The alignment of collagen fibrils and bone trabeculae relates directly to the direction of forces exerted on these tissues. The role of mechanical factors in development is covered in the text *Smith's Recognizable Patterns of Human Deformation*.

Normal Stages in Morphogenesis

The general steps in normal morphogenesis as set forth here are illustrated in Figures 3–1 to 3–16. The first week is a period of cell division without much enlargement, the conceptus being dependent on the cytoplasm of the ova for most of its metabolic needs. By seven to eight days, the zona pellucida is gone, and the outlying trophoblast cells invade the endometrium and form the early placenta that must function both to nourish the parasitic embryo and to maintain the pregnancy via its endocrine function. During this time, a relatively small inner cell mass

Figure 3–1. Two-cell specimen, within zona pellucida. (From the Department of Embryology, Carnegie Institution of Washington, D.C., Baltimore.)

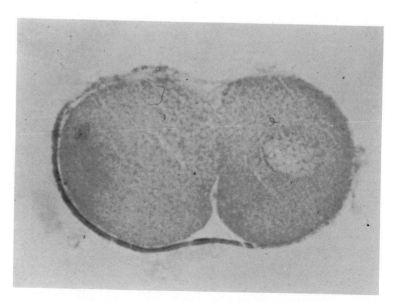

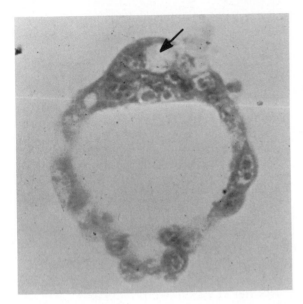

Figure 3–2. *Four to five day* blastocyst. The embryonic cell mass *(top)*. (From the Department of Embryology, Carnegie Institution of Washington, D.C., Baltimore.)

Figure 3–3. *Seven days.* The major part of the conceptus, the cytotrophoblast, has invaded the endometrium, and the embryo *(arrow)* is differentiating into two diverse cell layers, the ectoderm and endoderm. The amniotic cavity is beginning. (From the Department of Embryology, Carnegie Institution of Washington, D.C., Baltimore.)

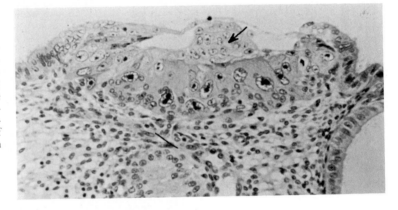

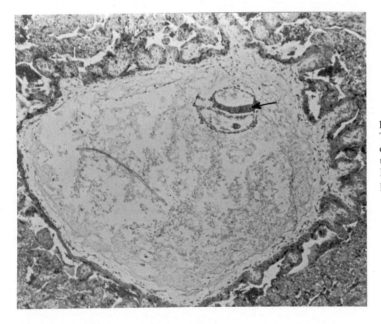

Figure 3–4. *Fourteen to sixteen days.* The thicker ectoderm *(arrow)* has its continuous amniotic sac, whereas the underlying endoderm has its yolk sac. Major changes will now begin to take place.

Figure 3–5. *Seventeen to eighteen days.* Mesoblast cells migrate from the ectoderm through the node (the hillock marked by the arrow) and the primitive streak to specific locations between the ectoderm and endoderm, there constituting the highly versatile mesoderm. Anterior to the node the notochordal process develops, providing axial support and influencing subsequent development such as that of the overlying neural plate.

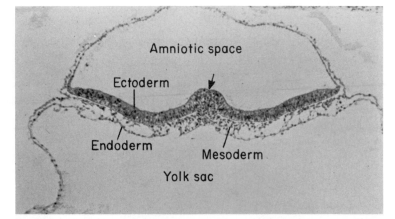

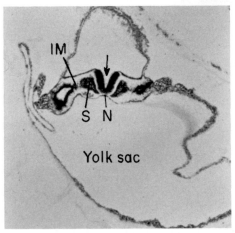

Figure 3–6. *Twenty-one to twenty-three days.* The midaxial ectoderm has thickened and formed the neural groove *(arrow)*, partially influenced by the underlying notochordal plate (N). Lateral to it, the mesoblast has now segmented into somites (S), intermediate mesoderm (IM), and somatopleure and splanchnopleure as intervening steps toward further differentiation. Vascular channels are developing in situ from mesoderm, blood cells are being produced in the yolk sac wall, and the early heart is beating. Henceforth, development is extremely rapid, with major changes each day.

Figure 3–7. *Twenty-four days.* The fore part of the embryo is growing rapidly, especially the anterior neural plate. The cardiac tube, under the developing face *(arrow)*, is functional. (From the Department of Embryology, Carnegie Institution of Washington, D.C., Baltimore.)

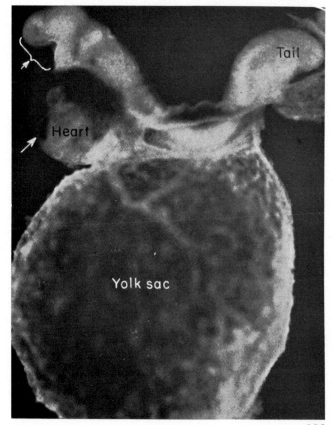

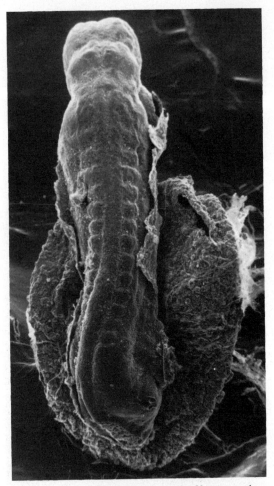

Figure 3–8. Scanning EM photograph of human embryo of about 23 to 25 days' gestation, with the amnion largely stripped away. This dorsal view beautifully shows the developing brain (anterior) and spinal cord just after neural tube formation and the orderly bilateral segmentation of the somites. (Courtesy of Dr. Jan E. Jirásek, Prague, Czechoslovakia.)

has become a bilaminar disc of ectoderm and endoderm, each with its own fluid-filled cavity, the amniotic sac and yolk sac, respectively. By the end of the second week, a small mound, a primitive node, has developed in the ectoderm, and behind it a primitive streak forms. The embryo now has an axis to which further morphogenesis will relate. Cells migrate forward from the node between the ectoderm and endoderm to form an elastic cord, the notochord, which temporarily provides axial support for the embryo as well as influencing the adjacent morphogenesis. Ectodermal cells migrate through the node and the primitive streak to specific areas between the ectoderm and endoderm, becoming the

mesoderm. One of the early mesodermal derivatives is a circulatory system; during the third week, the heart begins to develop, vascular channels form in situ, and blood cells are produced in the yolk sac. By the end of the third week, the heart is pumping, a neural groove has formed anterior to the node, the para-axial mesoderm has begun to be segmented into somites, the anterior and posterior regions of the embryo have begun to curl under, and the foregut and hindgut pouches become distinct. The stage is now set for the period of major organogenesis, which is best considered in relation to individual structures.

Early morphogenesis is set forth in the accompanying figures. As noted in the illustrations found on the inside front cover and inside back cover of this book, each stage of development represents a synchronous syndrome of characteristics.

ABNORMAL MORPHOGENESIS

As mentioned in the introduction, there are three general types of developmental pathology leading to structural defects. The first type is malformation, which is a poor formation of the tissue. The second is deformation due to altered mechanical forces on a normal tissue. Deformation may be secondary to extrinsic forces, such as uterine constraint on a normal fetus, or to intrinsic forces related to a more primary malformation. The third type of pathology is disruption, which is a result of the breakdown of a previously normal tissue. An example of the latter is porencephalic cyst of vascular causation.

Extrinsic deformation is set forth in a separate text, *Smith's Recognizable Patterns of Human Deformation*. A few disruption patterns of anomaly are considered in this book, with the major emphasis being on patterns of malformation, including malformation sequences. However, it is very important for the reader to appreciate that many of the anomalies in a given malformation sequence or syndrome are actually deformations that are engendered by the altered mechanical forces resulting from the more primary malformation. For example, most minor anomalies represent deformations, often secondary to a malformation.

Malformations may be broken down into a number of subcategories in terms of the nature of the poor formation.

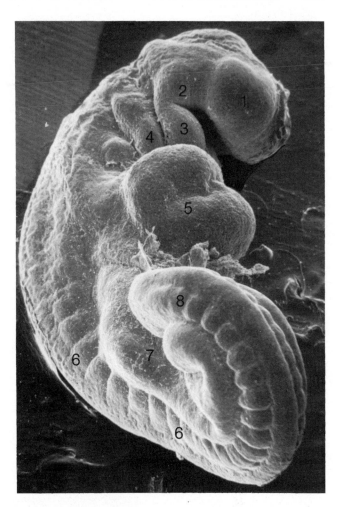

Figure 3–9. Scanning EM photograph of a 28 to 30 day human embryo with the amnion removed, showing the following features: (1) early optic vesicle outpouching, (2) maxillary swelling, (3) mandibular swelling, (4) hyoid swelling, (5) heart, (6) somites, with adjacent spinal cord, (7) early rudiments of upper limb bud, and (8) the tail. (Courtesy of Dr. Jan E. Jirásek, Prague, Czechoslovakia.)

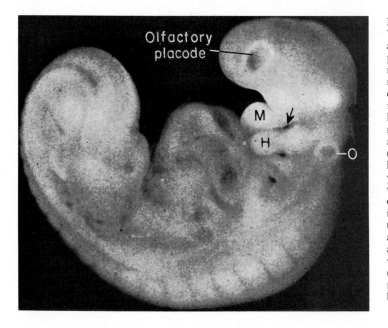

Figure 3–10. *Twenty-eight to thirty days.* The optic cup has begun to invaginate. Between it and the mandibular process is the area of the future mouth, where the buccopharyngeal membrane, with no intervening mesoderm, has broken down. Within the recess of the mandibular (M) and hyoid (H) processes, the future external auditory meatus will develop *(arrow)*, and dorsal to it the otic vesicle (O) forms the inner ear. The relatively huge heart must pump blood in the yolk sac and developing placenta as well as to the embryo proper. Foregut outpouchings and evaginations will now begin to form various glands and the lung and liver primordia. Foregut and hindgut are now clearly delineated from the yolk sac. The somites, which will differentiate into myotomes (musculature), dermatomes (subcutaneous tissue), and sclerotomes (vertebrae), are evident on into the tail bud.

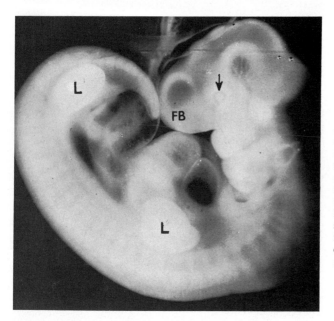

Figure 3–11. *About thirty to thirty-one days.* The brain is rapidly growing and its early cleavage into bilateral future cerebral hemispheres is evident in the telencephalic outpouching of the forebrain (FB). To the right of this is the developing eye with the optic cup *(arrow)* and the early invagination of the future lens from surface ectoderm. From the somatopleura the limb swellings (L) have developed. The loose mesenchyme of the limb bud, interacting with the thickened ectodermal cells at its tip, carries all the potential for the full development of the limb. The liver is now functional and will be a source of blood cells. The mesonephric ducts, formed in the mesonephric ridges, communicate to the cloaca, which is beginning to become septated, and the yolk sac is regressing.

Figure 3–12. *Thirty-six days.* The retina is now pigmented, still incompletely closed at its inferomedial margin. Closure of the retinal fissure is nearly complete. The auricular hillocks are forming the early auricle *(arrow)* from the adjacent borders of the mandibular and hyoid swellings. The hand plate (H) has formed with condensation of mesenchyme into the five finger rays. The lower limb lags behind the upper limb in its development. The ventricular septum is partitioning the heart. The ureteral bud from the mesonephric duct has induced a kidney from the mesonephric ridge, which is also forming gonad and adrenal. Cloacal septation is nearly complete; the infraumbilical mesenchyme has filled in all the cloacal membrane except

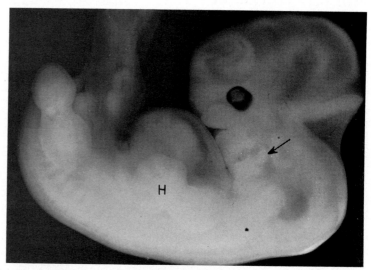

the urogenital area; and the genital tubercles are fused, whereas the labioscrotal swellings are unfused. The gut is elongating, and a loop of it may be seen projecting out into the body stalk.

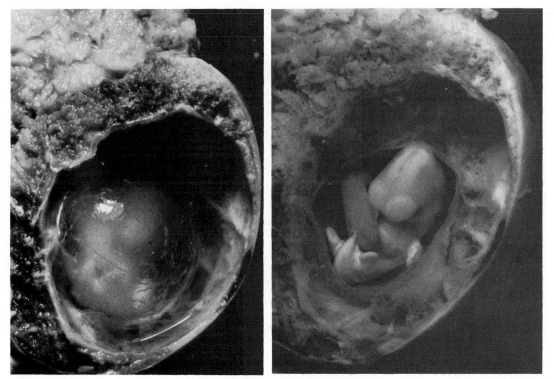

Figure 3–13. *Forty-two days.* In situ embryo *(left)* with the amnion removed *(right)* to show the phenomenal extent of early brain development with formation of the cerebral hemispheres, large heart, still "paddle-like" limbs, and the regressing tail. (Courtesy of Dr. Jan E. Jirásek, Prague, Czechoslovakia.)

Figure 3–14. *Forty-five days.* The nose (N) is relatively flat, and the external ear (E) is gradually shifting in relative position as it continues to grow and develop. A neck area is now evident, the anterior body wall has formed, and the thorax and abdomen are separated by the septum transversum (diaphragm). The fingers are now partially separated, and the elbow is evident. The major period of cardiac morphogenesis and septation is complete. The urogenital membrane has now broken down, yielding a urethral opening. The phallus and lateral labioscrotal folds are the same for both sexes at this age.

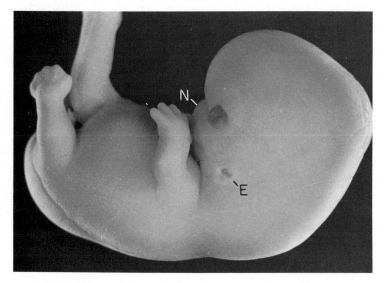

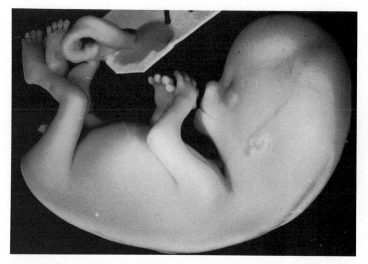

Figure 3–15. *Ten week male.* The eyelids have developed and fused, not to re-open until four or five months. Muscles are developed and functional, normal morphogenesis of joints is dependent on movement, and primary ossification is occurring in the centers of developing bones. In the male, the testicle has produced androgen and masculinized the external genitalia, with enlargement of the genital tubercle, fusion of the labioscrotal folds into a scrotum, and closure of the labia minoral folds to form a penile urethra, these structures being unchanged in the female. The testicle does not descend into the scrotum until eight or nine months.

Figure 3–16. *Three and one-half month male.* The fetus is settling down for the latter two thirds of prenatal life. The morphogenesis of the lung, largely solid at this point in development, will not have progressed to the capacity for aerobic exchange for another three to four months. The skin is increasing in thickness, and its accessory structures are differentiating. The form of the palmar surface of the hand and foot, especially the character of the prominent apical and other pads, will influence the patterning of parallel dermal ridges that form transversely to the relative lines of growth stress on the palms and soles between 16 and 19 weeks. Subcutaneous tissue is thin, and adipose tissue does not develop until seven to eight months.

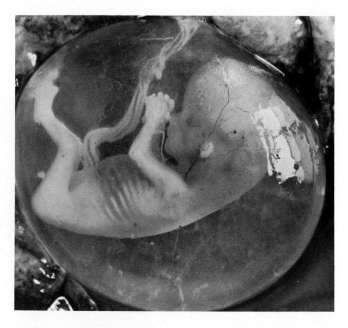

Types of Malformation

Incomplete Morphogenesis

These are anomalies that represent incomplete stages in the development of a structure; they include the following subcategories, with one example listed for each:

Lack of development: renal agenesis secondary to failure of ureter formation.

Hypoplasia: micrognathia.

Incomplete separation: syndactyly (cutaneous).

Incomplete closure: cleft palate.

Incomplete septation: ventricular septal defect.

Incomplete migration of mesoderm: exstrophy of bladder.

Incomplete rotation: malrotation of the gut.

Incomplete resolution of early form: Meckel diverticulum.

Persistence of earlier location: cryptorchidism.

Aberrant Form

An occasional anomaly may be interpreted as an aberrant form that never exists in any stage of normal morphogenesis. An example is the pelvic spur in the nail-patella syn-

Table 3–1. RELATIVE TIMING AND DEVELOPMENTAL PATHOLOGY OF CERTAIN MALFORMATIONS

Tissues	Malformation	Defect In	Cause Prior To	Comment
Central nervous system	Anencephaly	Closure of anterior neural tube	26 days	Subsequent degeneration of forebrain
	Meningomyelocele	Closure in a portion of the posterior neural tube	28 days	80% lumbosacral
Face	Cleft lip	Closure of lip	36 days	42% associated with cleft palate
	Cleft maxillary palate	Fusion of maxillary palatal shelves	10 weeks	
	Branchial sinus and/or cyst	Resolution of branchial cleft	8 weeks	Preauricular and along the line anterior to sternocleidomastoid
Gut	Esophageal atresia plus tracheoesophageal fistula	Lateral septation of foregut into trachea and foregut	30 days	
	Rectal atresia with fistula	Lateral septation of cloaca into rectum and urogenital sinus	6 weeks	
	Duodenal atresia	Recanalization of duodenum	7 to 8 weeks	
	Malrotation of gut	Rotation of intestinal loop so that cecum lies to right	10 weeks	Associated incomplete or aberrant mesenteric attachments
	Omphalocele	Return of midgut from yolk sac to abdomen	10 weeks	
	Meckel diverticulum	Obliteration of vitelline duct	10 weeks	May contain gastric and/or pancreatic tissue
Genitourinary system	Diaphragmatic hernia	Closure of pleuroperitoneal canal	6 weeks	
	Extroversion of bladder	Migration of infraumbilical mesenchyme	30 days	Associated müllerian and wolffian duct defects
	Bicornuate uterus	Fusion of lower portion of müllerian ducts	10 weeks	
	Hypospadias	Fusion of urethral folds (labia minora)	12 weeks	
	Cryptorchidism	Descent of testicle into scrotum	7 to 9 months	
Heart	Transposition of great vessels	Directional development of bulbus cordis septum	34 days	
	Ventricular septal defect	Closure of ventricular septum	6 weeks	
	Patent ductus arteriosus	Closure of ductus arteriosus	9 to 10 months	
Limb	Aplasia of radius	Genesis of radial bone	38 days	Often accompanied by other defects of radial side of distal limb
	Syndactyly, severe	Separation of digital rays	6 weeks	
Complex	Cyclopia, holoprosencephaly	Prechordal mesoderm development	23 days	Secondary defects of midface and forebrain
	Sirenomelia (sympodia)	Development of posterior axis	23 days	Associated defects of cloacal development

drome. Such an anomaly may be more specific for a particular clinical syndrome entity than anomalies of incomplete morphogenesis.

Accessory Tissue

Accessory tissue such as polydactyly, preauricular skin tags, and accessory spleens may be presumed to have been initiated at approximately the same time as the normal tissue, developing into finger rays, auricular hillocks of His, and spleen, respectively.

Hamartomata

These anomalies represent an organizational defect leading to an abnormal admixture of tissues, often with a tumor-like excess of one or more tissues. Some have malignant potential. Examples of hamartomata are hemangiomata, melanomata, fibromata, lipomata, adenomata, and some strange admixtures that defy traditional classification.

Functional Defects

Function is a necessary feature in joint development, and hence joint contractures such as clubfoot may be caused by functional deficit in the use of the lower limb resulting from a more primary malformation.

RELATIVE TIMING OF MALFORMATIONS

Malformations resulting from incomplete morphogenesis usually have their origin *prior to* the time when normal development would have proceeded beyond the form represented by the malformation. This type of developmental timing should not be construed as indicating that something hap-

pened *at* a particular time; all one can say is that a problem existed *prior to* a particular time.

Serious errors in early morphogenesis seldom allow for survival; hence, only a few malformation problems are seen that can be said to have occurred prior to 23 days. The cyclopia-cebocephaly and the sirenomelia-sympodia types of defect appear to be the consequence of defects in the prechordal and postaxial mesoderm, respectively, and presumably developed prior to 23 days. Aside from these examples, the vast majority of serious malformations represent errors that occur after three weeks of development.

Table 3–1 sets forth the relative timing as well as the presumed developmental error for some of the malformations that appear to represent incomplete stages in morphogenesis.

References

Ebert, J. D., and Sussex, I.: Interacting Systems in Development. New York, Holt, Rinehart, and Winston, 1970.

Graham, J. M.: Smith's Recognizable Patterns of Human Deformation, 2nd ed. Philadelphia, W. B. Saunders Co., 1988.

Hamilton, W. J., Boyd, J. D., and Mossman, H. W.: Human Embryology. Baltimore, Williams and Wilkins Co., 1962.

Langman, J.: Medical Embryology. Baltimore, Williams and Wilkins Co., 1985.

Millen, J. W.: Timing of human congenital malformations. Dev. Med. Child. Neurol., 5:343, 1963.

Moore, K. L.: The Developing Human: Clinically Oriented Embryology, 3rd ed. Philadelphia, W. B. Saunders Co., 1982.

Nilsson, L., Ingelman-Sundberg, A., and Wirsen, C.: A Child Is Born. New York, Dell Books, 1986.

Streeter, G. L.: Developmental Horizons in Human Embryos; Age Groups XI to XXIII. Washington, D.C., Carnegie Institute of Washington, 1951.

Willis, R. A.: The Borderland of Embryology and Pathology. Washington, Butterworth, 1962.

4

Genetics, Genetic Counseling, and Prevention via Early Fetal Recognition

relative to single defects and patterns of malformation

The basic process of morphogenesis is genetically controlled, being dependent on the environment for expression of the genetic potential.

Judging from the malformation problems for which a mode of etiology has been strongly indicated, the major cause is genetic aberration. There are three general genetic modes of determination for abnormal morphogenesis: polygenic determination, mutant genes in single or double dose, and gross genetic imbalance due to a chromosomal abnormality. Figure 4–1 provides a perspective as to the frequency of human disorders relative to each of these types of genetic determination. These are considered separately as

they relate to problems of malformation, especially multiple defect syndromes. The recommended genetic counsel is presented at the end of each section.

POLYGENIC DETERMINATION

Much of the usual variability among individuals as well as many common disorders within a species may be ascribed to minor differences in a number of gene loci involved in the determination of a particular characteristic. A polygenically determined abnormality is herein defined as one that is predominantly the consequence of minor dif-

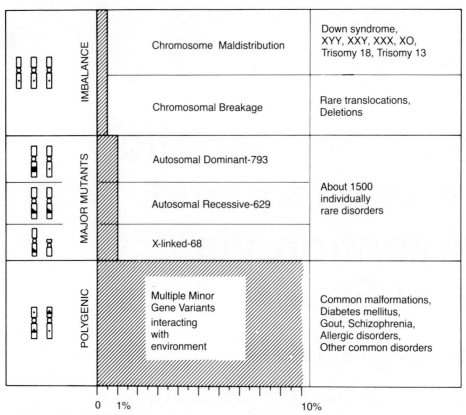

Figure 4–1. The scale at the base represents the percentage of individuals born who do have, or will have, a problem in life secondary to a genetic difference. The three categories of genetic aberrations are depicted to the left. The dots within the chromosomes represent "normal" genes, the bar represents a dominant mutant gene, the hash-bar represents a recessive mutant gene, and the triangles denote minor gene variants.

ferences at many gene loci, no one of which may be held fully responsible for the abnormality. Obviously, it is difficult to prove polygenic inheritance, but current evidence in the human indicates that this is the major mode in the etiology of many of the single localized defects in morphogenesis accounting for the majority of babies born with a malformation problem. The following indirect evidence for polygenic inheritance of the single common defects comes predominantly from the work of Carter[1] and has been partially summarized by Smith and Aase.[2]

Frequency of the Defect in Relatives

The frequency of *recurrence* of the same type of defect in offspring from unaffected parents ranges from 2 to 5 per cent (Table 4–1), 20 to 40 times the general frequency within that population group.

Concordance in Dizygotic Twins

The question asked in these surveys is the following: If one twin has a defect, with what frequency does the other twin have the same type of defect? If both twins have the defect, they are concordant for the anomaly; if one twin has the defect and the other does not, they are nonconcordant. The incidence of concordance in dizygotic twins is similar to that of siblings born of separate pregnancies and thereby gives no evidence toward a major environmental factor in the etiology for these defects.

Influence of Genetic Background

Sex. The difference between the XX and the XY genetic background is a major genetic one that has an appreciable effect on the occurrence of these major malformations, no

Table 4–1. **RECURRENCE RISKS FOR SOME DEFECTS**[1-4]

Defect	Normal Parents of One Affected Child	Recurrence Risk For	
		Future Males	*Future Females*
Cleft lip with or without cleft palate	4–5%*		
Cleft palate alone	2–6%		
Cardiac defect (common types)	3–4%		
Pyloric stenosis	3%	4%	2.4%
Hirschsprung anomaly	3–5%		
Clubfoot	2–8%		
Dislocation of hip	3–4%	0.5%	6.3%
Neural tube defects—anencephaly, meningomyelocele	3–5%		
Scoliosis	10–15%		

*Range of recurrence risks observed.

one of which has an equal sex incidence (Fig. 4–2).

Some of the sex differences in malformation occurrence may be explained as the direct effects of structural genital differences, such as hypospadias in the male. Similarly, the marked male predominance of the urethral obstruction malformation sequence may be explained by the fact that the most common site of urethral obstruction is in the prostatic urethra.[14] The humoral impact of testosterone, which makes connective tissue tougher in the male, may explain the relative preponderance of dislocation of the hip, related to connective tissue laxity, in the female. Also, testosterone, which is produced by the male during the first few postnatal months, may enhance the likelihood of muscle hypertrophy and thereby increase the tendency to develop hypertrophic pyloric stenosis.[14] The sex differences related to the incidence of other structural defects would appear to imply that genes on the X and/or Y chromosome may increase the likelihood of particular anomalies developing during morphogenesis.

One indirect manner in which the genetic background of XX versus XY may influence the frequency of structural defects at birth is

simply the growth rate in utero. Thus, with the exception of anomalies related to joint laxity, most late uterine constraint–induced deformations are more common in the male, who is normally growing faster in the last trimester of gestation than the female.[15]

These sex differences provide cogent evidence for polygenic inheritance. Taking pyloric stenosis as an example, Carter[1] reasoned as follows: If it takes more genetic factors to give rise to this anomaly in the female, then the affected female should pass on more of these genetic factors to her offspring, who would have a higher frequency of pyloric stenosis than would the offspring of affected males. This is precisely what Carter found, the incidence of pyloric stenosis from affected mothers being four times as high as the incidence from affected fathers (24 per cent vs. 6 per cent). This is the type of quantitative effect that would be expected with polygenic inheritance.

Race. Numerous subtle genetic differences exist between racial groups. Persistent genetic isolation increases the differences between groups, and genetic admixture obviously lessens these differences.

The types of minor genetic differences hypothesized as being the predominant cause for the foregoing malformations would presumably differ among racial groups. Therefore, the incidence of these anomalies would show racial variance. This is precisely what has been found, there being variability for the *types* of single malformation among racial groups.

Among particular racial groups or subgroups, the incidence of a particular anomaly may be relatively high. For example, club foot is a frequent anomaly among Polynesians, but is relatively rare in the Chinese.

PROPORTION OF MALES VS. FEMALES

PYLORIC STENOSIS	5:1
CLUBFOOT	2:1
CLEFT LIP +/− PALATE	2:1
CLEFT PALATE ALONE	1:1.3
MENINGOMYELOCELE	1:1.5
ANENCEPHALY	1:3
CONG. DISLOC. HIP	1:5.5

Figure 4–2. Relative sex incidence of single common malformations.

Admixture between Polynesian and Chinese individuals gave rise to an intermediary frequency of club foot, as might be anticipated for polygenic inheritance.[5] Another similar example is polydactyly, which has an incidence of 0.7 per cent in blacks, 0.24 per cent among whites, and 0.52 per cent among the mulatto racial admixture.[6]

Variation of Recurrence Risk in Relation to Severity of Malformation

In accordance with the hypothesis of polygenic inheritance for the foregoing anomalies, the more severe the degree of structural defect, the greater the adverse genetic influences involved and thereby the greater should be the chance for recurrence from the same parentage. Carter[1] has obtained data that support this hypothesis. The risk for recurrence in subsequent children when an offspring has a severe bilateral cleft lip and palate is 5.7 per cent, as contrasted with a 2.5 per cent recurrence risk when the offspring has a less severe degree of defect, such as a unilateral cleft lip.

Interaction Between Genetic and Environmental Factors

Environmental influences can play a role in the determination of these malformations. Some indications of environmental effects have been observed in Scotland and England in studies of anencephaly-meningomyelocele families, namely, seasonal variability[7] and social class differences.[8] Birth order influences have also been noted, congenital dislocation of the hip and pyloric stenosis being more likely to occur in first-born children.[1]

One obvious environmental factor is fetal in utero constraint leading to deformation. Such constraint is more common in the first-born,[15] who is the first to distend the uterus and abdominal wall. This probably explains the greater frequency of dislocation of the hip as well as most other deformations in the first-born.

The interaction between genetic and environmental factors is dramatically exemplified by certain studies that show that the genetic background may have a profound influence on the likelihood of a given environmental teratogen causing malformation. For example, Fraser[9] could regularly produce cleft palate in mouse embryos of the A/Jax strain by giving the mothers a high dosage of cortisone during early gestation, but the same treatment in a different strain gave rise to only 17 per cent affected offspring.

The search for environmental factors that can allow for expression of a single malformation obviously should continue. However, it should be appreciated that current evidence indicates a uterine constraint–induced deformation or a subtle polygenic mode as the predominant modes of causation for the more common single defects. Furthermore, just as the polygenic mode implies multiple minor genetic differences that are difficult to individualize, so environmental factors are likely to be multiple and subtle in character. The total factors combine to approach the subtle threshold for a particular defect in morphogenesis, a threshold predominantly set by the genetic makeup of the individual.

Counseling for Defects for Which Polygenic Inheritance Has Been Indicated

1. Explain the developmental pathology of the defect so that the parents can appreciate that there was only a single localized defect in the early development of their child. Then discuss the management of and prognosis for the child. When the single defect is of the type that—with repair—need not interfere with the social acceptance or function of the child, it is often helpful to tell the parents that the *child* is normal. For example, given a child with isolated cleft lip, the parents may be told, "Your *child* is normal; the *lip* did not close completely, and therefore we shall have a plastic surgeon bring about the closure." The purpose of this approach is to assist in the parental acceptance of the child by not branding the whole child as malformed, but localizing the defect to what it actually represents in an anatomic and functional sense.

2. Explain that the localized problem in development must have occurred *prior to* a particular time in gestation (see Table 3–1, Chapter 3), and reassure the parents that it was not related to any factor after that time.

3. Ask the parents if they have any ideas concerning the cause of the structural defect. Many of the parental concerns relative to etiology can be dispelled.

4. Explain that morphogenesis is a genetically determined process in which numerous genes play a role, as a team, in the development of a given structure. Then indicate that the "team of genes" derived from *both* parents did not allow for full normal development of the particular structure leading to the structural defect. Indicate how subtle the end point is, toward normal or malformation, for such single defects.

5. Indicate to the parents that the likelihood of a subsequent offspring having a similar set of genes allowing for a similar structural defect is of low magnitude, 3 to 5 per cent or less for most of the single common defects, with the exception of scoliosis. The more precise recurrence risk data are summarized in Table 4–1. In giving this counsel, the risk figures may be slightly increased when the defect is severe in degree and decreased when the anomaly is mild in degree. The risk figures may be separately stated for the sex of the offspring, especially for pyloric stenosis and congenital dislocation of the hip. If two offspring are affected, the risk for subsequent offspring being affected is two- to threefold greater than the previously mentioned figure, being approximately 10 to 15 per cent. The risk of an affected individual having affected offspring is of similar magnitude to that of the sibling recurrence risk, about 3 to 5 per cent.

Note: This counsel is obviously crude, being based on empiric data. However, the author believes that it is the most appropriate at our present state of knowledge and is thereby preferable to not giving the parents any perspective on etiology and recurrence risk. It is to be hoped that future knowledge will allow for more precise counseling relative to individuals with a single, localized structural defect.

MAJOR MUTANT GENE DETERMINATION

Genes located on the X chromosome are referred to as X-linked genes and those on the autosomes as autosomal-linked genes. Man is a diploid organism with two sets of chromosomes, one set being derived from each parent. Each pair of chromosomes will have comparable gene determinants located at the same position on each chromosome of the pair. The pair of genes may be referred to as *alleles*, or partners, which normally work together. Thus, with the exception of the genes of the X and Y chromosomes in the male, each genetic determinant is present in *two doses*, one from each parent. A *mutant* gene indicates a *changed* gene. A major mutant gene is herein defined as a genetic determinant that has changed in such a way that it can give rise to an abnormal characteristic. If a mutant gene in single dose produces an abnormal characteristic despite the presence of a normal allele (partner), it may be referred to as *dominant* because it causes abnormality even when counterbalanced by a normal gene partner. A mutant gene that causes an abnormal characteristic only when present in double dosage (or single dosage without a normal partner, as for an X-linked mutant gene in the male) is referred to as recessive. There are gradations, from a mutant gene that always causes an abnormal characteristic in single dosage (dominant) to one that occasionally causes some abnormality in single dosage (semidominant) to a gene that never causes any evident alteration except when present in double dosage (recessive). These principles are set forth in Figure 4–3.

Expression is a term used to indicate the extent of abnormality that is due to a genetic aberration. The expression may be stated as severe, usual, mild, or no expression, the latter being synonymous with lack of penetrance in an individual who has the genetic aberration. Individuals with the same genetic aberration frequently show variance in expression, especially with respect to structural defects.

Traditionally, the mutant gene disorders have been categorized into those due to genes located on the autosomes—autosomal dominant and autosomal recessive—and disorders due to genes on the X-chromosome—X-linked recessive and X-linked dominant.

Autosomal Dominant

Autosomal dominant disorders often show wide variation in expression among affected individuals, presumably because of minor differences in the normal allele (partner) of the mutant gene as well as other differences in the genetic or environmental background of the affected individual. Figure 4–4 demonstrates the variance in expression for an autosomal dominant disorder, ectrodactyly.

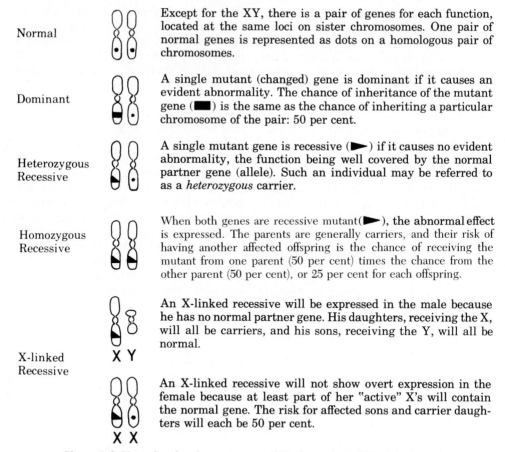

Normal

Except for the XY, there is a pair of genes for each function, located at the same loci on sister chromosomes. One pair of normal genes is represented as dots on a homologous pair of chromosomes.

Dominant

A single mutant (changed) gene is dominant if it causes an evident abnormality. The chance of inheritance of the mutant gene (■) is the same as the chance of inheriting a particular chromosome of the pair: 50 per cent.

Heterozygous Recessive

A single mutant gene is recessive (►) if it causes no evident abnormality, the function being well covered by the normal partner gene (allele). Such an individual may be referred to as a *heterozygous* carrier.

Homozygous Recessive

When both genes are recessive mutant(►), the abnormal effect is expressed. The parents are generally carriers, and their risk of having another affected offspring is the chance of receiving the mutant from one parent (50 per cent) times the chance from the other parent (50 per cent), or 25 per cent for each offspring.

An X-linked recessive will be expressed in the male because he has no normal partner gene. His daughters, receiving the X, will all be carriers, and his sons, receiving the Y, will all be normal.

X-linked Recessive   **X Y**

An X-linked recessive will not show overt expression in the female because at least part of her "active" X's will contain the normal gene. The risk for affected sons and carrier daughters will each be 50 per cent.

X X

Figure 4–3. Normal and major mutant gene inheritance (mendelian inheritance).

The risk of the single mutant gene being passed to a given offspring is 50 per cent, yet the risk of a severe defect of hand development is less than 50 per cent because of variance in expression. To utilize the example of the Waardenburg syndrome, the risk of inheritance of the mutant gene from an affected individual is 50 per cent, yet only about 20 per cent of affected individuals have deafness, the most disturbing expression of the mutant gene. Hence, the risk for deafness in offspring of a parent with the Waardenburg syndrome is the risk of receiving the mutant gene (50 per cent) times the likelihood of expression for deafness in the disorder (20 per cent), or 10 per cent. This dichotomy between the risk of receiving the gene and the risk of a particular expression of the disorder must be utilized in counseling, especially for autosomal dominant disorders.

The first question to ask oneself after making the clinical diagnosis of an autosomal dominant mutant gene disorder is: "When did the gene mutation occur?" If the disorder is one that always shows some expression, and the parents are quite normal, then this may be presumed to be a *fresh gene mutation* that happened in one of the germ cells that went to form the conceptus. The parents of a child who has a fresh gene mutation therefore have a negligible risk for recurrence. Actually, a high proportion of individuals with autosomal dominant patterns of malformation represent fresh gene mutations. Since the affected individuals often have limited capability of reproduction, the majority of cases seen are fresh mutations. For some conditions, such as the Apert syndrome, there have been only a few reported cases of offspring from affected individuals, but these demonstrated the autosomal dominant inheritance. Some of the sporadic syndromes of unknown etiology may also be single gene mutations, but lack of reproduction prevents a testing of the hypothesis. Fresh gene mutation is more likely at *older paternal age*, as has been shown for at least 12 autosomal dominant multiple malformation syndromes.[10] Hence, paternal age should always be noted in the evaluation of disorders that may be the consequence of a single mutant gene. There may even be the occurrence of different autosomal dominant disorders in the same sibship related to older paternal age. For example, Dr. David Rimoin recounted a family in which the father was 48 years of age when a child with achondroplasia was born and 52 years of age when a child with neurofibromatosis was born.

Counseling for Autosomal Dominant Disorders

1. Examine the parents and siblings and occasionally other relatives to determine whether any of them show features of the disorder in question. If neither parent shows any expression of an autosomal dominant disorder, which always shows some effect on the individual, the parents may be told, "A single gene was altered in one of the germ cells prior to the development of the child. This event is extremely unlikely to happen again, and therefore your risk for further affected children is negligible." They should also be reassured that relatives need have no concern of having affected children.

2. The risk for an *affected* individual having an affected child is 50 per cent for each offspring. When possible, be acquainted with the frequency of various features in affected individuals so that the counseling can include

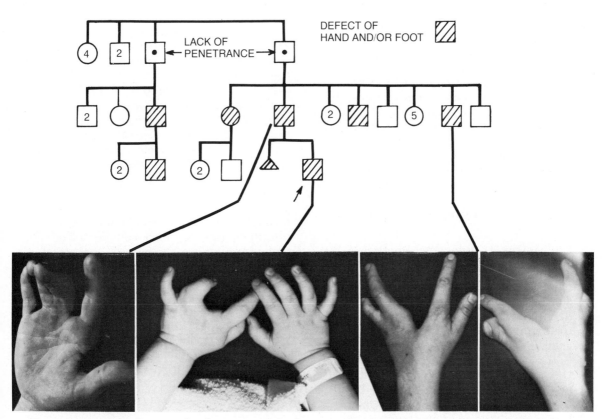

Figure 4–4. Variation in expression for autosomal dominant ectrodactyly among various related individuals. Note also the *intraindividual* asymmetry of expression in the propositus *(arrow)*. (From Smith, D. W.: J. Pediatr., *69:*1150, 1966).

not only the risk of a given offspring receiving the mutant gene but also the likelihood of any particular defect occurring.

3. Explain, when feasible, the developmental pathology and how all the aspects of altered development are secondary to the effects of the single altered gene. Outline the natural history of the condition and management for the child.

Autosomal Recessive

Autosomal recessive disorders generally have less variation in expression than do autosomal dominant syndromes. Possibly, this is because both genes of a pair are mutant, and therefore there is *no* normal partner gene to carry on the function of the particular gene. The inheritance is from clinically normal parents who both have the *same*, or an allelic, recessive mutant gene in *single dose*, the risk of which is obviously enhanced if the parents are related. Hence, consanguinity should always be asked about in disorders known to be autosomal recessive as well as when evaluating patterns of malformation of unknown cause.

The recurrence risk from the same parentage is 25 per cent for each subsequent offspring. The risk of any relative having an affected offspring may be calculated by multiplying their risk of being a heterozygote (carrier) times the risk of marrying a heterozygote (the general heterozygote frequency for that gene in the population) times one fourth (the chance of two heterozygotes having an affected offspring).

Counseling for Autosomal Recessive Disorders

1. Explain that the child has one pair of altered genes and that the disturbance in development is caused by that pair. Outline the natural history and management for the child.

2. Explain to the parents that most individuals have several altered genes that cause no problem, because each is counterbalanced by its normal gene partner. They happen to have one altered gene in common, and the chance of any given offspring receiving both of these altered genes and being affected is 25 per cent for each pregnancy.

3. Explain that the chance of their normal children having a single altered gene (carrier) is two out of three, but since the chance of randomly marrying another carrier is slight, their risk of having affected children should be quite small. The general risk of any unaffected relative having an affected child may be calculated as set forth above.

X-Linked Recessive

The X-linked genes in the XY male are present in but a single dose with no partner gene, and hence, the full recessive disorder is expressed with but a single recessive mutant gene. The frequency of X-linked recessive disease in the male is thereby a direct reflection of the frequency of X-linked recessive genes per X chromosomes in the population. The chance of an XX female having a pair of such X-linked recessive genes and expressing the same disorder as the male is very small. Hence, the following precepts are the important ones in detecting X-linked recessive inheritance:

1. With rare exception, only males are affected, and the transmission is through unaffected or mildly affected heterozygous (carrier) females.

2. There is no male to male transmission.

X-linked recessive disorders in the male, especially the more severe ones, may often represent a fresh gene mutation. These disorders present a problem in striving to determine at what level the gene mutation arose, for it could be in the patient alone or in the mother or even back one or two generations, having been silently passed through carrier females. For some X-linked disorders, this dilemma can be solved by demonstrating the presence or absence of a heterozygous (carrier) mild expression in the females in question. Such observations can also be of value in determining whether any related female at risk is a carrier. Older paternal age has been noted to be a factor in fresh X-linked mutation, at least for hemophilia A.[11] The older paternal age has been in the father of the mother of the first affected XY male, who cannot receive his X from his father.

Counseling for X-Linked Recessive Disorders

1. First, try to determine by family pedigree evaluation or observation of heterozy-

gous expression whether the mother is a carrier.

2. Explain the X-linked single mutant gene and how it caused trouble because the male has no normal partner gene to counter the mutant gene. Then relate the natural history of the disorder and management for the body.

3. If the mother is a carrier, she may be told that there is a 50 per cent risk of any future male being affected; that all daughters will be normal with a 50 per cent risk of being a carrier; that normal sons cannot transmit the disorder; and that affected sons would have normal sons who cannot transmit the disease, and all their daughters would be unaffected carriers.

4. If the mother is *not* a carrier, the risk for recurrence from the mother is negligible, and the affected boy's risk is as listed previously.

X-Linked Dominant

X-linked single gene *dominant* disorders show expression in the XX female, usually with a more severe effect in the XY male. This type of inheritance is most commonly confused with autosomal dominant inheritance, from which it may be discriminated in the following ways:

1. There is usually a more severe expression in affected males.

2. Affected males have normal sons (no male to male transmission), and all their daughters are affected.

The counseling is the same as for X-linked recessive except that all carrier females are affected.

Single Mutant Gene With Sex Limitation

Several disorders, such as the oral-facial-digital syndrome, are found almost exclusively in females and apparently cause early lethality in the affected male because there is a 50 per cent deficiency in sons as compared with daughters from affected females, with about 50 per cent of the daughters and none of the sons being affected. At present, it has not been possible to determine whether this disorder, for example, is an X-linked dominant with early lethality in the male or an autosomal dominant that has a lethal effect in the male.

Genetic Counseling for a Single Mutant Gene Defect With Presumed Early Lethality in the Affected Male

1. Explain that this is the result of a single altered gene and discuss the natural history and management.

2. Examine the parents, especially the mother. If they are quite normal, assume a fresh gene mutation with a negligible recurrence risk.

3. If the mother is affected, her risk would be one in four for a normal male, one in four for an affected male that would be a lethal, one in four for an affected female, and one in four for a normal female. The same risks would apply for any affected female.

GENETIC IMBALANCE DUE TO GROSS CHROMOSOMAL ABNORMALITIES

The 46 normal chromosomes consist of 22 homologous pairs of autosomes plus the XX pair of sex chromosomes in the female and the XY pair in the male. Normal development is not only dependent on the gene content of these chromosomes but on the gene balance as well. An altered number of chromosomes most commonly arises because of a fault in chromosome distribution at cell division. During the gametic meiotic reduction division (Fig. 4–5), one of each pair of autosomes and one of the sex chromosomes are distributed randomly to each daughter cell, whereas during mitosis (Fig. 4–6), each replicated chromosome is separated longitudinally at the centromere such that each daughter cell receives an identical complement of genetic material.

Figure 4–7 shows the natural appearance of the stained chromosomes at early, middle, and later stages of mitosis. It would obviously be difficult to count these chromosomes or to distinguish their individual structure from such preparations. In order to obtain adequate preparations for the study of chromosome number and morphology, the cultured cells are treated with a toxic agent such as colchicine, which blocks the spindle formation and thus leads to the accumulation of

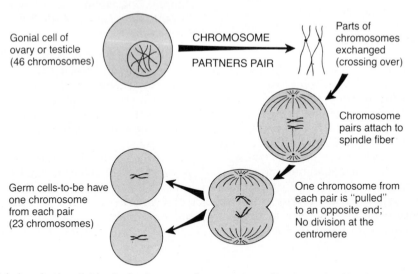

Figure 4–5. Meiotic reduction division in development of gametes (sex cells). One pair of 21 chromosomes is followed through the cycle.

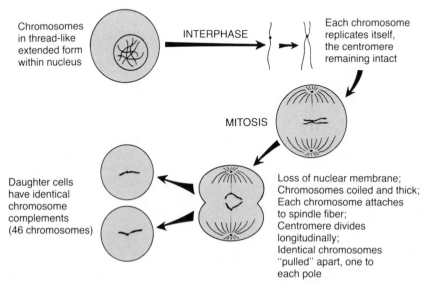

Figure 4–6. Usual cell cycle. One chromosome 21 is followed through the cycle.

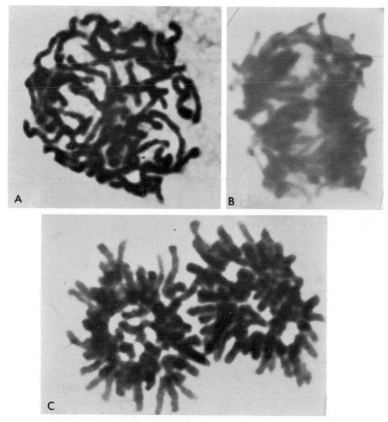

Figure 4–7. Chromosomes of untreated mitotic cells. *A,* Prophase cell. *B,* Metaphase cell with chromosomes attached to the spindle fibers and beginning to separate. *C,* Anaphase cell, with identical chromosomal complements having been "pulled apart" toward the development of two daughter cells.

cells at the metaphase of mitosis. These cells are then exposed to a hypotonic solution that spreads the unattached chromosomes, allowing for such preparations as that shown in Figure 4–8. Various techniques can be employed to allow for the identification of individual chromosomes. For example, trypsin treatment and Giemsa staining bring out the banding patterns in chromosomes, as shown in Figure 4–8.

Abnormal morphogenesis may result from genetic imbalance. Figure 4–9 illustrates some of the types of chromosomal abnormalities that can lead to gross genetic imbalance.

Chromosomal maldistribution leading to an altered number of chromosomes occurs in at least 4 per cent of recognized pregnancies (Fig. 4–10). Most of the genetic imbalances have such an adverse effect on morphogenesis that the conceptuses do not survive. Figure 4–10 summarizes the frequency and types of chromosomal abnormal-

ities found in spontaneous abortuses, about 50 per cent of which have a chromosomal abnormality and, in live-born babies, 0.5 per cent of whom have an altered number of chromosomes. The majority of the latter are sex chromosome aneuploidies or trisomy 21, because these are the least likely to have an early lethal effect. However, only about one in 500 XO conceptuses survive to term. It is estimated by Dr. Patricia Jacobs that about 4 per cent of 18 trisomy and 13 trisomy conceptuses survive, whereas about 21 per cent of conceptuses with 21 trisomy survive to term.

Though little is known about the etiology of faulty chromosomal distribution, one recognized factor is the increased likelihood of such errors at older maternal age. This applies especially to the autosomal trisomy syndromes and to a lesser extent to some of the sex chromosome aneuploidies. Figure 4–11 shows the progressive increase in the frequency of the Down syndrome during the

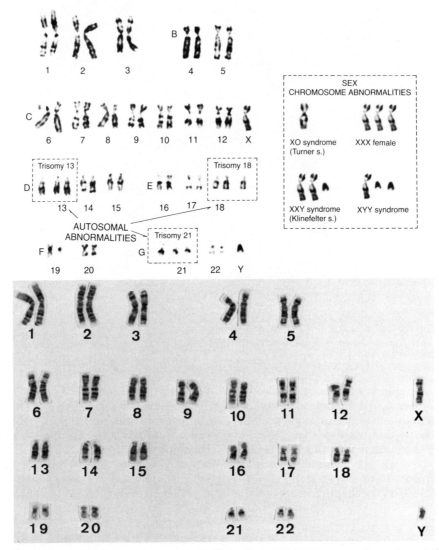

Figure 4—8. *Above,* Giemsa-stained chromosomes arranged into a karyotype by letter grouping and number designation on the basis of length of the chromosome, position of the centromere, and banding patterns. The common types of aneuploidy in newborn babies are shown within boxes. *Below,* Excellent banded karyotype. (Courtesy of Dr. Albert Schinzel, Human Genetics Institute, University of Zurich.)

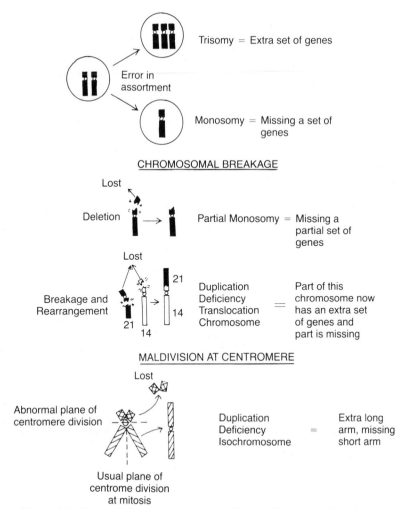

Figure 4–9. Types of chromosomal abnormalities leading to genetic imbalance.

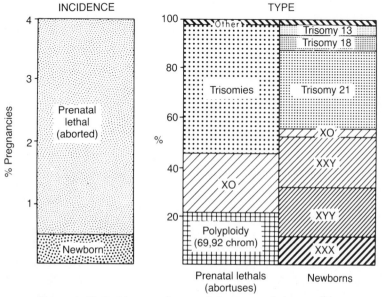

Figure 4–10. Incidence and types of chromosomal abnormalities.

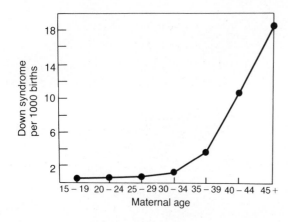

Figure 4–11. Increasing incidence of the Down syndrome during the latter period of a woman's reproductive period. (From Smith, D. W.: Am. J. Obstet. Gynecol., *90:*1055, 1964.)

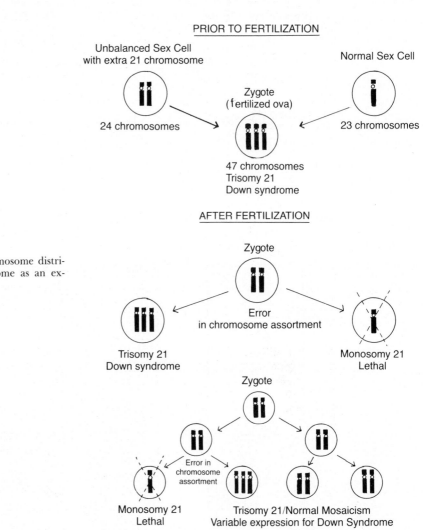

Figure 4–12. Faulty chromosome distribution, with 21 chromosome as an example.

latter period of a woman's reproductive life. The figure delineates the frequency of the disorder in uninterrupted pregnancies. The frequency of aneuploidy detected by amniocentesis at 14 to 16 weeks of gestation is appreciably higher, because some of the aneuploid conceptuses detected at this early stage in gestation would normally have been aborted or stillborn.

The timing of the error in chromosome distribution seldom can be stated with assurance, for it could occur prior to meiosis, during the first or second division of meiosis, or even during the first division of the zygote and still result in an aneuploid individual (Fig. 4–12).

Errors in the assortment of chromosomes that occur during postzygotic cell division can give rise to mosaic individuals having at least two different cell populations from the standpoint of chromosomal number (Fig. 4–12). Those who are mosaics for XO/XX often have less abnormality than the wholly XO individual, and in similar fashion, trisomy 21–normal mosaic individuals show every gradation, from the Down syndrome to near-normal appearance and function. The mosaic aneuploid line of cells may become over-

grown in a competitive population of cells, such as in leukocytes. Hence, when mosaic XO, mosaic autosomal trisomy, or mosaic triploidy is suspected and the cultured leukocytes (blood culture) are "normal," a skin biopsy for cultured fibroblast cells should also be obtained. The latter will usually persist in showing the aneuploid cell line.

Less commonly, genetic imbalance can result from chromosomal breakage (see Fig. 4–9). A broken piece of a chromosome may be lost. With more than one break, rearrangement of chromosomal pieces may take place between the broken chromosomes, a phenomenon referred to as translocation. An individual can have a translocation chromosome with no evident problem as long as he or she still has a balanced set of genes. However, a balanced carrier of a translocation chromosome has a significant risk of producing unbalanced germ cells during meiotic reduction division (Fig. 4–13). Should a germ cell receive a translocation chromosome containing a large part of a 21 chromosome and also receive the normal 21 chromosome from that same parent, the resulting zygote would have partial trisomy 21. Such individuals generally have the Down syndrome. About 6 per

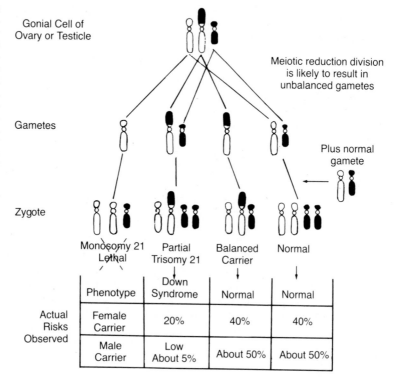

Figure 4–13. Potential inheritance from "balanced" translocation carrier; 21/"14" translocation carrier example, showing only the 21 and "14" chromosomes. The translocation could be a fresh occurrence in the development of this gonial cell. The above example occurred in a past generation, and this individual is a balanced translocation carrier. The lower risk of Down syndrome from the carrier male may be due to reduced likelihood of an unbalanced sperm reaching the ova first! This is a good example of how it is difficult to predict the actual outcome in offspring of translocation carriers.

Gonial Cell of Ovary or Testicle

Meiotic reduction division is likely to result in unbalanced gametes

Gametes

Plus normal gamete

Zygote

Monosomy 21 Lethal

Partial Trisomy 21

Balanced Carrier

Normal

	Phenotype	Down Syndrome	Normal	Normal
Actual Risks Observed	Female Carrier	20%	40%	40%
	Male Carrier	Low About 5%	About 50%	About 50%

cent of the Down syndrome patients have 46 chromosomes, with the extra dose of 21 chromosome being attached to another chromosome. Similarly, a small proportion of patients with the trisomy 18 syndrome or the trisomy 13 syndrome have the extra set of genes attached as part of a translocation chromosome.

The major reason for doing chromosome studies on individuals with autosomal trisomy syndromes, beyond confirmation of the clinical diagnosis, is to determine whether the patient has a translocation chromosome rather than the more usual full trisomy. This applies predominantly to babies with genetic imbalance disorders who are born to younger mothers, since the vast majority of such babies born to older mothers have full trisomy. If it is a translocation case, then both parents should be studied to determine whether either of them is a balanced translocation carrier with a consequent high risk of having affected offspring. Fortunately, only about one third of the patients with partial translocation trisomy will be found to have a translocation carrier parent, because most of them represent fresh occurrences for which there is a negligible recurrence risk.

Summitt[12] has estimated that one in 520 normal individuals has a balanced structural chromosomal rearrangement, whereas one in 1700 individuals has an unbalanced chromosomal rearrangement.

Chromosomal breakage with or without rearrangement allows for a wide variety of individual rare genetic imbalances with extra or missing segments of chromosomes. Many of these fetuses do not survive prenatal life. Among undiagnosed mentally deficient children with multiple defects, Summitt[12] found 8 per cent to have a chromosomal abnormality, most of whom had a small extra piece of autosome and/or a piece missing. Our own experience with 145 such unknown multiple defect cases revealed three (2 per cent) with a chromosomal abnormality, and these three died early in life. The utilization of the banding techniques for specific chromosome identification should allow for more accurate identification of such disorders, in terms of the piece that is missing or extra.

The clinical phenotype may allow the clinician to recommend that the cytogeneticist scrutinize a particular chromosome segment with special care, ideally in early prophase preparations that better allow for the recognition of a missing or small extra piece. Examples of focused cytogenetics studies (terminology utilized by Dr. Vincent Riccardi) include 13q− in instances of retinoblastoma and associated defects, 11q− in cases of aniridia and Wilms tumor, and 15q− in some instances of Prader-Willi syndrome. The clinical recognition of 4 p− syndrome may allow for recognition of the cytogenetic aberration that might be *very* difficult to detect in a general, unfocused assessment of the karyotype.

Another type of chromosomal abnormality that can lead to genetic imbalance is maldivision or breakage at the centromere during mitosis, leading to the formation of an isochromosome, as depicted in Figure 4–9. The cell receiving the isochromosome has an extra dose of the long arm of the altered chromosome and is missing the set of genes on the short arm of that chromosome. Occasional cases of the autosomal trisomy syndromes may be found to have a presumed isochromosome of the long arm of 21, 13, or 18 chromosome causing the genetic imbalance. Also, X isochromosome-X has not been infrequent in individuals who have partial expression of the XO syndrome.

Counseling for Chromosomal Abnormalities

Autosomal Trisomy Syndromes

1. If there is any question as to assurance of the diagnosis, if the mother is young (generally less than 30 years), or if there are other cases of the same syndrome in the family pedigree, chromosomal studies should be carried out on the patient in order to determine whether it is a full trisomy or a translocation case. If it is a full trisomy, the future risk for younger mothers is less than 1 per cent, and for older mothers it is about the same as for any mother of that age (see Fig. 4–11). Should it be a translocation case, both parents should be studied to determine whether either parent is a balanced translocation carrier, a finding in about one third of such cases. The recurrence risk from chromosomally normal parents is apparently very small, certainly less than 1 per cent. The recurrence risk from a translocation carrier parent is obviously greater, but often less

than the theoretic possibilities might indicate (see Fig. 4–12).

2. Inform the parents that the chromosome abnormality amounts to a gross genetic imbalance that upsets the pattern of development. Emphasize that there is no implication of a *gene* abnormality; rather, there is a genetic imbalance with extra or missing genes. Also emphasize that, with unusual exception, the chromosomes of the parents are normal. Then explain what is *usual* for the genetic imbalance—the natural history for the syndrome.

3. For the trisomy 18 or 13 syndromes, the parents may be told that most affected individuals with these trisomies are so seriously affected that they do not survive the first few months of pregnancy and that the parents "must have a good genetic background" and/or the mother "must be very good at carrying babies" in order for a baby with such a genetic imbalance to have survived to be born. Thus, the parents may be helped to view the situation as a "late miscarriage." This sets the stage for informing them of the limited capacity for postnatal survival, the outcome if the baby should survive early infancy, and the indications for providing comfort without medical intervention toward survival, if they are in agreement with this approach. Whether the parents take the baby home or have the baby taken care of elsewhere is their decision; they simply should be reassured that survival will be limited no matter where the baby is being cared for.

Other Chromosomal Disorders

XO Syndrome. Suspicion of XO syndrome should lead to a chromosome study. An appreciable proportion of cases with partial expression of the full XO syndrome are found to be XO/XX mosaic, X iso-X, XX/X iso-X mosaic, or X deleted-X. The recurrence risk for these conditions is apparently very low to negligible, and older maternal age has not been a significant factor. In fact, X-linkage studies have more commonly indicated a lack of paternal rather than maternal sex chromosome in the XO cases.

Any Case With Deletion or a Translocation Chromosome. Both parents should have chromosomal studies. The majority of them will be found to be normal, and their recurrence risk is negligible. If a parent is a bal-

anced translocation carrier, there is a significant recurrence risk. This may be figured out on a theoretic basis in terms of the possible meiotic products. However, the theoretic and the actual risks may not coincide, as is evident in Figure 4–13 for translocation carrier males.

PREVENTION OF SERIOUS GENETIC DISORDERS THROUGH EARLY FETAL RECOGNITION AND TERMINATION OF AFFECTED PREGNANCIES

It is becoming increasingly possible to evaluate the developing fetus in an attempt to detect serious disorders early enough to allow for termination of affected pregnancies when there is a significant risk, often a recurrence risk, of a serious disorder.[13] The following are some of the techniques of early fetal evaluation and indications for their application, especially for single defects and patterns of malformation.

Chromosomal Abnormalities

Chromosome studies on the developing fetus can be done on cultured amnion cells at 14 to 16 gestational weeks and currently represent the most common indication for amniocentesis. Such studies should be considered for

1. Older pregnant women. The overall incidence of aneuploidy climbs progressively after 35 years. Beyond 40 years, the incidence of aneuploidy is about one in 40 pregnancies, the most common being trisomy 21.

2. Young pregnant women (under 30) who have had a trisomy 21 child. The recurrence risk is close to 1 per cent.

3. A potential parent who is a balanced translocation carrier and has a significant risk of having a genetically unbalanced offspring.

4. The pregnant woman who is a carrier for a serious X-linked recessive disorder. Determination of genetic sex allows for termination of XY male fetuses who would have a 50 per cent risk of being affected by a serious X-linked recessive disorder.

5. Women who have had an offspring with trisomy 18, trisomy 13, or XXY syndrome. Although the actual recurrence risk is not

known and is apparently low, early amniocentesis and fetal chromosomal studies are often considered for these women. At least a part of the reason is psychologic. Some women may have such a fear of repetition of the problem that they would not consider a future pregnancy without diagnostic amniocentesis, even though they might desperately wish to have a normal child.

Biochemical Studies

These may be performed on amniotic fluid or cells.

1. Certain autosomal recessive inborn errors of metabolism, such as Tay-Sachs disease, can be detected by enzyme studies on cultured amnion cells. Hopefully, the mucopolysaccharidoses may be accurately diagnosed in utero also.

2. Alpha-fetoprotein has been detected in about 90 per cent of early pregnancies in which the fetus has either anencephaly or meningomyelocele, presumably because of leakage of cerebrospinal fluid into the amniotic space.

Radiography and Ultrasonograph Studies

1. The dimensions of the fetal head can be outlined and measured by sonography by 14 to 16 weeks of fetal life, allowing for early termination of affected fetuses with primary microcephaly (often autosomal recessive) and anencephaly.

2. Roentgenographic studies of the fetal skeleton may allow for early detection of an affected fetus with a gross skeletal defect. One example is the radial aplasia-thrombocytopenia syndrome, an autosomal recessive disorder. The radius is ossified by 16 weeks, and visualization of the ulna with no radius by 16 weeks could be used as evidence to detect a recurrence of this disorder.

Direct Fetosocopy

Fiberoptic fetoscopes are now being developed with the hope that they may provide direct visualization of the fetus for evidence of external malformation and also permit fetal blood samples to be obtained.

References

1. Carter, C. O.: The inheritance of common congenital malformations. Progr. Med. Genet., 4:59, 1965.
2. Smith, D. W., and Aase, J. M.: Polygenic inheritance of certain common malformations. J. Pediatr., 76:653, 1970
3. Nora, J. J.: Etiologic factors in congenital heart disease. Pediatr. Clin. North Am., 18:1059, 1971.
4. Riseborough, E. J., and Wynne-Davies, R.: A genetic survey of idiopathic scoliosis in Boston. J. Bone Joint Surg. [Am.], 55:974, 1973.
5. Ching, G. H. S., Chung, C. S., and Nemechek, R. S.: Genetic and epidemiological studies of clubfoot in Hawaii. Am. J. Hum. Genet., 21:566, 1969.
6. Saldanha, P. H., Cavalcanti, A. A., and Lemos, M. S.: Incidencia de defeitos congenitos na populacao de Sao Paulo. Rev. Paul. Med., 63:211, 1963.
7. McKeown, T., and Record, R. G.: Seasonal incidence of congenital malformation of the central nervous system. Lancet, 1:192, 1951.
8. Edwards, J. H.: Congenital malformations of the central nervous system in Scotland. Br. J. Prev. Soc. Med., 12:115, 1958.
9. Fraser, F. C.: The Use of Teratogens in the Analysis of Abnormal Developmental Mechanisms. First International Conference on Congenital Malformations. Philadelphia, J. B. Lippincott Co., 1961.
10. Jones, K. L., et al.: Older paternal age and fresh gene mutation. J. Pediatr., 86:84, 1975.
11. Herrmann, J.: Ein Einfluss des zeugungsalters auf die Mutationen zu Hämophilie A. Humangenetik, 3:1, 1966.
12. Summitt R.: Cytogenetics in mentally retarded children with anomalies: A controlled study. J. Pediatr., 74:58, 1969.
13. Milunsky, A.: The Prenatal Diagnosis of Hereditary Disorders. Springfield, Ill., Charles C Thomas, 1973.
14. Arenas, F., and Smith, D. W.: Sex liability to single structural defects. Am. J. Dis. Child, 132:970, 1978.
15. Graham, J. M.: Smith's Recognizable Patterns of Human Deformation, 2nd ed. Philadelphia, W. B. Saunders Co., 1988.

The Psychologic Adaptation
to the child with structural anomalies

During pregnancy the prospective parents anticipate a normal child, but many have a lingering fear that the baby may be abnormal. When told that the baby does have a structural anomaly, their initial response is often denial, mixed with such feelings as guilt, anxiety, self-pity, and sadness. The last-named emotion may partially represent a grief response to the "loss" of the anticipated normal child. The situation can present a smashing blow to the ego of one or both parents and may become a major threat to their marriage. The knowledge and counseling approach of the physician can play an integral role in the realistic adaptation of the parents to this unexpected problem. The physician's knowledge is important in arriving at the correct diagnosis, prognosis, management plan, and genetic counsel. Ideally, the approach involves informing *both* parents of the facts and indicating probable consequences of the situation for the baby and the family. Once the parents have been given an honest perspective of the problem, it is important to involve them integrally in any decisions that need to be made. In fact, given adequate knowledge and counseling, it is the parents who should make the paramount decisions. Depending on the nature of the disorder and the desires of the parents, management may vary from no medical intervention with the anticipation of limited survival at one extreme to full intervention in terms of survival and functional adaptation at the other.

ONE EXTREME: OPTION OF NO MEDICAL INTERVENTION

The author's approach includes giving the parents the option of no medical intervention for disorders in which there is a severe defect in brain development and function and also for those problems that will severely limit the capacity of the baby to survive and function, even with full medical intervention. Examples include anencephaly and some of the other more severe neural tube defects, hydranencephaly, holoprosencephaly, the trisomy 18 syndrome, the trisomy 13 syndrome, the 4p− syndrome, and the Meckel-Gruber syndrome. The parental counseling approach is set forth for two of these disorders:

1. *Anencephaly as an isolated defect.* The parents are informed about the neural groove and how it usually closes by 28 days of development to form the neural tube, the fore-

runner of the brain. Failure of this neural groove closure has resulted in the severe problem in early brain morphogenesis for their baby. They are then told that about 1 per cent of developing fetuses have such a neural tube defect, of which 90 per cent do not survive to be born and are spontaneously aborted. The mother can be told: "You must be well-suited for carrying children to have carried a baby with this problem to full term. Having survived intrauterine life, its capacity for continued survival is limited. If we intervene to maintain survival, the baby's function will be severely limited. We feel that the kindest approach is that of no medical intervention. Do we have your permission for such an approach?" The anomaly is thus explained from a developmental viewpoint, the situation is interpreted as a late miscarriage, and the parents are given the option of no medical intervention.

2. *The trisomy 18 or trisomy 13 syndromes.* The parents are told that normal development is dependent on a balanced set of genes and that the baby has a genetic imbalance due to an extra 18 or 13 chromosome. They are then told, "At least 4 per cent of recognized pregnancies begin with such an extra chromosome. Most of those with an extra 18 or 13 chromosome do not survive early fetal life and are miscarried. You must be very well-suited for carrying babies to have had a baby with this extra chromosome who survived to be born. Although the baby survived intrauterine life, its capacity to survive outside of you is limited. If we intervene and try to prolong life, the baby's function will be extremely limited. We feel the kindest approach is to let nature take its course by not intervening from the medical standpoint. Do we have your permission for this approach?" Thus, the parents are told the basic cause of the problem, helped to interpret the situation as a late miscarriage, and given the option of no medical intervention.

THE OTHER EXTREME: INTERPRETATION AS A "NORMAL CHILD"

At the other extreme are those babies with a structural disorder that can be adequately managed so that it need not impair the child's capacity to lead a normal life. It is especially important to make the distinction between deformation and malformation in this counseling. For deformations, overwhelming emphasis may be placed on the normalcy of the child while explaining that the late fetal constraint caused a mild to moderate transient molding that may now be restored to normal form.[1] A somewhat similar approach may be utilized for certain malformations. Included are otherwise normal infants with a single defect such as cleft lip, pyloric stenosis, polydactyly, and some instances of cardiac anomalies. The following is the author's approach in counseling parents about such defects, using isolated cleft lip as an example. "Your *baby* is normal. There was a problem in the full closure of the lip. This is a normal stage in development of the lip, which usually closes by 35 days in utero. A plastic surgeon can bring about complete closure, and the result is usually quite acceptable. The reason I stated that your *baby* is normal is that I do not believe that this problem in closure of the *lip* need interfere with your child's leading a normal life." Thus the anomaly is explained from a developmental viewpoint, its management is discussed, and its impact on the child is explained. Major emphasis is placed on stating that the baby is normal and localizing the problem in realistic terms of what it represents—a correctable anomaly that need not handicap the child. It is hoped that such counsel will be of value in bringing about a realistic acceptance of the baby by the parents. Hence, *acceptance* of the whole child becomes the key to the approach. Until there is acceptance, the normal flow of affection between parents and child may be warped in the unfortunate direction of either rejection or overprotection.

THE INTERMEDIATE SITUATION: THE CHRONICALLY HANDICAPPED CHILD

There are a number of structural disorders that fall in between the previously mentioned extremes with regard to counseling. The approach for these conditions is usually an individualized one, depending on the nature and severity of handicap engendered by the disorder. The parents should be given facts relative to the cause of the problem, the *usual* range of functional limitations for the disorder, and what can be done to help the child to adapt. For these conditions, the approach is to help the parents accept the child *with his or her problem*. It is often worthwhile to have the family meet with other families or groups of individuals who have the same type of problem. For example, the Little People of America can help individuals with shortness of stature, and the National Association for Retarded Citizens may be supportive to a family that has a child with mental deficiency.

The physician who provides counseling for problems of malformation should be prepared to devote considerable time to the effort. The parents may comprehend and retain only part of the initial counsel, at least partly because of the emotional shock of the situation. The physician should also realize that there may be initial resentment toward the counselor because the information he or she is presenting has not yet been accepted by the parents. Finally, it is important to appreciate that there is great variability in the acceptance of a child with a malformation problem. Some individuals seem almost incapable of accepting a handicapping disorder; others can develop a genuine bond of deep parental love for a handicapped child.

References

1. Graham, J. M.: Smith's Recognizable Patterns of Human Deformation, 2nd ed. Philadelphia, W. B. Saunders Co., 1988.
2. Miller, L. G.: Toward a greater understanding of the parents of the mentally retarded child. J. Pediatr., 73:699, 1968.

6

Minor Anomalies
as clues to more serious problems and toward the recognition of malformation syndromes

Minor anomalies are herein defined as unusual morphologic features that are of no serious medical or cosmetic consequence to the patient. The value of their recognition is that they may serve as indicators of altered morphogenesis in a general sense or may constitute valuable clues in the diagnosis of a specific pattern of malformations.

Regarding the general occurrence of minor anomalies detectable by surface examination (except for dermatoglyphics), Marden et al.[1] found that 14 per cent of newborn babies had a single minor anomaly. This was of little concern because the frequency of major defects in this group was not appreciably increased. However, only 0.8 per cent of the babies had two minor defects, and in this subgroup, the frequency of a major defect was five times that of the general group. Of special importance were the findings in babies with three or more minor anomalies. This was found in only 0.5 per cent of babies (20), and 90 per cent of them had one or more major defects as well, as depicted in Figure 6–1. In summary, the finding of several minor anomalies in the same individual is unusual and often indicates that a more

serious problem in morphogenesis has occurred.

These minor external anomalies are most common in areas of complex and variable features, such as the face, auricles, hands, and feet. Before ascribing significance to a given minor anomaly in a patient, it is important to note whether it is found in other family members. Almost any minor defect may occasionally be found as a usual feature in a particular family, as noted in Figure 6–2.

The following figures illustrate certain minor anomalies and allude to their developmental origin and relevance (Figs. 6–3 to 6–8). Many, if not most, minor anomalies represent deformations due to altered mechanical forces affecting the development of otherwise normal tissue. The reason for the deformation may be purely external uterine constraint. Thus, most minor anomalies of external ear formation at birth are constraint-induced. However, the minor deformational anomaly may be the result of a more primary malformation, and this is the presumed reason for the association between minor anomalies and major malformations. Also de-

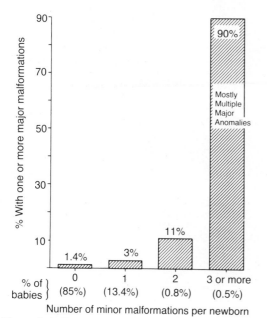

Figure 6–1. Frequency of major malformations in relation to the number of minor anomalies detected in a given newborn baby. (From Marden, P. M., Smith, D. W., and McDonald, M. J.: J. Pediatr., *64*:357, 1964.)

specific indicator of a general lag in osseous maturation. It may, for example, lead to the detection of congenital hypothyroidism in the newborn or young infant, as shown in Figure 6–10. The finding of a large posterior fontanel is especially helpful in this regard, since the posterior fontanel is normally fingertip size or smaller in 97 per cent of full-term neonates. Large fontanels may also be a feature in certain skeletal dysplasias and can, of course, be a sign of increased intracranial pressure.

DERMAL RIDGE PATTERNS
(Dermatoglyphics)

The parallel dermal ridges on the palms and soles form between the thirteenth and nineteenth fetal weeks. Their patterning appears to be dependent on the surface contours at the time, and the parallel dermal ridges tend to develop transversely to the planes of growth stress.[6] Curvilinear arrangements occur when there was a surface mound, for example, over the fetal pads that are prominently present during early fetal life on the fingertips, on the palm between each pair of fingers, and occasionally in the hypothenar area. Indirect evidence suggests that a high fetal fingertip pad tends to give rise to a whorl pattern, a low pad yields an arch pattern, and an intermediate pad produces a loop, as illustrated in Figure 6–11*B*.

The dermal ridge patterning thereby provides an indelible historical record that indicates the form of the early fetal hand (or

Text continued on page 669

picted, for the purpose of perspective, are some minor variants found in newborn babies with sufficient frequency that they should not be classed as anomalies (Fig. 6–9).

CALVARIUM

The presence of unusually *large fontanels* (see standards in Chapter 7) may be a non-

Figure 6–2. An otherwise normal mother *(left)* and daughter with clinodactyly of the fifth finger. A family history should be obtained before ascribing significance to a given minor anomaly.

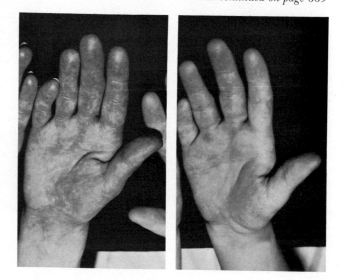

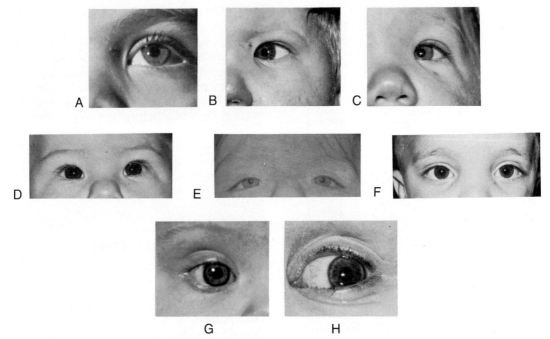

Figure 6–3. Minor anomalies of the ocular region. *A* to *C, Inner epicanthal folds* appear to represent redundant folds of skin, secondary to either low nasal bridge (most common) or excess skin, as in cutis laxa. Minor folds are frequent in early infancy, and as the nasal bridge becomes more prominent, they are obliterated. *D, E,* Telecanthus is the consequence of lateral displacement of the inner canthi, which partially obscures the medial portion of the eye and gives a false impression of strabismus and of hypertelorism. *Slanting of the palpebral fissures* seems to be secondary to the early growth rate of the brain above the eye versus that of the facial area below the eye. For example, the patient with upslanting *(D)* had mild microcephaly with a narrow frontal area, resulting in the upslant; the patient with downslanting *(E)* had maxillary hypoplasia, resulting in the downslant. Mild degrees of upslant were noted in 4 per cent of 500 normal children. *F, Ocular hypertelorism* refers to widely spaced eyes. A low nasal bridge will often give rise to a visual impression of ocular hypertelorism. This should always be determined by measurement. Measurement of inner canthal distance, coupled with the visual distinction of whether telecanthus is present, is usually sufficient. *G, H, Brushfield spots* are speckled rings about two thirds of the distance to the periphery of the iris. There is relative lack of patterning beyond the ring. These spots are found in about 20 per cent of normal newborn babies, but they are found in 80 per cent of babies with Down syndrome.

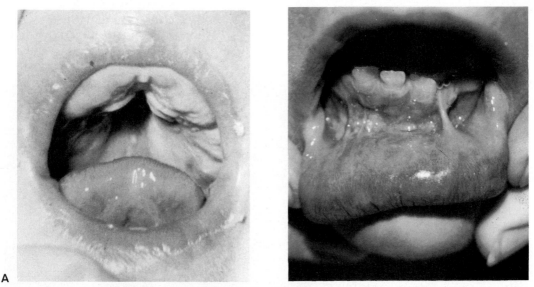

Figure 6–4. Minor anomalies of the oral region. *A, Prominent lateral palatal ridges* may be secondary to a deficit of tongue thrust into the hard palate, allowing for relative overgrowth of the lateral palatal ridges. Such a ridge may be a feature in a variety of disorders, especially those with hypotonia and with serious neurologic deficits related to sucking. As such, it can be a useful sign of a long-term deficit in function. *B, Aberrant frenula.*

664

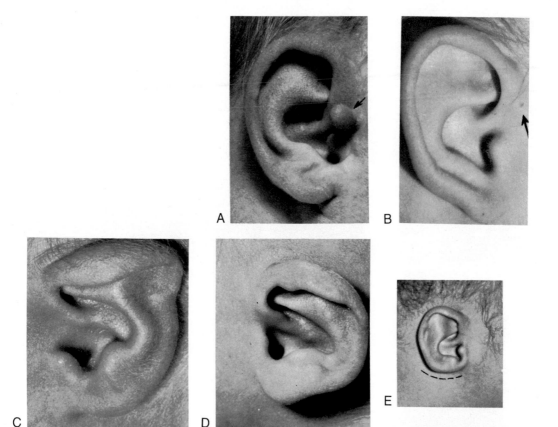

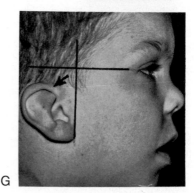

Figure 6–5. Minor anomalies of the auricular region. *A, Preauricular tags,* which often contain a core of cartilage, appear to represent accessory hillock of His, the hillocks that normally develop in the recess of the mandibular and hyoid arches and coalesce to form the auricle. *B, Preauricular pits* may be familial, are twice as common in females as in males, and are more common in blacks than in whites. *C, D, Incomplete development of the scapha helix* is, in minor degrees, not an unusual finding in infants (see Fig. 6–9, *D* and *E*). *E, Lack of lobulus. F, Protruding ear* is usually due to lack of development or function of the posterior auricular ear muscle. *G, Low-set ears:* This designation is made when the helix meets the cranium *(arrow)* at a level below that of a horizontal plane with the corner of the orbit. This latter plane may relate to the lateral vertical axis of the head. More ideally, the horizontal plane may be an extension of a line through both inner canthi, such as can be done with a pliable strip of x-ray film. *Ears slanted:* When the angle of the slope of the auricle exceeds 15 degrees from the perpendicular. Note: The findings of low placement and slanted auricle often go together and usually represent a lag in morphogenesis, since the auricle is normally in that position in early fetal life. It is important to appreciate that deformation of the head secondary to in utero constraint may temporarily distort the usual landmarks.

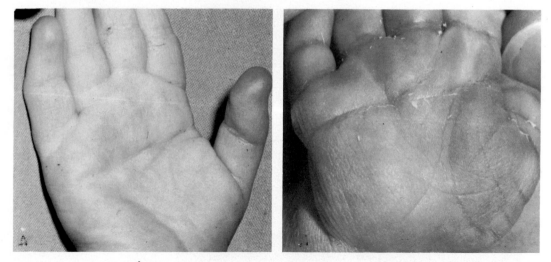

A

B

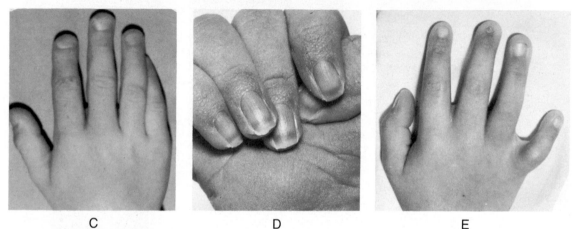

C

D

E

Figure 6–6. Minor anomalies of the hands. *A, B, Creases* represent the planes of folding (flexion) of the thickened volar skin of the hand. As such, they are simply deep wrinkles. The finger creases relate to flexion at the phalangeal joints, and if there has been no flexion, there is no crease. Hypoplasia of the middle phalanx may result in only one plane of flexion on that finger *(A)*. The thenar crease is the consequence of oppositional flexion of the thumb. Hence, if there is no oppositional flexion, there will be no crease. The slanting upper palmar crease reflects the palmar plane of folding related to the slope of the third, fourth, and fifth metacarpal-phalangeal joints. The midpalmar crease is the plane of skin folding between the upper palmar crease and the thenar crease. Any alteration in the slope of the third, fourth, and fifth metacarpal-phalangeal planes of flexion, or relative shortness of the palm, may give rise to but a single midpalmar plane of flexion and thereby the *simian crease (A)*. The latter is found unilaterally in about 4 per cent of normal infants and bilaterally in 1 per cent. Davies[4] found the incidence to be 3.7 per cent in newborn babies and noted that the simian crease is twice as common in males as in females. All degrees are found between normal and *simian crease*, including the *bridged palmar crease (B)*. The creases are evident by 11 to 12 weeks of fetal life; hence, any gross alteration in crease patterning is usually indicative of an *abnormality in form and/or function of the hand prior to 11 fetal weeks.*[5] *Clinodactyly (curved finger) (A)* is most common in the fifth finger and is the consequence of hypoplasia of the middle phalanx, normally the last digital bone to develop. Up to 8 degrees of inturning of the fifth finger is within normal limits. Regardless of which digits are affected (fingers or toes), there is usually incurvature toward the area between the second and third digits. Partial *cutaneous syndactyly (A)* represents an incomplete separation of the fingers and most commonly occurs between the third and fourth fingers and between the second and third toes. *C to E*, The *nails* generally reflect the size and shape of the underlying distal phalanx. Hence, the *short, broad nail (C)*, the *narrow hyperconvex nail (D)*, and the *hypoplastic nail (E)* reflect the relative dimensions of the underlying respective phalanges. *Asymmetric length (E)* of fingers is usually the result of hypoplasia of one or more fingers. *Camptodactyly (E)* most commonly affects the fifth, fourth, and third digits in decreasing order of frequency. It is presumably the consequence of relative shortness in the length of the flexor tendons with respect to the growth of the hand.

Illustration continued on opposite page

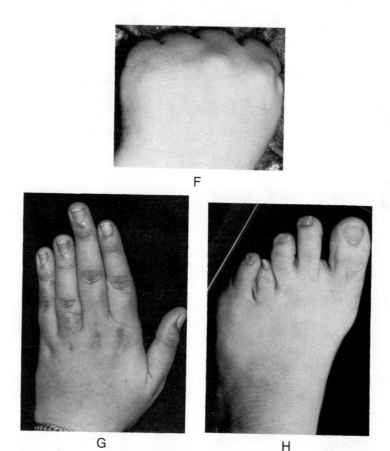

Figure 6–6 *Continued F* to *H, Malproportionment* or disharmony in the length of particular segments of the hand is not uncommon. The most common is a short middle phalanx of the fifth finger with clinodactyly. Another is relative shortness of the fourth and/or fifth metacarpal or metatarsal bone *(H)*. This is best appreciated in the hand by having the patient make a fist and observing the position of the knuckles as shown in *F*. The altered alignment of these metacarpal-phalangeal joints may result in an altered palmar crease, especially the simian crease. It may also yield the impression of partial syndactyly between the third, fourth, and fifth fingers. Such relative shortness of the fourth and fifth metacarpals *may develop* postnatally by there being earlier than usual fusion of the respective metacarpal-epiphyseal plates. When this happens, it tends to occur in the center of the epiphyseal plate first, yielding the radiographic appearance of a "coned-down" epiphysis. This is a nonspecific anomaly that may occur by itself or as one feature of a number of syndromes.

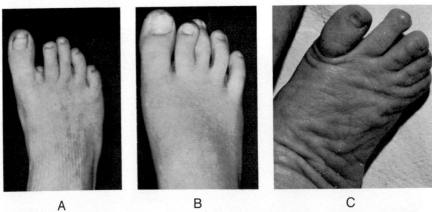

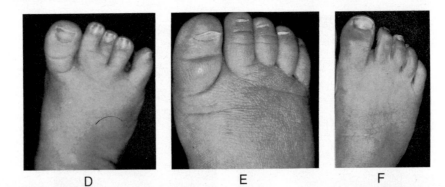

Figure 6–7. Minor anomalies of the feet. *A,* Asymmetric length of toes. *B,* Clinodactyly of second toe with overlapping. *C,* Short first metatarsal with dorsiflexion of hallux. *D,* Syndactyly (most commonly between digits 2 and 3). *E,* Hypoplasia of nails (in two and one-half year old). *F,* Short, broad toenail. *G,* Deep crease between hallux and second toe. *H,* Wide gap between hallux and second toe.

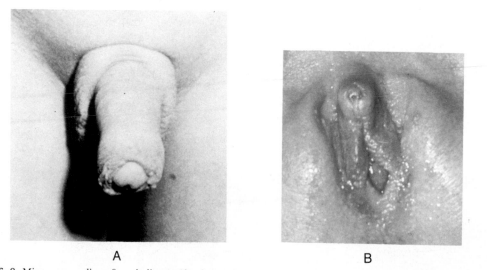

A   B

Figure 6–8. Minor anomalies of genitalia. *A, Shawl scrotum* appears to represent a mild deficit in the full migration of the labial-scrotal folds and as such may be accompanied by other signs of incomplete masculinization of the external genitalia. This photo shows a patient with the Aarskog syndrome. *B, Hypoplasia of the labia majora* may give rise to the false visual impression of a large clitoris, as in this patient with the trisomy 18 syndrome.

foot). Mild to severe alterations in hand morphology occur in a variety of syndromes, and hence it is not surprising that dermatoglyphic alterations have been noted in numerous dysmorphic syndromes. These alterations have seldom been pathognomonic for a particular condition. Rather, they simply provide additional data that, viewed in relation to the total pattern of malformation, may enhance the clinician's capacity to arrive at a specific overall diagnosis.

Dermal ridge patterning may be evaluated utilizing a seven-power illuminated magnifying device such as an otoscope or a stamp collector's flashlight, which has a wider field of vision. Permanent records may be obtained by a variety of techniques.[7-9]

There are two general categories of dermatoglyphic alterations: an *aberrant pattern* and *unusual frequency* and/or *distribution of a particular pattern on the fingertips*.

Aberrant Patterning

Distal Axial Palmar Triradius (Fig. 6–11A). Triradii occur at the juncture of three sets of converging ridges. There are usually no triradii between the base of the palm and the interdigital areas of the upper palm. However, patterning in the hypothenar area often gives rise to a distal axial triradius located, by definition, greater than 35 per cent of the distance from the wrist crease to

the crease at the base of the third finger. This alteration, found in about 4 per cent of whites, is a frequent feature in a number of patterns of malformation.

Open Field in Hallucal Area (Arch Tibial) (Fig. 6–11A). Open field simply means that there is a relative lack of complexity in patterning and thereby implies a low surface contour in that area at the time ridges developed. The hallucal area of the sole usually has a loop or whorl pattern, and a lack of such a pattern is unusual in the normal individual but is found in about 50 per cent of patients with the Down syndrome and as an occasional feature in other syndromes.

Lack of Ridges. The failure of development of ridges in an area, most commonly the hypothenar region of the palm, is an occasional but nonspecific feature in the de Lange syndrome.

Other Patterns. There are a number of other unusual patterns, especially in the upper palmar, hypothenar, and thenar areas, which may be of clinical significance, but these are so rarely of value in an individual case that they will not be discussed.

Unusual Frequency or Distribution of Patterns on the Fingertips

A quantitation of the overall extent of patterning on the ten fingertips may be achieved by obtaining fingerprints and re-

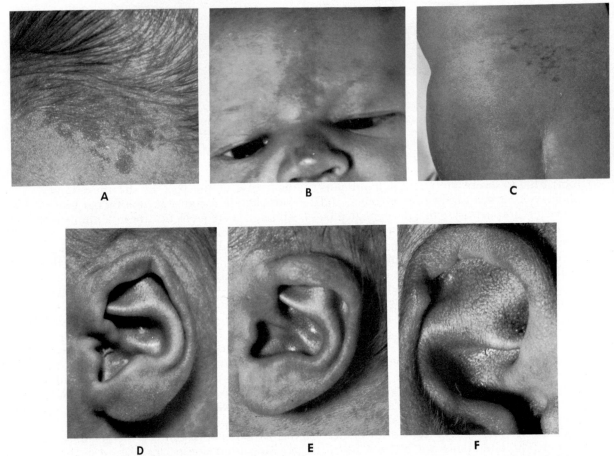

Figure 6–9. Minor variants in the newborn that should *not* be classed as anomalies. *A* to *C,* Fine nonelevated pink to red capillary hemangiomata at nape of neck *(A),* over central forehead and eyelids *(B),* and in lumbosacral area *(C). D, E,* Incompletely outfolded scapha helix (see Fig. 6–5, *C* and *D). F,* Darwinian tubercle.

Illustration continued on opposite page

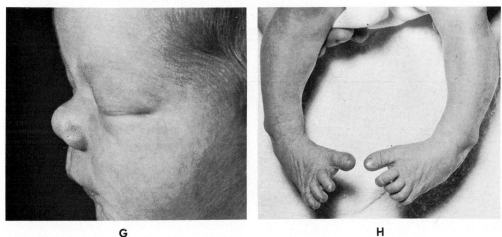

G   H

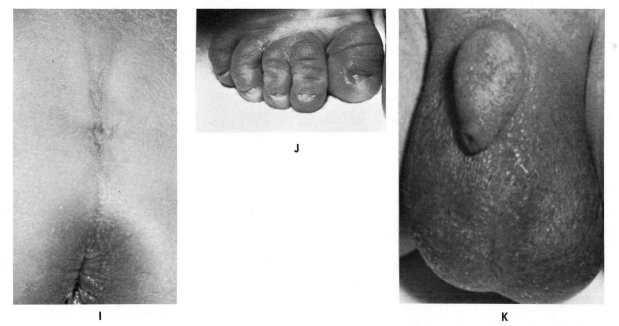

I   K

J

Figure 6–9 *Continued G,* "Saddle" nose, mildly upturned nares. *H,* Mild to moderate inbowing of lower leg, with tibial torsion. *I,* Sacral dimple, not deep. *J,* Mild syndactyly of second and third toes; also, toenail hypoplasia in newborn. *K,* Hydrocele of testicle.

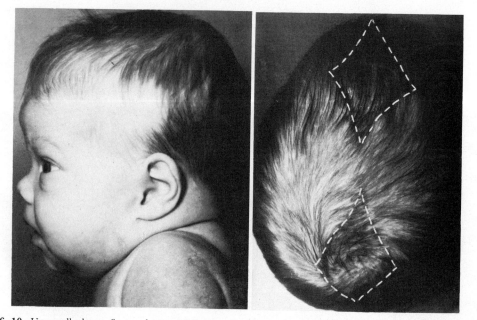

Figure 6–10. Unusually large fontanels, especially the posterior fontanel, in a six week old baby with athyrotic hypothyroidism. The fetal onset of retarded osseous maturation is also evident in the immature facial bone development. (From Smith, D. W., and Popich, G.: J. Pediatr., *80*:753, 1972.)

cording the total fingertip ridge count, as illustrated in Figure 6–11*C*.

High Frequency of Low Arch Configurations. It is unusual to find a normal person with more than six of ten fingertips having a low arch configuration; however, this is a frequent feature in the trisomy 18 syndrome and the XXXXY syndrome, presumably reflecting hypoplasia of the fetal fingertip pads in these disorders. High frequency of low arches is nonspecific, being an occasional finding in certain other syndromes and in about 0.9 per cent of normal individuals.

High Frequency of Whorl Patterning. It is unusual to find nine or more fingertip whorls in an individual (3 per cent in normal persons). Excessive patterning, presumably reflecting prominent fetal pads, is more likely to be found in the XO syndrome, the Smith-Lemli-Opitz syndrome, occasionally in other patterns of malformation, and in some normal individuals.

Unusual Distribution, Especially of Radial Loop Patterns. Loops opening to the radial side of the hand are unusual on the fourth and fifth fingers. Radial loop patterns on these fingers are more common in people with Down syndrome (12.4 per cent) than in individuals who are normal (1.5 per cent).

HAIR: ORIGIN AND RELEVANCE OF ABERRANT SCALP AND UPPER FACIAL HAIR PATTERNING AND GROWTH

The origin and relevance of hair directional patterning and aberrant hair growth[10, 11] will be considered individually.

Hair Directional Patterning

Normal Development and Relevance. The origin of the sloping angulation of each hair follicle, which determines the surface hair directional patterning, is derived from the direction of stretch on the surface skin during the time the hair follicle is growing down from it into the loose underlying mesenchyme, as shown in Figure 6–12. Over the scalp and upper face, this directional patterning reflects the plane of growth stretch on the surface skin that was exerted by the growth of underlying structures during the period of hair follicle downgrowth, which takes place from ten to 16 weeks of fetal life. Thus the parietal hair whorl, or crown, is interpreted as representing the focal point from which the posterior scalp skin was un-

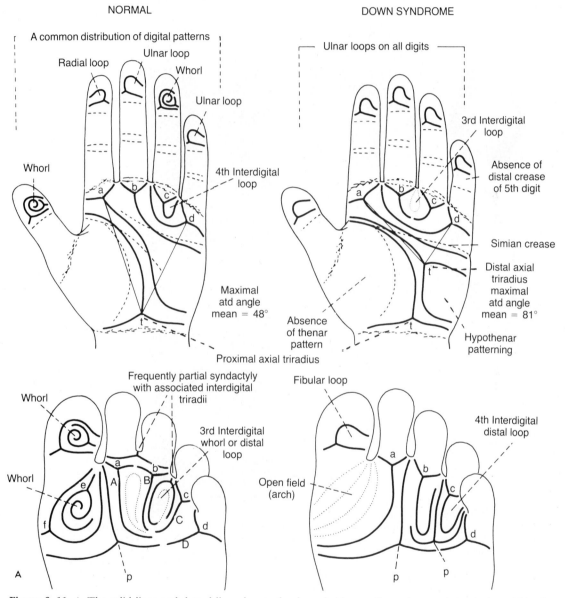

Figure 6–11. *A,* The solid lines and dotted lines denote the dermal ridge configurations, and the dashes within the palm represent the creases. (Courtesy of Dr. M. Bat-Miriam; prepared by Mr. R. Lee of the Kennedy-Galton Center near St. Albans, England.)

Illustration continued on following page

Ridge Count

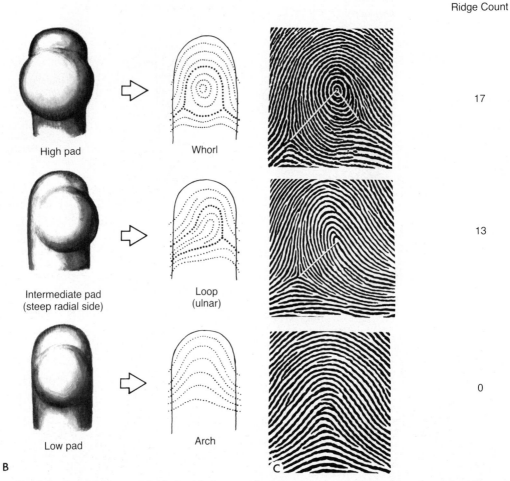

High pad

Whorl

17

Intermediate pad
(steep radial side)

Loop
(ulnar)

13

Low pad

Arch

0

B

C

Figure 6–11 *Continued B,* Presumed relationship between fetal fingertip pads at 16 to 19 weeks of fetal life and the fingertip dermal ridge pattern, which develops at that time. *C,* Technique for dermal ridge counting: A line is drawn between the center of the pattern and the more distal triradius, and the number of ridges that touch this line is the fingertip ridge count. The sum of the ten fingertip ridge counts is the total ridge count; this average is 144 in the male and 127 in the female. (From Holt, S.: Br. Med. Bull., *17*:247, 1961.)

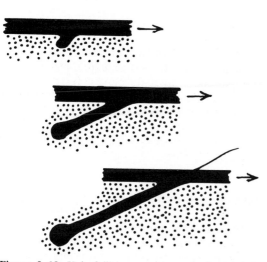

Figure 6–12. Hair follicles over the scalp begin their downgrowth into the loose underlying mesenchyme at ten fetal weeks. The slope of each hair follicle and thereby the hair directional patterning is determined by the direction of growth stretch *(arrows)* exerted on the surface skin by the development of underlying tissues. For the scalp hair, the patterning relates to the growth in size and form of the underlying brain during the period of 10 to 16 weeks. By 18 weeks, when hairs are extruded onto the surface, their patterning is set. (From Smith, D. W., and Gong, B. T.: Teratology, *9*:17, 1974.)

der growth tension exerted by the dome-like outgrowth of the early brain during this fetal period (Fig. 6–13). Its location is normally several centimeters anterior to the position of the posterior fontanel. Fifty-six per cent of single parietal hair whorls are located to the left of the midline, presumably because the left side of the brain tends to be slightly larger than the right; 30 per cent are right-sided, and 14 per cent are midline in location. Five per cent of normal individuals have bilateral parietal hair whorls. From the posterior whorl, the parietal hair stream flares out progressively, sweeping anteriorly to the forehead. Over the frontal region, the growth of the forebrain and the upper face results in bilateral frontal hair streams that emanate from the fixed points of the ocular puncta and tend to arc outward in a lateral direction, thereby affecting eyebrow hair directional patterning (Fig. 6–14). The anterior parietal hair stream normally converges with the upsweeping frontal hair stream on the forehead, resulting in a variety of forehead hair patterning, such as converging whorls and quadriradial patterns. If the frontal hair stream meets with the parietal hair stream above the forehead, there may be an anterior upsweep of the scalp hair, known as a "cowlick." Mild to moderate lateral upsweep or central upsweep of the scalp hair occurs in 5 per cent of normal individuals.

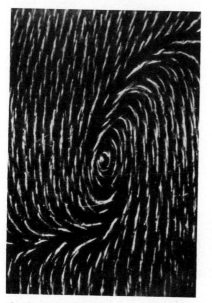

Figure 6–13. Parietal hair whorl at 18 weeks. This appears to be the fixed focal point from which the skin is being stretched by the dome-like outgrowth of the brain between 10 and 16 weeks. (From Smith, D. W., and Gong, B. T.: Teratology, *9*:17, 1974.)

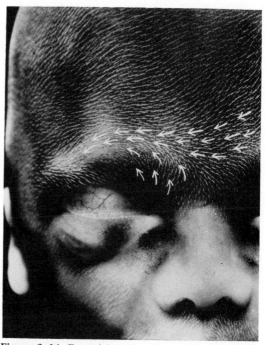

Figure 6–14. Frontal hair stream at 18 weeks, arcing laterally from the ocular punctum to meet with the downsweeping parietal hair stream. The frontal hair stream has been influenced by the growth of the underlying upper facial structures and the forebrain. (From Smith, D. W., and Gong, G. T.: Teratology, *9*:17, 1974.)

Defects of the calvarium, such as primary craniosynostosis, have not been noted to affect hair patterning, since the calvarium is not yet developed at the time of hair follicle downgrowth.

Relevance and Nature of Aberrant Scalp and Upper Facial Hair Directional Patterning. Abnormal size and/or shape of the brain and upper facial area during the ten to 16 week fetal period can apparently result in aberrant hair patterning. Severe microcephaly may lead to a lack of a parietal hair whorl (25 per cent) and/or a frontal upsweep of the scalp hair (70 per cent), as shown in Figure 6–15. The latter feature appears to relate to the individual who has a narrow and smaller frontal area of the brain. The parietal whorl is more likely to be midline and posteriorly located in patients with microcephaly, as shown in Figure 6–16. In a variety of other gross defects of early brain development, the hair directional patterning may be secondarily altered. In each case, the aberrant scalp hair patterning reflects the altered shape and/or growth of the early fetal brain. Gross aberrations of hair patterning often imply a serious degree of mental deficiency, since the brain is at such an early stage of development at ten to 16 weeks (Fig. 6–17).

Abnormal eyebrow patterning, such as the unusual outflaring of the medial eyebrows of the patient shown in Figure 6–18, implies that there was abnormal shape and/or growth in the upper midface prior to or during the period of hair follicle downgrowth, which occurs from ten to 16 weeks of fetal development.

Hair Growth Patterns

Normal Development and Relevance. At 18 fetal weeks, when hair first emerges, it grows on the entire face and scalp, as noted in Figure 6–19. Later, the eyebrows and scalp hair predominate, and the growth of hair over the remainder of the face is apparently suppressed. Studies imply that there is a periocular zone of hair growth suppression.

Nature and Relevance of Aberrant Facial Hair Growth Patterns. The V-shaped midline, downward projection of the scalp hair, known as the "widow's peak," is considered to represent an upper forehead intersection

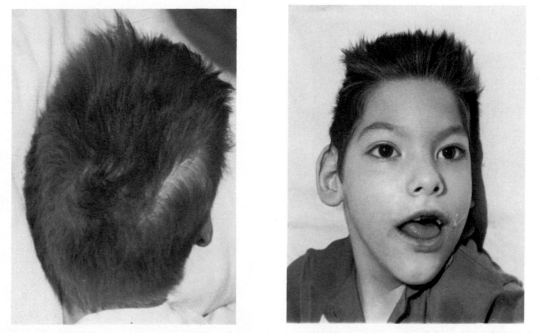

Figure 6–15. Hair patterning in a patient with primary microcephaly. The posterior scalp shows a lack of a concise whorl, and the anterior scalp shows a marked frontal upsweep. These findings are interpreted as being the consequence of a deficit in growth of the brain prior to and during the period of hair follicle development and thus imply an early defect in morphogenesis of the brain, prior to 10 to 16 weeks. (From Smith, D. W., and Gong, B. T.: Teratology, 9:17, 1974.)

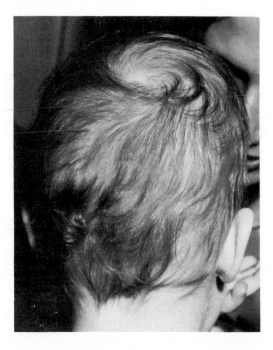

Figure 6–16. Posterior scalp hair patterning of the type more commonly found in mild microcephaly, in this instance, the Down syndrome. The parietal whorl tends to be more central and posterior than usual, being over the former position of the posterior fontanel. This is considered secondary to the brain having been smaller and more symmetric than usual at 10 to 16 weeks, the time when the hair follicles develop. (From Smith, D. W., and Gong, B. T.: Teratology, 9:17, 1974.)

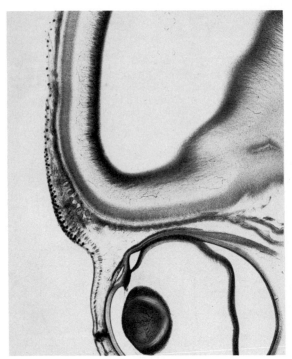

Figure 6–17. Sagittal section of forebrain area of a ten week fetus, showing the early stage of cerebral cortical development and the lack of any organized calvarium at the time the hair follicles are beginning their downgrowth. (From Smith, D. W., and Gong, B. T.: Teratology, 9:17, 1974.)

Figure 6–18. Aberrant mideyebrow patterning, which implies an aberration in growth and/or form of underlying facial structures by 10 to 16 fetal weeks. This patient has the Waardenburg syndrome, in which aberrant mid-uppper facial development is a usual feature.

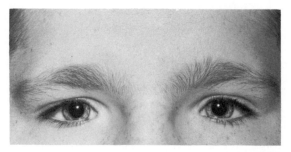

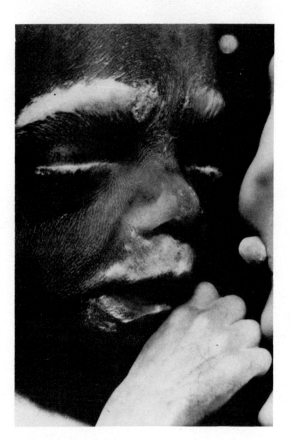

Figure 6–19. Hair growth on the face at 18 weeks, shortly after the hairs have been extruded onto the surface skin. (From Nilsson, L., Ingelman-Sundberg, A., and Wirsen, C.: A Child Is Born. New York, Delacorte Press, 1966.)

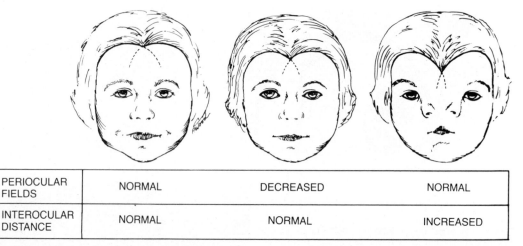

PERIOCULAR FIELDS	NORMAL	DECREASED	NORMAL
INTEROCULAR DISTANCE	NORMAL	NORMAL	INCREASED

Figure 6–20. If the eyes are widely spaced, or the area of periocular hair growth suppression is smaller than usual, the bilateral zones of periocular hair growth suppression may overlap at a lower point than usual, allowing for the presence of a widow's peak. The drawing on the right is of a patient with the frontonasal dysplasia anomaly. (From Smith, D. W., and Cohen, M. M., Jr.: Lancet, 2:1127, 1973.)

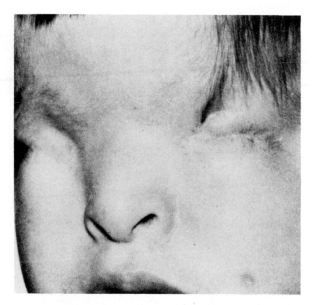

Figure 6–21. Aberrant growth of hair in lateral forehead area, related to the cryptophthalmos anomaly. (From Bergsma, D., and McKusick, V. A. (eds.): National Foundation—Birth Defects. Baltimore, Williams and Wilkins Co., 1973, p. 27.)

of the bilateral fields of periocular hair growth suppression. This may occur because the fields are widely spaced, as in ocular hypertelorism, or because the ocular fields of hair growth suppression are smaller with a low scalp hairline and low position of intersection, as illustrated in Figure 6–20. In the presence of cryptophthalmos, there may be an abnormal projection of scalp-like hair growth toward the ocular area (Fig. 6–21).

The auricle appears to influence hair growth in the region anterior to the ear. With absence of the auricle, there is usually absence of hair growth in the sideburn area (Fig. 6–22) anterior to the ear. When there is a rudimentary ear, such as is often found in the Treacher Collins syndrome, there may be an aberrant tongue of hair growth projecting onto the cheek area.

Usually, a short neck or webbed neck may

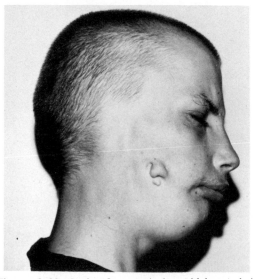

Figure 6–22. Lack of preauricular (sideburn) hair growth in relation to a deficit of auricular development.

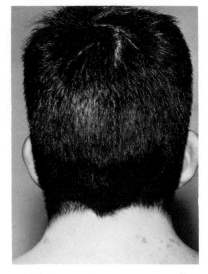

Figure 6–23. Low posterior hairline, usually related to either a short or webbed neck.

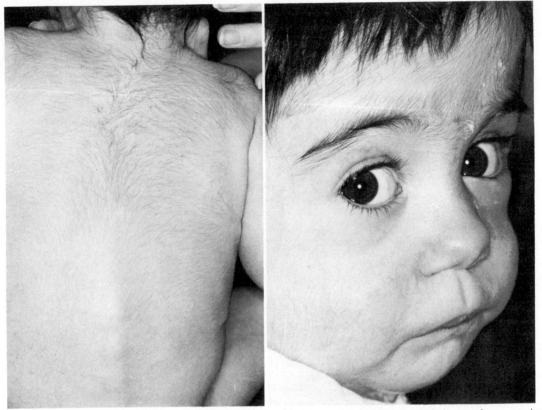

Figure 6–24. General facial and body hirsutism, presumably secondary to a general deficit in hair growth suppression in areas in which the hair growth is usually suppressed, especially over the forehead and upper back.

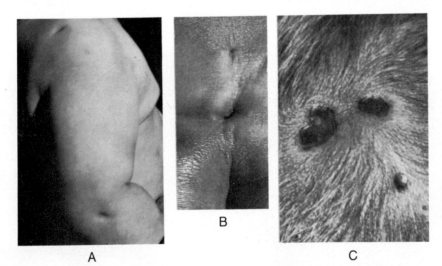

Figure 6–25. Unusual *dimples (A, B)* may occur at a location where there has been a closer than usual proximity between the skin and underlying bony structures during fetal life, resulting in deficient development of subcutaneous tissue at that locus. Such dimples may be secondary either to a deficit in early subcutaneous tissue or to an aberrant bony promontory. They tend to occur at the elbows, knees, over the acromion promontories, and over the lower sacrum, as shown above. In the latter location, they often have subsidiary creases and pits and should be distinguished from a pilonidal sinus. *(C) Punched-out scalp lesions* are most commonly found toward the midline in the posterior parietal scalp area. The skin is usually totally lacking, but the crater becomes covered with scar tissue postnatally. The developmental pathology for these lesions is unknown.

be associated with the secondary feature of a low posterior hairline, especially at the lateral borders, as shown in Figure 6–23.

Whether the facial and body hirsutism (Fig. 6–24) found in patients with the de Lange syndrome and in a variety of failure to thrive growth deficiency disorders represents a more generalized failure of normal growth suppression in these conditions remains to be determined.

OTHER CUTANEOUS ANOMALIES

Cutaneous features such as unusual dimples and punched-out scalp lesions are shown in Figure 6–25.

References

1. Marden, P. M., Smith, D. W., and McDonald, M. J.: Congenital anomalies in the newborn infant, including minor variations. J. Pediatr., *64*:357, 1964.

2. Popich, G. A., and Smith, D. W.: Fontanels: Range of normal size. J. Pediatr., *80*:479, 1972.

3. Smith, D .W., and Popich, G. A.: Large fontanels in congenital hypothyroidism: A potential clue toward earlier recognition. J. Pediatr., *80*:753, 1972.

4. Davies, P.: Sex and the single transverse crease in newborn singletons. Dev. Med. Child Neurol., *8*:729, 1966.

5. Popich, G. A., and Smith, D. W.: The genesis and significance of digital and palmar hand creases: Preliminary report. J. Pediatr., 77:1917, 1970.

6. Mulvihill, J., and Smith, D. W.: Genesis of dermal ridge patterning. J. Pediatr., *75*:1969.

7. Ford-Walker, N.: Inkless methods of finger, palm and sole printing. J. Pediatr., *50*:27, 1957.

8. Uchida, I. A., and Soltan, H. C.: Evaluation of dermatoglyphics in medical genetics. Pediatr. Clin. North Am., *10*:409, 1963.

9. Aase, J. M., and Lyons, R. B.: Technique for recording dermatoglyphics. Lancet, *1*:432, 1971.

10. Smith, D. W., and Gong, B. T.: Scalp hair patterning as a clue to early fetal brain development. J. Pediatr., *83*:374, 1973 and Teratology, *9*:17, 1974.

11. Smith, D. W., and Cohen, M. M., Jr.: Widow's peak scalp anomaly, origin and relevance to ocular hypertelorism. Lancet, *2*:1127, 1973.

12. Graham, J. M.: Recognizable Patterns of Human Deformation, 2nd ed. Philadelphia, W. B. Saunders Co., 1988.

13. Smith, D. W., and Takashima, H.: Protruding auricle, a neuromuscular sign. Lancet, *1*:747, 1978.

7

Normal Standards

The following compilation of normal measurements is set forth as an aid in determining whether or not a given feature is abnormal. Such data may be especially useful when the visual impression is potentially misleading. For example, when the nasal bridge is low-set, the visual impression may falsely suggest ocular hypertelorism, and when the patient is obese, the hands may *appear* to be small. Besides comparing patient measurements with these normal cross-sectional population standards, it may be important to contrast the findings of the patient with those of his parents and/or siblings in an attempt to determine whether or not a given feature is unusual for that particular family.

These measurements have been predominantly obtained from whites and hence may not be accurate for other racial groups. Separate data are presented for males and females, except for features that do not show significant differences between the sexes. For paired structures, the measurements are given for the right side. Many of the charts were kindly supplied by Dr. Murray Feingold from his Boston study of normal measurements.

STANDARDS FOR HEIGHT AND WEIGHT*

The growth charts for young children (Figs. 7–1 to 7–4) were developed by J. M.

*Obtainable from Creaseys Ltd., Print Division, Bull Plain, Hertford, England.

Tanner and R. H. Whitehouse at the University of London Institute of Child Health. The data on means and standard deviations (Tables 7–1 and 7–2) relate to the four growth charts for young children. The subsequent four charts, which concern growth from birth through adolescence (Figs. 7–5 to 7–8), are from Tanner et al.[1]

Notes on Use

1. *Weight* is preferably taken in the nude; otherwise, the estimated weight of clothing is subtracted before plotting.

2. When a child is born earlier than 40 weeks' gestation preterm, the birth weight is plotted at the appropriate number of weeks on the chart. Subsequent weights are plotted in relation to this "conception age"; thus for a child born at 32 weeks, the 8-weeks-after-birth weight is plotted at B (birth) on the scale, the 12-week weight at 4 weeks after B, and so on. Length is plotted in the same manner.

3. *Supine length* (up to age 2.0 years) should be taken with the infant lying on a measuring table constructed for this purpose. One person holds the infant's head so that he looks straight upward (the lower borders of the eye sockets and the external auditory meati should be in the same vertical plane) and pulls very gently to bring the top of the head into contact with the fixed measuring board. A second person, the measurer, presses the infant's knees down into contact with the board, and, also pulling gently to stretch the infant out, holds the infant's feet, with the

toes pointing directly upward. He brings the movable footboard to rest firmly against the infant's heels and reads the measurement to the last completed 0.1 cm.

4. *Standing height* should be taken without shoes, the child standing with heels and back in contact with an upright wall or preferably a stadiometer made for this purpose.* His head is held so that he looks straight forward, with the lower borders of the eye sockets on the same horizontal plane as the external auditory meati (i.e., head not with nose tipped upwards). A right-angled block (preferably counterweighted) is slid down the wall until its bottom surface touches the child's head, and a scale fixed to the wall is read. During the measurement, the child should be told to stretch his neck to be as tall as possible, though care must be taken to prevent his heels from coming off the ground. The measurer should apply gentle but firm upward pressure under the mastoid processes to help the child stretch. In this way, the variation in height from morning to evening is minimized. Standing height should be recorded to the last completed 0.1 cm.

5. The sources of the standards on young children are (a) weight from 32 to 40 weeks

*Obtainable from Holtain Ltd., Crymmych, Pembrokeshire, England.

gestation, Tanner-Thomson standards (published by Creaseys, 1970 and in Arch. Dis. Child., *45*:566, 1970) from Aberdeen data; (b) length from 32 to 40 weeks estimated from West European and North American data, not available for England; and (c) weight and length after 40-week birth, same sources as Tanner-Whitehouse 0 to 18 year old standards (published by Creaseys, 1966 and detailed in Arch. Dis. Child., *41*:454, 613, 1966.)

OTHER STANDARDS

The reader will find charts showing normal measurements for head circumference, chest, hand, foot, inner and outer canthal distances, palpebral fissure, length, fontanel, ear, penis, and testis (Figs. 7–9 to 7–21) after the growth charts.

Reference

1. Tanner, J. M., Whitehouse, R. H., and Takaishi, M.: Standards from birth to maturity for height, weight, height velocity, and weight velocity. Arch. Dis. Child., *41*:613, 1966.

LINEAR GROWTH
MALES, FIRST 5 YEARS

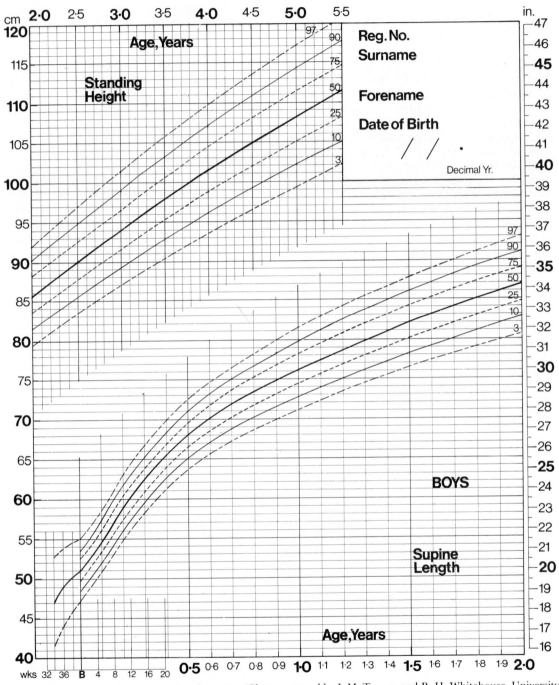

Figure 7–1. Linear growth, males, first five years. (Chart prepared by J. M. Tanner and R. H. Whitehouse, University of London Institute of Child Health, for the Hospital for Sick Children, Great Ormond Street, London, W. C.1. Printed by Creaseys of Hertford, Ltd. No. Ref SHWB28. For information on sources used to develop standards, see text, item 5.)

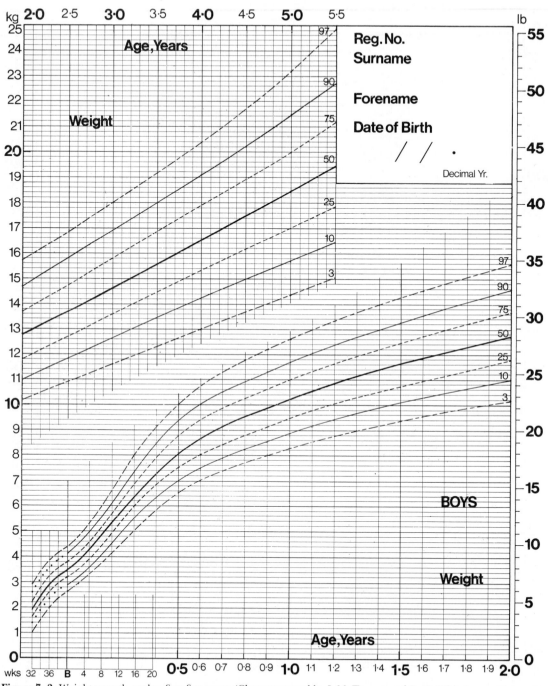

Figure 7–2. Weight growth, males, first five years. (Chart prepared by J. M. Tanner and R. H. Whitehouse, University of London Institute of Child Health, for the Hospital for Sick Children, Great Ormond Street, London, W. C. 1. Printed by Creaseys of Hertford, Ltd. No. Ref SHWB28. For information on sources used to develop standards, see text, item 5.)

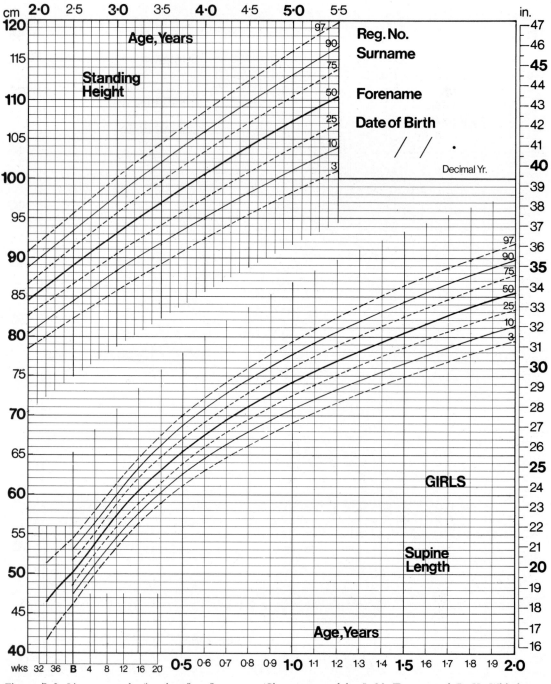

Figure 7–3. Linear growth, females, first five years. (Chart prepared by J. M. Tanner and R. H. Whitehouse, University of London Institute of Child Health, for the Hospital for Sick Children, Great Ormond Street, London, W. C.1. Printed by Creaseys of Hertford, Ltd. No. Ref SHWB28. For information on sources used to develop standards, see text, item 5.)

WEIGHT GROWTH
FEMALES, FIRST 5 YEARS

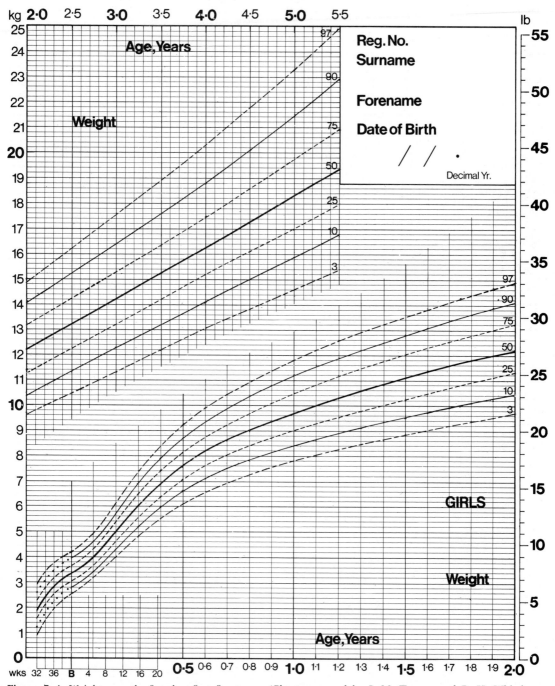

Figure 7–4. Weight growth, females, first five years. (Chart prepared by J. M. Tanner and R. H. Whitehouse, University of London Institute of Child Health, for the Hospital for Sick Children, Great Ormond Street, London, W. C.1. Printed by Creaseys of Hertford, Ltd. No. Ref SHWB28. For information on sources used to develop standards, see text, item 5.)

Table 7–1. **MEANS AND STANDARD DEVIATIONS—MALES***

Weight		Head Circumference		Length Velocity	Height Velocity	Weight Velocity		Triceps Skinfold		Subscapular Skinfold	
Mean	SD	Mean	SD	Mean	SD	Mean	SD	Mean	SD	Mean	SD
3.50	0.53	36.00	1.97	47.00	3.00	8.93	1.80	175.0	12.56	172.0	14.8
5.93	0.66	40.20	1.70	36.00	2.63	9.85	2.38	193.0	12.10	182.0	14.8
7.90	0.80	43.65	1.60	24.00	2.34	6.80	1.61	201.0	12.00	184.8	15.0
9.20	1.15	45.60	1.60	16.25	2.15	4.30	1.22	202.0	12.50	184.0	15.2
10.20	1.01	46.65	1.60	13.40	1.98	3.33	0.93	201.0	12.70	182.0	15.8
11.60	1.17	48.10	1.49	10.50	1.75	2.44	0.71	198.3	12.90	173.0	15.6
12.70	1.33	49.03	1.49	8.90/9.00	1.48/1.64	2.10	0.63	195.8	13.10	168.0	15.2
14.70	1.61	50.37	1.41	7.88	1.34	1.96	0.69	191.0	10.40	162.0	15.5
16.60	1.90	51.12	1.36	7.00	1.12	1.90	0.77	187.0	13.50	158.3	16.2
18.50	2.17	51.60	1.33	6.48	1.03	1.92	0.85	183.5	13.90	155.2	16.6
20.50	2.44	51.88	1.33	6.09	0.91	2.07	0.94	181.4	14.70	153.4	16.8
22.60	2.75	52.12	1.33	5.79	0.87	2.31	1.02	180.3	15.60	153.0	17.5
25.00	3.12	52.29	1.33	5.55	0.77	2.47	1.14	180.0	17.00	153.8	18.3
27.50	5.98	52.43	1.36	5.35	0.76	2.67	0.88	180.8	18.70	155.5	19.9
30.30	7.04	52.70	1.49	5.16	0.70	2.87	1.60	182.4	20.70	158.0	23.4
33.30	7.78	53.10	1.46	5.01	0.68	3.08	1.70	184.4	22.40	162.0	26.0
36.50	8.48	53.60	1.54	4.98	0.79	3.50	1.75	186.0	23.00	165.8	26.5
40.70	8.47	54.10	1.54	6.55	1.03	5.13	1.78	184.4	23.70	187.0	25.2
48.40	9.42	54.59	1.54	9.45	1.20	9.06	1.95	181.0	23.50	186.0	23.1
56.30	9.52	54.85	1.49	5.86	1.13	5.68	1.89	178.4	23.20	188.0	20.7
60.20	9.63	55.00	1.46	2.65	0.91	2.60	1.00	178.8	23.40	179.6	18.7
62.10	9.60			1.00	0.50			182.0	21.70	185.7	17.8
63.00	9.69			0.05	0.40			185.7	21.50	190.4	17.5
								188.8	21.20	192.3	17.5

*Adapted from data in Forfar, J. O., and Arneil, G. C.: Textbook of Paediatrics, Second Edition. Edinburgh, Scotland, Churchill Livingstone, 1978, and from Tanner, J. M., and Whitehouse, R. H.: Personal communication.

Table 7–2. **MEANS AND STANDARD DEVIATIONS—FEMALES***

Weight		Head Circumference		Length Velocity	Height Velocity	Weight Velocity		Triceps Skinfold		Subscapular Skinfold	
Mean	SD	Mean	SD	Mean	SD	Mean	SD	Mean	SD	Mean	SD
3.40	0.57	34.00	1.60	41.00	3.00	7.42	1.91	175.7	10.9	173.2	12.3
5.56	0.64	39.60	1.52	32.00	2.63	9.25	2.69	189.7	10.5	183.0	12.9
7.39	0.80	42.60	1.44	22.50	2.34	6.60	1.55	196.3	11.9	186.0	14.1
8.72	0.90	44.62	1.44	16.45	2.15	4.29	1.32	198.8	12.9	184.8	14.4
9.70	1.01	45.45	1.41	14.70	1.98	3.37	0.99	199.5	13.6	182.0	14.0
11.10	1.12	46.90	1.38	11.20	1.75	2.44	0.72	199.4	13.8	177.3	14.4
12.20	1.33	47.90	1.37	9.15/9.30	1.43/1.64	2.08	0.57	198.7	13.7	173.8	14.8
14.30	1.54	49.33	1.25	7.90	1.34	2.00	0.73	196.8	13.6	169.0	16.3
16.30	1.69	50.20	1.28	7.03	1.15	2.00	0.78	194.7	13.4	166.0	17.5
18.30	2.65	50.80	1.28	6.48	1.09	2.05	1.10	192.5	13.9	163.4	18.5
20.40	3.39	51.20	1.28	6.09	0.95	2.17	1.22	190.7	14.7	162.0	19.1
22.60	4.23	51.50	1.28	5.82	0.87	2.30	1.34	190.0	16.1	162.1	20.7
25.10	5.24	51.70	1.28	5.55	0.80	2.54	1.38	191.7	17.6	164.2	23.2
27.70	6.34	51.90	1.28	5.47	0.78	2.81	0.96	194.6	18.7	167.8	25.5
30.70	7.72	52.15	1.30	5.47	0.83	3.16	1.56	197.0	19.4	172.2	27.7
34.20	8.68	52.65	1.33	6.50	1.01	4.05	1.65	198.7	19.8	178.0	28.0
39.60	9.52	53.20	1.33	8.33	1.10	7.43	1.42	199.8	20.1	184.0	26.5
47.80	9.79	53.62	1.28	5.50	1.05	7.25	1.40	201.5	19.9	188.3	24.7
53.00	9.79	53.97	1.20	2.36	0.84	3.55	1.30	205.3	19.2	193.0	22.6
55.20	9.79	54.18	1.14	0.60	0.52	1.48	1.41	209.8	18.2	198.7	19.9
56.00	9.79	54.27	1.14	0.20	0.52	0.22	1.11	213.4	17.4	201.5	19.0
56.40	9.79			0.00	0.50			215.0	16.6	202.8	18.3
56.60	9.79			0.00	0.40			215.5	16.4	203.0	18.7
								215.5	16.4	203.0	18.7

*Adapted from data in Forfar, J. O., and Arneil, G. C.: Textbook of Paediatrics, Second Edition. Edinburgh, Scotland, Churchill Livingstone, 1978, and from Tanner, J. M., and Whitehouse, R. H.: Personal communication.

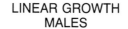

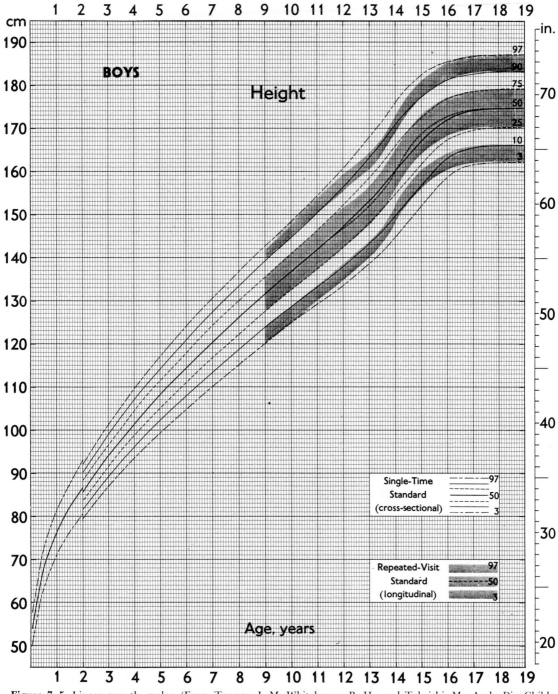

Figure 7–5. Linear growth, males. (From Tanner, J. M. Whitehouse, R. H., and Takaishi, M.: Arch. Dis. Child., *41*:613, 1966.)

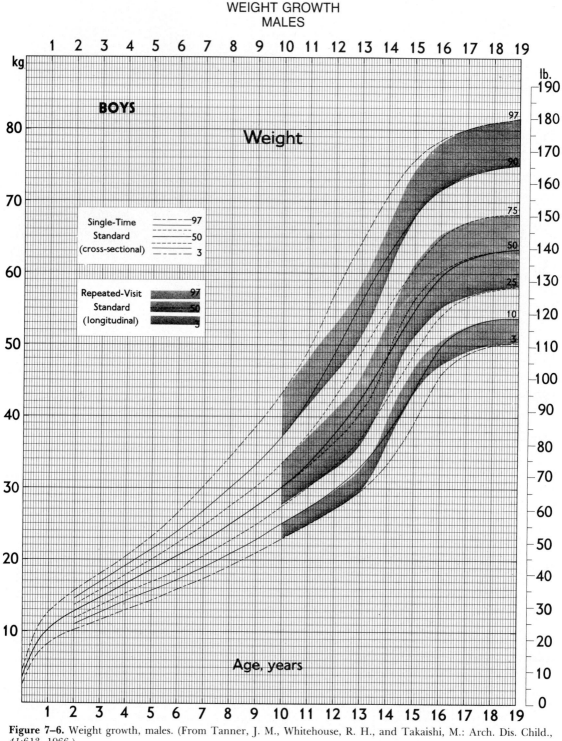

Figure 7–6. Weight growth, males. (From Tanner, J. M., Whitehouse, R. H., and Takaishi, M.: Arch. Dis. Child., *41*:613, 1966.)

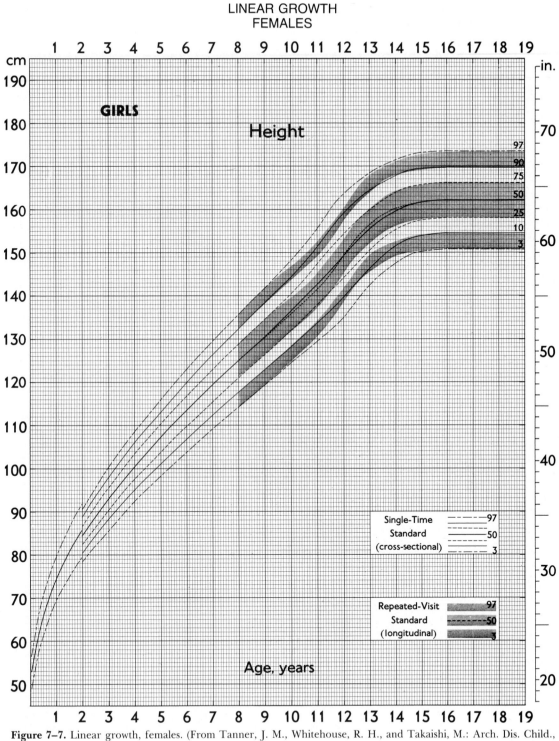

LINEAR GROWTH
FEMALES

Figure 7–7. Linear growth, females. (From Tanner, J. M., Whitehouse, R. H., and Takaishi, M.: Arch. Dis. Child., *41*:613, 1966.)

WEIGHT GROWTH
FEMALES

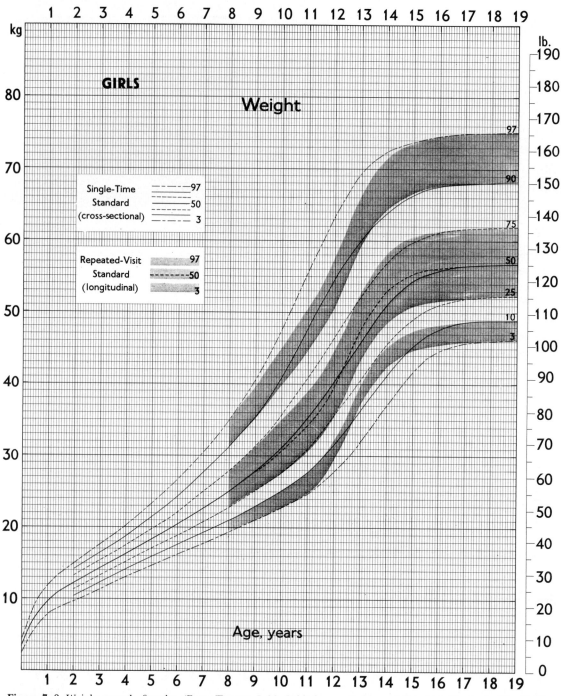

Figure 7–8. Weight growth, females. (From Tanner, J. M., Whitehouse, R. H., and Takaishi, M.: Arch. Dis. Child., *41*:613, 1966.)

HEAD CIRCUMFERENCES

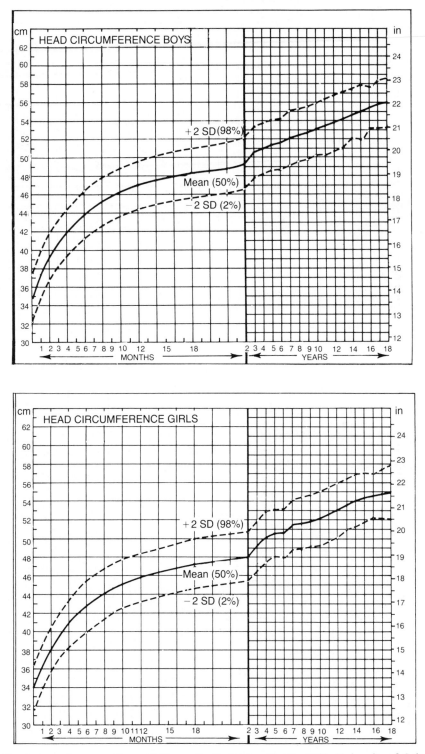

Figure 7–9. Head circumferences. (From Nellhaus, G.: Pediatrics, *41*:106, 1968. University of Colorado Medical Center Printing Services.)

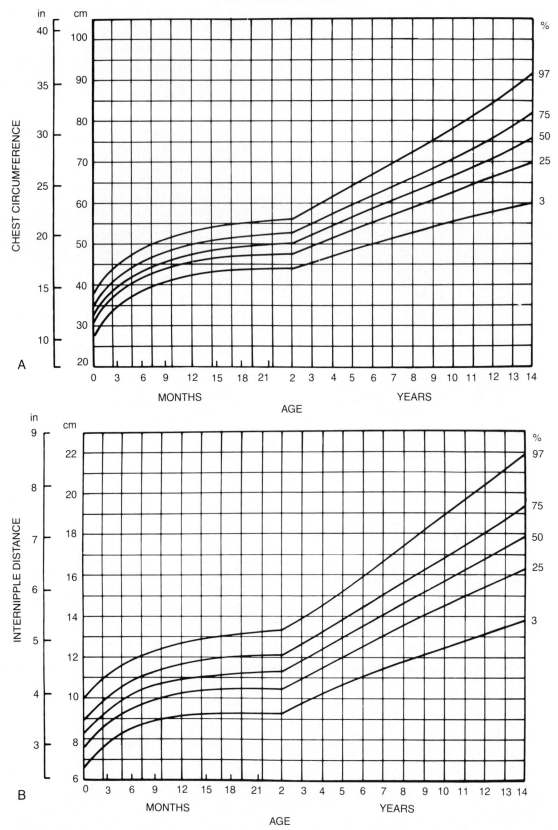

Figure 7–10. Chest circumference *(A)* and internipple distance *(B)*. (From Feingold, M., and Bossert, W. H.: Birth Defects, *10*:Supplement 13, 1974.)

694

HAND MEASUREMENTS

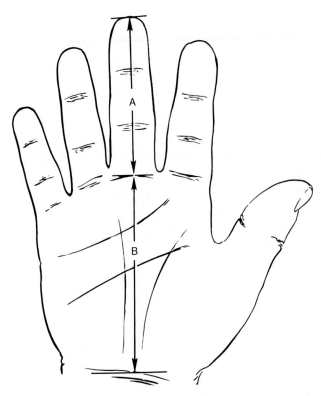

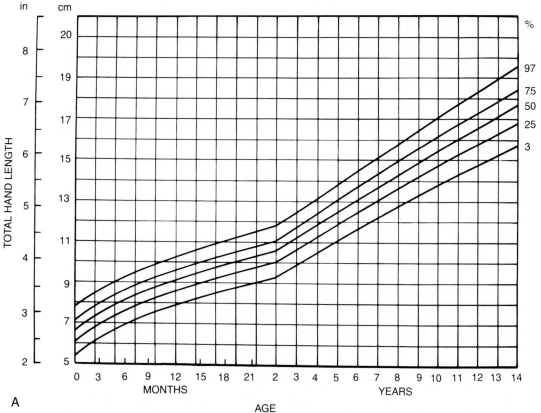

Figure 7–11. Hand length *(A)*, middle finger length *(B)*, and palm length *(C)*. (From Feingold, M., and Bossert, H. W.: Birth Defects, *10*:Supplement 13, 1974.)

Illustration continued on following page

HAND MEASUREMENTS

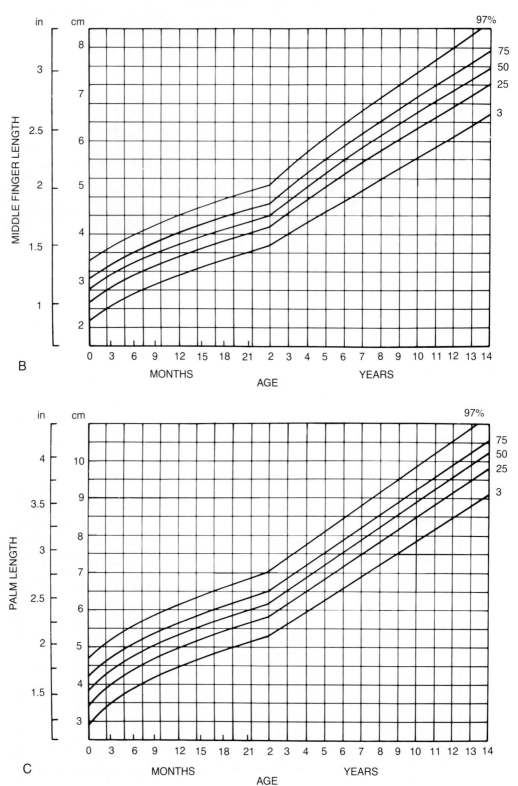

B

C

HAND MEASUREMENTS

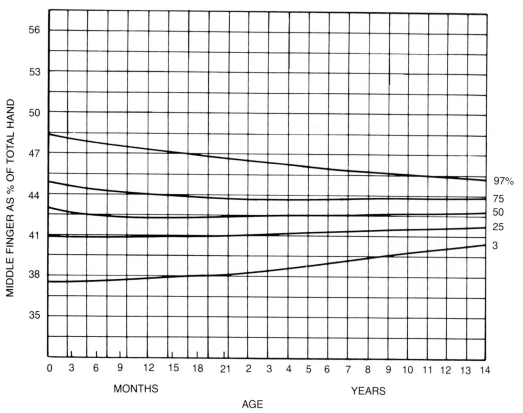

Figure 7–12. Proportion (per cent) of middle finger to hand length. (From Feingold, M., and Bossert, W. H.: Birth Defects, *10*:Supplement 13, 1974.)

FOOT LENGTH

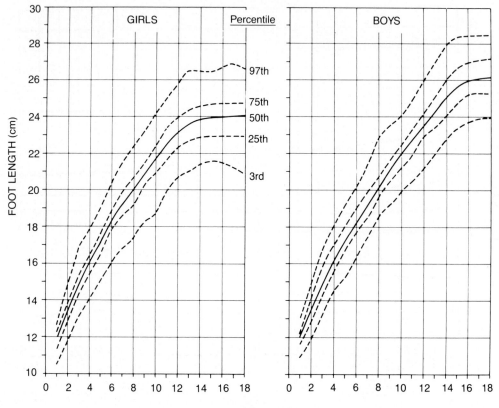

Figure 7–13. Mean and percentile values for foot length. Note: The adolescent growth spurt of the foot usually begins prior to the general linear growth spurt and ends before final height attainment. Thus, the foot growth spurt is a good early indicator of adolescence. (Adapted from Blais, M. M., Green, W. T., and Anderson, M.: J. Bone Joint Surg., *38-A*:998, 1956.)

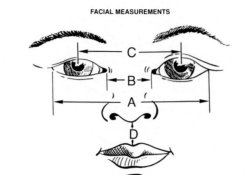

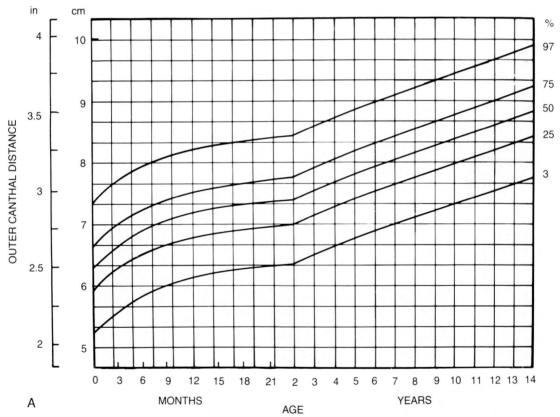

A

Figure 7–14. Outer canthal *(A)*, inner canthal *(B)*, and interpupillary *(C)* measurements. (From Feingold, M., and Bossert, W. H.: Birth Defects, *10*:Supplement 13, 1974.)

Illustration continued on following page

FACIAL MEASUREMENTS

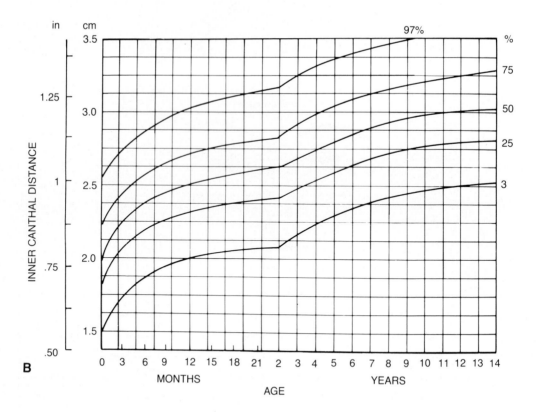

B

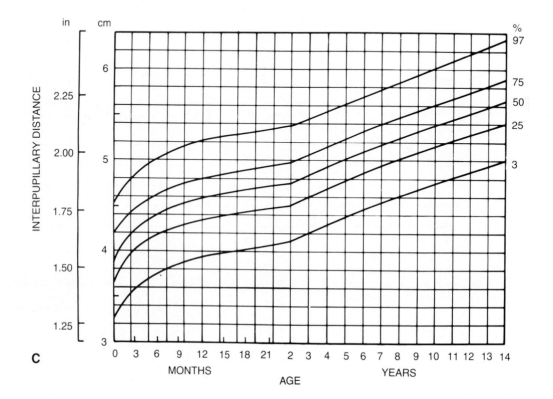

C

EYE MEASUREMENTS

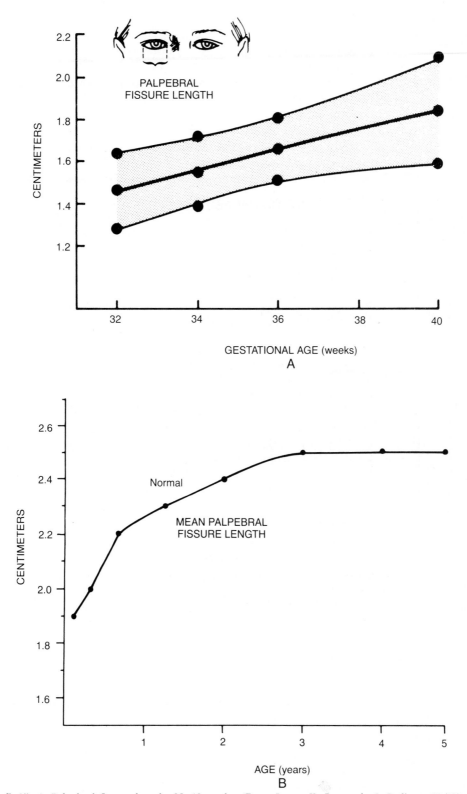

Figure 7–15. *A*, Palpebral fissure length, 32–40 weeks. (From Jones, K. L., et al.: J. Pediatr., *92*:787, 1978.) *B*, Palpebral fissure length, from inner to outer canthus, one to five years. (Data from Chouke, K. S.: Am. J. Phys. Anthropol., *13*:255, 1929.)

FONTANEL MEASUREMENTS

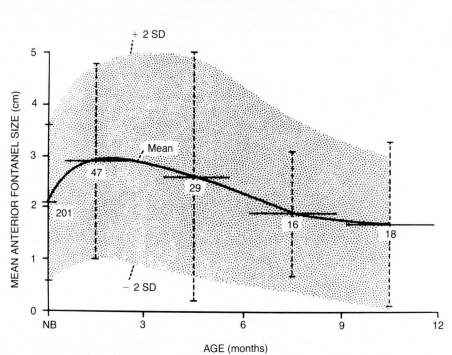

Figure 7–16. Mean anterior fontanel measurement (length plus width divided by two) during the first year. The numbers below the mean line indicate the number of normal infants measured at each age. Note: The posterior fontanel was fingertip size or smaller in dimension in 97 per cent of newborn infants. (From Popich. G., and Smith, D. W.: J. Pediatr., *80*:749, 1972.)

EAR LENGTH

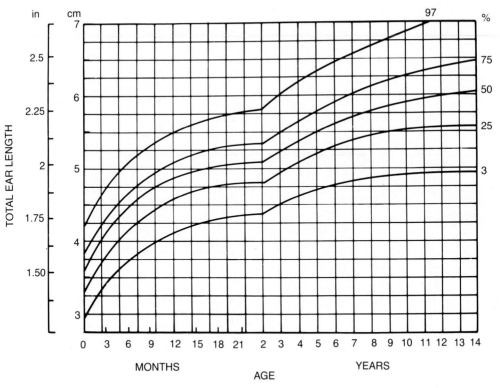

Figure 7–17. Maximum ear length. (From Feingold, M., and Bossert, W. H.: Birth Defects, *10*:Supplement 13, 1974.)

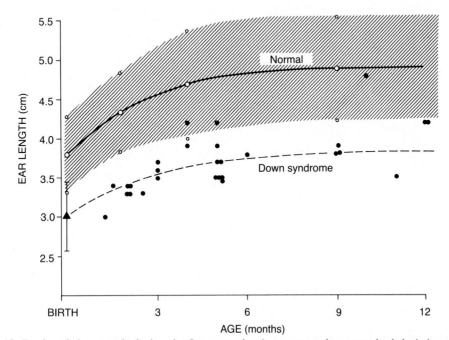

Figure 7–18. Ear length in normals during the first year, showing mean and two standard deviations in hatched area, as contrasted with ear length in the Down syndrome, showing mean and two standard deviations for 26 affected newborns and individual values (black dots) during first year. (From Aase, J. M., et al.: J. Pediatr., *82*:845, 1973.)

PENILE LENGTH

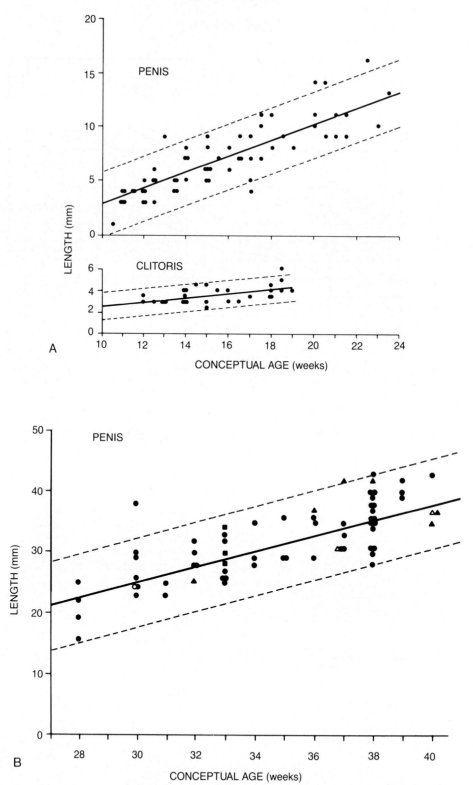

Figure 7–19. *A,* Growth of the penis contrasted with growth of the clitoris from formalin-fixed fetuses. *B,* Penile stretched length (from pubic bone to tip of glans) in the newborn. The mean full-term length is 3.5 cm with a 2 standard deviation range, from 2.8 to 4.2 cm. The solid line approximates the mean values, and the broken lines the two standard deviation values. (From Feldman, K. W., and Smith, D. W.: J. Pediatr., *86*:395, 1975.)

PENILE AND TESTICULAR GROWTH

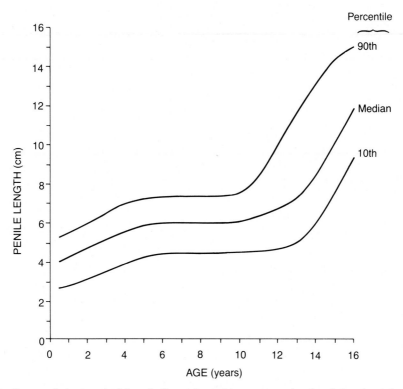

Figure 7–20. Penile growth in stretched length (from the pubic ramus to the tip of the glans) from infancy into adolescence. (From Schonfeld, W. A.: Am. J. Dis. Child., *65*:535, 1943.)

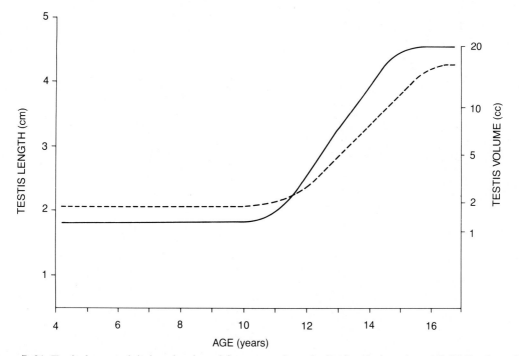

Figure 7–21. Testicular growth in length, adapted from normal standards of testicular volume. (Solid line from data of A. Prader, Zurich; broken line from data of Laron, A., and Zilka, E.: J. Clin. Endocrinol. Metab., *29*:1409, 1969.)

APPENDIX:
PATTERN OF MALFORMATION
DIFFERENTIAL DIAGNOSIS
BY ANOMALIES

The following lists were developed from the syndromes delineated in Chapter One. Listed for each anomaly are the syndromes in which this defect is a frequent feature, as well as those syndromes in which it is an occasional feature. Characteristics such as mental or growth deficiency are not considered because they are frequent features in a large number of disorders.

The anomalies are set forth under the following headings:

1. Central Nervous System Dysfunction other than Mental Deficiency
2. Deafness
3. Brain: Major Anomalies
4. Cranium
5. Scalp and Facial Hair Patterning
6. Facies
7. Ocular Region
8. Eye
9. Nose
10. Maxilla and Mandible
11. Oral Region and Mouth
12. Teeth
13. External Ears
14. Neck, Thorax, and Vertebrae
15. Limbs
16. Limbs: Nails, Creases, Dermatoglyphics
17. Limbs: Joints
18. Skin and Hair
19. Cardiac
20. Abdominal
21. Renal
22. Genital
23. Endocrine and Metabolic
24. Immune Deficiency
25. Hematology-Oncology
26. Unusual Growth Patterns

1. CENTRAL NERVOUS SYSTEM DYSFUNCTION OTHER THAN MENTAL DEFICIENCY

Hypotonicity

Frequent in

Occasional in

Hypertonicity

Frequent in

Occasional in

Ataxia

Frequent in

Occasional in

Seizures

Frequent in

Occasional in

2. DEAFNESS

Frequent in

Occasional in

3. BRAIN: MAJOR ANOMALIES

Encephalocele

Frequent in

Occasional in

Hydrocephalus

Frequent in

Occasional in

Microcephaly

Frequent in

Occasional in

Macrocephaly

Frequent in

Occasional in

4. CRANIUM

Craniosynostosis

Frequent in

Occasional in

Occiput, Flat or Prominent

Frequent in

Occasional in

Delayed Closure of Fontanels

Frequent in

Occasional in

Frontal Bossing or Prominent Central Forehead

Frequent in

Occasional in

5. SCALP AND FACIAL HAIR PATTERNING

Anterior Upsweep, Scalp

Frequent in

Occasional in

Shallow Orbital Ridges

Frequent in

Occasional in

Prominent Supraorbital Ridges

Frequent in

Prominent Eyes

Frequent in

Strabismus

Frequent in

Occasional in

Nystagmus

Frequent in

Occasional in

8. EYE

Myopia

Frequent in

Iris, Unusual Patterning or Coloration

Frequent in

Occasional in

Glaucoma

Frequent in

Occasional in

Large Cornea

Frequent in

Keratoconus, Microcornea

Frequent in

Occasional in

Corneal Opacity

Frequent in

Occasional in

Cataract, Lenticular Opacities

Frequent in

Occasional in

Lens Dislocation

Frequent in

Occasional in

Retinal Pigmentation

Occasional in

9. NOSE

Low Nasal Bridge

Frequent in

Occasional in

Prominent Nasal Bridge

Frequent in

Occasional in

Broad Nasal Bridge

Frequent in

Broad Nasal Root

Frequent in

Small or Short Nose, with or without Anteverted Nostrils

Frequent in

Occasional in

Hypoplasia of Nares and/or Alae Nasi

Frequent in

Occasional in

Prominent Nose (Relative)

Frequent in

Occasional in

Choanal Atresia

Frequent in

10. MAXILLA AND MANDIBLE

Malar Hypoplasia

Frequent in

Occasional in

Maxillary Hypoplasia, often with Narrow or High Arched Palate

Frequent in

Occasional in

Micrognathia

Frequent in

Occasional in

Prognathism

Frequent in

Occasional in

11. ORAL REGION AND MOUTH

Cleft Lip with or without Cleft Palate

Frequent in

Occasional in

Abnormal Philtrum

Frequent in

Prominent Full Lips

Frequent in

Hurler S. 406
Hurler-Scheie Compound S. 410
Hypohidrotic Ectodermal Dysplasia
    S. 476
Leprechaunism S. 537
Maroteaux-Lamy
    Mucopolysaccharidosis S. 418
Marshall S. 212
Multiple Neuroma S. 466
Neu-Laxova S. 150
Scheie S. 408
Trisomy 8 S. 26
Waardenburg S. 208
Williams S. 106

Occasional in

Fabry S. 540

Lower Lip Pits

Frequent in

Popliteal Web S. 262
Van de Woude S. 200

Occasional in

Oral-Facial-Digital S. 220, 222

Downturning Corners of Mouth

Frequent in

de Lange S. 80
Escobar S. 264
Robinow S. 112
Russell-Silver S. 88
Trisomy 9p S. 42
4p− S. 38
18p− S. 56
18q− S. 58

Microstomia

Frequent in

Fetal Valproate Effects 502
Hallermann-Streiff S. 102
Hecht S. (limited opening) 190
Oto-Palato-Digital S., type I 232
Oto-Palatal-Digital S., type II 234
Pena-Shokeir Phenotype 144
Rapp-Hodgkin Ectodermal
    Dysplasia S. 481

Robinow S. 112
Ruvalcaba S. 226
Trisomy 18 S. 16

Occasional in

Oromandibular-Limb Hypogenesis
    Spectrum 588
Treacher Collins S. 210

Macrostomia

Frequent in

Angelman S. 168
Facio-Auriculo-Vertebral Spectrum .. 584
Morquio S. 416
Neu-Laxova S. 150
Scheie S. 408
18p− S. 56

Occasional in

Beckwith-Wiedemann S. 136
Treacher Collins S. 210
Williams S. 106
18q− S. 58

Cleft Palate or Bifid Uvula without Cleft in Lip

Frequent in

Cerebro-Costo-Mandibular S. 534
Dubowitz S. 92
Escobar S. 264
Femoral Hypoplasia—Unusual Facies
    S. 268
Fibrochondrogenesis 282
Hay-Wells S. 254
Kneist Dysplasia 312
Meckel-Gruber S. 152
Nager S. 216
Oral-Facial-Digital S. 220, 222
Oto-Palato-Digital S., type I 232
Oto-Palatal-Digital S., type II 234
Partial Trisomy 10q S. 50
Popliteal Web S. 262
Retinoic Acid Embryopathy 508
Robin Sequence 196
Short Rib—Polydactyly, Majewski
    type 286
Shprintzen S. 224
Spondyloepiphyseal Dysplasia
    Congenita 310

Microglossia

Frequent in

Occasional in

Hypertrophied Alveolar Ridges

Frequent in

Occasional in

Broad Secondary Alveolar Ridge

Frequent in

Abnormalities of Larynx

Frequent in

Occasional in

12. TEETH

Anodontia (Aplasia)

Frequent in

Occasional in

Hypodontia (Including Conical Teeth)

Frequent in

Occasional in

Enamel Hypoplasia

Frequent in

Occasional in

Carious

Frequent in

Early Loss of Teeth

Frequent in

Occasional in

Irregular Placement of Teeth

Frequent in

13. EXTERNAL EARS

Low-Set Ears

Frequent in

Occasional in

Malformed Auricles

Frequent in

Occasional in

Preauricular Tags or Pits

Frequent in

Occasional in

14. NECK, THORAX, AND VERTEBRAE

Web Neck or Redundant Skin

Frequent in

Occasional in

Short Neck

Frequent in

Occasional in

Nipple Anomaly

Frequent in

Occasional in

Hypoplasia of Clavicles

Frequent in

Occasional in

Other Clavicular Anomalies

Frequent in

Occasional In

Scoliosis

Frequent in

Occasional in

Other Vertebral Defects

Frequent in

Occasional in

Odontoid Hypoplasia

Frequent in

Occasional in

15. LIMBS

Arachnodactyly

Frequent in

Occasional in

Fractures

Frequent in

Achondrogenesis type IA 278
Hypophosphatasia 346
Maffucci S. 460
Osteochondromatosis S. 461
Osteogenesis Imperfecta S., type I ... 432
Osteogenesis Imperfecta S., type II .. 436
Osteopetrosis: Autosomal Recessive—
  Lethal 353
Pseudo-Vitamin D Deficiency
  Rickets 344
Pyknodysostosis 360

Occasional in

Amyoplasia Congenita Sequence
  (delivery) 140
Antley-Bixler S. (prenatal, femur) 378
Cleidocranial Dysostosis 362
Dyskeratosis Congenita S 474
Hajdu-Cheney S. 348
Homocystinuria S. 426
Klippel-Feil Sequence (neck) 558
Langer-Giedion S. 248
Lowe S. 180
McCune-Albright S. 454
Menkes S. 166
Pena-Shokeir Phenotype 144
Pyle-Metaphyseal Dysplasia 352
X-Linked Hypophosphatemic
  Rickets (pseudofractures) 342

Short Limbs

Frequent in

Achondrogenesis Syndromes 278, 280
Achondroplasia 298
Acrodysostosis 392
Acromesomelic Dysplasia 308
Atelosteogenesis 284
Brachydactyly S., type E 396
Chondrodysplasia Punctata,
  Conradi-Hünermann type (short
  femur and/or humerus) 338
Chondroectodermal Dysplasia 324
Diastrophic Dysplasia 326
Femoral Hypoplasia–Unusual
  Facies S. 268
Fetal Aminopterin Effects
  (forearms) 506
Fetal Varicella Effects 514
Fibrochondrogenesis 282

Grebe S. 258
Hypochondroplasia 304
Jeune Thoracic Dystrophy 292
Kniest Dysplasia 312
Langer Mesomelic Dysplasia 390
Leri-Weill Dyschondrosteosis
  (forearm) 388
Melnick-Needles S. (upper arms) 528
Metatropic Dysplasia 318
Mietens S. (forearms) 228
Neu-Laxova S. 150
Osteogenesis Imperfecta S., type II .. 436
Pallister-Hall S. (arms) 154
Pseudoachondroplastic
  Spondyloepiphyseal Dysplasia 306
Rhizomelic Chondrodysplasia
  Punctata S. (short humerus
  and/or femur) 340
Robinow S. (forearms) 112
Ruvalcaba S. 226
Schinzel-Giedion S. (forearms) 188
Short Rib—Polydactyly, Majewski
  type 286
Thanatophoric Dysplasia 290

Occasional in

Coffin-Siris S. 522
de Lange S. 80
Early Urethral Obstruction
  Sequence 562
Fetal Warfarin Effects 504
Hypophosphatasia 346
Meckel-Gruber S. 152
Nager S. (forearms) 216
Osteogenesis Imperfecta S., type I ... 432

Limb Reduction, Moderate to Gross

Frequent in

Adams-Oliver S. 270
CHILD S. 266
Early Amnion Rupture Sequence 576
EEC S. (ectrodactyly) 252
Grebe S. 258
Holt-Oram S. 272
Miller S. 214
Oromandibular-Limb Hypogenesis
  Spectrum 588
Roberts-SC Phocomelia S. 256
Sirenomelia Sequence 574

Occasional in

de Lange S. 80
Early Urethral Obstruction 562

Small Hands and Feet, including Brachydactyly

Frequent in

Occasional in

Clinodactyly of Fifth Fingers

Frequent in

Occasional in

Thumb Hypoplasia to Aplasia, Triphalangeal Thumb

Frequent in

Occasional in

Radius Hypoplasia to Aplasia

Frequent in

Occasional in

Metacarpal Hypoplasia—All Metacarpals

Frequent in

Occasional in

Metacarpal Hypoplasia—Third, Fourth, and/or Fifth

Frequent in

Occasional in

Metacarpal Hypoplasia–First Metacarpal with Proximal Placement of Thumb

Frequent in

Occasional in

Elbow Dysplasia and Cubitus Valgus

Frequent in

Occasional in

Patella Dysplasia

Frequent in

Occasional in

Neurofibromatosis S. (absence) 452
Popliteal Pterygium S. 262
Trisomy 8 S. 26

XO S. 74
4p − S. (hyperconvex) 38
9p − S. 46

16. LIMBS: NAILS, CREASES, DERMATOGLYPHICS

Nail Hypoplasia or Dysplasia

Frequent in

Acromesomelic Dysplasia (short) 308
Adams-Oliver S. (small) 270
Antley-Bixler S. (narrow) 378
CHILD S. 266
Chondroectodermal Dysplasia 324
Clouston S. 484
Coffin-Siris S. 522
Dyskeratosis Congenita S. 474
EEC S. 252
Fetal Alcohol Effects 491
Fetal Hydantoin Effects 495
Fetal Valproate Effects
    (hyperconvex) 502
Fetal Warfarin Effects 504
Fibrochondrogenesis 282
Goltz S. 472
Hajdu-Cheney S. 348
Hay-Wells S. 254
Jugular Lymphatic Obstruction
    Sequence 560
Langer-Giedion S. (brittle) 248
Larsen S. 246
Melnick-Needles S. 528
Metaphyseal Chondrodysplasia,
    McKusick type 334
Nail-Patella S. 386
Oto-Palato-Digital S., type I (short) .. 232
Pachyonychia Congenita S. (thick) 486
Pallister-Hall S. 154
Popliteal Pterygium S. 262
Progeria S. 118
Pyknodysostosis 360
Rapp-Hodgkin Ectodermal
    Dysplasia S. 481
Schinzel-Giedion S. (hyperconvex) ... 188
Sclerosteosis 356
Tricho-Dento-Osseous S. (brittle) 482
Tricho-Rhino-Phalangeal S. 250
Trisomy 4p S. 36
Trisomy 9p S. 42
Trisomy 13 S. (hyperconvex) 20
Trisomy 18 S. 16
Weaver S. 130
Williams S. 106

Occasional in

Autosomal Recessive Hypohidrotic
    Ectodermal Dysplasia S. 480
Hypohidrotic Ectodermal
    Dysplasia S. 476
Incontinentia Pigmenti S. 448
Leprechaunism S. 537
Rothmund-Thomson S. 124
Senter S. 490

Single Crease (Simian), Upper Palm

Frequent in

Aarskog S. 110
Carpenter S. 370
Cohen S. 174
de Lange S. 80
Down S. 10
Fetal Alcohol Effects 491
Fetal Hydantoin Effects 495
Fetal Trimethadione Effects 500
Saethre-Chotzen S. 364
Schinzel-Giedion S. 188
Seckel S. 100
Smith-Lemli-Opitz S. 104
Triploidy S. 32
Trisomy 8 S. 26
Trisomy 13 S. 20
Zellweger S. 178
4p − S. 38
5p − S. 40
18q − S. 58

Occasional in

Coffin-Lowry S. 236
Killian/Teschler-Nicola S. 176
Langer-Giedion S. 248
Larsen S. 246
Meckel-Gruber S. 152
Noonan S. 108
Pallister-Hall S. 154
Rubinstein-Taybi S. 84
Trisomy 18 S. 16
XXXXX S. 73
XXXXY S. 70
Zellweger S. 178
18p − S. 56

Distal Palmar Axial Triradius

Frequent in

Occasional in

Low Arch Dermal Ridge Pattern on Majority of Fingertips

Frequent in

Occasional in

Whorl Dermal Ridge Pattern on Majority of Fingertips

Frequent in

Occasional in

Prominent Fingertip Pads

Occasional in

17. LIMBS: JOINTS

Joint Limitation and/or Contractures; Inability to Fully Extend (Other than Foot)

Frequent in

Occasional in

Club Foot—Especially Equinovarus Deformity, including Metatarsus Adductus

Frequent in

Occasional in

Clenched Hand; Index Finger Tending to Overlie the Third and the Fifth Finger Tending to Overlie the Fourth

Frequent in

Occasional in

Joint Hypermobility and/or Lax Ligaments

Frequent in

Occasional in

Joint Dislocation

Frequent in

Occasional in

18. SKIN AND HAIR

Loose, Redundant Skin

Frequent in

Edema of Hands and Feet

Frequent in

Occasional in

Altered Skin Pigmentation, Melanomata

Frequent in

Occasional in

Photosensitive Dermatitis

Frequent in

Occasional in

Deep Sacral Dimple, Pilonidal Cyst

Frequent in

Occasional in

Other Dimples

Frequent in

Unusual Acne

Frequent in

Occasional in

Alopecia (sparse to absent hair)

Frequent in

Occasional in

Hirsutism

Frequent in

Occasional in

Assorted Abnormalities of Hair

Frequent in

20. ABDOMINAL

Inguinal or Umbilical Hernia or Omphalocele

Frequent in

Occasional in

Umbilical Anomaly

Frequent in

Occasional in

Hepatomegaly

Frequent in

Occasional in

Pyloric Stenosis

Occasional in

Incomplete Rotation of Colon (Malrotation)

Frequent in

Occasional in

Renal Insufficiency

Frequent in

Occasional in

Hypertension

Occasional in

22. GENITAL

Hypospadias or Ambiguous External Genitalia, including Bifid Scrotum

Frequent in

Occasional in

Micropenis, Hypogenitalism, Other than Conditions Cited Above

Frequent in

Occasional in

Cryptorchidism

Frequent in

Occasional in

Hypoplasia of Labia Majora

Frequent in

Occasional in

Bicornuate Uterus and/or Double Vagina

Frequent in

Occasional in

Vaginal Atresia

Frequent in

Occasional in

Anal Defects or Anorectal Malformations

Frequent in

Occasional in

23. ENDOCRINE AND METABOLIC

Hypogonadism

Frequent in

Occasional in

Hypothyroidism

Frequent in

Occasional in

Other Endocrine Abnormalities

Frequent in

Occasional in

Diabetes Mellitus

Frequent in

Occasional in

Hypocalcemia

Frequent in

Hypercalcemia

Occasional in

Vicarious Calcification

Frequent in

Occasional in

Cockayne S. (intracranial) 122
Klippel-Trenaunay-Weber S.
(cranial) 456
Smith-Lemli-Opitz S. (epiphyseal) 104

Lipoatrophy (Loss or Lack of Subcutaneous Fat)

Frequent in

Berardinelli Lipodystrophy S. 538
Cockayne S. 122
Fetal Alcohol Effects 491
Lenz-Majewski Hyperostosis S. 537
Leprechaunism S. 118
Progeria S. 118
Werner S. 120

Hyperlipemia

Frequent in

Arteriohepatic Dysplasia
(cholesterol) 526
Berardinelli Lipodystrophy S. 538

Occasional in

Chédiak-Higashi S. 542

Hyperthermia

Frequent in

Autosomal Recessive Hypohidrotic
Ectodermal Dysplasia S. 480
Hypohidrotic Ectodermal
Dysplasia S. 476

Occasional in

Noonan S. (malignant) 108
Oromandibular-Limb Hypogenesis
Spectrum 588
Rapp-Hodgkin Ectodermal
Dysplasia S. 481
Schwartz-Jampel S. (malignant) 186

24. IMMUNE DEFICIENCY

Immunoglobulin Deficiency

Frequent in

Ataxia-Telangiectasia S. (IgA, IgE) ... 164
Dyskeratosis Congenita S. 474
Shwachman S. 337

Occasional in

Bloom S. (IgA, IgM) 94
Kartagener S. (IgA) 545
18p− S. (IgA) 56
18q− S. (IgA) 58

Thymic Defect

Frequent in

Ataxia-Telangiectasia S. 164
DiGeorge Sequence 556
Dyskeratosis Congenita S. 474
Metaphyseal Chondrodysplasia,
McKusick type 334

Occasional in

Beckwith-Wiedemann S. 136
CHARGE Association 606
Fraser S. 204
Marshall-Smith S. 134
Smith-Lemli-Opitz S. 104

25. HEMATOLOGY-ONCOLOGY

Anemia

Frequent in

Aase S. 277
Chédiak-Higashi S. 542
Dyskeratosis Congenita S. 474
Fanconi Pancytopenia S. 274
Osteopetrosis: Autosomal Recessive—
Lethal 353
Peutz-Jeghers S. 462
Radial Aplasia—Thrombocytopenia
S. 276

Occasional in

Fabry S. 540
Fetal Rubella Effects 510
Hypophosphatasia 346
Kenny S. 345
Langer-Giedion S. 248
Metaphyseal Chondrodysplasia,
McKusick type 334
Shwachman S. 337
Trisomy 8 S. 26

Thrombocytopenia

Frequent in

Chédiak-Higashi S. 542
Dyskeratosis Congenita S. 474

26. UNUSUAL GROWTH PATTERNS

Obesity

Frequent in

Occasional in

Hydrops Fetalis

Frequent in

Occasional in

Chondrodysplasia Punctata,
  Conradi-Hünermann type 338
Lethal Multiple Pterygium S. 148
Short Rib—Polydactyly, Majewski
  type 286

Early Macrosomia, Overgrowth

Frequent in

Beckwith-Wiedemann S. 136
Berardinelli Lipodystrophy S. 538
Marshall-Smith S. 134
Ruvalcaba-Myhre S. 463
Sotos S. 128
Weaver S. 130

Occasional in

Killian/Teschler-Nicola S. 176
Sclerosteosis 356

Asymmetry

Frequency in

CHILD S. (limbs) 266
Chondrodysplasia Punctata,
  Conradi-Hünermann type (limbs) .. 338

Facio-Auriculo-Vertebral Spectrum .. 584
Klippel-Feil Sequence (facial) 558
Klippel-Trenaunay-Weber S. 456
Osteochondromatosis S. (limb) 461
Proteus S. 458
Russell-Silver S. 88
Saethre-Chotzen S. (facial) 364
Sclerosteosis (mandible) 356
Triploid/Diploid Mixoploidy S.
  (limbs) 32

Occasional in

Beckwith-Wiedemann S.
  (hemihypertrophy) 136
Goltz S. 472
Incontinentia Pigmenti S.
  (hemiatrophy) 448
McCune-Albright S. (facial) 454
MURCS Association (facial) 604
Neurofibromatosis S. (segmental
  hypertrophy) 452
Noonan S. (head) 108
Opitz S. (cranium) 114
Oromandibular-Limb Hypogenesis
  Spectrum (facial) 588
Seckel S. (facial) 100
XYY S. (facial) 64
4p− S. (cranial) 38
13q− S. (facial) 54

Index

Page numbers in *italics* refer to illustrations; page numbers followed by "t" refer to tables.

765

FETAL DEVELOPMENT

AGE weeks	LENGTH cm		WT gm	GROSS APPEARANCE	CNS	EYE, EAR	FACE, MOUTH	CARDIO-VASCULAR	LUNG
	C–R	Tot.							
7½	2.8				Cerebral hemisphere / Infundibulum, Rathke's	Lens nearing final shape	Palatal swellings / Dental lamina, Epithel	Pulmonary vein into left atrium	
8	3.7				Primitive cereb. cortex / Olfactory lobes / Dura and pia mater	Eyelid / Ear canals	Nares plugged / Rathke's pouch detach. / Sublingual gland	A–V bundle / Sinus venosus absorbed into right auricle	Pleuroperitoneal canals close / Bronchioles
10	6.0				Spinal cord histology / Cerebellum	Iris / Ciliary body / Eyelids fuse / Lacrimal glands / Spiral gland different	Lips, Nasal cartilage / Palate		Laryngeal cavity reopened
12	8.8				Cord—cervical & lumbar enlarged, Cauda equina	Retina layered / Eye axis forward / Scala tympani	Tonsillar crypts / Cheeks / Dental papilla	Accessory coats, blood vessels	Elastic fibers
16	14				Corpora quadrigemina / Cerebellum prominent / Myelination begins	Scala vestibuli / Cochlear duct	Palate complete / Enamel and dentine	Cardiac muscle condensed	Segmentation of bronchi complete
20						Inner ear ossified	Ossification of nose		Decrease in mesenchyme / Capillaries penetrate linings of tubules
24		32	800		Typical layers in cerebral cortex / Cauda equina at first sacral level		Nares reopen / Calcification of tooth primordia		Change from cuboidal to flattened epithelium / Alveoli
28		38.5	1100		Cerebral fissures and convolutions	Eyelids reopen / Retinal layers complete / Perceive light			Vascular components adequate for respiration
32		43.5	1600	Accumulation of fat		Auricular cartilage	Taste sense		Number of alveoli still incomplete
36		47.5	2600						
38		50	3200		Cauda equina, at L–3 / Myelination within brain	Lacrimal duct canalized	Rudimentary frontal maxillary sinuses	Closure of foramen ovale, ductus arteriosus, umbilical vessels, ductus venosus	
First postnatal year +					Continuing organization of axonal networks / Cerebrocortical function, motor coordination / Myelination continues until 2–3 years	Iris pigmented, 5 months / Mastoid air cells / Coordinate vision, 3–5 months / Maximal vision by 5 years	Salivary gland ducts become canalized / Teeth begin to erupt 5–7 months / Relatively rapid growth of mandible and nose	Relative hypertrophy left ventricle	Continue adding new alveoli